Comprehensive Virology 14

Comprehensive Virology

Edited by Heinz Fraenkel-Conrat
University of California at Berkeley

and Robert R. Wagner
University of Virginia

Editorial Board

Volume 1:   *Descriptive Catalogue of Viruses* – by Heinz Fraenkel-Conrat

Reproduction

Volume 2:   *Small and Intermediate RNA Viruses* – Contributors: J.T. August,
           L. Eoyang, A. Siegel, V. Hariharasubramanian, L. Levintow,
           E. R. Pfefferkorn, D. Shapiro, and W. K. Joklik

Volume 3:   *DNA Animal Viruses* – Contributors: L. Philipson, U. Lindberg, J.A. Rose,
           N.P. Salzman, G. Khoury, B. Moss, B. Roizman, and D. Furlong

Volume 4:   *Large RNA Viruses* – Contributors: P.W. Choppin, R.W. Compans,
           R.R. Wagner, and J.P. Bader

Volume 7:   *Bacterial DNA Viruses* – Contributors: D.T. Denhardt, D.S. Ray, and
           C.K. Mathews

Structure and Assembly

Volume 5:   *Virions, Pseudovirions, and Intraviral Nucleic Acids* – Contributors:
           T.I. Tikchonenko, John T. Finch, Lionel V. Crawford, and H. Vasken Aposhian

Volume 6:   *Assembly of Small RNA Viruses* – Contributors: K.E. Richards,
           R.C. Williams, L. Hirth, P.P. Hung, Y. Okada, T. Ohno, and R.R. Rueckert

Volume 13: *Primary, Secondary, Tertiary, and Quaternary Structures* – Contributors:
           G. Air, R. W. Compans, F. A. Eiserling, W. Fiers, R. V. Gilden, J. King,
           H.-D. Klenk, S. Oroszlan, and W. B. Wood

Regulation and Genetics

Volume 8:   *Bacterial DNA Viruses* – Contributors: D. Rabussay, E. P. Geiduschek,
           R. A. Weisberg, S. Gottesman, M. E. Gottesman, A. Campbell, R. Calendar,
           J. Geisselsoder, M.G. Sunshine, E.W. Six, and B.H. Lindqvist

Volume 9:   *Genetics of Animal Viruses* – Contributors: H. S. Ginsberg, C. S. H. Young,
           W. Eckhart, J. H. Subak-Sharpe, M. C. Timbury, C.R. Pringle, E.R. Pfefferkorn,
           P. D. Cooper, L. K. Cross, B. N. Fields, P. K. Vogt, M. A. Bratt,
           and L. E. Hightower

Volume 10: *Viral Gene Expression and Integration* – Contributors: A. J. Shatkin,
           A. K. Banerjee, G. W. Both, A. S. Huang, D. Baltimore, D. H. L. Bishop,
           W. Doerfler, and H. Hanafusa

Volume 11: *Plant Viruses* – Contributors: L. Van Vloten-Doting, E. M. J. Jaspars,
           G. Bruening, J. G. Atabekov, H. Fraenkel-Conrat, M. Salvato, L. Hirth,
           I. Takebe, T. O. Diener, and A. Hadidi

Additional Topics

Volume 12: *Newly Characterized Protist and Invertebrate Viruses* – Contributors: T. W. Tinsley,
           K. A. Harrap, K. N. Saksena, P. A. Lemke, L. A. Sherman, R. M. Brown, Jr.,
           T. I. Tikchonenko, and L. Mindich

Volume 14: *Newly Characterized Vertebrate Viruses* – Contributors: P.E. McAllister,
           F.L. Schaffer, D.W. Verwoerd, A. Granoff, W.S. Robinson, J.A. Robb,
           D.H.L. Bishop, and W.E. Rawls

Virus-Host Interactions

Volume 15: *Immunity to Viruses* – Contributors: M. B. A. Oldstone, B. Mandel, N. R. Cooper,
           R. M. Zinkernagel, E. De Maeyer, and J. De Maeyer-Guignard

Comprehensive

Edited by

Heinz Fraenkel-Conrat

Department of Molecular Biology and Virus Laboratory
University of California, Berkeley, California

and

Robert R. Wagner

Department of Microbiology
University of Virginia, Charlottesville, Virginia

Virology

14

Newly Characterized Vertebrate Viruses

PLENUM PRESS · NEW YORK AND LONDON

Library of Congress Cataloging in Publication Data

Main entry under title:

Newly characterized vertebrate viruses.

(Comprehensive virology, edited by H. Fraenkel-Conrat and R. R. Wagner; v. 14)
1. Viruses. 2. Vertebrates—Diseases. 3. Fishes—Diseases. I. Fraenkel-Conrat, Heinz,
1910-   II. Wagner, Robert R., 1923-   III. Series: Fraenkel-Conrat, Heinz,
1910-   Comprehensive virology; v. 14
QR357.F72 vol. 14 [QR360]   576'.64'08s
ISBN 0-306-40231-7   [636.089'601'94]   79-810

© 1979 Plenum Press, New York
A Division of Plenum Publishing Corporation
227 West 17th Street, New York, N.Y. 10011

Printed in the United States of America

Foreword

The time seems ripe for a critical compendium of that segment of the biological universe we call viruses. Virology, as a science, having passed only recently through its descriptive phase of naming and numbering, has probably reached that stage at which relatively few new—truly new—viruses will be discovered. Triggered by the intellectual probes and techniques of molecular biology, genetics, biochemical cytology, and high resolution microscopy and spectroscopy, the field has experienced a genuine information explosion.

Few serious attempts have been made to chronicle these events. This comprehensive series, which will comprise some 6000 pages in a total of about 18 volumes, represents a commitment by a large group of active investigators to analyze, digest, and expostulate on the great mass of data relating to viruses, much of which is now amorphous and disjointed, and scattered throughout a wide literature. In this way, we hope to place the entire field in perspective, and to develop an invaluable reference and sourcebook for researchers and students at all levels.

This series is designed as a continuum that can be entered anywhere, but which also provides a logical progression of developing facts and integrated concepts.

Volume 1 contains an alphabetical catalogue of almost all viruses of vertebrates, insects, plants, and protists, describing them in general terms. Volumes 2–4 deal primarily, but not exclusively, with the processes of infection and reproduction of the major groups of viruses in their hosts. Volume 2 deals with the simple RNA viruses of bacteria, plants, and animals; the togaviruses (formerly called arboviruses), which share with these only the feature that the virion's RNA is able to act as messenger RNA in the host cell; and the reoviruses of animals and plants, which all share several structurally singular features, the

vii

most important being the double-strandedness of their multiple RNA molecules.

Volume 3 addresses itself to the reproduction of all DNA-containing viruses of vertebrates, encompassing the smallest and the largest viruses known. The reproduction of the larger and more complex RNA viruses is the subject matter of Volume 4. These viruses share the property of being enclosed in lipoprotein membranes, as do the togaviruses included in Volume 2. They share as a group, along with the reoviruses, the presence of polymerase enzymes in their virions to satisfy the need for their RNA to become transcribed before it can serve messenger functions.

Volumes 5 and 6 represent the first in a series that focuses primarily on the structure and assembly of virus particles. Volume 5 is devoted to general structural principles involving the relationship and specificity of interaction of viral capsid proteins and their nucleic acids, or host nucleic acids. It deals primarily with helical and the simpler isometric viruses, as well as with the relationship of nucleic acid to protein shell in the T-even phages. Volume 6 is concerned with the structure of the picornaviruses, and with the reconstitution of plant and bacterial RNA viruses.

Volumes 7 and 8 deal with the DNA bacteriophages. Volume 7 concludes the series of volumes on the reproduction of viruses (Volumes 2–4 and Volume 7) and deals particularly with the single- and double-stranded virulent bacteriophages.

Volume 8, the first of the series on regulation and genetics of viruses, covers the biological properties of the lysogenic and defective phages, the phage-satellite system P 2–P 4, and in-depth discussion of the regulatory principles governing the development of selected lytic phages.

Volume 9 provides a truly comprehensive analysis of the genetics of all animal viruses that have been studied to date. These chapters cover the principles and methodology of mutant selection, complementation analysis, gene mapping with restriction endonucleases, etc. Volume 10 also deals with animal cells, covering transcriptional and translational regulation of viral gene expression, defective virions, and integration of tumor virus genomes into host chromosomes.

Volume 11 covers the considerable advances in the molecular understanding of new aspects of virology which have been revealed in recent years through the study of plant viruses. It covers particularly the mode of replication and translation of the multicomponent viruses and others that carry or utilize subdivided genomes; the use of protoplasts in such studies is authoritatively reviewed, as well as the nature of viroids, the smallest replicatable pathogens. Volume 12 deals with special groups of viruses of protists and invertebrates which show properties that set them apart from the main virus families. These are the lipid-containing phages and the viruses of algae, fungi, and invertebrates.

Volume 13 contains chapters on various topics related to the structure and assembly of viruses, dealing in detail with nucleotide and amino acid sequences, as well as with particle morphology and assembly, and the structure of virus membranes and hybrid viruses. The first complete sequence of a viral RNA is represented as a multicolored foldout.

The present volume contains chapters on special and/or newly characterized vertebrate virus groups: bunya-, arena-, corona-, calici-, and orbiviruses, icosahedral cytoplasmic deoxyriboviruses, fish viruses, and hepatitis viruses.

Several subsequent volumes will deal with virus–host relationships and with methodological aspects of virus research.

Contents

Chapter 1

Bunyaviridae

David H. L. Bishop and Robert E. Shope

1. Introduction 1
   1.1. Characteristics of the Bunyaviridae............. 3
   1.2. Isolation and Relationships of Members and
        Possible Members of the Bunyaviridae Family . 5
2. Structural Components and Their Functions 68
   2.1. Virus Particle Morphology and Morphogenesis .. 68
   2.2. Composition and Properties of Bunyavirus
        Particles 78
   2.3. Diagrammatic Representation of Bunyavirus
        Virions 105
3. Replication of Bunyaviruses...................... 106
   3.1. Adsorption and Penetration 106
   3.2. Primary Transcription: Early Viral Messenger
        RNA Synthesis 107
   3.3. Viral Protein Synthesis 108
   3.4. Virus RNA Replication 110
   3.5. Secondary Transcription: Amplified Messenger
        RNA Synthesis 111
   3.6. Virus Assembly and Budding................. 113
4. Genetics 114
   4.1. Isolation and Characterization of Temperature-
        Sensitive, Conditional Lethal Bunyavirus
        Mutants 114
   4.2. High-Frequency Homologous Virus Genetic
        Recombination 119

     4.3.   Complementation Analyses 123
     4.4.   Group I/II Double Mutants 125
     4.5.   High-Frequency Heterologous Recombination
            between Certain Bunyaviruses 125
     4.6.   Summary of the Bunyavirus Genetics Studies 130
  5. Defective Interfering Virus 131
  6. Conclusions 131
  7. References 132

Chapter 2

Arenaviruses

William E. Rawls and Wai-Choi Leung

  1. Introduction 157
  2. Historical Considerations 158
  3. Pathobiology 160
  4. Morphologic and Physical Properties 164
  5. Proteins.. 168
     5.1.   Polypeptides............................. 168
     5.2.   Antigens 170
  6. Nucleic Acids 172
  7. Internal Components of the Virus 175
     7.1.   Virus-Associated Ribosomes 175
     7.2.   Ribonucleoprotein Core 176
     7.3.   Virus-Associated Enzymes 177
  8. Replication in Cultured Cells 178
  9. Interference and Defective Interfering Particles........ 182
 10. Concluding Remarks.............................. 184
 11. References 185

Chapter 3

Coronaviridae

James A. Robb and Clifford W. Bond

  1. Introduction 193
     1.1.   Summary 193
     1.2.   Definition and Members of the Coronavirus Family   194

2. Virions 195
    2.1. Morphology 195
    2.2. Composition............................. 197
    2.3. Fine Structure and Arrangement of Virion
          Components 201
3. Growth Properties in Cell and Organ Culture 204
    3.1. Infectivity Assays 204
    3.2. Growth Curves and Multiplication Kinetics 205
    3.3. Modification of Infectivity 207
4. Multiplication of Virus 207
    4.1. Adsorption 207
    4.2. Penetration and Uncoating 208
    4.3. Biosynthesis of Viral Macromolecules 209
    4.4. Assembly 215
    4.5. General Comments 215
5. Alteration in Host Cell Metabolism 216
6. Defective Virus and Viral Interference 217
    6.1. Defective Virus 217
    6.2. Interference by Defective Virus 217
    6.3. Other Forms of Interference 218
7. Pathogenesis of Coronavirus Disease 218
    7.1. Spectrum of Disease 218
    7.2. Route of Infection 219
    7.3. Animal Response to Infection 225
    7.4. Summary of Pathogenesis 230
8. Persistent Infections 231
9. Genetics 236
10. Conclusion 237
11. References 237

Chapter 4

Caliciviruses

Frederick L. Schaffer

1. Introduction and Classification 249
2. Natural History and Disease Aspects 250
    2.1. Vesicular Exanthema of Swine Virus (VESV) 250
    2.2. San Miguel Sea Lion Virus (SMSV) 250

2.3.   Relationship between VESV and SMSV   251
2.4.   Feline Calicivirus (FCV)......................   252
2.5.   Human Calicivirus   252
3.   Antigenic Aspects   253
3.1.   VESV and SMSV   253
3.2.   FCV   254
3.3.   Relation between FCV and VESV/SMSV.......   255
4.   Caliciviruses in Cultured Cells   255
4.1.   Growth and Host Range.....................   256
4.2.   Cytopathology   257
4.3.   Genetics   259
4.4.   Viral RNA   259
4.5.   Viral Protein   261
5.   The Virion   264
5.1.   Purification   264
5.2.   Morphology and Structure....................   264
5.3.   Sedimentation   266
5.4.   Buoyant Density   267
5.5.   Inactivation and Stability   268
5.6.   Virion RNA................................   269
5.7.   Virion Protein   272
5.8.   Virion Mass   274
6.   Defective Interfering Virus   275
7.   Concluding Remarks...........................   275
8.   Addendum   276
9.   References   278

Chapter 5

Orbiviruses

D. W. Verwoerd, H. Huismans, and B. J. Erasmus

1.   Introduction   285
2.   Propagation and Assay Systems   286
2.1.   Primary Isolation   286
2.2.   Cultivation   288
2.3.   Cytopathology   289
2.4.   Assay Systems..............................   290

3. The Virion 290
   3.1. Morphology 290
   3.2. Physicochemical Properties 294
   3.3. The Viral Genome......................... 298
   3.4. The Viral Capsid 303
   3.5. Viral Enzymes 307
4. Replication...................................... 309
   4.1. Adsorption and Penetration 309
   4.2. Site of Replication......................... 309
   4.3. Synthesis of Viral Nucleic Acids 310
   4.4. Synthesis of Viral Proteins 312
   4.5. Mutants and Defective Particles 316
   4.6. Effect of Viral Infection on Cellular Functions ... 317
5. Antigenic Properties 318
   5.1. Serological Reactions 318
   5.2. Serological Classification 322
   5.3. Antigens Involved in Antigenic Variation 323
   5.4. Immunity 324
6. Epizootiology.................................. 325
   6.1. Host Range 325
   6.2. Transmission 327
   6.3. Ecological Factors......................... 329
   6.4. Pathogenesis............................. 329
7. Concluding Remarks.............................. 331
8. References 332

Chapter 6

Icosahedral Cytoplasmic Deoxyriboviruses

Rakesh Goorha and Allan Granoff

1. Introduction 347
2. Classification and General Biological Properties of
   Icosahedral Cytoplasmic Deoxyriboviruses 348
3. Size, Morphology, and Structure.................... 349
   3.1. Size 349
   3.2. Morphology and Structure.................... 353
4. Physical Properties 356

5. Chemical Composition 356
   5.1. DNA 356
   5.2. Proteins and Enzyme Activities 358
   5.3. Lipids 360
6. Replication 361
   6.1. Replication of Frog Virus 3 364
   6.2. Nuclear Requirement for ICDV Replication 385
7. Conclusions and Prospects for the Future 390
8. References 392

Chapter 7

Fish Viruses and Viral Infections

Philip E. McAllister

1. Introduction 401
2. Fish Herpesviridae................................ 401
   2.1. Biology of the Diseases 402
   2.2. Biology of the Viruses 404
3. Fish Iridoviridae 409
   3.1. Biology of the Diseases 409
   3.2. Biology of the Viruses 410
4. Fish Reoviridae 414
   4.1. Biology of the Diseases 415
   4.2. Biology of the Viruses 417
5. Fish Rhabdoviridae 426
   5.1. Biology of the Diseases 426
   5.2. Biology of the Viruses 430
6. Fish Retroviridae................................. 440
   6.1. Biology of the Diseases 441
   6.2. Evidence of Putative Virus 444
7. Unclassified and Putative Fish Viruses Associated with
      Neoplasia 446
   7.1. Stomatopapilloma of Eel–Associated Viruses 446
   7.2. Brown Bullhead Papilloma–Associated Virus 447
   7.3. Atlantic Salmon Papilloma–Associated Virus 448
   7.4. Pleuronectid Epidermal Papilloma–Associated
         Virus 449
8. Unclassified and Putative Fish Viruses 451
   8.1. Bluegill Virus 451
   8.2. Grunt Fin Agent 452

8.3. Ulcerative Dermal Necrosis–Associated Virus ... 454
8.4. Gill Necrosis of Carp–Associated Virus 454
9. References 455

Chapter 8

Viruses of Human Hepatitis A and B

William S. Robinson

1. Introduction: Recognition of Hepatitis Viruses 471
2. Hepatitis B Virus (HBV) 473
    2.1. Infectious HBV 473
    2.2. Hepatitis B Surface Antigen 474
    2.3. Hepatitis B Virion and Its DNA 477
    2.4. Incomplete Hepatitis B Viral Forms 484
    2.5. Hepatitis B Core Antigen (HB_cAg) 485
    2.6. Hepatitis B_e Antigen (HB_eAg) 486
    2.7. Synthesis of HBV Antigens in Infected Liver 487
    2.8. Current Estimate of the Number of HBV Genes
          and the Total Virus-Specified Polypeptide 488
3. Course of HBV Infection 489
    3.1. Self-Limited HBV Infection 489
    3.2. Persistent HBV Infection 491
4. Disease Associated with HBV Infection 492
    4.1. Acute and Chronic Hepatitis B 492
    4.2. Hepatocellular Carcinoma 493
    4.3. Other Disease Syndromes Associated with HBV
          Infection 493
5. Epidemiology of HBV 494
    5.1. Total Viral Hepatitis in the United States 494
    5.2. HBV Infections in the United States 495
    5.3. HBV Infections in Other Parts of the World 495
    5.4. Persistent HBV Infection 495
    5.5. HBV Transmission 498
6. Hepatitis A Virus (HAV) 500
    6.1. Infectious HAV 500
    6.2. Hepatitis A Antigen (HAAg) Forms in Feces,
          Liver, and Bile 502
    6.3. Viral Antigen Synthesis in Infected Liver 504
7. Course of HAV Infection 505

8.   Immunity to HAV   507
9.   Disease Associated with HAV Infection   507
10.   Epidemiology of HAV Infections   507
      10.1.   Incidence of HAV Infection   508
      10.2.   Routes of HAV Transmission   509
11.   References   512

Index   527

CHAPTER 1

Bunyaviridae

David H. L. Bishop

Department of Microbiology, The Medical Center
University of Alabama in Birmingham
Birmingham, Alabama 35294

and

Robert E. Shope

Yale Arbovirus Research Unit (YARU)
Department of Epidemiology and Public Health
Yale University School of Medicine
New Haven, Connecticut 06510

1. INTRODUCTION

The Bunyaviridae are a relatively newly defined family of arthropod-borne viruses. Of the viruses that have been registered as of 1978 in the published and working *International Catalogue of Arboviruses* (Berge, 1975; Taylor, 1967; see Berge *et al.*, 1970, 1971; Karabatsos, 1978), 95 have been proposed as members of the genus Bunyavirus (Table 1), formerly known as the "Bunyamwera supergroup of viruses" (Calisher *et al.*, 1973; Casals, 1963, 1971; Fenner, 1976*a,b*; Murphy *et al.*, 1973; Porterfield *et al.*, 1973/1974, 1975/1976). Other genera of bunyaviruses have not yet been defined, although another 63 registered viruses are considered as possible members of the family. On serological criteria they have not been placed in the Bunyavirus genus (Table 2) (Porterfield *et al.*, 1975/1976). In addition, there are currently

TABLE 1

Proposed Serological Classification of Viruses of Family Bunyaviridae, Genus Bunyavirus

Anopheles A group[a]
Anopheles A[b]
  CoAr 3624[c]
Lukuni
ColAn 57389[c]
Tacaiuma (SP Ar 2317[c])
  CoAr 3627[c] (CoAr 1071[c])

Bunyamwera Group
Bunyamwera
Germiston
Shokwe[c]
Batai (Calovo)
Ilesha
Birao
Tensaw
Cache Valley (Tlacotalpan)
Maguari
Northway
Santa Rosa
Lokern
Wyeomyia
Taiassui[c]
Anhembi
Sororoca
Main Drain
Kairi
Guaroa

Bwamba group
Bwamba
Pongola

C group
Caraparu
  Caraparu (BeH 5546[c])
  Caraparu/Trinidad[c]
  Ossa
Apeu
Madrid
Marituba
  Murutucu
  Restan
  Nepuyo
  Gumbo Limbo
Oriboca
  Itaqui

California group
California encephalitis
  Tahyna (Lumbo[c])
  Inkoo
San Angelo
La Crosse (snowshoe hare)
Melao
  Serra do Navio
Keystone
Jamestown Canyon (South River[c], Jerry Slough)
Trivittatus

Capim group
Capim
Guajara (Gu 71 u 350[c])
Bushbush
  BeAn 84381[c]
  Gu 71 u 344[c]
Juan Diaz

Capim group (cont.)
Acara
Moriche
BeAn 153564[c]

Guama group
Guama
  Moju
  BeAn 109303[c]
  Mahogany Hammock
Bimiti
  BeAn 116382[c]
Catu
Bertioga

Koongol group
Koongol
Wongal

Mirim group
Mirim
Minatitlan

Olifantsvlei group
Olifantsvlei
  Bobia[c]
Botambi

Patois group
Patois
Shark River
Zegla
Pahayokee

Simbu group
Akabane
  Yaba-7[c]
  Facey's Paddock[c]
Shamonda
  Sango
  Sabo
Sathuperi
  Shuni
  Aino (Kaikalur, Samford)
Simbu
Thimiri
Nola
Peaton[c]
Manzanilla
Ingwavuma
Mermet
  Inini[c]
Buttonwillow
Oropouche
  Utinga[c]

Tete group
Tete
Bahig
Matruh
Tsuruse
Batama[c]

Unassigned members
Gamboa
Guaratuba
Jurona
Kaeng Khoi

[a] The Anopheles A group was proposed as a group in the genus Bunyavirus (Calisher *et al.*, 1973); the group has not yet been officially accepted in the Bunyavirus genus.
[b] Viruses are classified in three steps indicated by degrees of indentation—complex, virus, subtype; viruses in parentheses are varieties.
[c] These viruses are not in the published or working *International Catalogue of Arboviruses* (Berge, 1975; Karabatsos, 1978).

at least 34 viruses which are under study and consideration for candidacy (Tables 1 and 2).

1.1. Characteristics of the Bunyaviridae

The assignments of viruses to the Bunyaviridae family were initially made by serological studies (Casals, 1963). Such assignments were later confirmed by additional serological and morphological criteria (Berge, 1975; Casals, 1971; Murphy and Coleman, 1967; Murphy *et al.*, 1973). These assignments have been substantiated by molecular analyses which indicate that bunyaviruses are categorically different than other arthropod-borne viruses.

The principal characteristics of members of the Bunyavirus genus include the following:

1. The virus particles are spherical (90–100 nm in diameter) and enveloped.
2. The viruses have a single-stranded, three-segment, negative-sense RNA genome of total molecular weight of between 4 and 6×10^6. The viruses are capable of genetic reassortment. The viral RNA segments are designated according to their sizes, large (L), medium (M), and small (S).
3. Three circular, helical, viral nucleocapsids can be isolated from virus preparations. Each is composed of nucleocapsid protein (N) and a single RNA species (L, M, or S). The RNA species have 5′ and 3′ ends but can be extracted from nucleocapsids (or virus particles) as noncovalently closed circles.
4. Two virus-specific glycoproteins (designated G1 and G2) have been identified in all bunyaviruses so far analyzed; they are located on the outer surface of the virus particles.
5. Virus replication occurs in the cytoplasm of infected cells.
6. Virus particles are formed by budding primarily into the Golgi cisternae. Virions are liberated from infected cells by fusion of the intracellular vacuoles with the cellular plasma membrane and virus egestion, or by cell membrane disruption and discharge of the cell contents.

From the limited amount of available information, the same structural and genetic characteristics are attributable to at least some of the other possible members of the Bunyaviridae family.

TABLE 2

Proposed Serological Classification of Bunyaviruslike Viruses (Other Possible Members of Family Bunyaviridae)

Anopheles B group	Phlebotomus fever group	Thogoto group
Anopheles B[b]	Candiru	Thogoto
Boraceia	Itaituba	SiAr 126[c]
	Nique	
Bakau group	Punta Toro	Turlock group
Bakau	CoAr 3319[c]	Turlock
Ketapang	Saint-Floris	Umbre
	Gordil	M'Poko
Crimean hemorrhagic fever–Congo	Aguacate	Barmah Forest[c]
group	Anhanga	Marweh[c]
Crimean hemorrhagic fever–Congo	Arumowot	
Hazara	Bujaru	Uukuniemi group
	Cacao	Uukuniemi
Kaisodi group	Caimito	Oceanside[c]
Kaisodi	Chagres	Grand Arbaud
Lanjan	Chilibre	Manawa
Silverwater	Frijoles	Zaliv Terpeniya
	Icoaraci	Ponteves
Mapputta group	Itaporanga	EgAn 1825-61[c]
Mapputta	Karimabad	
Maprik	Pacui	Unassigned viruses
Gan Gan[c]	Rio Grande	Belmont[a]
Trubanaman	Salehabad	Bhanja
	SudAn 754-61[c]	Khasan[a]
Nairobi sheep disease group	SF-Naples	Kowanyama
Nairobi sheep disease (Ganjam)	Iss. Phl. 3[c]	Lone Star
Dugbe	SF-Sicilian	Razdan
	Urucuri	Rift Valley fever
		Sunday Canyon
	Sakhalin group[a]	Tamdy[a]
	Sakhalin	Tataguine
	Tillamook[c]	Witwatersrand
	Taggert	
	Clo Mor	
	Avalon	

[a] These viruses are proposed but not yet officially accepted as other possible members of the family.

[b] Viruses are classified in three steps indicated by degrees of indentation—complex, virus, and subtype; viruses in parentheses are varieties.

[c] These viruses are not in the published or working *International Catalogue of Arboviruses* (Berge, 1975; Karabatsos, 1978).

Historically, before a universal system of virus classification was devised, Casals and Brown (1954) divided the arboviruses into groups A and B on the basis of serological relationships. Casals and Whitman (1961) subsequently recognized a third grouping, which they called group C, now known to be a grouping in the genus Bunyavirus. As many new serological groupings became evident, the alphabetical system was no longer proliferated and groups were called by the name of a prominent virus within the serogroup.

In their study of group C viruses, Casals and Whitman (1961) defined serological characteristics which still apply generally to the bunyaviruses:

1. The neutralization test and hemagglutination-inhibition (HI) test reactions coincide in specificity and are as a rule interchangeable in defining the serotype of a given isolate.
2. The complement-fixation (CF) test reaction coincides sometimes, *but not always*, in specificity with the neutralization/HI test reactions.

The fact that two isolates of the same serotype (*as defined by the neutralization test*) may each express the major complement-fixing antigen of totally different viruses (see later discussion of group C viruses) is an intriguing observation that may be explained by ancestral genetic reassortment of RNA segments coding for different antigenic determinants.

The gene products which relate to the neutralization/hemagglutinin (H) and the CF determinants of bunyaviruses are not known, although the principal CF antigen probably represents the major virion nucleocapsid protein (Lindsey *et al.*, 1977), while the neutralization/H determinants are probably resident in the viral glycoproteins (Obijeski *et al.*, 1976a). It is believed that the nucleocapsid protein and viral glycoproteins are coded for by different bunyavirus RNA segments (Gentsch and Bishop, 1978; Gentsch *et al.*, 1977b). If correct, then divergence of the neutralization/H and CF determinants could be explained by ancestral reassortment.

1.2. Isolation and Relationships of Members and Possible Members of the Bunyaviridae Family

The Bunyaviridae family of arthropod-borne viruses is the largest taxonomic subset of arboviruses, the other major subsets being the alphaviruses and flaviviruses (family Togaviridae), orbiviruses (family Reoviridae), and rhabdoviruses (family Rhabdoviridae) (Casals, 1963, 1971; Fenner, 1976a,b; Fenner *et al.*, 1974; Porterfield *et al.*, 1975/1976). Members of the Bunyaviridae family have been isolated from various arthropods and vertebrates as well as from all continents of the world, except Antarctica.

Serological analyses have categorized most of the accepted, possible, and candidate bunyaviruses into groups which, together with some unassigned viruses, give a current total of 188 viruses (Tables 1 and 2).

The viruses in the Bunyavirus genus are given in Table 1. Another term previously used for the genus is "Bunyamwera supergroup," so named because of the serological interrelationships that were detected between particular members of the various serogroups. Thirteen interrelated groups of viruses, as well as four unplaced viruses, form the supergroup (Table 1). Most of the serogroups shown in Table 1 have registered members which are either closely or distantly related to other members of the serogroup, as shown by one or more of the tests usually employed to relate and categorize viruses (CF, neutralization, HI, and immunodiffusion). In addition to the registered members, there are other bunyavirus isolates which, although not yet registered members of a particular serogroup, are under study and consideration for candidacy on the basis of either molecular or certain serological similarities to accepted supergroup members. Some of these isolates are described in this text.

The basis for the serological classification of bunyaviruses is the neutralization test and, where applicable, the HI test. The CF test has been especially useful in placing bunyaviruses in groups, where these viruses would otherwise have remained ungrouped if only the neutralization and HI test reactions were considered.

A system of classification of bunyaviruses has been proposed by the Subcommittee on Interrelationships among Catalogued Arboviruses (Berge, 1975) based on how closely the viruses can be related serologically. Five categories were suggested: group, complex, virus (or serotype), subtype, and variety. These categories reflect the degree of serological relatedness of different viruses. This degree is indicated in Tables 1 and 2 by progressive indentations indicating complex, virus, and subtype and by parentheses for viruses which are considered as varieties. The term "variety" is applied to those viruses which are only just distinguished in HI, CF, and/or neutralization tests; "subtype" applies to those viruses which can be more easily differentiated by one or more of the tests; "serotype" (or virus) is used for isolates which can be readily differentiated by these tests; "complex" is used for viruses which, although readily differentiated, show significant cross-reactivities; and "group" is used for the assemblage of virus complexes which have low cross-reactivities. Although the terms are arbitary and reflect only the serological tests employed, they are useful in describing the serological relationships of the multitude of bunyaviruses that have been recognized. Consequently these terms are used in the following text. Another term which is used in the text is "virus variant." We consider a variant as being serologically indistinguishable from another virus. At the molecular level the term is used to describe a recent evolutionary event whereby genome RNA fingerprinting studies indicate that a variant is almost identical to another virus isolate. At the molecular level a virus variety is one which has an easily distinguished genome sequence (El Said *et al.*, 1979).

The reader should understand that the connotations associated with the use of the above terms for some serogroups of viruses are not necessarily exactly the same as for other serogroups of viruses. For example, in the California group some recognized serotypes are more closely related by the neutralization test than are analogous members of other groups of bunyaviruses.

The 63 registered arboviruses which are proposed as members of the Bunyaviridae family, but which are not in the Bunyavirus genus, have been described as "bunyaviruslike viruses" or "other possible members" (Porterfield *et al.*, 1975/1976). They are enumerated in Table 2. The same basis of classification of these viruses has been applied in this text to that described above for members of the Bunyavirus genus. The definition of other genera of the family awaits definitive molecular proof that these possible members are genetically equivalent to the accepted Bunyaviridae. Most of the groups of possible bunyaviruses are candidates of the family only on morphological (electron microscopic) evidence.

In this chapter the serological, biological, and molecular attributes of the registered, certain candidate, and other possible members of the Bunyaviridae family will be discussed.

1.2.1. Serological and Biological Characteristics of the Members of the Bunyavirus Genus (Bunyamwera Supergroup Viruses)

The serological and biological properties of Bunyamwera super-group viruses are discussed below in order to set the framework in which the molecular and genetic attributes of the viruses can be considered. Since Bunyamwera virus is the prototype of the genus and the family, the Bunyamwera group viruses will be discussed first.

Most of the members of the genus have been isolated from mosquitoes. Few have come from ticks. Although overall an extremely diverse set of vertebrates appear from serological and isolation studies to be the normal hosts for members of the genus, particular groups of bunyaviruses and/or particular virus serotypes appear to be quite limited in their vertebrate host tropisms. For many members of the genus it has been shown that mosquito vectors can experimentally transmit the agent (Theiler and Downs, 1973).

1.2.1a. Bunyamwera Group

The Bunyamwera group of viruses was recognized as a distinct group of arboviruses by Casals and Whitman in 1960. The 21 currently accepted and proposed members of the group are given in Table 1. Calovo virus, although registered as a member, is now considered as a subtype or variety of Batai virus (see later). Five of the viruses have been isolated from humans, while eight (Bunyamwera, Batai (Calovo), Germiston, Guaroa, Ilesha, Maguari, Tensaw, and Wyeomyia), have been associated with naturally occurring clinical or overt human infections (Theiler and Downs, 1973).

Bunyamwera virus was originally obtained from *Aedes* mosquitoes collected in 1943 in Bwamba County, Uganda, and isolated by Smithburn *et al.* (1946) at the Entebbe East African Virus Research Institute, Uganda. The virus has subsequently been reisolated from *Aedes*, *Mansonia*, and *Culex* mosquitoes, as well as from viremic humans in Uganda and/or Cameroon, Kenya, Nigeria, Central African Empire, and South Africa (Berge, 1975). Antibodies reactive to the virus have been detected in human sera obtained from various parts of the African continent with up to 80% of inhabitants in certain areas being recorded as seropositive (Berge, 1975).

Although some early studies reported Bunyamwera reactive antibodies in human sera from North Borneo, Colombia, the South American Amazon Delta, and North and West Africa (Berge, 1975; Smithburn, 1954), it is now considered unlikely that such antibodies were specific to Bunyamwera virus since the known geographic distribution of Bunyamwera virus isolation encompasses only regions of East, Central, and South Africa. It is currently believed that the Bunyamwera antibodies found in the other geographic regions were due to infection by other members of the group which are now known to be present in those regions but which were unavailable for the earlier studies (Berge, 1975; Smithburn, 1954).

Serological studies have demonstrated Bunyamwera antibodies in a high percentage of sera obtained from chimpanzees (in the Congo) and domestic animals (in many regions of South, East, and Central Africa). Only rarely have antibodies been found in rodent and avian sera in different regions of Africa (Berge, 1975; Paterson et al., 1957; Smithburn et al., 1946).

Experimental infection of a variety of animals by Bunyamwera virus has been documented, with results ranging from death to seroconversion depending on the species, route of inoculation, dose and age of the host, etc. (Berge, 1975). Attenuation of the virus after 100 serial intracerebral mouse passages has been reported (Smithburn et al., 1946). Human infection by the virus can result in prostration, fever, stiff neck, rash, and a variety of other signs and symptoms (Berge, 1975). One of the first reported natural infections of humans involved a 13-year-old mosquito catcher in Tongaland (South Africa) who contracted a Bunyamwera virus infection (Kokernot et al., 1958). Virus was recovered from the patient's blood and he later seroconverted and recovered. Bunyamwera virus was also isolated from *Aedes* mosquitoes collected during the same period and from the same locality where the boy acquired his infection.

Experimental transmission of Bunyamwera virus by mosquitoes (including *Aedes aegypti*, *Culex fatigans*, and *Anopheles quadrimaculatus*) has been demonstrated (Berge, 1975; Ogunbi, 1968; Smithburn et al., 1946).

Five of the 21 viruses belonging to the Bunyamwera serogroup came originally from Africa (Birao, Bunyamwera, Germiston, Ilesha, and Shokwe viruses). Birao virus, isolated in 1969 from *Anopheles pharoensis* collected at Birao in the Central African Empire, has been reisolated a few times, all the isolates coming from *Anopheles* species in that country (Berge, 1975). Germiston virus was reported by Kokernot et al. (1960) to have come from *Culex* mosquitoes taken from human bait at Germiston, South Africa, in an urban area where febrile illnesses of unexplained etiology had previously occurred. Subsequent isolates of Germiston virus from insects have been made in Natal and Transvaal (South Africa), Ethiopia, Uganda, and Rhodesia. Isolates from vertebrates have come from sentinel hamsters in South Africa and Mozambique and wild rodents in Uganda (Berge, 1975; Monath et al., 1972). Laboratory-acquired human infections by Germiston virus have been documented (Kokernot et al., 1960). Antibodies to Germiston virus have been detected in wild rodent, human, and domestic animal sera collected in various parts of Africa, even as far north as Ethiopia (Berge, 1975; Theiler and Downs, 1973).

Ilesha virus has been isolated several times from human samples (in Uganda, Senegal, Cameroon, Ethiopia, and the Central African Empire), the first isolate having been made from a febrile 9-year-old human in Nigeria (Yaba Annual Report, 1957). One virus isolate has been made from *Anopheles gambiae* (Berge, 1975). Antibodies believed to be specific to Ilesha virus have been found in human, goat, and bovine sera but not in sheep or pigs from Nigeria, Liberia, Ghana, Ethiopia, and Uganda (Berge, 1975; Theiler and Downs, 1973). Shokwe virus was isolated by B. M. McIntosh at Ndumu, South Africa, from *Aedes cumminsi* mosquitoes.

An Asian Bunyamwera group virus, Batai virus, was initially isolated in 1955 from *Culex* species collected in Kuala Lumpur, Malaya, although other Batai isolates have been reported from insects collected in Thailand, India (topotype Chittoor), the Ukrainian S.S.R., Czechoslovakia (topotype Calovo), Yugoslavia, Japan, and Sarawak (Berge, 1975). Antibodies to the virus have been found in human sera (Malaya), various animal sera, particularly domestic animals in each of the above countries, in addition to a variety of avian sera collected in Thailand (Berge, 1975). Calovo virus, which is considered as a subtype or variety of Batai virus (Berge, 1975), has been repetitively isolated from anopheline mosquitoes collected in Central Europe following its initial isolation in 1960 in Czechoslovakia (Bardos and Cupkova, 1962; Bardos and Danielova, 1961). Human and animal serological surveys (see Brummer-Korvenkontio, 1973*b*) indicate that Calovo virus infections are widespread throughout Central Europe, particularly among large domestic animals (horses, cattle, sheep, pigs, etc.). An association of Calovo virus infections with hospitalized febrile patients has been reported. However, Calovo virus has not yet been isolated from man (Berge, 1975).

Anhembi, Guaroa, Kairi, Maguari, Santa Rosa, Sororoca, Taiassui, Tlacotalpan, and Wyeomyia viruses were originally isolated in various countries of the Caribbean and/or in Central and South America (Berge, 1975). Anhembi virus came from pooled *Phoniomyia* and *Trichoprosopon* mosquitoes collected in 1965 in Casa Grande, Brazil (Lopes *et al.*, 1975). An isolate of Anhembi virus from a spiny rat has also been reported (Lopes *et al.*, 1975). Guaroa virus was initially recovered in 1956 by Groot *et al.* (1959) from the serum of a 75-year-old man at Guaroa, Bogota, Colombia, in a region where a febrile disease of unknown etiology was prevalent. Other human isolates and human antibodies have been reported from Colombia and Brazil, in one case from an afebrile, partially paralyzed individual who had lost his hair (Berge, 1975; Causey *et al.*, 1962). Mosquito isolates from *Anopheles* species in Panama and Colombia have been made (Berge, 1975). Human Guaroa virus infections appear to be widespread in the Amazon Valley as well as in Central and South America. Birds have been implicated from serological surveys to be possible hosts for the virus (Theiler and Downs, 1973). Kairi virus originally came from *Aedes* species collected in 1955 in the Melajo forest, Trinidad (Anderson *et al.*, 1960*a*). Other isolates of the virus have been made from a *Saimiri* monkey at Belem, Brazil, and various insects collected in Colombia, Argentina, Trinidad, and Brazil (Berge, 1975). Antibodies against the virus have been found in human, donkey, and monkey sera in Trinidad and human sera in Colombia. Maguari virus is another Bunyamwera group virus isolated from mosquitoes in Brazil (Causey *et al.*, 1961). Serological studies indicate that Maguari virus frequently infects humans and various large animals in different parts of South America (particularly the Amazon valley, Brazil, French Guiana, Trinidad, Guatemala, Argentina, Peru, and Colombia). Although not isolated from human sources, the virus has been isolated from horses in French Guiana and Colombia and several times from sentinel mice in Brazil (Berge, 1975). Many Maguari virus isolates have come from a variety of insects (Brazil, Trinidad, Ecuador, Colombia, Argentina), with the original isolate having been made from mixed mosquitoes collected in the Utinga forest in Brazil (Berge, 1975). Santa Rosa virus, a recent addition to the Bunyamwera group, was isolated by Sudia and Newhouse from *Aedes* mosquitoes collected in 1972 at Santa Rosa, Mexico (Sudia *et al.*, 1975). Sororoca and Taiassui viruses are Brazilian isolates which have been isolated only from *Aedes* and *Sabethini* mosquitoes (Berge, 1975; Woodall, 1967).

Although antibodies to Tlacotalpan virus have been detected in Mexican human, pig, and cattle sera, the virus has been isolated only from *Mansonia* and other mosquitoes (Scherer *et al.*, 1967). Wyeomyia virus is a Bunyamwera group virus obtained by Roca-Garcia (1944) from *Wyeomyia melanocephala* caught in 1940 in Villavicencio in Colombia. Other strains have been isolated from various mosquitoes in Colombia, Panama, Trinidad, the Amazon Valley, Brazil, and French Guiana (Berge, 1975). A human Wyeomyia virus isolate and human antibodies to the virus (27% seropositive in some regions) have been reported from Panama (Berge, 1975; Srihongse and Johnson, 1965).

Five Bunyamwera group viruses (Cache Valley, Lokern, Main Drain, Northway, and Tensaw viruses) have come from the southern continental United States, Canada, and Alaska. Cache Valley virus was reported by Holden and Hess (1959) to have come from *Culiseta inornata* mosquitoes collected in 1956 in Cache Valley, Utah, United States. Other isolates have been reported from various mosquitoes (*Culiseta*, *Aedes*, *Psorophora*, and *Anopheles* species) in different areas of the United States (Anslow *et al.*, 1969), Argentina, Mexico, and Canada, as well as from *Aedes* and *Anopheles* species in Jamaica (Berge, 1975). Antibodies to the virus have been detected in the sera of hoofed animals (various), rodents, racoons, and foxes in the United States, horses and primates in Trinidad, and humans in Trinidad, Guyana, and the United States (Berge, 1975). Lokern virus was originally isolated from *Culex tarsalis* obtained in Kern County California, and reisolated from hares, rabbits, and midges in the same area (Berge *et al.*, 1970). Antibodies to the virus have been found in human and a variety of vertebrate sera (from birds, rodents, and domestic animals) in California (Berge *et al.*, 1970).

Main Drain virus was initially isolated from *Culicoides variipennis* collected in 1964 in Kern County, California (Berge *et al.*, 1970; Nelson and Scrivani, 1972). Other isolates have come from hares in the same region. Equine, bovine, ovine, hare, rabbit, and various rodent (but not human) serum samples collected in California have been reported to have antibodies against the virus (Berge, 1975; Berge *et al.*, 1970). Northway virus was obtained in 1972 by Ritter and associates (Calisher *et al.*, 1974; Ritter and Feltz, 1974) from mosquitoes collected in 1971 in Northway, Alaska. Other isolates have been recovered from sentinel rabbits and various mosquitoes in different parts of Alaska and the Yukon (Berge, 1975; Calisher *et al.*, 1974). Tensaw virus was reported by Chamberlain *et al.* (1969) and Coleman (1969) to have come from *Anopheles crucians* collected in 1960 at Baldwin City, Alabama. The virus has been isolated many times from mosquitoes in various states of the United States (Alabama, Georgia, Florida, and Wisconsin), and a few times from various vertebrates (a dog, cotton rats, and marsh rabbits) (Anslow *et al.*, 1969; Chamberlain, 1963; Berge, 1975). Antibodies to the virus have been found in human (up to 25% seropositive in some areas), racoon, bovine, and chicken serum samples (Berge, 1975). A human case of encephalitis possibly due to Tensaw virus infection has been described.

The serological relationships of the group have been documented by CF, neutralization and HI tests. HI test reactions among members of the Bunyamwera group viruses are shown in Table 3. Casals and Whitman (1960) demonstrated that Bunyamwera, Cache Valley, Kairi, and Wyeomyia were related but distinct viruses. Okuno (1961) con-

TABLE 3

Hemagglutination-Inhibition Reactions of Bunyamwera Group Viruses[a]

	Antibody										
Antigen	Bunyam-wera	Germis-ton	Batai	Ilesha	Tensaw	Cache Valley	Maguari	Lokern	Main Drain	Kairi	Sororoca
Bunyamwera	0[b]	>64	>16	>16	>64	>32	>32	>64	>16	>16	>32
Germiston	2	0	8	0	64	>32	32	16	>16	8	8
Batai	32	>64	0	8	32	32	4	16	>16	16	>32
Ilesha	>32	>64	>16	0	>64	>32	>32	>64	>16	>16	>32
Tensaw	>32	>64	2	4	0	32	4	2	16	>16	>32
Cache Valley	>32	32	4	8	32	0	4	16	>16	>16	>32
Maguari	>32	>64	8	16	32	32	0	8	>16	>16	>32
Lokern	>32	>64	16	>16	64	>32	<8	0	>16	>16	>32
Main Drain	>32	>64	>16	>16	>64	>32	>32	>64	0	>16	>32
Kairi	32	>64	>16	>16	64	>32	>32	>64	16	0	>32
Sororoca	>32	>64	>16	>16	>64	>32	32	>64	>16	>16	0

[a] Data from R. Anslow and R. W. Shope (unpublished).
[b] Fold difference from homologous. This system of expressing serological results (this and other tables), although not conventional, permits comparison of data from one source with those of other sources in the same table.

shares a common CF antigen with CoAr 3624; Lukuni virus shares the antigen of CoAn 57389. Anopheles A is related to Lukuni virus and Tacaiuma to CoAr 3627 virus, but each can be distinguished from the other.

Calisher *et al.* (1973) have reported HI cross-reactions of CoAn 57389 virus with La Crosse virus of the California group and Tensaw virus of the Bunyamwera group. Because of this, the Anopheles A group has been proposed to belong to the Bunyavirus genus of the Bunyaviridae family (Calisher *et al.*, 1973).

1.2.1c. Bwamba Group

Both Bwamba and Pongola viruses, the two known members of the Bwamba group, have been isolated from mosquitoes in various parts of the African continent (Berge, 1975; Kokernot *et al.*, 1957a; Ota *et al.*, 1976; Smithburn *et al.*, 1941). Bwamba virus was originally isolated from the plasma of nine laborers in Bwamba County, Uganda, who developed a fever, headache, epigastric pain, and myalgia. Pongola virus came from *Aedes* species in Tongaland (South Africa), and later from mosquitoes captured in Uganda and Nigeria. Since its initial isolation, Bwamba virus has been repeatedly recovered from the blood of febrile human patients in East Africa as well as in Nigeria and the Central African Empire. Human disease, but no deaths or lasting or severe illnesses, has been associated with Bwamba virus infections. Bwamba virus has been recovered from *Anopheles funestus* in both Uganda and Nigeria, as well as from *Aedes circumluteolus*. Antibodies reactive to these viruses have been detected widely throughout Africa (south of the Sahara) in human, monkey, domestic animal, and avian (but not in rodent) sera, with neutralizing antibodies in up to 97% of the human serum samples obtained from people in certain regions of Tanzania and Uganda (Berge, 1975). Although serologically closely related to each other (Kokernot *et al.*, 1957a), and perhaps distantly to viruses of the California group (Casals, 1963), Bwamba and Pongola viruses are, for practical reasons, considered to form a separate group with two subtypes—Bwamba and Pongola (Berge, 1975; Casals, 1963).

1.2.1d. Group C Viruses

The initial members of the group C viruses were recognized by Casals and Whitman in 1961 as a separate serogroup of culicine mos-

quito-transmitted viruses, serologically distinct from the group A
viruses (alphaviruses) and the group B viruses (flaviviruses). Ten of
the viruses (Apeu, Caraparu, Itaqui, Madrid, Marituba, Murutucu,
Nepuyo, Oriboca, Ossa, and Restan) have been isolated from man as
well as from various insects (Berge, 1975). Many of the viruses have
also been obtained from rodents and/or marsupials in South, Central,
and North America (Berge, 1975), indicating that these small mammals
and mosquitoes probably constitute the principal virus cycle in nature.

Apeu virus, recovered initially from a sentinel *Cebus apella* in 1955
in the Oriboca Forest, Brazil (Causey *et al.*, 1961), has been subsequently isolated from sentinel mice and *Cebus* species, from natural
and laboratory-acquired human infections, and from wild-caught
Caluromys philander and *Marmosa cinerae* in Para, Brazil (Berge,
1975). The virus has been isolated from *Aedes* and *Culex* species from
the same region. Antibodies reactive to Apeu and Caraparu viruses
have been detected in human and various rodent sera in parts of Brazil
(Berge, 1975). Serologically, Apeu virus is closely related to Caraparu
virus, the latter also having come from a naturally infected sentinel
Cebus apella in 1956 in the Instituto Agronomico do Norte Forest,
Brazil (Causey *et al.*, 1961). Other isolates of Caraparu virus have been
made from sentinel *Oryzomys* and wild mouse species in Trinidad
(Trinidadian subtype) and Brazil and from various wild-caught rodents
in both countries. Human and mosquito isolates of Caraparu virus have
been reported from Brazil, Trinidad, and Surinam (Berge, 1975).
Human antibodies to Caraparu virus have been detected in residents of
those countries and French Guiana (Theiler and Downs, 1973).

Gumbo Limbo virus, isolated from *Culex* mosquitoes collected in
the Everglades National Park, Florida, in 1963, has been recovered also
from *Aedes* mosquitoes as well as a cotton rat in the same area (Berge,
1975; Henderson *et al.*, 1969). Itaqui virus originally came in 1959 from
a sentinel Swiss mouse in Brazil (Shope *et al.*, 1961). Other isolates
have come from sentinel mice, hamsters, and *Cebus* species, wild
rodents and marsupials, and various *Culex* mosquitoes in Para, Brazil
(Berge, 1975; Shope *et al.*, 1961). One human isolate of the virus has
been recorded. Antibodies to the virus have been detected in rodent but
rarely in marsupial sera in Brazil (Berge, 1975).

Madrid virus was isolated in 1961 by De Rodaniche *et al.* (1964)
from the plasma of a 36-year-old Panamanian mosquito catcher who
developed a fever, chills, headache, prostration, and body pains. Other
isolates of the virus have come from sentinel mice and hamsters and
Culex mosquitoes in Panama (Berge, 1975; De Rodaniche *et al.*, 1964).

Human antibodies to the virus have been detected in Panama (Berge, 1975). Marituba virus, the first group C agent to be isolated, came from a sentinel *Cebus apella* in 1954 in Oriboca Forest (Causey *et al.*, 1961). Additional isolates in Brazil have come from a laboratory-acquired human infection, a naturally infected *Didelphis marsupialis*, sentinel *Cebus* and mice species, and various *Culex* mosquitoes. Arboreal *Caluromys* and *Marmosa* have been shown to have higher antibody titers than forest floor-dwelling rodents and marsupials (Berge, 1975).

Murutucu virus, although it has been isolated a few times from human samples in Para, Brazil, came originally from a sentinel *Celus apella* in the Instituto Agronomico do Norte Forest in Brazil (Causey *et al.*, 1961). Many other virus isolates have been obtained from various wild and sentinel rodents and *Culex* mosquitoes (in Brazil) as well as from insects obtained in French Guiana (Berge, 1975). Human and rodent antibodies to Murutucu virus have been documented both in Brazil and in French Guiana (Berge, 1975). Nepuyo virus was isolated from *Culex* mosquitoes collected in 1957 in southeastern Trinidad (Spence *et al.*, 1966). Other isolates of the virus have been made from man (Scherer *et al.*, 1976a), wild rodents in Brazil and Panama, sentinel mice in Brazil and Trinidad, mosquitoes and fruit-eating bats in Honduras, *Culex* species in Trinidad and Brazil, and mosquitoes and sentinel rodents in Mexico (Berge, 1975). Human antibodies reactive to Nepuyo virus have been reported (Berge, 1975; Calisher *et al.*, 1971).

Ossa virus originally was isolated in 1961 from the serum of a mosquito catcher who developed a fever, chills, and headaches in the Bocas del Toro Province of Panama (De Rodaniche *et al.*, 1964). A few other isolates of the virus have been made from mosquitoes and sentinel animals in the Republic of Panama (Berge, 1975; Galindo and Srihongse, 1967). Restan virus came from *Culex* mosquitoes collected in the Bush Bush Forest of eastern Trinidad (Jonkers *et al.*, 1967). Human isolates of the virus have been obtained both in Trinidad and in Surinam, and human antibodies to the virus have been found in human sera collected in Surinam (Berge, 1975).

Oriboca virus, which has been partially characterized at the molecular level (see later), was originally isolated from a sentinel *Cebus apella* monkey in the Oriboca Forest, Brazil (Causey *et al.*, 1961). The virus has been reisolated from sentinel mice, other rodents, and marsupials in Brazil and Trinidad, as well as from man both in Brazil and in Surinam (Berge, 1975; Metselaar, 1966). Hemagglutination inhibition tests have shown that about 3% of the human population and between 5% and 19% of the rodents and marsupials tested in and around Para and Amazonas, Brazil, have antibodies against Oriboca virus (Berge, 1975). The virus has been repetitively isolated from *Culex*, *Aedes*, *Psorophora*, and *Mansonia* mosquitoes (Berge, 1975). Some 14 natural and laboratory-acquired Oriboca virus infections have been documented, with signs and symptoms including fever, myalgia, headaches, and conjunctival inflammation (Berge, 1975). No severe illnesses or human deaths have been attributed to Oriboca virus infections (Berge, 1975).

The group C viruses are separated into four complexes, each of which has from one to five virus types and subtypes (Table 1). This proposed classification is based on neutralization (Karabatsos and Henderson, 1969; Berge, 1975) and HI test data (De Rodaniche *et al.*, 1964; Shope, 1965; Shope and Whitman, 1966; Jonkers *et al.*, 1967; Casals and Whitman, 1961; Shope *et al.*, 1961; Berge, 1975). The group C viruses, of all the bunyavirus groups, illustrate most clearly the divergence of the CF reaction from the neutralization and HI reactions. In a single forest near Belem, Brazil, there exist six viruses which can be categorized into three pairs; each pair has closely related surface (HI and neutralization) antigens—Caraparu and Apeu, Marituba and Murutucu, and Oriboca and Itaqui. However, the members of the pairs can be shown to differ from each other by the CF test (Casals and Whitman, 1961; Shope *et al.*, 1961; Shope and Whitman, 1966; Berge, 1975) and share an antigen with a member of the other pairs—Caraparu with Itaqui, Apeu with Marituba, and Murutucu with Oriboca (Shope and Causey, 1962). This divergence of the reactivity of the surface antigen(s) from that of the CF antigen might be explained genetically if genome segment reassortment has occurred, presuming that the segment expressing the surface antigen differs from that expressing the major CF antigen—as indicated by *in vitro* genetic studies (see later). A variety of Caraparu virus, BeH 5546, has been isolated infrequently in Brazil. It too may be a natural recombinant, since it has the surface antigen of Caraparu virus and the CF antigen of Oriboca and Murutucu viruses.

1.2.1e.   California Group

The isolates of the California group viruses include Lumbo virus from Mozambique, Tahyna virus from Central Europe, Inkoo virus from Finland, Melao virus from Port of Spain, Trinidad, and Serra do

Navio from Brazil. The other recognized members of the group were all obtained from various parts of the North American continent (Sudia *et al.*, 1971). South River virus (Sudia *et al.*, 1971), an additional candidate member of the group, has also come from North America. The viruses in this group have been isolated from various mosquitoes and vertebrates (including man) but rarely from rodents. Reviews of the epidemiological and serological literature concerning the California group arboviruses have been published by Sudia *et al.* (1971), Hammon and Sather (1966), Sather and Hammon (1967), and Parkin *et al.* (1972).

Several studies into the transmission and serological, molecular, and genetic properties of California group viruses have been undertaken over the past decade. Six of the viruses have been implicated or associated with naturally occurring human infections (Tahyna, California encephalitis, Jamestown Canyon, Inkoo, La Crosse, and snowshoe hare viruses).

The original California encephalitis virus isolate was implicated in the early 1940s to cause human encephalitis (Hammon and Reeves, 1952), although no isolates were made from humans. Certain enzootic, disease-associated regions of the United States have since been identified by both serological and virus isolation studies (Berge, 1975; Henderson and Coleman, 1971; Masterson *et al.*, 1971; Sudia *et al.*, 1971). Each year in the United States many cases of human encephalitis have been shown to be associated with infection by La Crosse virus, particularly in the midwestern and eastern states of the United States (W. Thompson and M. Grayson, personal communication; Cramblett *et al.*, 1966; Monath *et al.*, 1970; Thompson and Evans, 1965; Vianna *et al.*, 1971; Wong *et al.*, 1973). Many of the cases described each year occur in three major enzootic areas of the United States (i.e., the Wisconsin–Iowa–Minnesota tristate area, Ohio, and Albany, N.Y.), although the disease has been documented in other regions of the country, such as Florida (Quick *et al.*, 1965), Indiana (Young, 1966), and Georgia (Hilty *et al.*, 1972).

California Encephalitis Virus

The prototype California encephalitis virus isolate, BFS-283, was recovered from *Culex tarsalis* mosquitoes in 1943 by Hammon and Reeves in Kern County, San Joaquin Valley, California; a second isolate, BFS-91, was obtained from *Aedes melanimon* (*dorsalis*) (Hammon and Reeves, 1952; Hammon *et al.*, 1952; Reeves and Hammon,

1952). The virus was implicated from serological evidence as the cause of three cases of human encephalitis in California in 1945. The virus has been subsequently isolated from a variety of mosquitoes [*Culex tarsalis*, *Aedes melanimon* (*dorsalis*), *Aedes vexans*, *Aedes nigromaculis*, *Psorophora signipennis*, *Culiseta inornata*, and *Aedes dorsalis*] collected in California, New Mexico, Texas, and Utah (Berge, 1975; Sudia *et al.*, 1971). Recently, transovarial transmission of California encephalitis virus by the mosquito *Aedes dorsalis* has been reported (Crane *et al.*, 1977). No isolates of this virus have been made in South America, Europe, Asia, Africa, or Australia. Neutralizing and HI antibodies have been found in human and other vertebrate sera in the United States (Berge, 1975).

Since the initial isolation of the virus in 1943, several thousand other California group virus isolates have been obtained from mosquitoes and vertebrates in many parts of the United States, Canada, the Caribbean, Brazil, Europe, and Africa. Many have come from arctic and subarctic zones.

Serological tests have been used to categorize the 14 accepted or candidate members of the California complex (Table 1) (Berge, 1975; Hammon and Sather, 1966; Murphy and Coleman, 1967). Some of the virus isolates can barely be distinguished from other members in particular serological tests, and are therefore considered as varieties of a recognized subtype of the group.

The results of the California intragroup neutralization relationships are described by Lindsey *et al.* (1976), Whitman and Shope (1962), Sather and Hammon (1967), Jennings *et al.* (1968), De Foliart *et al.* (1969), Issel (1973), and Brummer-Korvenkontio *et al.* (1973). HI relationships are shown in Table 4.

Divergence of the complement-fixation reaction (Sprance and Shope, 1977; Casals, cited in Brummer-Korvenkontio *et al.*, 1973; Sather and Hammon, 1967) and the neutralization reaction are not recognized among the California group viruses, quite in contrast to the group C viruses. This may mean that natural reassortant viruses have not been recovered or that if viruses with antigenic divergence occur they have not yet been recognized.

Serological tests between California encephalitis antigen (or antibodies) with the antibodies (or antigens) of members of other bunyavirus groups have provided evidence of minor cross-reactivities with members of the Bunyamwera, group C, Bwamba, Simbu, Anopheles A, and Patois group viruses. As discussed in Section 1.2.1a, Guaroa virus has been shown to be related to several members of the

TABLE 4
Hemagglutination-Inhibition Reactions of California Group Viruses[a]

Antigen	Antibody									
	CE	LAC	SSH	JC	KEY	SA	TVT	MEL	TAH	INK
California encephalitis	0[b]	2	2	4	4	32	32	>64	8	
La Crosse	4	0	4	32	0	32	16	>64	>4	2
Snowshoe hare	4	2	0	32	8	32	8	>64	>4	
Jamestown Canyon	16	0	2	0	0	64	8	16	4	
Keystone	>16	16	>16	16	0	>128	16	16	>4	
San Angelo	0	0	2	64	2	0	8	>64	>4	
Trivittatus	4	4	8	32	2	32	0	64	16	
Melao	16	4	2	4	0	16	8	0	4	
Tahyna	2	0	2	8	2	16	4	>64	0	2
Inkoo									>2	0

[a] Data from Whitman and Shope (1962), Sather and Hammon (1967), Brummer-Korvenkonitio *et al.* (1973), Whitman (1963, unpublished), and Clarke and Ardoin (1969, unpublished).
[b] Fold difference from homologous titer; see Table 3.

California group when both HI and neutralization of infectivity tests are used but not when CF tests are used (Whitman and Shope, 1962). Guaroa virus is, however, related to members of the Bunyamwera group by CF tests but not by HI or neutralization of infectivity tests (Whitman and Shope, 1962).

Tahyna and Lumbo Viruses

Although no isolates of Tahyna virus have been obtained in the United States, numerous isolates have been made from mosquitoes as well as from viremic human sera in Europe (Berge, 1975; Likar and Casals, 1963). Tahyna virus was originally isolated in 1958 from *Aedes caspius* mosquitoes collected at Tahyna Village, Czechoslovakia (strain 92, Bardos and Danielova, 1959). Although it has been isolated only twice from man, many isolates of the virus have been reported from various mosquitoes collected in Czechoslovakia, Yugoslavia (topotype Trojica), France (topotype Souche D), Italy, Kenya, Mozambique, Austria, the German Federal Republic, the U.S.S.R., and Romania, as well as from sentinel rabbits in Austria and Czechoslovakia (Berge, 1975). Hares have been implicated as a major vertebrate host in at least parts of Europe. The virus has been recovered from first generation larvae of *Culiseta annulata* in southern Moravia, suggesting that larval survival or transovarial transmission may be an overwintering mechanism for this virus (Bardos *et al.*, 1975; Thompson, 1977). Parts of Central Europe are recognized focal enzootic areas for Tahyna virus as documented by serological, human illness, and isolation studies (Berge, 1975). However, the virus does not appear to be present in some parts of Southern Europe (e.g., south Italy).

Lumbo virus was isolated in 1959 from *Aedes pembaensis* mosquitoes collected at Lumbo, Mozambique (Kokernot *et al.*, 1962). Based on the close serological relationship to Tahyna virus, it is considered as a variety of that virus, although certain serological tests can distinguish the two viruses (Kunz and Aspock, 1967; Kunz *et al.*, 1964). Some serological relationship of Lumbo to Bwamba virus (the prototype of the Bwamba group) has been documented (Kokernot *et al.*, 1962).

Antibodies against Tahyna virus have been reported in human sera collected in almost all countries of Europe (Berge, 1975), in south-central U.S.S.R. (D. Lvov, personal communication), and (Lumbo variety) widely in South and West Africa (Berge, 1975). Antibodies have been found in sera obtained from European hares, rabbits, horses, cows, pigs, a ground squirrel, a fox, a wild boar, roe deer, and hedgehogs but not birds in many of those regions.

Experimental infection of hamsters, chick embryos, suckling white rats, and newborn or young mice by Tahyna virus induces either death or seroconversion, depending on the dose, route of inoculation, age of the animals, etc. Tahyna infection of humans causes a febrile illness, with nausea, headaches, anorexia, encephalitis, and eventual recovery with seroconversion.

The highest levels of human Tahyna virus infections have been reported from Central Europe, where up to 96% of particular populations have been shown to have antibodies against the virus. In a study undertaken in the Moravia and Slovakia areas of Czechoslovakia (Bardos *et al.*, 1962), it was found that children under 1 year old had antibodies (22% of the sera tested), although no antibodies were found in sera obtained from 1-year-old children. Fifty percent of children between 1 and 5 years old were found to have antibodies, while 85% of sera obtained from young adolescents over 15 years old were seropositive. For older people, the percentages of positive sera have been reported to be higher, with values of up to 96% in certain areas of Czechoslovakia.

Some evidence has been obtained with different isolates of Tahyna virus that there may be different varieties of the virus in different ecological niches throughout Europe (Cupkova, 1971; Malkova and Reddy, 1975).

Jamestown Canyon, Jerry Slough, and South River viruses

Jamestown Canyon virus was obtained from *Culiseta inornata* insects collected in the Jamestown Canyon north of Boulder, Colorado, in 1961 (Berge, 1975). The virus has also been isolated from *Aedes* species obtained in Canada (Iversen *et al.*, 1969, 1973) and from both *Aedes* and *Psorophora* species in several states in the United States (e.g., Utah, Texas, California, and Wisconsin), as well as from horseflies, deerflies, and sentinel white-tailed deer in Wisconsin (Berge, 1975; De Foliart *et al.*, 1969; Issel, 1973; Sudia *et al.*, 1971). Jerry Slough virus, which apparently is serologically almost identical to Jamestown Canyon virus and is considered as a variety of the latter, was isolated twice in 1963 from *Culiseta inornata* mosquitoes collected in California, close to where the original California encephalitis virus isolate was made (Berge, 1975). Neutralizing antibodies specific to Jamestown Canyon virus have been detected in white-tailed deer in both Wisconsin and Texas (Issel *et al.*, 1972, 1973).

The New Jersey isolate South River (NJO-94F) is identical to Jamestown Canyon virus in cross-complement fixation tests, although minor differences have been detected by neutralization tests (Sprance and Shope, 1977) and immunodiffusion tests (Murphy and Coleman, 1967). South River virus is considered a variety of Jamestown Canyon virus.

La Crosse Virus

La Crosse virus was isolated in 1964 from autopsy brain tissue of a 4-year-old girl who died in 1960 from meningoencephalitis at La Crosse, Wisconsin, after suffering from fever, headache, vomiting, convulsions, and pleocytosis (Thompson *et al.*, 1965). The child had lived in a hardwood deciduous forested area of the Upper Mississippi Valley. It was subsequently determined that her mother, father, and three of the eight other children in the family had antibodies against La Crosse virus.

La Crosse virus has been isolated in different parts of the United States from a variety of mosquitoes (*Aedes triseriatus*, *Aedes trivittatus*, *Aedes communis*, *Aedes vexans*, *Aedes atlanticus tormentor*, *Aedes sollicitans*, *Aedes dorsalis*, *Aedes canadensis*, *Culex pipiens*, *Anopheles crucians*, *Anopheles punctipennis*, and *Psorophora howardii*), as well as from *Hybomitra lasiophthalma* (Macq.) horseflies (Sudia *et al.*, 1971; Thompson *et al.*, 1972; Wright *et al.*, 1971). The virus has been isolated in the early spring and summer in Wisconsin from *Aedes triseriatus* larvae obtained from basal tree holes, old tires, and other environmentally protected oviposition sites (Beaty and Thompson, 1975; Grimstad *et al.*, 1977; Pantuwatana *et al.*, 1974; Watts *et al.*, 1974). La Crosse virus has been recovered from mosquito larvae collected in Ohio (Berry *et al.*, 1974) and mosquito eggs and larvae in Minnesota (Balfour *et al.*, 1975, 1976). Virus has been obtained from the blood of sentinel rabbits, squirrels, and chipmunks caged in forested areas in Wisconsin (Ksiazek and Yuill, 1977; Pantuwatana *et al.*, 1974; Watts *et al.*, 1974).

Neutralizing antibodies to La Crosse virus have been detected in the summer months in various forest-dwelling small mammals trapped in Wisconsin, particularly animals such as chipmunks (up to 100% seropositive in some endemic areas), tree squirrels, cottontails, and flying squirrels (Gauld *et al.*, 1974; Moulton and Thompson, 1971; Thompson *et al.*, 1967). Antibodies have been detected in Wisconsin foxes (T. Yuill, personal communication). Since viremias are produced in experimentally inoculated small mammals such as chipmunks, and La Crosse virus isolates have been obtained from wild-caught chipmunks (Gauld, *et al.*, 1975), these semihibernating animals are considered to be one of the probable summer season enhancing hosts for the virus cycle in the Wisconsin–Iowa–Minnesota region.

Transovarial, venereal, and oral transmissions of La Crosse virus by *Aedes triseriatus* have been demonstrated (Beaty and Thompson, 1975; Pantuwatana *et al.*, 1972; Thompson, 1977; Thompson and Beaty, 1978; Watts *et al.*, 1972, 1973, 1974). Transovarial transmission of La Crosse virus has also been demonstrated with *Aedes albopictus* (Tesh and Gubler, 1975). Oral transmission of La Crosse virus by various *Aedes* species which were infected by feeding on viremic hosts (or through a membrane) has been demonstrated (Watts *et al.*, 1973). The observation by Watts *et al.* (1973) that different *Aedes* species exhibited vastly different transmission efficiencies to a secondary host is of interest when one considers the question of possible insect tropisms for arboviruses. These investigators found that 70% of their *Aedes triseriatus* transmitted La Crosse virus, whereas no transmission was observed with *Aedes stimulans*, *Aedes hendersoni*, and *Anopheles punctipennis* (Watts *et al.*, 1973, 1975). Highest venereal transmission rates to *Aedes triseriatus* have been obtained after females have taken a previous blood meal (W. Thompson, personal communication).

After female mosquitoes have ingested a viremic blood meal, viral antigens have been demonstrated initially in their midgut tissues on the seventh day of extrinsic incubation (Beaty and Thompson, 1976, 1977). Viral antigens have been detected in most insect tissues by 2 weeks after engorgement, suggesting that disseminated infections develop (possibly involving hemolymph transmission). Viral antigens in ovarian tissues and infectious virus in eggs have been reported (Beaty and Thompson, 1976, 1977). Viral antigens in gonad, salivary, and other tissues of transovarially infected pupae and emerging adults have been recorded, indicating that female mosquitoes may be able to infect animals immediately after emergence (Beaty and Thompson, 1976, 1977). Eight successive *Aedes triseriatus* transovarial passages of La Crosse virus to offspring (71% infected) have been demonstrated experimentally (Miller *et al.*, 1977).

The distribution of *Aedes triseriatus* mosquitoes in relation to the known virus enzootic areas, and the close association of the insect with the natural habitats of chipmunks and tree squirrels (Gauld *et al.*, 1974), has led to the suggestion that the maintenance of La Crosse virus in the Wisconsin region of the midwestern United States involves both horizontal transmission (male to female mosquitoes, infected females to mammals, infected mammals to female mosquitoes) and vertical transmission (female mosquitoes to offspring) (Grimstad *et al.*, 1977; Thompson, 1977).

Experimental infection of newborn or young mice by La Crosse virus leads to encephalitis and death, while infection of chipmunks and tree squirrels leads to a viremia and eventual production of neutralizing antibodies (Berge, 1975; Pantuwatana *et al.*, 1972; Watts *et al.*, 1972).

Serological studies have indicated that at least 800 human La Crosse virus infections have occurred in the United States since 1960, mostly in the midwestern and eastern United States (Berge, 1975; M. Grayson, 1978, personal communication; Henderson and Coleman, 1971; Sudia *et al.*, 1971; W. Thompson, 1978, personal communication; Thompson and Evans, 1965). The signs and symptoms usually associated with severe La Crosse virus infections include headaches, fever, convulsions and seizures, lethargy, and vomiting. Mild infections may just involve low-grade fever and headaches (T. Monath, personal communication). Seroconversions with neutralizing antibody titers of up to 10^3 TCID$_{50}$ units have been reported by 2 weeks after the onset of the disease. Human infections have principally been recorded for 7-month-old to 20-year-old males and females in rural and suburban areas of the United States where La Crosse virus is enzootic.

Snowshoe Hare Virus

Snowshoe hare virus was originally isolated in 1959 from the blood of an emaciated sluggish *Lepus americanus* (snowshoe hare) trapped in Bitterroot Valley, Montana (Burgdorfer *et al.*, 1961). Other isolates of the virus have been made from snowshoe hares, lemmings, sentinel rabbits, many *Aedes* species, other mosquito species, and a few ticks taken off small mammals collected in different parts of the northern United States, Alaska, and Canada (Hoff *et al.*, 1971a; Iversen *et al.*, 1973; Karabatsos, 1978; McKiel *et al.*, 1966; McLean *et al.*, 1970, 1972, 1975a; Newhouse *et al.*, 1963; Sudia *et al.*, 1971; Wagner *et al.*, 1975; Whitney *et al.*, 1969; Yuill *et al.*, 1969). Virus has also been obtained from a blackfly (Sommerman, 1977) and from larvae of *Aedes* species (McLean *et al.*, 1975a,b; McLintock *et al.*, 1976), indicating that transovarial transmission and overwintering of the virus in eggs occur. The isolation of snowshoe hare virus from regions of the United States where La Crosse, Jamestown Canyon, and Trivittatus viruses have been obtained indicates that at least certain of the California group bunyaviruses are sympatric in nature.

Antibodies to snowshoe hare virus have been detected in up to 92% of the snowshoe hares trapped in various parts of North America, including Montana, the Canadian Northern and Yukon Territories, Nova Scotia, British Columbia, and Alaska (Embil *et al.*, 1978; Karabatsos, 1978; Newhouse *et al.*, 1963). Antibodies against the virus, associated in some cases with subclinical infections, have been reported in human serum samples collected in British Columbia, Alberta, and New York State (Karabatsos, 1978). Also, antibodies have been found in a single sentinel rabbit in New York State, as well as in 5% of the hares trapped in Montana (Karabatsos, 1978; Newhouse *et al.*, 1971). Other species reported to have snowshoe hare viral antibodies include *Citellus* species from the Yukon and Montana, in addition to *Marmota monax* and deer in New York State (Karabatsos, 1978).

Keystone Virus

Keystone virus was first isolated in 1962 in Clearwater, Florida, and again in 1964 from engorged *Aedes atlanticus-tormentor* mosquitoes (considered now as the primary vector) collected in Florida (Bond *et al.*, 1966). The virus has been obtained from various *Aedes* species as well as various *Culex* species and *Anopheles crucians* (Berge, 1975; Parkin *et al.*, 1972; Sudia *et al.*, 1971; Wellings *et al.*, 1972) with most of the isolates coming from states in the south and southeastern part of the United States (Florida, Georgia, Mississippi, Louisiana, Texas, Virginia, and North Carolina, Parkin *et al.*, 1972). The virus has been isolated from first generation larvae of *Aedes atlanticus*, which again indicates that transovarial transmission occurs (Le Duc *et al.*, 1975a).

Keystone virus has been recovered from sentinel rabbits and cotton rats in the Tampa Bay area of Florida (Bond *et al.*, 1966; Jennings *et al.*, 1968) and from cotton rats in Georgia (Sudia *et al.*, 1971). Neutralizing antibodies specific to Keystone virus have been detected in the sera of rice rats, cottontail rabbits, horses, and man in Florida (Bond *et al.*, 1966; Parkin *et al.*, 1972) and white-tailed deer in Texas (Issel *et al.*, 1973). No human diseases have been associated with Keystone virus infections, even though around 20% of human sera have been shown to be positive for Keystone virus antibodies in some regions of Florida (Parkin *et al.*, 1972). Experimental transovarial transmission of Keystone virus in *Aedes albopictus* has been observed (R. Tesh, personal communication).

Isolations of both Trivittatus and Keystone viruses have been made from pooled collections of mosquitoes collected in the Tampa Bay area, indicating that these two viruses are sympatric in nature (Bond *et al.*, 1966). Studies undertaken on the DelMarVa Peninsula in 1971 and 1972, and reported by Le Duc *et al.* (1975*b*), yielded 96 California group bunyaviruses, 94 of which were identified as Keystone virus. Two of the isolates were identified as Jamestown Canyon virus. These two viruses were recovered from *Aedes canadensis* mosquitoes. One of the Keystone isolates also came from *Aedes canadensis* mosquitoes while the other 93 Keystone viruses came from *Aedes atlanticus* mosquitoes. Here again evidence was obtained for two viruses isolated from the same species of mosquito in the same locality. Studies in other areas of the southeastern United States (e.g., Georgia) have yielded both La Crosse and Keystone viruses in the same locality and from the same species of insect (T. Monath, personal communication).

Inkoo Virus

The North European California group isolate, Inkoo virus, was originally obtained in 1964 from unengorged *Aedes communis* and *Aedes punctor* mosquitoes taken off human bait in a swampy deciduous forest at Inkoo, southern Finland (Brummer-Korvenkontio, 1969; Brummer-Korvenkontio *et al.*, 1973). Inkoo virus has not been isolated from vertebrates, although serological evidence suggests that the virus is widespread throughout Finland and Lapland (Berge, 1975). Neutralizing antibodies have been detected in human samples (up to 68% in some areas) as well as in sera taken from cows, reindeer, snow hares, red foxes, moose, and hazel grouse (Berge, 1975; Brummer-Korvenkontio, 1973*a*). A few cases of human clinical illness with seroconversion to Inkoo antibodies have been recorded (Berge, 1975).

Comparative neutralization of infectivity studies and other serological tests (Brummer-Korvenkontio *et al.*, 1973) indicate that Inkoo virus is quite closely related to Tahyna virus, the other known European California group isolate.

Melao Virus

Isolated in 1955 from *Aedes* (*Ochlerotatus*) *scapularis* mosquitoes collected in Melajo Forest in northeast Trinidad (Spence, *et al.*, 1962*b*), Melao virus has been isolated from other *Aedes* species as well as from *Psorophora ferox* collected in Brazil (Woodall, 1967) and in mosquito samples collected in Panama (C. H. Calisher, personal communication). No vertebrate isolations of Melao virus have been made, nor have serological surveys detected Melao virus antibodies in human or monkey sera.

A newly registered virus, Serra do Navio, isolated from *Aedes fulvus* mosquitoes in 1966 from the Amapa Territory of Brazil (F. Pinheiro and J. P. Woodall, unpublished data), is serologically grouped as a subtype of Melao virus (Table 4).

San Angelo Virus

San Angelo virus was obtained from engorged *Anopheles p. pseudopunctipennis* mosquitoes collected in 1958 from the inside walls of a chickenhouse near San Angelo, Texas (Grimes *et al.*, 1962). Limited serological surveys have detected San Angelo antibodies in a coyote, a racoon, and a few opossums, as well as white-tailed deer (Berge, 1975; Grimes *et al.*, 1962; Issel *et al.*, 1973). Isolates of San Angelo-type viruses have been obtained from *Psorophora confinnis* collected elsewhere in Texas (Houston, San Benito, and Lubbock) and in Arizona, and these isolates have been shown to be serologically quite similar to San Angelo virus; however, whether they are identical is not known (Berge, 1975). Experimental transovarial transmission of San Angelo virus in *Aedes albopictus* mosquitoes has been observed (R. Tesh, personal communication).

Trivittatus Virus

Trivittatus virus was originally isolated in 1948 from *Aedes* species collected near Bismarck, North Dakota (Taylor, 1967). The virus has been reisolated many times from *Aedes*, *Culex*, *Culiseta*, *Mansonia*, and *Anopheles* species collected in various parts of the United States (Berge, 1975; Sudia *et al.*, 1971) and from insects in Santa Rosa,

Mexico (Sudia *et al.*, 1975). Field-collected *Aedes trivittatus* larvae have also yielded virus (Andrews *et al.*, 1977). Watts *et al.* (1976) have demonstrated experimental transmission of Trivittatus virus by *Aedes trivittatus* mosquitoes. Trivittatus virus has been shown to be capable of experimentally infecting chipmunks and squirrels (Pantuwatana *et al.*, 1972), and the virus has been recovered from the blood of a cotton rat and a sentinel rabbit, and neutralizing antisera have been obtained from white-tailed deer, cottontail rabbits, fox squirrels, and racoons (Issel *et al.*, 1972; Pringer *et al.*, 1975).

Summary of the California Group Viruses

Serological and virus isolation studies have provided evidence for several distinguishable California group members. The viruses have been obtained from Central and Northern Europe, Africa, the Caribbean, South America, and the North American continent. At least four members of the group (California encephalitis, La Crosse, Tahyna, and Inkoo viruses) have been associated with human clinical diseases, and enzootic areas have been defined for some of these arboviruses. Transmission studies have clearly defined mechanisms of vertical and horizontal transmission for many of the viruses and indicate means whereby the viruses can overwinter. The observation that overwintered eggs may hatch periodically through the next spring and summer, or even in successive later years, provides means for persistence not only of an insect species but also of the virus in an ecologic niche (T. Yuill, personal communication). In certain places, particular, if not preferred, vector–host relationships have been identified (e.g., in Wisconsin for La Crosse virus: *Aedes triseriatus*–chipmunks and tree squirrels). Even so, in enzootic regions both isolation and serological studies indicate that other vectors and hosts become infected (Sudia *et al.*, 1971). This and the fact that in the North American continent there are many places where several California group members coexist (as well as with other bunyaviruses) would in theory allow the possibility for dual virus infections of vector or vertebrate hosts to generate recombinant viruses. Whether this has happened in nature remains to be determined.

1.2.1f.   Capim Group

The six registered viruses in the Capim group (Table 1) have been isolated from wild rodents or marsupials, sentinel animals, and/or various culicine mosquitoes collected in Central and South America.

Both antibody and virus isolation studies indicate that members of this group commonly infect rodents, suggesting that these animals play an important role as the vertebrate hosts of Capim group viruses. No evidence has been obtained that any member of this group causes human disease.

Acara virus came from a sentinel mouse in 1961 in Para (Brazil). It has been subsequently isolated from sentinel mice, *Culex* species, *Nectomys* rodents, and marsupials in Para (Woodall, 1967), as well as from *Culex* mosquitoes in Panama (Berge, 1975). Antibodies reactive to the virus have been reported only in various rodent sera collected in Para State, Brazil. Bushbush virus was originally isolated from *Culex* mosquitoes collected in 1959 in the Bush Bush Forest, eastern Trinidad (Spence *et al.*, 1967). The virus was subsequently isolated from sentinel mice and *Culex* species in Brazil (Berge, 1975). J. P. Woodall (personal communication) has shown that the Brazilian isolates (BeAn 20076) are antigenically slightly different from the Trinidad prototype. Serological studies have indicated that Bushbush virus is cross-reactive in neutralization of infectivity tests (but not in CF tests) with Bimiti and Catu viruses of the Guama group of bunyaviruses (Berge, 1975).

Capim virus, which was first recovered from a trapped woolly opossum, *Caluromys philander*, in 1958 at Utinga Forest, Para State, Brazil, has also been isolated from sentinel mice, *Proechimys*, and *Culex* mosquitoes in Brazil (Berge, 1975). Antibodies to the virus have been detected in *Proechimys* sera but not in human sera in Para State. Guajara virus is another member of the Capim group which was originally isolated from a sentinel Swiss mouse in Para State, and later from other sentinel mice in Brazil and Panama in addition to *Proechimys* species and *Culex* and *Limatus* mosquitoes collected in Brazil. Brazilian *Proechimys* rodents have been shown to often have antibodies against Guajara virus. Juan Diaz virus, isolated from a sentinel mouse in Panama in 1962, has not been obtained from any other animal or insect and therefore is categorized as a possible arbovirus (Berge *et al.*, 1970). Moriche virus has been isolated only once from *Culex* species collected in 1964 in Bush Bush Forest, Trinidad. No other isolates have been obtained (Berge, 1975).

Serological studies indicate that there are four Capim virus complexes, each containing from one to three types or subtypes (Tables 5–7). As in group C, the Capim group demonstrates marked antigenic diversity. A virus from Guatemala, GU 71 u 350, is indistinguishable by HI test from Guajara virus yet has a CF antigen in common with Acara virus. This may be an example of a naturally occurring recom-

TABLE 5

Neutralization Reactions of Capim Group Viruses[a]

				Antibody			
Virus	Capim	Guajara	Bushbush[b]	Acara	BeAn 84381	BeAn 153564	Juan Diaz
Capim	0[c]	1.4	>3.6				>2048[d]
Guajara	>2.4	0	>4.0				>2048
Bushbush[b]	>1.3	>1.5	0				2048
Acara	>2.3	5.3	5.2	0	>5.0	>5.0	>2048
BeAn 84381	4.0	4.0	1.0	>5.0	0	>5.0	>2048
BeAn 153564				>5.0	>5.0	0	
Juan Diaz	>64[d]	>32	512	>8	>64		0

[a] Data from Andrade, Travassos, and Shope (1976, unpublished), Andrade and Woodall (1965, 1966, 1969, unpublished), Andrade and Shope (1964, unpublished), and Berge (1975).
[b] The Bushbush strain used in these studies was BeAn 20076, which is not identical with the Trinidadian prototype (J. P. Woodall, personal communication).
[c] Difference in log neutralizing index from homologous; see Table 3.
[d] Difference in serum titer from homologous (data for Juan Diaz only); see Table 3.

binant virus. The proposed classification of the Capim group, presented in Table 1, includes two unregistered and unpublished viruses (BeAn 84381, isolated by the staff of the Belem Virus Laboratory in Brazil, and GU 71 u 344, isolated by W. Scherer in Guatemala) as well as a new distinct type from Brazil, BeAn 153564. While the Brazilian isolates may be considered as subtypes of Bushbush virus, *Proechimys*

TABLE 6

Hemagglutination-Inhibition Reactions of Capim Group Viruses[a]

					Antibody				
Antigen	Capim	Guajara	Bushbush	Moriche	Acara	BeAn 84381	BeAn 153564	71 u 344	71 u 350
Capim	0[b]	>8	>8	>16	>4	>8	>4		
Guajara	>8	0	>8	>16	>4	>8	>4		
Bushbush	>8	>8	0	>16	>4	4	>4		
Moriche	>8	>8	>8	0	>4	>8	>4		
Acara	>8	>8	>8	4	0	>8	>4	>32	>32
BeAn 84381	>8	>8	4	>16	>4	0	>4	8	>32
BeAn 153564	>8	>8	>8	>16	>4	>8	0	>32	>32
71 u 344	>8	>8	8	>16	>4	2	>4	0	>32
71 u 350	>8	0	>8	>16	>4	>8	>4	>32	0

[a] Data from Andrade, Travassos, and Shope (1976, unpublished).
[b] Fold difference from homologous titer; see Table 3.

TABLE 7

Complement-Fixation Reactions of Capim Group Viruses[a]

Antigen	Antibody			
	Capim	Guajara	Bushbush	Acara
Capim	0[b]	8	>8	>8
Guajara	32	0	4	>8
Bushbush (Moriche, Juan Diaz)[c]	>64	4	0	>8
Acara (BeAn 84381, BeAn 153564, GU71 u 350)	>16	>8	>8	0

[a] Data from Andrade, Travassos, and Shope (1976, unpublished), Andrade and Shope (1960, unpublished), and Berge (1975).
[b] Fold difference from homologous titer; see Table 3.
[c] The viruses in parentheses react indistinguishably from Bushbush by complement-fixation test.

and *Nectomys* species immune to BeAn 84381 often show no cross-protection with Bushbush virus (J. P. Woodall, personal communication). The unregistered viruses are not formally described, and their mention here is not intended to constitute priority.

1.2.1g. Guama Group

Serological and virus isolation studies suggest that rodents in parts of Central and South America as well as in Florida (United States) are the most common vertebrates that become infected with Guama group viruses. Two of the viruses, Guama and Catu, have been associated with human illnesses.

Of the six registered viruses in this group (Table 1), Mahogany Hammock virus was recovered from *Culex* species collected in 1964 in the Everglades National Park, Florida (Coleman *et al.*, 1969). Additional isolates have been obtained from *Culex* mosquitoes and a cotton rat in the same region (Berge, 1975). Guama virus, the prototype of this serogroup, was isolated from a sentinel *Cebus apella* in the Oriboca Forest, Para State, Brazil (Causey *et al.*, 1961). Many other isolates of the virus have been obtained both from sentinel mice and from other sentinel vertebrates in Brazil, Surinam, Colombia, Trinidad, and Panama (Berge, 1975). Additional isolates have come from various wild rodents and marsupials in Brazil and/or Trinidad, as well as a bat in Para State and fledgling wrens in Utinga Forest, Brazil (Berge, 1975). A variety of mosquitoes collected in Brazil, Trinidad, French Guiana, and Panama have yielded Guama virus strains (Berge, 1975). At least seven Guama virus isolates have been made from human sera in Brazil, with signs and symptoms associated with the virus infection including fever, headaches, myalgia, and leukopenia (Berge, 1975).

Catu virus is another member of the group which was isolated from various sentinel mice and *Cebus* monkeys; however, the original virus isolate came from a human serum sample taken from a 17-year-old man with fever, headaches, and muscle pains (Causey *et al.*, 1961; Berge, 1975). Human, rodent, and marsupial samples in Trinidad and Brazil, as well as a bat sample in Brazil, have yielded Catu virus strains (Berge, 1975; Causey *et al.*, 1961; Tikasingh *et al.*, 1974). Mosquito isolates of the virus have been made from *Culex* species in Brazil, Trinidad, and French Guiana and from *Anopheles* species in Brazil. Antibody surveys have detected antibodies reactive to Catu virus in both rodent and marsupial sera in Brazil (Berge, 1975).

Bertioga virus, recovered twice from sentinel mice in 1962 at Bertioga Beach, Sao Paulo, Brazil, has not been isolated elsewhere (Lopes *et al.*, 1975). Since no arthropod isolates have been made, Bertioga virus is classified as a possible arbovirus. Bimiti virus, obtained in 1955 from *Culex* species in Melajo Forest, northeast Trinidad (Spence *et al.*, 1962a), has been isolated from various *Culex* species in Trinidad, Brazil, French Guiana, and Surinam, as well as from rodent and marsupial samples collected in Trinidad and Brazil (Berge, 1975). Antibodies to the virus have been reported from single human and single donkey serum samples in Trinidad (Berge, 1975). Moju virus was recovered in 1959 from *Culex* mosquitoes in Para,

TABLE 8

Neutralization Reactions of Guama Group Viruses[a]

Virus	Antibody						
	Guama	Moju	BeAn 109303	Mahogany Hammock	Bimiti	Catu	Bertioga
Guama	0[b]	>4.3	2.1	2.6	>4.3	>4.3	>3.9
Moju	2.3	0	3.6	0	>4.4	>4.0	
BeAn 109303	1.9	>4.3	0	1.0	>5.0	5.3	
Mahogany Hammock	3.0	>3.5	>1.3	0	>5.2	5.3	
Bimiti	>3.2	>2.7	>4.3	1.7	0	>3.8	
Catu	>3.6	>4.9	>4.3	>3.1	>4.4	0	>3.9
Bertioga	>4.4	>4.9		>2.1	1.8	>3.9	0

[a] Data from Coleman *et al.* (1969), Andrade, Tavassos, and Shope (1976, unpublished), and Lopes *et al.* (1975).
[b] Difference in log neutralizing index from homologous; see Table 3.

TABLE 9

Hemagglutination-Inhibition Reactions of Guama Group Viruses[a]

Virus	Antibody							
	Guama	Moju	BeAn 109303	Mahogany Hammock	Bimiti	BeAn 116382	Catu	Bertioga
Guama	0[b]	>32	8	>8	>8	>8	>4	>4
Moju	16	0	>16	≥2	>8	>8	>4	>4
BeAn 109303	8	32	0	>8	>8	>8	>4	>4
Mahogany Hammock	16	16	8	0	8	>8	>4	>4
Bimiti	>32	>32	>16	>16	0	>8	>4	>4
BeAn 116382	>32	32	>16	>4	8	0	>4	>4
Catu	>32	>32	>16	>16	4	>8	0	>4
Bertioga	>32	>32	>16	>16	>8	>8	>4	0

[a] Data from Andrade and Shope (1968, unpublished).
[b] Fold difference from homologous titers; see Table 3.

Brazil; other isolates have come from sentinel mice and *Cebus* species, in addition to wild rodents and marsupials in Brazil (Woodall, 1967). Both phlebotomine and various mosquito isolates, mainly from *Culex* and *Mansonia* species, have also been reported (Berge, 1975). Antibodies to Moju virus have been detected in certain rodent sera in Brazil (Berge, 1975).

The results of serological studies with members of the Guama group indicate that there are five viruses which are nearly completely distinct from each other. One of these, Guama, is more closely related to Moju, BeAn 109303, and Mahogany Hammock than to other members of the group (Tables 8 and 9). By complement fixation all members of the group cross-react (Whitman and Casals, 1961). Catu, Guama, Moju, Mahogany Hammock, Bimiti, and BeAn 109303 are virtually identical by CF. BeAn 116382 and Bertioga differ reciprocally from other Guama group viruses by at least eightfold. BeAn 116382 and Bertioga have not been tested with each other. The proposed scheme of classification is shown in Table 1. BeAn 109303 and BeAn 116382 are unpublished isolates made from sentinel mice at the Belem Virus Laboratory, Brazil; their mention here is not intended to constitute priority of publication.

1.2.1h. Koongol Group

The two members of the Koongol group, Koongol and Wongal, were both isolated in 1960 in Queensland, Australia, from *Culex annulirostris* (Doherty *et al.*, 1963). No isolates of these viruses have been made from vertebrates. The viruses have not been associated with human disease. Serologically identical viruses have been recovered principally from *Culex annulirostris* collected in North Western Australia, Queensland, New South Wales, and Northern Victoria. Koongol virus has been obtained from *Ficalbia* species in New Guinea (Berge, 1975). It has been suggested from hemagglutination-inhibition tests on cattle and other vertebrate sera that both viruses may be widespread in Australia (Berge, 1975; Doherty *et al.*, 1970). Serologically, the two viruses are indistinguishable by CF test and are closely related to each other by HI and neutralization tests (Berge, 1975); weak cross-reactivities have been detected by HI test with Bwamba, Tahyna, and Guaroa viruses of the Bwamba, California, and Bunyamwera groups, respectively (Casals, 1963). Koongol and Wongal are classified as separate viruses in the Koongol group.

1.2.1i. Mirim Group

Neither virus in the Mirim group has been associated with human disease. Mirim virus was isolated in 1957 from a sentinel *Cebus apella* in Brazil (Woodall, 1967) and later from various insects and other sentinel animals (Berge, 1975). Antibodies to the virus have been found in various vertebrates in Brazil. Some relationship of Mirim to Moju and Guama viruses (both members of the Guama group) has been reported when HI tests were used but not when CF tests were used (Berge, 1975).

Minatitlan virus was isolated once from a sentinel hamster at Minatitlan, Veracruz, Mexico, in 1967 (Berge *et al.*, 1971) and again from mosquitoes in Guatemala in 1970 (Scherer *et al.*, 1976*b*). A reactivity of Minatitlan virus antigens with group C polyvalent mouse ascitic fluid has been reported (Berge *et al.*, 1971).

Recent CF and neutralization tests carried out by D. Hassinger at YARU indicate that Mirim and Minatitlan are related. These two viruses form a previously unrecognized serological group in the genus *Bunyavirus*; the Mirim group containing Mirim and Minatitlan viruses is therefore proposed.

1.2.1j. Olifantsvlei Group

The viruses in the Olifantsvlei group, Bobia, Botambi, and Olifantsvlei, have not been associated with human illnesses. Olifantsvlei virus was isolated in 1963 from *Culex pipiens* collected in baited traps at Olifantsvlei, Johannesburg, South Africa (Karabatsos, 1978). Other insect isolates have been obtained in the Sudan and Ethiopia (Karabatsos, 1978; Ota *et al.*, 1976). Botambi virus was isolated from *Culex guiarti* collected in 1968 in the Central African Empire (Berge, 1975). Bobia virus also came from arthropods collected in the Central African Empire. No serological surveys have been reported. Serological tests conducted at the Institut Pasteur in Dakar, Senegal, and YARU in the United States have shown a close antigenic relationship between Olifantsvlei and Bobia viruses (Table 10), cross-reactivity with Bunyamwera grouping sera (Karabatsos, 1978), and a distant relationship to Botambi virus, leading to the proposed classification scheme shown in Table 1.

1.2.1k. Patois Group

The four viruses in the Patois group, Pahayokee, Patois, Shark River, and Zegla, were isolated in Central or North America (Berge, 1975). Rodents may be the major vertebrate hosts of these viruses. Both Pahayokee and Shark River viruses were originally obtained in 1964 from *Culex* species captured in the Everglades National Park in Florida, United States, from *Culex* (*Melanoconion*) species (Berge, 1975; Fields *et al.*, 1969). Shark River-like viruses have been obtained from sentinel hamsters in Guatemala and Mexico (Scherer *et al.*, 1972). Patois and Zegla viruses came initially from wild cotton rats (*Sigmodon hispidus*) in Panama (Srihongse *et al.*, 1966). They have also been recovered from wild or sentinel rodents in Honduras and/or Mexico, Guatemala, and British Honduras (Berge, 1975; Scherer *et al.*, 1976a). Antibody surveys have shown that Patois group virus infections of man are rare.

TABLE 10

Neutralization Relationships of the Olifantsvlei Group[a]

Virus	Antibody		
	Olifantsvlei	Bobia	Botambi
Olifantsvlei	0[b]	0.2	2.6
Bobia	1.4	0	Not done
Botambi	4.0	Not done	0

[a] Data from Berge (1975), J.-P. Digoutte (1978, unpublished), and P. Bres (1970, unpublished).
[b] Difference in log neutralizing index from homologous; see Table 3.

Patois virus has been transmitted from wild-caught *Culex* mosquitoes (captured in Panama) to hamsters as evidenced by seroconversion of the hamsters, although no virus isolation was achieved (Galindo and Srihongse, 1967). Despite the fact that Zegla virus has not been obtained from insect sources, its close serological relationship with Patois virus (which has been recovered from various *Culex* species) suggests that Zegla virus should be considered as a possible arbovirus (Berge, 1975).

No human disease has been associated with any virus of this group, although antibodies against Zegla and Patois viruses have been detected in human, pig, and/or rat sera in various countries of Central America (Berge, 1975; Scherer *et al.*, 1972), and Shark River neutralizing antibodies have been detected in Mickosukee and Seminole Indians from the Everglades region of Florida (J. Nuckolls, personal communication).

Serological comparisons of this group of bunyaviruses to members of other groups have indicated cross-reactivities between Patois virus and members of groups C, Guama, Capim, Bunyamwera, and California. The proposed classification (Table 1), based on neutralization test data (Scherer *et al.*, 1972; Fields *et al.*, 1969) and HI test data (Srihongse and Shope, 1968), reflects the closer relationship of Patois to Shark River virus and Zegla to Pahayokee virus than to other members of the group. The Patois group viruses are indistinguishable by CF.

1.2.11. Simbu Group

The viruses that have been assigned to the Simbu group have been obtained from widely different zoogeographic regions, including Africa (Akabane, Ingwavuma, Nola, Sabo, Sango, Sathuperi, Shamonda, Shuni, Simbu, Thimiri, and Yaba-7 viruses), Asia (Aino, Akabane, Ingwavuma, Kaikalur, Sathuperi, and Thimiri viruses), Australia [Akabane, Aino (Samford), Facey's Paddock virus, Peaton, and Thimiri viruses], South America (Inini, Manzanilla, Oropouche, and Utinga viruses), and North America (Buttonwillow and Mermet viruses). Two of the viruses have been associated with natural or laboratory-acquired human diseases (Oropouche and Shuni viruses, Berge, 1975).

Aino (Takahashi *et al.*, 1968) and Akabane (Oya *et al.*, 1961) viruses were originally isolated in Japan from *Culex tritaeniorhynchus* and *Aedes vexans nipponii*, respectively. Both viruses have also been isolated in Australia. Akabane virus has been shown to be associated with severe disease epizootics causing congenital defects in cattle, sheep, and goats in Japan (since World War II) as well as in Australia (Blood, 1956; Hartley *et al.*, 1975; Inaba *et al.*, 1975; Kurogi *et al.*, 1975, 1976, 1977; Parsonson *et al.*, 1975, 1977).

Studies in Japan have indicated that Akabane infections of cattle have been spreading in recent years (Y. Inaba and A. Oya, personal communication) with estimated losses of more than 50,000 calves since 1972. Most animal losses occur in Japan in the autumn and winter months (A. Oya, personal communication). Calf losses due to Akabane virus infections in Australia are put in at several thousand over the past two decades (T. St. George, personal communication). Aino virus (topotype Samford) has also been shown to cause congenital abnormalities in calves in Australia, and neutralizing antibodies have been detected in calves born with congenital defects as well as in older cattle in Japan and Australia (Coverdale *et al.*, 1978; Muria *et al.*, 1974). Infection by Samford virus appears to be less frequent than that induced by Akabane virus (T. St. George, personal communication).

In Australia the virus has been isolated twice from, and is probably transmitted by, the biting midge *Culicoides brevitarsis*: the vector in Japan has not been identified.

An Akabanelike isolate (MP 496) has been isolated from *Culex brevitaris* collected in 1972 in a coastal forest in Kenya. Serologically it has been shown to be very closely related to prototype Akabane virus (Metselaar and Robin, 1976).

If ewes are infected by Akabane virus in the first month or two of pregnancy, deformed newborn lambs can be produced having locked limbs (arthrogryposis), hydranencephaly and anencephaly (with part of the cerebellum replaced by fluids), and other developmental defects (Inaba *et al.*, 1975; Parsonson, *et al.*, 1975, 1977). These deformities are similar to those observed for Akabane or Aino congenitally infected calves (Coverdale *et al.*, 1978; Hartley *et al.*, 1975; Inaba *et al.*, 1975; Kurogi *et al.*, 1975, 1976, 1977). In the North, Center, and Eastern regions of Australia, sheep and cows develop an early immunity, and disease is not observed in their offspring, whereas farther south (at the limits of the distribution of *Culicoides brevitarsis*) nonimmune pregnant animals are susceptible to infection and produce congenitally deformed offspring after virus infection.

Virus isolation and/or serological studies suggest that Akabane virus may also be present in Vietnam, Philippines, Thailand, Indonesia,

Israel, Malaya, and Taiwan (Berge, 1975; Kalmar *et al.*, 1975; Y. Inaba and T. St. George, personal communication). A killed tissue culture (hamster cell) vaccine for Akabane virus has been developed and is being tested in Japan (Y. Inaba, personal communication).

Samford virus, which was initially registered as a distinct virus serotype in the *International Catalogue of Arboviruses*, was subsequently withdrawn when serological studies indicated that it was indistinguishable from Aino virus. It was obtained in Queensland, Australia, from *Culicoides* midges taken off cattle (Doherty *et al.*, 1972). Facey's Paddock virus, obtained in 1974 from *Culex annulirostris* collected in Queensland, is a recently proposed member of the Simbu group viruses. Serologically it is distantly related to Oropouche, Mermet, and Utinga viruses by CF tests. Peaton virus, another proposed Simbu group virus which is serologically distinct from Akabane and Aino viruses, has been isolated several times from *Culicoides brevitarsis* collected in 1976 in Queensland (T. D. St. George, personal communication). Antibodies to Peaton virus have been detected in various large domestic animals in the North, Center, and Eastern regions of Australia.

Ingwavuma virus was originally isolated from the spectacled weaver bird *Hyphanturgus ocularius* and subsequently from other birds (and *Culex* mosquitoes) in South Africa, Nigeria, Central Africa, and Cyprus (Berge, 1975; Causey *et al.*, 1972; McIntosh *et al.*, 1965). The virus has been recovered from viremic pigs in Thailand and Taiwan as well as from birds and mosquitoes in India and various other parts of Asia (Berge, 1975; Top *et al.*, 1974). The Cyprus and Thai isolates are considered as geographic varieties of Ingwavuma virus. Serological studies of both domestic animals and birds have shown a high incidence of Ingwavuma virus infection in Thailand (Top *et al.*, 1974).

Sathuperi virus was first obtained in 1957 from *Culex vishnui* mosquitoes captured near Vellore Madras, India (Dandawate *et al.*, 1969). The virus has been isolated from cattle in Nigeria (Causey *et al.*, 1972). Kaikalur, a subtype of Shuni virus, was isolated in 1971 from *Culex tritaeniorhynchus* collected in the town of Kaikalur, Krishna District, Andhra Pradesh, India (Rodriques and Dandawate, 1977). Thimiri virus, recovered in 1963 from paddy birds (*Ardeola grayii*) in India, has been isolated from other birds (*Sylvia* species) trapped in Egypt (Causey *et al.*, 1969). No human disease has been associated with either Sathuperi, Kaikalur, or Thimiri virus. A Thimiri virus isolate has been obtained from *Culicoides histris*, a bird-feeding midge, collected in 1974 in the Northern Territories, Australia; antibodies to the virus have been detected in migratory birds from North Australia (H. A. Standfast, personal communication).

Of the African Simbu group isolates, Nola virus was obtained once in 1970 from *Culex perfuscus* collected in the Central African Empire (Berge, 1975). Sabo virus was recovered first in 1966 from a viremic goat and later from viremic cattle and *Culicoides* midges in Nigeria (Causey *et al.*, 1972). Serological studies have detected Sabo virus antibodies in cattle, goat, sheep, and pig sera (Berge *et al.*, 1970). Sango virus has been obtained from cattle sera and midges in Nigeria as well as from mosquitoes in Kenya (Berge *et al.*, 1970; Causey *et al.*, 1972). Serological surveys have detected Sango virus antibodies in both cattle and goat sera (Berge *et al.*, 1970). Sathuperi virus has been isolated from cattle and *Culicoides* species in Nigeria (Causey *et al.*, 1972). Shamonda and Shuni were both recovered from viremic cattle in addition to *Culicoides* species (Berge *et al.*, 1970; Causey *et al.*, 1972; Kemp *et al.*, 1971). A single human isolate of Shuni virus has been reported as well as isolates from cattle, sheep, and *Culicoides* in Nigeria (Causey *et al.*, 1972) and *Culex* species in South Africa (Berge, 1975). Yaba-7 virus (Theiler and Downs, 1973) was isolated only once from *Mansonia africana* mosquitoes in Nigeria.

Simbu virus, the prototype of the group, was isolated in 1955 from *Aedes* species collected at Lake Simbu, Northern Natal, South Africa (Weinbren *et al.*, 1957a). Other isolates have been obtained in the Central African Empire and Cameroon. Human antibodies to Simbu virus have been recorded for sera taken in Botswana and South Africa.

Manzanilla virus, isolated in 1954 from the serum of a howler monkey *Alouatta seniculus insularis* (Anderson *et al.*, 1960b), and Oropouche virus, isolated from a febrile charcoal burner in 1955 (Anderson *et al.*, 1961), both were initially obtained in Trinidad (Berge, 1975). Manzanilla virus antibodies have been detected in howler monkey sera but only rarely in human sera from some regions of Trinidad. Oropouche virus has been associated with large human epidemics in Brazil involving thousands of persons in 1961, 1967, 1968, 1972, and 1975 (Pinheiro *et al.*, 1962, 1976). The midge *Culicoides parensis* is considered the probable vector during these epidemics. The virus has been recovered many times from febrile Brazilians as well as several times from various midges and mosquitoes in Trinidad and Brazil, and *Bradypus tridactylus* in Brazil (Berge, 1975). Antibodies to Oropouche virus have been found in Trinidad human, avian, and primate sera (Berge, 1975; Pinheiro *et al.*, 1976). Utinga virus was isolated in 1965 from the blood of a three-toed sloth (*Bradypus tridactylus*) near

Belem, Brazil (Theiler and Downs, 1973), while Inini virus came from a bird (*Pteroglossus* sp.) caught in French Guiana.

Buttonwillow virus, one of the North American Simbu group viruses, has been obtained from several species of rabbits in addition to various midges collected in California (Hardy *et al.*, 1970). The virus was initially isolated in 1962 from the serum of a rabbit shot in 1961 (Berge, 1975; Reeves *et al.*, 1970). Antibodies to the virus have been detected in sheep, rabbit, and various rodent sera in California, Utah, Montana, Arizona, and Canada (Berge, 1975). No human disease has been associated with either Buttonwillow or Mermet virus infections. Mermet virus was isolated in 1964 from the blood of a purple martin netted in Illinois and has been obtained from other birds in Illinois and Texas (Calisher *et al.*, 1969) and from Ohio and Tennessee. Serologically it is very closely related to, but distinguishable from, Ingwavuma and Manzanilla viruses when both CF and neutralization of infectivity tests are used (Calisher *et al.*, 1969).

Although not all the tests have been completed (particularly with the newer isolates), neutralization tests (Table 11) and CF tests (Table 12) have been used extensively by one of the authors (R. E. S.) to study the Simbu group viruses. The proposed classification scheme shown in Table 1 indicates ten virus complexes with one or two viruses each. Mermet and Ingwavuma are quite closely related to Manzanilla and are considered subtypes. Aino, Samford, and Shuni viruses are not distinguishable in tests to date, but whether they are identical has not been determined. Inini virus has not been investigated in these analyses.

1.2.1m. Tete Group

Many of the viruses in the Tete group (Table 1) have been retrieved from birds (Berge, 1975). Both Bahig and Matruh viruses have each been isolated over 40 times from more than ten species of birds trapped in Egypt and/or Cyprus (Berge *et al.*, 1970, 1971). Bahig virus was isolated from ticks collected in Italy and Egypt (Converse *et al.*, 1974a), while Matruh virus was isolated from ticks obtained in Egypt (Moussa *et al.*, 1974). Evidence has been obtained for transovarial transmission of Bahig virus by the isolation of the virus from tick larvae (Converse *et al.*, 1974a). A few isolates of both viruses have been obtained from birds in Italy (Balducci *et al.*, 1973). Antibodies against the viruses have been detected in avian sera collected in Cyprus as well as in other parts of Europe (Berge *et al.*, 1971; Berge, 1975). Batama

TABLE 11

Neutralization Test Relationships of Simbu Group Viruses[a]

Virus	AKA	Yaba-7	SHA	SAN	Sabo	SAT	SHU	Aino	Simbu	THI	ING	MAN	MER	BUT	ORO	UTI
Akabane	0[b]	1.9	2.4	3.1	>2.6	>4.1	3.1	>1.4	>2.2	>1.8	>3.5	>2.7	2.3	2.8	>2.6	>1.8
Yaba-7	<3.2	0	2.8	>3.7	>2.4	>3.9	2.5	>1.2	>2.0	1.4	3.1	2.5	2.5	>2.6	>2.4	1.5
Shamonda	4.1	3.1	0	2.6	3.2	4.8	3.4	>1.7	2.8	2.3	4.1	3.0	3.4	3.4	3.1	2.4
Sango	2.4	1.5	1.7	0	4.8	4.2	2.0	>0.2	>1.1	>0.7	2.4	1.6	1.4	>1.7	>1.5	1.6
Sabo	<3.4	2.2	3.1	3.9	0	>4.1	3.1	>1.3	2.2	1.8	>3.5	2.7	2.5	2.8	2.5	>1.8
Sathuperi	>3.5	1.9	>2.5	>3.2	>1.9	0	3.6	>1.0	>1.5	1.0	>2.8	>2.0	2.4	>2.1	>1.9	1.6
Shuni	5.0	3.4	4.0	3.6	3.4	>2.9	0	0	3.0	2.6	4.3	3.5	<4.2	3.6	3.4	2.6
Aino	>4.6	>3.1	>3.7	>4.0	>3.0	>3.0	0	0	>2.6		>4.7	>3.6	>3.9	>3.2	>3.1	>2.2
Simbu	>3.9	>2.3	2.7	>3.6	>2.3		>2.8	>0.7	0	1.5	>3.2	>2.6	2.8	>2.5	>2.3	1.5
Thimiri										0						
Ingwavuma	>3.8	>2.2	>2.8	>3.5	>2.2	<2.9	2.6	>1.0	1.7	0.8	0	1.9	0	1.6	1.8	1.6
Manzanilla	3.8	2.7	3.3	3.5	2.7	3.7	3.1	>1.6	2.2	1.8	1.4	0	<0.4	2.3	2.2	1.6
Mermet	4.1	>2.5	3.0	>3.8	2.3	>4.0	<2.2	>1.2	>2.1	1.1	2.8	0.3	0	2.0	2.5	>1.5
Buttonwillow	4.0	>2.4	3.0	>3.7	>2.4	3.8	2.9	>1.2	2.0	>1.6	2.5	1.6	1.6	0	>2.4	>1.6
Oropouche	3.9	>2.3	>2.9	>3.6	>2.3	>3.8	>2.8	>1.1	>1.9	>1.5	>3.4	>2.4	2.8	>2.5	0	1.0
Utinga	3.5	2.0	>2.7	>3.4	>2.1	>3.6	>2.6	>0.9	1.7	>1.3	2.9	1.8	2.9	2.1	1.4	0

[a] Data from Shope (1969, unpublished) and Berge (1975).

[b] Difference in log neutralizing index from homologous; see Table 3.

TABLE 12

Complement-Fixation Relationships of Simbu Group Viruses[a]

Antigen	Antibody									
	Aka-Bane	Sabo	Shuni	Sathu-peri	Simbu	Thi-miri	Manza-nilla	Button-willow	Oro-pouche	Utinga
Akabane	0[b]	8	2	4	8	>256	>64	>2	>32	128
Sabo (Yaba-7)	0	0	8	>2	2	>256	>64	>2	>32	32
Shuni (Sango)	4	4	0	8	8	>256	>64	>2	>32	64
Sathuperi (Shamonda)	4	4	4	0	4	>256	>64	>2	>32	32
Simbu	2	>32	4	16	0	128	>64	>2	>32	32
Thimiri						0				
Manzanilla (Mermet, Ingwavuma)	>32	>32	>8	>32	>128	>256	0	2	32	32
Buttonwillow	>32	>32	>8	32	128	64	16	0	32	32
Oropouche	32	>32	>8	>8	32	32	32	64	0	4
Utinga	>32	>32	>8	32	64	>256	64	>2	16	0

[a] Data from Zachary and Shope (1967, unpublished) and Berge (1975).
[b] Fold difference from homologous; see Table 3.

virus, isolated by J. P. Digoutte and J. Moindrot from three species of birds in the Central African Empire, has been proposed as a new member of the Tete group.

Tsuruse virus, isolated from a nestling blue magpie in Japan (Schaffer and Scherer, 1972), and Tete virus, obtained in 1959 from a spotted backed weaver bird collected in Natal, South Africa (Berge *et al.*, 1970), are serologically cross-reactive with each other as well as with the other members of the group, as shown by reciprocal CF tests (Berge *et al.*, 1970). No member of the group has been associated with a human disease.

The serological reactions in the Tete group reflect very close relationships by neutralization, HI, and CF tests (Berge, 1975). The neutralization results are shown in Table 13. It is proposed that the five viruses be considered as subtypes in the Tete group.

1.2.1n. Unassigned Viruses

The unassigned viruses in the Bunyamwera supergroup are Gamboa, Guaratuba, Jurona, and Kaeng Khoi. These viruses are not serologically related to each other and are only weakly serologically cross-reactive with particular members of the different serogroups described above. Because of this, they have not been assigned to any particular group. None of the viruses has been associated with human disease.

A relationship of Gamboa virus, isolated on several occasions from *Aedeomyia squamipennis* in Panama, was initially reported with Capim virus when HI tests were used (Berge *et al.*, 1970). Transovarial transmission of Gamboa virus by *Aedeomyia squamipennis* has been demonstrated by P. Galindo and P. Peralta (personal communication). Guaratuba virus, retrieved from the brain of a sentinel suckling white mouse in Brazil, and later from other sentinel mice and hamsters, as well as *Aedes* species and a bird, has been shown to be distantly related to Bertioga virus of the Guama group when reciprocal complement-fixation and neutralization of infectivity tests are used (Berge, 1975).

Jurona virus was isolated in 1962 in Brazil from *Hemagogus* mosquitoes (Woodall, 1967). Forest birds have been reported to have antibodies to this virus, although neutralizing antibodies were not detected (Shope *et al.*, 1966). Hemagglutination of goose erythrocytes by Jurona virus has been reported to be inhibited by Oropouche, Simbu, and Bunyamwera grouping sera. Complement-fixation tests have not, however, picked up Jurona cross-reactivities with those viruses or other known arboviruses. Kaeng Khoi virus, intially isolated in 1969 from a dead suckling wrinkle lipped bat (*Tadarida plicata*) in a central Thailand cave, has been subseqeuntly isolated from bedbugs and several hundred other bats in Thailand (Williams *et al.*, 1976). Neutralizing antibodies to the virus have been detected in rats and guano miners in Thailand, although no disease has been ascribed to Kaeng Khoi virus

TABLE 13

Neutralization Relationships of Tete Group Viruses[a]

Virus	Antibody				
	Tete	Batama	Bahig	Matruh	Tsuruse
Tete	0[b]	2.2	>2.2	2.1	>0.9
Batama	0.8	0	>2.0	1.4	
Bahig	1.4	3.3	0	1.5	>0.5
Matruh	1.4	3.0	>0.4	0	
Tsuruse	1.7		0.4		0

[a] Data from Digoutte (1978, unpublished) and Downs (1973, unpublished).
[b] Difference of log neutralizing index from homologous; see Table 3.

infections of man. Using hyperimmune mouse ascitic fluid raised
against Kaeng Khoi virus in HI tests with Batai virus (Bunyamwera
group), a cross-reaction at a 1:10 dilution has been observed (R. E.
Shope, unpublished data).

1.2.1o. Summary of the Bunyamwera Supergroup Viruses

The recognized and proposed members of the Bunyamwera
supergroup have been placed into 13 interrelated serogroups with some
five unassigned members. Overall the viruses have been recovered from
all continents of the world except Antarctica. Many of the viruses have
been shown to infect humans, and 27 are implicated as the cause of
human diseases as shown either by direct virus isolation from febrile
patients or from serological evidence. All but two of the 12 group C
viruses have been associated with human disease. Almost all members
of the supergroup have been recovered from various mosquitoes and/or
midges; few have been obtained from ticks. A few viruses have been
isolated from phlebotomine insects.

1.2.2. Serological and Biological Characteristics of Possible Members of the Bunyaviridae Family

Most of the serogroups of possible members of the Bunyaviridae
family are candidates of the family on the basis of morphological
properties. Whether this will be substantiated by molecular analyses
remains to be determined.

1.2.2a. Anopheles B Group

The two members of the Anopheles B group, Anopheles B and
Boraceia, were isolated from *Anopheles* species collected in South
America. Anopheles B virus is serologically unrelated to the Anopheles
A group viruses but, like Anopheles A virus, was obtained in 1940 from
Anopheles species collected in Colombia (Roca-Garcia, 1944). Boraceia
virus was recovered from *Anopheles cruzii* collected in 1962 in Brazil
(Lopes *et al.*, 1966); it has also been obtained from *Phoniomyia* species
(Lopes and Sacchetta, 1974). Antibodies to Boraceia virus have been
reported in 24% of human serum samples obtained in Casa Grande,
Brazil (Lopes and Sacchetta, 1974). The neutralization and CF test

results of Lopes *et al.* (1966) indicate that Boraceia virus is a subtype of Anopheles B virus.

1.2.2b. Bakau Group

The two viruses which make up the Bakau group, Bakau and Keta-pang, both came from *Culex* species collected in Malaya in 1956 (Berge, 1975). Isolates of Bakau virus have been obtained from ticks (*Argas abdussalami*) in Pakistan and a primate (*Macaca* species) in Malaysia (Berge, 1975). Although not associated with a human disease, antibodies to Bakau and Ketapang viruses have been detected in human sera from various parts of Malaya.

Bakau and Ketapang viruses are very closely related by CF tests but are distinct virus serotypes by neutralization and HI tests (Berge, 1975).

1.2.2c. Crimean Hemorrhagic Fever–Congo Group

The etiological agent of a sometimes severe human disease often involving epidemics in the Crimean regions of the U.S.S.R. and other parts of Eastern Europe, Iran, and Pakistan is a virus (Crimean hemor-rhagic fever virus) which was originally isolated from *Hyalomma plum-beum plumbeum* (Panz) ticks collected in the Crimea in 1945 and sub-sequently from the blood of patients (Chumakov, 1946, 1947, 1963, 1969*a*, 1973).

A similar virus (Congo virus), isolated in 1956 from the serum of a 13-year-old boy in Kisangani (Stanleyville, Zaire, Simpson *et al.*, 1967; Woodall *et al.*, 1967), is serologically very closely related to Crimean hemorrhagic fever virus, although probably not so severe a disease agent. Because the two isolates cannot be serologically distinguished, they are considered together and are called Crimean hemorrhagic fever–Congo virus (Casals, 1969; Chumakov *et al.*, 1969). Whether the virus isolates should be considered as varieties or variants is an unre-solved issue.

Other human virus isolates have been made in the U.S.S.R., Eastern Europe, Republic of the Congo, Uganda, and certain Eurasian countries (Berge *et al.*, 1970; Berge, 1975; Chumakov *et al.*, 1969*a*, 1970; Horvath, 1976).

Animals from which virus isolates have been made include trade animals (cattle, sheep, goats, and pigs) in Kenya and Nigeria (Kemp *et al.*, 1971), hedgehogs and a goat in Nigeria (Causey *et al.*, 1970), and hedgehogs in the U.S.S.R. (Berge *et al.*, 1970; Berge, 1975).

Many isolates of the virus have been reported from a variety of ticks (*Hyalomma* and other species) collected in Nigeria, Senegal, and Uganda (Berge *et al.*, 1970; Berge, 1975; Institut Pasteur de Dakar, Annual Report, 1971, 1972). Isolates of the virus have been reported from *Culicoides* species obtained in Nigeria (Berge *et al.*, 1970). Virus isolation has been documented from ticks collected in various European countries (Yugoslavia, Greece, Turkey, Bulgaria, U.S.S.R., Hungary) and Eurasian countries (including Central U.S.S.R., Iran and Pakistan) (Begum *et al.*, 1970*b,c*; Perelatov *et al.*, 1972).

Transmission of Crimean hemorrhagic fever virus from infected donor *Hyalomma*, *Rhipicephalus*, and *Dermacentor* ticks to susceptible animals has been demonstrated (Kondratenko, 1976). Since a variety of ticks are known to be carried by migratory birds, and Crimean hemorrhagic fever–Congo viruses have been isolated in widely separated regions of Africa, Europe, and Eurasia, it has been suggested that the intercontinental passage of infected migratory birds, or ticks carried by such birds, may be or may have been involved in the process of dissemination (see Chumakov, 1969*b*; Kaiser *et al.*, 1974).

Neutralizing antibodies to the virus have been found in human sera collected in certain regions of the U.S.S.R., Nigeria, Bulgaria, Hungary, Rumania, Turkey, India, Pakistan, Iran, and Yugoslavia, and in the sera of cattle, horses, sheep, goats, hedgehogs, and hares in those regions (Chumakov, 1969*b*; David-West *et al.*, 1974; Horvath, 1975, 1976; Perelatov *et al.*, 1972; Saidi *et al.*, 1975; Shanmugan *et al.*, 1976; O. Papadopoulos, D. Serter, and J. Vesenjak-Hirjan, personal communications).

It has been suggested that infection of man by the virus probably occurs directly from ticks, including ticks associated with cattle (Pak, 1972; Perelatov *et al.*, 1972). Nosocomial outbreaks of Crimean hemorrhagic fever have also been documented (Donchev *et al.*, 1974). The symptoms and signs recorded for human disease associated with Crimean hemorrhagic fever–Congo virus infections include fever, headaches, nausea, vomiting, backaches, joint pains, photophobia, thrombocytopenia, and leukopenia, as well as gastrointestinal, subcutaneous, and skin hemorrhages. Genital, CNS, kidney, cardiac, and liver pathological changes occur often associated with organ hemorrhages and necroses (Berge *et al.*, 1970; Chumakov, 1969*a*; Radev and Bakardjiev, 1975; Zeitlenok *et al.*, 1957). Epidemics of virus infection have been documented in the U.S.S.R., Pakistan, Rumania, and Yugoslavia (see Casals, 1978; Casals *et al.*, 1966; Chumakov, 1963).

Crimean hemorrhagic fever–Congo viruses are distinguishable by neutralization, HI, and CF tests from Hazara virus—the other recognized virus in the group (Buckley, 1974; Casals, 1969; Casals and Tignor, 1974). Hazara virus, which was obtained from the tick *Ixodes redikorzevi* collected from a high mountain vole on subarctic terrain (at 12,000 ft) in Pakistan (Begum *et al.*, 1970*a*), is not known to be the etiological agent of any human disease, although antibodies reactive to the virus have been detected in human sera collected from adults in Hazara District as well as Karachi, Lahore, and Dacca in Pakistan (Berge *et al.*, 1970). Other isolates of Hazara virus have been obtained from ticks collected in semidesert regions of Pakistan (Begum *et al.*, 1970*a,b,c*).

A distant CF relationship between the Semunya strain of Congo virus and Ganjam virus (believed to be a variety of Nairobi sheep disease virus) of the Nairobi sheep disease group has been detected by Shope (1967, unpublished data). Casals (1978) and Davies (cited in Casals, 1978) detected a similar distant relationship by indirect fluorescent antibody and indirect hemaglutination tests between Nairobi sheep disease virus and both Hazara and the IbAr 10200 strain of Congo virus. These intergroup relationships are not deemed close enough to propose that the Crimean hemorrhagic fever–Congo group should be merged with the Nairobi sheep disease group.

1.2.2d.   Kaisodi Group

Kaisodi, Lanjan, and Silverwater viruses have all been obtained from ticks either in Mysore, India, in 1957 (Kaisodi virus: Bhatt *et al.*, 1966; Pavri and Casals, 1966), Kuala Lumpur in 1960 (Lanjan virus: Tan *et al.*, 1967), or Canada in 1960 (Silverwater virus: McLean, 1961). Other than the initial isolate from *Haemaphysalis spinigera*, Kaisodi virus has been recovered from a ground thrush in Mysore (Berge, 1975). No human disease, human virus isolations, or human antibodies to the virus have been recorded. Lanjan virus has been obtained from *Haemaphysalis* species (Berge, 1975), although the original isolate came from *Dermacentor auratus* taken off rats and squirrels (Tan *et al.*, 1967). The only vertebrates found occasionally to have antibodies against Lanjan virus in Malaya are various species of *Rattus* (Berge, 1975).

Silverwater virus was obtained from *Haemaphysalis leporis-palustris* ticks removed from snowshoe hares shot on Manitoulin island near Silverwater, Ontario,Canada (McLean, 1961). Other virus isolates from different *Haemaphysalis* species, including their eggs, larval, nymph, and adult forms (Hoff *et al.*, 1971*b*), have been obtained in various parts of Alberta, Ontario, Wisconsin, and Alaska (Ritter and Felz, 1974). Isolates of the virus have also been obtained from snowshoe hares (*Lepus americanus*) in Alberta, Canada (Hoff *et al.*, 1971*b*). Antibodies to the virus have been detected in snowshoe hares, squirrels, chipmunks, coyotes, domestic rabbits, and cattle in Alberta and Wisconsin, but not in human sera tested from Manitoulin Island (Berge, 1975; Hoff *et al.*, 1971*c*).

The group relationships have been established only by CF tests, although Pavri and Casals (1966) reported that Lanjan virus antibodies inhibit its own hemagglutinin at a 1:320 dilution while Kaisodi antibodies inhibit it at a 1:160 dilution. Definitive classification must await further serological studies.

1.2.2e. Mapputta Group

The four registered viruses in the Mapputta group, Gan Gan, Mapputta, Maprik, and Trubanaman, were each obtained from mosquitoes collected in Australasia. None of the viruses in the group has been associated with human illness. Mapputta virus was isolated twice by Doherty *et al.*, (1963) from *Anopheles meraukensis* in 1960 at the Mitchell River Mission, Queensland, Australia. Other isolates of the virus from *Anopheles* species have been obtained from New South Wales (I. D. Marshall, personal communication) and Northern Territory, Australia (T. St. George, personal communication) Maprik virus, obtained by I. D. Marshall and G. M. Woodroofe in 1966 from *Aedes* species in New Guinea, has subsequently been obtained from various places in the Sepik District of New Guinea from *Mansonia*, *Ficalbia*, and other culicine and anopheline mosquitoes (Berge, 1975). No vertebrate isolates or antibody surveys have been recorded. Trubanaman virus was initially isolated at the Queensland Institute of Medical Research, Brisbane, from *Anopheles annulipes* collected in 1966 at the Mitchell River Mission, Queensland, Australia (Doherty *et al.*, 1968). It has been subsequently isolated from other *Anopheles* collected in Northern New South Wales (I. D. Marshall, personal communication), and antibodies to the virus have been detected in human and domestic and wild animals in various parts of Queensland (Doherty *et al.*, 1968, 1970), the highest percentage of animals with neutralizing antibodies being horses, wallabies, and kangaroos (40–50% incidence).

Gan Gan virus has been recently registered as a new serotype from Australia; the virus was originally isolated in Nelson Bay, New South Wales, from *Aedes vigilax* collected in 1970 (Gard *et al.*, 1973). Subsequent isolates have come from *Culex* and *Aedes* species in Southern Queensland (I. D. Marshall, personal communication). Gan Gan virus is indistinguishable from Maprik virus by CF tests but different by neutralization tests (Tables 14 and 15). A proposed classification scheme shown in Table 2 reflects that Gan Gan virus is more closely related to Maprik than to Mapputta or Trubanaman viruses.

1.2.2f. Nairobi Sheep Disease Group

The prototype of the Nairobi sheep disease group, Nairobi sheep disease virus, was identified as a disease entity in a blood sample taken in 1910 by R. E. Montgomery (1917) in Nairobi, Kenya, from a diseased Persian fat tail sheep which was suffering from severe gastroenteritis. It was shown that the blood sample could induce disease in other sheep on inoculation (Montgomery, 1917). Numerous virus isolates have been made from sheep and goats in Kenya, sheep and sheep ticks in Uganda (Weinbren *et al.*, 1958), and sheep in the Republic of the Congo. Apparently only domestic animals and ticks are infected by the virus. Viral antibodies in sheep, goats, and human sera in those regions (Berge, 1975), and in northern Somalia (Edelsten, 1975), have been reported. Limited serological surveys have shown that

TABLE 14
Neutralization Relationships of Mapputta Group Viruses[a]

		Antibody		
Virus	Maprik	Gan Gan	Trubanaman	Mapputta
Maprik	0[b]	1.6	4.5	5.3
Gan Gan	4.4	0	>4.3	>4.2
Trubanaman	4.8	2.7	0	>2.9
Mapputta	4.5	2.7	>3.9	0

[a] Data from Berge (1975), Doherty *et al.* (1968), and I. Marshall (1978, unpublished).
[b] Difference in log neutralizing index from homologous; see Table 3.

TABLE 15

Complement-Fixation Relationships of Mapputta Group
Viruses[a]

Antigen	Antibody			
	Mapputta	Trubanaman	Maprik	Gan Gan
Mapputta	0[b]	32	16	32
Trubanaman	64	0	32	16
Maprik	>128	256	0	4
Gan Gan	>128	128	4	0

[a] Data from I. Marshall (1978, unpublished).
[b] Fold difference from homologous titer; see Table 3.

antibodies to the virus can be detected in domestic animals as far south as Botswana, the Kalahari Desert, Mozambique, and various parts of South Africa (Berge, 1975). Human illness association with either natural or laboratory-acquired infections is often mild, with arthralgia and fever as two of the associated signs and symptoms. In sheep, where mortalities of up to 73% of a flock can occur, the disease produces glomerulonephritis, marked leukopenia, and a drop in total serum protein (Weinbren *et al.*, 1958).

Many isolates of Nairobi sheep disease virus have been obtained from the tick *Rhipicephalus appendiculatus* (Berge, 1975). An attenuated strain of the virus has been obtained which confers a lasting protective immunity in sheep (Berge, 1975).

Ganjam virus is now considered to be a strain of Nairobi sheep disease virus; it was isolated in 1954 from *Haemaphysalis* ticks taken off goats in Bhanjanagar, Ganjam District of Orissa, India (Boshnell *et al.*, 1970; Casals, 1968; Dandawate and Shah, 1969). It has also been recovered from other ticks taken from birds, *Culex* mosquitoes, and febrile human sera collected in India (Berge, 1975; Rajagopalan *et al.*, 1970).

Dugbe virus, the other virus of the group, has been retrieved from ticks and humans, and is associated with a febrile human illness. Dugbe virus, in addition to its initial isolation in 1964 from *Amblyomma variegatum* ticks in Ibadan, Nigeria (Causey *et al.*, 1971), has been isolated several times from various ticks and the sera of febrile patients in Nigeria, Cameroon, and the Central African Empire (Berge *et al.*, 1970; Berge, 1975; Converse *et al.*, 1974a). Isolates of the virus have been obtained from trade animals (cattle, sheep, goats, and pigs, Kemp *et al.*, 1971), a giant pouched rat, *Culicoides* midges, and (once) from

Aedes aegypti. Virus antibodies have been reported in cattle, goat, and sheep sera (Berge *et al.*, 1970). Dugbe virus has been shown to infect ticks under experimental conditions, producing a long-lasting infection.

The group serological relationships were established by CF tests (Berge, 1975). Until neutralization tests are done, it is premature to propose a definitive classification scheme. There are definite but distant intergroup relationships between the Nairobi sheep disease group and the Crimean hemorrhagic fever–Congo group (see above).

1.2.2g. Phlebotomus Fever Group

Thirteen of the 23 registered members of the Phlebotomus fever group have been isolated from phlebotomine arthropods. Five of the viruses, Candiru, Chagres, Punta Toro, and the Naples and Sicilian sandfly fever viruses, have been isolated from human samples and shown to be associated with human disease by both isolation and serological studies (see Tesh *et al.*, 1976). Many of the viruses have been obtained from wild rodents. Epidemiological studies suggest that in many cases the normal virus cycle in nature probably involves rodents and phlebotomine flies.

Aguacate virus was obtained by R. Tesh and associates in 1969 (Tesh *et al.*, 1974) from *Lutzomyia* species in Panama. Other isolates of the virus have come from various phlebotomine insects collected in central Panama and the Canal Zone, Panama (Tesh *et al.*, 1974). Anhanga virus, which was obtained in 1962 from a sloth in Para, Brazil, has not been isolated from arthropods and therefore is considered as a possible arbovirus on account of its serological cross-reactivity with the arboviruses Icoaraci and Chagres (Berge, 1975). Bujaru virus, obtained from the rodent *Proechimys guyannensis oris* trapped in 1962 in the Utinga Forest in Brazil (Woodall, 1967), also has not been isolated from arthropods and is likewise considered as a possible arbovirus. Bujaru virus antibodies have been detected in both human and rodent sera collected in various parts of Brazil (Berge, 1975). Cacao, Caimito, Chilibre, Frijoles, and Nique viruses were obtained initially by R. Tesh and P. Peralta (Tesh *et al.*, 1974, 1975) from *Lutzomyia* insects in central Panama. Cacao virus was recovered from various *Lutzomyia* species in central Panama and the Canal Zone of Panama (Tesh *et al.*, 1974). Neutralizing antibodies to Cacao virus have been detected in human sera collected in Panama (Tesh *et al.*, 1974). Candiru virus has been obtained once in 1960 in Brazil from a febrile human serum sample (Woodall, 1967). The signs and symptoms of the associated illness were fever, headaches, dizziness, back pains, and pains in muscles and joints (Berge, 1975). No other isolates of the virus have been obtained from Brazil, although antibodies have been detected in human serum samples as well as a single bird serum sample collected in Brazil (Berge, 1975).

Chagres virus was initially isolated in 1960 from a human serum sample taken from a man who was suffering from headaches, fever, retroorbital pains, dizziness, anorexia, and nausea (Peralta *et al.*, 1965). Other isolates have come from human samples and phlebotomine insects (*Lutzomyia* species) in Panama (Srihongse and Johnson, 1974; Tesh *et al.*, 1974). Antibodies to Chagres virus have been detected in both human and sentinel animal sera obtained in Panama (Srihongse and Johnson, 1974; Tesh *et al.*, 1974).

Icoaraci virus, which was recovered in 1960 from a rodent in Brazil, has also been isolated from a spiny rat (*Proechimys guyannensis oris*) trapped in Para, Brazil, as well as from sentinel mice and various mosquitoes (including both *Aedes* and *Anopheles* and other mosquitoes) in Sao Paulo, Brazil (Berge, 1975; Causey and Shope, 1965). An additional Brazilian isolate of Icoaraci virus has been retrieved from *Lutzomyia* insects (Berge, 1975). Antibodies to Icoaraci virus have been detected in sera obtained from various rodents and marsupials in Para, Brazil (Berge, 1975; Causey and Shope, 1965).

Itaporanga virus was originally recovered from a dead sentinel Swiss mouse at Itaporanga, Sao Paulo State, Brazil, in 1962 (Trapp *et al.*, 1965). The virus has been isolated at Belem, Brazil, from sentinel Swiss mice (Woodall, 1967), a *Caluromys* marsupial, and the bird *Thamnophilus aethiops* (Berge, 1975). Other Itaporanga virus isolates have been made in Trinidad, Brazil, and French Guiana from various *Culex* mosquitoes (Berge, 1975). Antibodies to Itaporanga virus have been detected in human, marsupial, and various forest bird and bat sera collected near Belem, Brazil (Berge, 1975; Shope *et al.*, 1966). Both the isolation and antibody studies are interpreted as indicating that, at least in 1964, the natural transmission of Itaporanga virus in the Utinga Forest, Belem, was limited to vertebrates such as bats, forest birds, and *Caluromys* and *Marmosa* species which inhabited the forest canopy. Antibody surveys of the animals which were present in the neighboring forest floors (terrestrial marsupials such as *Didelphis* and *Philander*) gave uniformly low titers (Berge, 1975; Shope *et al.*, 1966).

Pacui virus, which was obtained in 1961 from *Oryzomys* rodents near Belem in Brazil, has subsequently been isolated from other *Oryzomys* species both in Brazil and in Trinidad (Aiken *et al.*, 1975;

Jonkers *et al.*, 1968). Many isolates of the virus have been obtained from *Lutzomyia flaviscutellata* phlebotomine flies in Brazil (Aitken *et al.*, 1975). In Brazil, neutralizing antibodies to Pacui virus have been detected in sera collected from various bait and wild rodents in addition to marsupials, but not in human or bat sera collected in the same localities (Aitken *et al.*, 1975). Punta Toro virus was obtained in 1967 from a human serum sample collected in 1966 from a patient in Pittsburgh, Pennsylvania, who had recently returned from Panama and who had a fever and back, sacral and retroorbital pains in addition to headaches, chills, and an enlarged spleen (Berge *et al.*, 1970). The virus has been isolated from another man in Panama (Tesh *et al.*, 1974), as well as from *Lutzomyia* species in Panama (Berge, 1975). Antibodies to the virus have been detected in human sera in Panama (Berge *et al.*, 1970; Tesh *et al.*, 1974).

Arumowot virus was recovered from *Culex antennatus* mosquitoes collected from the east bank of the Nile River in Sudan in 1963 and isolated at NAMRU-3 in Cairo, Egypt (Schmidt *et al.*, 1966). Other isolates of the virus have been obtained from insects in Nigeria, Rhodesia, and South Africa and from both rodents (rats, gerbils, shrews, etc.) and insects in the Central African Empire (Berge *et al.*, 1971; Berge, 1975; McIntosh *et al.*, 1976). Gordil virus was obtained from the striped grass mouse *Lemnyscomys striatus* in 1971 in the Central African Empire (Annual Report Pasteur Institut de Bangui, 1971). Saint-Floris virus was isolated simultaneously from the same individual animal. This mixed infection exemplifies the opportunities in nature for possible recombination between bunyaviruses. The only other isolate of Gordil virus came from a gerbil also trapped in the Central African Empire (Berge, 1975).

Two Phlebotomus fever group viruses, Karimabad and Salehabad, were originally obtained in Iran in 1960 from phlebotomine insects collected in 1959 (Taylor, 1967). Although both viruses have been isolated only once, serological studies in Iran (for Karimabad) and Pakistan and Bangladesh (for Karimabad and Salehabad) have indicated that antibodies reactive to the viruses are present in human sera in those countries (Berge, 1975). Antibodies to Karimabad virus have been found in quail and sparrow sera collected in Pakistan, while Salehabad antibodies have been detected in sheep sera collected in that country (Berge, 1975).

The Sicilian and Naples sandfly fever viruses orginially isolated by A. B. Sabin (1951, 1955) from human sera obtained during epidemics among American troops in Italy in 1943 and 1944 (respectively). In both cases the epidemics were associated with a high prevalence of *Phlebotomus papatasi* sandflies. Epidemics of the disease in countries bordering the Mediterranean have been traced back to the Napleonic wars (pappataci fever). In the beginning of this century a filterable agent in the blood of patients was shown to be the cause of the disease and *Phlebotomus* flies the vector (Doerr *et al.*, 1909). The Sicilian sandfly fever virus isolate obtained in 1943 came from Palermo, Sicily; however, many other isolates have been made from children and adult sera in Egypt, Bangladesh, Pakistan, and Iran (Barnett and Suyemoto, 1961; Berge, 1975; Taylor, 1967). Other isolates of the virus have come from various *Phlebotomus* species obtained in Egypt, India, and Pakistan (Schmidt *et al.*, 1960, 1970; Berge, 1975).

Antibodies to the Sicilian sandfly fever virus have been detected in cattle and sheep sera in Yugoslavia and human sera in Pakistan, Iran, Bangladesh, Yugoslavia, Tunisia, Turkey, and Egypt (Berge, 1975). Experimental infection of primates by the virus has been reported (Behbehani *et al.*, 1967). Sandfly fever epidemics have been reported from Bangladesh, Cyprus, Egypt, Greece, India, Iraq, Iran, Jordan, Lebanon, Malta, Sudan, Pakistan, Syria, Turkey, and also the U.S.S.R.—west of the Central Asian Republics (J. Hatem, D. Lvov, J. Vessenjak, personal communications; Theiler and Downs 1973; Sabin, 1955).

The Naples sandfly fever virus was originally isolated in Naples, Italy (Sabin, 1951, 1955). The virus has been recovered from human sources in the Nile Delta, Egypt, India, and Pakistan (Berge, 1975; George, 1971; Goverdhan *et al.*, 1976; Taylor, 1967), in Ashkhabad in Turkestan during an epidemic of sandfly fever (Gaidamovich *et al.*, 1974), as well as from *Phlebotomus* species collected in Egypt, India, and Iran (Berge, 1975; Barnett and Suyemoto, 1961; Goverdhan *et al.*, 1976; Schmidt *et al.*, 1960, 1966, 1970). Neutralizing antibodies to this virus have been detected in human sera obtained in Turkey, Egypt, Pakistan, Bangladesh, Iran, human and rodent sera in south-central U.S.S.R. and cattle and sheep sera in Yugoslavia (Berge, 1975).

Studies on the incidence of sandfly fever by testing for the prevalence of antibodies to both sandfly fever viruses in Greece have established that insecticide-spraying programs (instituted after the war to reduce malaria-transmitting agents) substantially reduced the incidence of human sandfly fever, to the extent that in Greece it became uncommon (Tesh and Papaevangelou, 1977). Similar observations have been made in Italy, where insect-spraying instituted after the war also reduced the incidence of the Naples and Sicilian sandfly fever virus infections of humans as evidenced by the relative lack of antibodies to these agents among those born after that period (i.e., since 1950, P. Verani, personal communication). Antibodies among the young in central Italy to the related ISS. Phl. 3 virus isolate (see below) have, however, been detected (P. Verani, personal communication).

Serological studies have shown that both Naples and Sicilian sandfly fever virus infections are highly prevalent in various countries of the Middle East and Central Europe (Berge, 1975). The disease associated with human infections most commonly involves such symptoms as anorexia, myalgia, headaches, fever, conjunctival inflammation, photophobia, and back and neck pains (Berge, 1975; Bartelloni and Tesh, 1976). Other signs and symptoms which have been recorded are vomiting, arthralgia, and respiratory problems (Berge, 1975).

Since the original suggestion by Doerr and Russ (1909) that sandfly fever is transmitted from one generation of *Phlebotomus* flies to another, Whittingham (1924) showed that the offspring of infected flies could induce the disease, implicating transovarial transmission in the maintenance of the agent among phlebotomine flies.

Two new Phlebotomus fever group members, Urucuri (Tesh *et al.*, 1975) and Rio Grande (Calisher *et al.*, 1977) viruses, have recently been described. A third unregistered isolate (ISS. Phl. 3) obtained by P. Verani and associates from central Italy in 1977 is related to, but distinguishable from, the Naples sandfly fever virus in CF, HI, and plaque reduction neutralization tests (P. Verani, personal communication).

Urucuri virus was isolated from the blood of a *Proechimys guyannensis* rodent captured in Utinga Forest, Para State, Brazil, in 1966. Additional isolates of the virus have been made from other *Proechimys* in Utinga and Embrapa as well as Serra do Navio, Amapa, Brazil. No isolates have been obtained from insects, so that Urucuri virus is described as a possible arbovirus on account of the serological crossreactivity to Phlebotomus grouping sera (Tesh *et al.*, 1975). Antibodies to Urucuri virus have been detected in rodent sera and occasionally in primate, edentate, and avian sera in different areas of Para State in Brazil (Karabatsos, 1978; Tesh *et al.*, 1975).

Two unregistered, candidate group members (CoAr 3319, SudAn 754-61) have been described by Tesh *et al.* (1975). The Sudan isolate (754-61) has been recovered from hedgehogs, rats, gerbils, mice, and a small monkey in different regions of Central and West Africa.

Rio Grande virus was isolated in 1974 from a pack rat (*Neotoma micropus*) trapped in 1973 in south Texas (Calisher *et al.*, 1977). Apart from pack rat isolates, no other isolates have been recorded so that the virus is classified as a possible arbovirus because of its serological cross-reactivity with known arboviruses of the Phlebotomus fever group (Karabatsos, 1978; Calisher *et al.*, 1977; Tesh *et al.*, 1975). Antibodies to the virus have been detected in various rodents, opossums, Texas tortoises, horses, a sheep, various birds, and a horned toad in south Texas (Calisher *et al.*, 1977).

The serological reactions of the Phlebotomus fever group differ in several features from those of other bunyavirus groups. Most of the viruses in the group are only distantly related to each other, usually requiring a very high-titered hyperimmune serum to demonstrate cross-reaction; this is true by neutralization tests and, in direct contrast to most bunyavirus groups, by CF tests, also (Tesh *et al.*, 1975). Cross-reactions are usually most readily detected by HI tests (Tesh *et al.*, 1975).

Until recently, it was believed that Phlebotomus fever group viruses which shared common CF antigens did not exist; however, BeAn 213452, an isolate from a Brazilian Amazon rodent, shares a common CF antigen with Candiru virus, but is readily distinguished by neturalization test (Andrade and Travassos, 1977, unpublished).

The proposed classification scheme shown in Table 2 is based on the data of Tesh *et al.* (1975), which in turn confirmed the studies of several individual viruses in the group in many laboratories throughout the world (Berge, 1975). Three additional agents, BeAn 213452, Saint-Floris, and Rio Grande, which are as yet incompletely studied, appear to be new serotypes.

1.2.2h.   Sakhalin Group

The four registered viruses in the Sakhalin group (Table 2) have been obtained from widely separated geographic regions: eastern U.S.S.R. (Sakhalin), Newfoundland (Avalon), Cape Wrath, Scotland (Clo Mor), and Macquarie Island, 800 miles southeast of Tasmania (Taggert). Tillamook, an unregistered virus (Yunker, 1975), was isolated from *Ixodes uriae* in coastal Oregon, United States. None of these viruses is known to cause human disease; all have been isolated from ticks.

The prototype of the group, Sakhalin virus, was originally obtained from *Ixodes (Ceratixodes) putus* tick nymphs collected in 1969 from rocky nesting grounds of sea birds on Tyuleniy Island, Sea of Okhotsk, off the Pacific coast of the U.S.S.R. (Lvov *et al.*, 1972, 1974). Antibodies (CF) to the virus have been detected in serum samples obtained from common guillemots trapped on the Tyuleniy and neighboring Kurile Islands, but not from sera taken fron snipes, ducks, cormorants, and storm petrels inhabiting these islands (Lvov *et al.*, 1972). Subsequent surveys of male and female ticks collected from Tyuleniy and Iona Islands (Sakhalin region), Ariy Kaman Island (Commodore Islands, Kamchatka region), and the southeast coast of Chukotka (Magadansk region) resulted in several Sakhalin virus isolates (Lvov *et al.*, 1974). Antibodies reactive to the virus have been identified in sera obtained from various sea birds (Lvov *et al.*, 1974). An isolate of Sakhalin virus has been made from *Ixodes uriae* collected from coastal Oregon of the United States (Thomas *et al.*, 1973).

Avalon virus was originally isolated from engorged adult *Ixodes uriae* ticks taken from a young herring gull collected in 1972, in a common puffin colony on Great Island, Newfoundland (Main *et al.*, 1976). Virus was isolated from the blood of the herring gull (Main *et al.*, 1976). Antibodies reactive to the virus were identified in sera obtained from both adult *Fratercula arctica* and *Oceanodroma leucorhoa*.

Clo Mor virus was isolated from a pool of engorged *Ixodes uriae* nymphs collected in a Common Murre colony at Clo Mor, Cape Wrath, Scotland in 1973.

Taggert virus, a recently registered Sakhalin group isolate, was obtained from *Ixodes* ticks collected in 1972 near a Royal Penguin rookery, Macquarie Island, South Ocean, southwest of New Zealand. The virus was subsequently isolated from ticks collected from the same region in 1976 and 1977 (T. St. George and J. G. Carley, personal communication). Neutralizing antibodies against the virus have been detected in the blood of penguins from Macquarie Island (Doherty *et al.*, 1975).

There are five distinct viruses in the Sakhalin group by CF test (Main *et al.*, 1976). The neutralization test confirms the distinctness of Taggert and Avalon viruses (Main *et al.*, 1976), but tests with Sakhalin, Tillamook, and Avalon have not been technically satisfactory. It is therefore premature to propose a definitive classification.

1.2.2i. Thogoto Virus

Thogoto virus was isolated in 1960 from the ticks *Boophilus* and *Rhipicephalus* by Haig *et al.* (1965), at Kabete, near Nairobi, Kenya. Isolates of the virus have been obtained from humans in Nigeria (Causey *et al.*, 1969) suffering from optic neuritis and fatal meningoencephalitis. Other isolates have been obtained from ticks in the

Central African Empire (Sureau *et al.*, 1976), trade animals in Nigeria (Kemp *et al.*, 1971), a camel in Nigeria, and various ticks recovered in Kenya, Sicily, Nigeria, and Egypt (Albanese *et al.*, 1972; Kemp *et al.*, 1971; Srihongse *et al.*, 1974). Antibodies to the virus have been detected in the sera of camels in Uganda and Kenya, as well as in sheep and goat sera in Kenya (Berge, 1975; Haig *et al.*, 1965). Thogoto virus is antigenically related to a virus obtained in Sicily. The Sicilian isolate (SiAr 126) represents a distinct subtype of Thogoto virus (Srihongse *et al.*, 1974).

1.2.2j. Turlock Group

The viruses in the Turlock group have all been isolated from culicine mosquitoes obtained either in Africa and Europe (M'Poko virus), or Asia (Umbre virus) and Australia (Barmah Forest virus), or North and South America (Turlock virus). None of the viruses is associated with a known human disease.

The Yaba-1 variety of M'Poko, obtained by C. C. Draper in Nigeria from *Culex* mosquitoes (Theiler and Downs, 1973), and the BA 365 variety, isolated subsequently from *Culex* species by Digoutte *et al.* (1970) near Bangui, Central African Empire, have been shown to be serologically essentially indistinguishable (Berge, 1975). Malkova *et al.* (1972) reported another M'Poko isolate from *Culex modestus* captured in South Moravia, Czechoslovakia, in 1963. Other than a few isolates from culicine mosquitoes, no other isolates of the virus have been recorded, although antibodies to M'Poko virus have been detected in human sera from the Central African Empire (Berge *et al.*, 1971).

Turlock virus was recovered from *Culex tarsalis* by Lennette *et al.* (1957) in 1954 near Sutter City, California. Additional isolates of the virus have come from wild birds in Belem, Brazil (Shope *et al.*, 1966; Berge, 1975), house finches in Kern County, California, and *Lepus californicus* and *Passer domesticus* obtained in Hale County, Texas (Hayes *et al.*, 1967). Other isolates of the virus have come from sentinel mice in Brazil and chicks in Kern County, Texas, as well as from various *Culex* species in many parts of the United States, Alberta (Canada), Equador, Trinidad, and Brazil (Berge, 1975; Wong *et al.*, 1971). Antibodies against the virus have been found in the sera of various wild mammals, birds, and horses in California and wild birds in Brazil (Berge, 1975).

Umbre virus was isolated from *Culex bitaeniorhynchus* in 1955 at Poona, India (Taylor, 1967). Other than isolates from Bombay State and South India (from *Culex vishnui*), and various *Culex* species in Malaysia, one other strain has been obtained from the blood of a bird caught in South India (Carey *et al.*, 1968). Antibodies to Umbre virus have been detected in serum samples collected from wild birds and sentinel chickens in Malaysia. Recently Barmah Forest virus has been obtained from *Culex* mosquitoes collected in Australia (G. M. Woodroofe and I. D. Marshall, personal communication). Marweh virus, which came from *Culex annulirostris* collected in 1974, appears to be serologically related to, but distinguishable from, Barmah Forest virus (J. G. Carley, personal communication).

Turlock, Umbre, and M'Poko viruses are closely related by both neutralization and CF tests. The neutralization data are presented in Table 16. They are proposed as three subtypes comprising the Turlock group. Although not all the tests have been completed, Barmah Forest virus appears to be a more distant relative of Umbre virus.

Digoutte *et al.* (1970) described a one-way cross-reaction by neutralization tests between the BA 365 and Yaba-1 strains of M'Poko virus, results which differ from those given in Berge (1975). It would be prudent to consider the Yaba-1 strain as a variety of M'Poko virus until these differences can be resolved. The same authors described significant neutralization of Yaba-1 virus by Ingwavuma (Simbu group) serum, indicating intergroup cross-reaction between the Turlock and Simbu groups.

1.2.2k. Uukuniemi Group

The viruses of the Uukuniemi group have all been obtained from various ticks in various parts of the world including Asia (Manawa and

TABLE 16

Neutralization Relationships of Turlock Group Viruses[a]

Virus	Antibody			
	Turlock	Umbre	M'Poko	Barmah Forest
Turlock	0[b]	>1.0	3.4	
Umbre	0.6	0	1.8	5.4
M'Poko	1.2	>0.6	0	
Barmah Forest		4.5		0

[a] Data from Shope (1970, unpublished) and I. D. Marshall (1978, personal communication).
[b] Difference in log neutralizing index; see Table 3.

Zaliv Terpeniya viruses), Europe (Grand Arbaud, Ponteves, and Uuku-niemi viruses), Africa (EgAn 1825-61 virus), and America (Oceanside). None of the viruses is known to cause human disease.

The prototype virus of the group, Uukuniemi virus, came from engorged *Ixodes ricinus* ticks taken from cows in 1960 at Uukuniemi, southeast Finland (Oker-Blom *et al.*, 1964). Many virus isolates have been obtained from *Ixodes ricinus* in south Finland (Saikku and Brummer-Korvenkontio, 1973), Norway (Traavik *et al.*, 1974), Czechoslovakia (Kolman *et al.*, 1966; Kolman and Husova, 1971), Poland (Wroblewska-Mularczykowa *et al.*, 1970), south-central U.S.S.R. (Sumakh and Potepli strains, Gaidamovich *et al.*, 1971*a,b*), the Soviet Far East (Klisenko *et al.*, 1973), western and northern Moravia (Kozuch *et al.*, 1970*a*), and Lithuania and the United States (from *Ixodes uriae*, Thomas *et al.*, 1973). Isolates of the virus from vertebrates have been recorded from passerine birds in the summer in an endemic region of southeast Finland (Saikku and Brummer-Korvenkontio, 1973; Saikku, 1974), Poland (Wroblewska-Mular-czykowa *et al.*, 1970), a blackbird in Azerbaijan, U.S.S.R. (Sumakh strain, Gaidamovich *et al.*, 1971*a*), and a yellow-necked mouse *Apodemus flavicollis* trapped in Czechoslovakia (Kozuch *et al.*, 1970*b*). Human antibodies to Uukuniemi virus have been found in parts of Czechoslovakia (Sekeyova *et al.*, 1970) and Hungary (Berge, 1975). Antibodies have been detected in cattle sera in Finland (Saikku, 1973) and avian sera collected in the Estonian S.S.R. (Gaidamovich *et al.*, 1973).

Grand Arbaud and Ponteves viruses came from southern France, where they were initially isolated from *Argas reflexus* nymph and imago ticks collected in 1966 from pigeonhouses in the Rhone Delta (Hannoun *et al.*, 1970). Other than additional isolates from the same region, including a Ponteves isolate from newborn tick larvae, no other isolates of these two viruses have been documented (Hannoun *et al.*, 1970). No vertebrate serological surveys for either Grand Arbaud or Ponteves virus have been reported.

Manawa virus was isolated from adult *Argas abdussalami* ticks in Lahore and from *Rhipicephalus* species in other parts of Pakistan (Begum *et al.*, 1970*b*; Berge *et al.*, 1970). No vertebrate antibodies against the virus have been found in limited serological surveys (Berge *et al.*, 1970).

Zaliv Terpeniya virus was initially isolated from female imago *Ixodes* (*Ceratixodes*) *putus* ticks collected in 1969 from Tyulenily Island, Zaliv Terpeniya (Patience Bay), in the Pacific Coast sea of

Okhotsk, U.S.S.R. (Lvov *et al.*, 1973*a*). Other isolates have been obtained from the Commodore and Kurshin Islands off the Pacific coast of the U.S.S.R. (Lvov *et al.*, 1973*a,b*). A closely related virus, Oceanside, was isolated from the Pacific Coast of the United States (Yunker, 1975).

An unregistered member of the group, EgAn 1825-61, was isolated from the blood of a southward-migrating palearctic bird caught in Egypt by J. Schmidt.

A complete serological comparison of viruses in the Uukuniemi group by HI or neutralization tests has not been done. Uukuniemi virus is distinct from Grand Arbaud and Zaliv Terpeniya by neutralization tests (Berge, 1975) and from Grand Arbaud and Manawa viruses by the HI test (Casals, 1972). The CF test results (Berge, 1975) indicate that the various members of the group are probably distinct, although not all of them have been compared. Tentatively it is proposed that the group contains six-subtypes of Uukuniemi virus.

1.2.21. Unassigned Viruses

The 11 registered or candidate viruses which have not been assigned to the Bunyavirus genus or to the serogroups of the possible members of the Bunyaviridae family are Belmont, Bhanja, Khasan, Kowanyama, Lone Star, Razdan, Rift Valley fever, Sunday Canyon, Tamday, Tataguine, and Witwatersrand viruses. Their membership in the family has, like that of the other possible members of the family, been proposed on electron microscopic evidence, and in some cases from limited molecular studies.

Belmont virus was obtained from *Culex annulirostris* collected in 1968 in Queensland, Australia (Doherty *et al.*, 1972). It has been subsequently isolated in 1978 from *Culex* species collected in the Northern Territory of Australia (T. St. George and J. G. Carley, personal communication).

Bhanja virus was retrieved from *Haemaphysalis* ticks taken off a paralyzed goat in 1954 at Poona, India (Shah and Work, 1969). The virus has been isolated many times from various ticks obtained in India, Italy, Nigeria, Cameroon, the Armenian S.S.R., and Yugoslavia (Institute Pasteur de Dakar, 1972; Matevosyan *et al.*, 1974; Sacca *et al.*, 1969; Vinograd *et al.*, 1975), as well as from a hedgehog, a ground squirrel, and the blood of cattle and sheep in various parts of Africa (Berge, 1975; Kemp *et al.*, 1971). Antibody surveys have suggested that the virus infects domestic animals and humans in parts of Yugoslavia (J. Vesenjak-Hirjan, personal communication), goats in Italy and Sicily (Albanese *et al.*, 1971; Verani *et al.*, 1970), and probably various mammals in India (Berge, 1975). Laboratory-acquired Bhanja virus infections have been documented (Calisher and Goodpasture, 1975; J. Vesenjak-Hirjan, personal communication).

Khasan virus, a recently registered virus, was isolated by D. K. Lvov and associates from *Haemaphysalis longicornis* ticks collected in 1977 from a spotted deer nursery in the Khasansk region, Primorye Territory, U.S.S.R.

Kowanyama virus was isolated by Doherty *et al.* (1968) from *Anopheles* species collected in 1963 at the Mitchell River Mission, Australia, and isolated in 1964 in Brisbane. Kowanyama virus isolates have come only from *Anopheles* species; however, antibodies to the virus have been detected in domestic fowl, horse, and kangaroo sera as well as the sera of adult Aborigines in north Queensland (Doherty *et al.*, 1970). Antibodies have also been found in sera collected from cattle, horses, sheep, pigs, kangaroos, wallabies, bandicoots, rats, and wild birds in Queensland (Doherty *et al.*, 1970).

Lone Star virus was obtained by Kokernot *et al.* (1969) from a tick removed from a woodchuck in western Kentucky in 1967. No other isolates of the virus have been made, although antibodies to Lone Star virus have been detected in a human serum sample from New York state (Kascsak *et al.*, 1978) and in racoons (40% incidence) trapped in Kentucky (Kokernot *et al.*, 1969).

Razdan virus, another recently registered virus, was isolated by D. K. Lvov and associates from ticks (*Dermacentor marginatus*) collected from sheep in the Razdansk Region of the Armenian S.S.R.

Rift Valley fever virus was isolated in 1930 by Daubney and Hudson (1931) in Kenya. The virus was obtained from the blood of a newborn lamb and has been subsequently isolated many times from lambs, sheep, and cattle (Alexander, 1951; Daubney *et al.*, 1931; Gear *et al.*, 1955; Kokernot *et al.*, 1957b), as well as from human sera samples—particularly those taken from veterinarians and laboratory workers who became infected while handling diseased animals (Berge, 1975). Many human infections, some fatal, have been documented in Kenya, Uganda, Zaire, Sudan, Rhodesia, Ethiopia, South Africa (Berge, 1975), and more recently Egypt, where in 1977 some 600 deaths were recorded in a 3-month period (M. Darwish, personal communication).

Among the various signs and symptoms associated with natural and laboratory-acquired human Rift Valley fever infections are the sudden onset of the disease 3–7 days after exposure, severe headaches, fever, shivering, nausea and vomiting, myalgia, jaundice, hemorrhages, and lymphadenopathy (Berge, 1975). Other recorded signs and symptoms include eye pains, conjunctival and facial inflammation, detachment of the retina, and central blindness often associated with retinitis and macular exudates. Hemorrhagic complications have been documented in association with fatal gastrointestinal hemorrhages; encephalitis also occurs in a certain percentage of severe cases (van Velden et al., 1977). A prolonged convalescence is usual. Many Rift Valley fever virus epidemics have occurred among sheep flocks and cattle herds in various parts of Central and South Africa and more recently in Egypt, causing considerable economic losses. The disease in these animals is characterized by loss of appetite and listlessness, as well as abortion and high mortalities, especially among young lambs. The disease in sheep frequently involves generalized hepatic necrosis.

Numerous isolations of the virus have been made from various species of mosquitoes, including *Eretmapodites*, *Aedes*, and *Culex* species (Berge, 1975; Weinbren et al., 1957b), and from *Culicoides* (V. H. Lee, personal communication).

In Egypt, Rift Valley fever virus was isolated from *Culex pipiens* during the 1977 and 1978 outbreaks (M. Darwish, personal communication). It is believed that the primary vertebrate hosts for the virus are probably sheep, cattle, and buffalo, and possibly certain antelopes and rodents (see Davies, 1975; Berge, 1975), although no virus isolates or antibodies to the virus have been detected among wild rodents in Uganda (Henderson et al., 1972). Alternate possible hosts are camels and pigs (Scott et al., 1963; Scott, 1963), all of which can be infected by virus-bearing mosquitoes (Berge, 1975). Man is often infected while handling sick or dead animals during an epizootic, and also when bitten by infected arthropods such as mosquitoes (and possibly midges).

Rift Valley fever virus is of considerable economic importance when epizootics occur (see Swanepoel, 1976) since considerable losses of domestic animals (sheep and cattle) occur, as in Egypt in the fall of 1977. Because of the importance of Rift Valley fever virus in various parts of Africa (and now the Middle East), vaccines for the virus have been developed. A live and inactivated neuroadapted (neurotropic) virus vaccine has been used with considerable success in the South African Veterinary Service (Barnard and Botha, 1977; Berge, 1975; Weiss, 1962). A mouse brain passaged virus vaccine has also been developed in Nigeria and shown to be effective in raising antibodies (Fagbami et al., 1975). A killed neurotropic virus vaccine has been prepared in the United States (Randall et al., 1962) and shown in man to be capable of evoking an antibody response. One vaccinated laboratory worker, however, developed only a low-titer antibody reponse and was not protected against subsequent infection by the pantropic strain of Rift Valley fever (Binn *et al.*, 1963). Pregnant ewes inoculated with Rift Valley fever vaccine have been shown to produce offspring with hydranencephaly and arthrogryposis (Coetzer and Barnard, 1977).

Experimental transmission of Rift Valley fever virus has been demonstrated using *Aedes*, *Culex*, and *Eretmapodites* species (Berge, 1975; Gear *et al.*, 1955; McIntosh *et al.*, 1973; Smithburn *et al.*, 1949). Since the original virus isolation, many alternate virus strains have been obtained in different parts of Africa and Egypt. Human and vertebrate serological surveys indicate that Kenya, Uganda, the Sudan, Egypt, Ethiopia, French Equatorial Africa, Rhodesia, Mozambique, and South Africa are areas where virus infection have occurred (Kokernot *et al.*, 1956; M. Darwish, personal communication; Johnson *et al.*, 1978).

The ability of Rift Valley fever virus to infect domestic pets has been studied, with not only fatal infections being documented for kittens and pups (but not adult cats or dogs) but also kitten-to-kitten and kitten-to-cat transmission observed (Walker *et al.*, 1970).

No serological relatives of Rift Valley fever virus have been identified.

Sunday Canyon virus came from *Argas* ticks collected in Texas in 1969 (Yunker *et al.*, 1977). No other isolates of the virus have been made (Karabatsos, 1978).

Tamdy virus was recovered from *Hyalomma asiaticum* ticks collected in 1971 in the Tamdynsk Region, Bukharsk Province, Uzbek S.S.R. Other isolates have been made from the Marvisk Province, Turkmen S.S.R.

Tataguine virus was obtained in 1962 from pooled *Culex* and *Anopheles* species in Senegal (Bres *et al.*, 1966). It has subsequently been obtained from various *Anopheles* and *Mansonia* mosquitoes collected in Ethiopia, Senegal, Cameroon, and Nigeria (Berge, 1975; Fagbami *et al.*, 1972; Ota *et al.*, 1976; Rickenbach *et al.*, 1976). Many isolates of the virus have been recovered from human samples in Senegal, Nigeria, Cameroon, and the Central African Empire (Berge, 1975), as well as from patients in the Cameroon affected by an exanthematic fever—the so-called *fievre rouge congolaise* (Digoutte *et al.*, 1969). Antibodies to the virus have been detected in human, domestic animal, rodent, and monkey sera collected in the Cameroon, Nigeria, Senegal (Berge, 1975; Digoutte *et al.*, 1969; Fagbami *et al.*, 1972).

Witwatersrand virus was isolated by McIntosh *et al.* (1960) from *Culex rubinotus* obtained in 1958 at Germiston, Transvaal, South Africa, during an epidemic of febrile illnesses. Other isolates of the virus have been obtained from culicine mosquitoes collected in South Africa and Uganda, as well as from sentinel hamsters in South Africa and Mozambique and various rodents trapped in Uganda. Antibodies to the virus have been detected both in human sera in South Africa (McIntosh *et al.*, 1960) and Mozambique and in rodent sera collected in Uganda (Berge, 1975). McIntosh *et al.* (1972) have reported serological reactions between Witwatersrand virus and Bunyamwera group viruses.

1.2.2m. Summary of the Bunyaviruslike Viruses, Other Possible Members of the Bunyaviridae Family

The fact that most of the possible members of the Bunyaviridae family are candidates of the family only on the basis of electron microscopic evidence, and not through serological relatedness with accepted members, raises two issues. First, are these viruses bunyaviruses, and, second, should other genera of bunyaviruses be formed?

The criteria for establishing other genera of bunyaviruses have yet to be defined. At the genetic level, viruses with three negative-sense RNA segments whose gene products perform similar functions to those of accepted members of the family would meet the established criteria for bunyaviruses (Section 1). Morphological and morphogenetic criteria have also been established (Section 1). For representatives of all of the proposed serogroups, the morphological and morphogenetic criteria appear to be met by the candidate members, although some studies need confirmation.

Only a limited number of molecular studies have been reported for bunyaviruslike viruses. These, and unpublished work (see later), indicate that at least the Phlebotomus fever virus group viruses, the Uukuniemi group viruses, Belmont virus, and Rift Valley fever virus meet the genetic and morphological criteria for candidacy. The criteria for forming other bunyavirus genera have yet to be established.

Many of the bunyaviruslike viruses are transmitted by ticks. These include the viruses belonging to the Bakau, Crimean hemorrhagic fever–Congo, Kaisodi, Nairobi sheep disease, Sakhalin, Thogoto, and Uukuniemi serogroups, as well as Bhanja, Khasan, Lone Star, Razdan, Sunday Canyon, and Tamdy viruses of the unassigned bunyaviruslike viruses. At least some of the tick-borne virus serotypes have been recovered from widely separated geographic regions of the world and have been associated with both avian and mammalian host infections (e.g., Crimean hemorrhagic fever–Congo virus). The transport of infected ticks and/or intercontinental passage of infected birds may well be involved in the dissemination of virus infections, and, through the ages, may have led to the establishment of different foci of virus infections. Tick survival without feeding over many years has been reported (e.g., in northern U.S.S.R.), which together with evidence indicating that transovarial passage of virus and persistent infections occur in ticks, suggests mechanisms for the maintenance and transmission of certain bunyaviruslike viruses.

At least 12 of the bunyaviruslike viruses cause human disease; two are responsible for severe human diseases that occur in epidemic proportions (Crimean hemorrhagic fever–Congo viruses and Rift Valley fever virus). Epizootics associated with bunyaviruslike virus infections of domestic animals are of economic importance in certain parts of the world (e.g., Nairobi sheep disease and Rift Valley fever viruses). The recent introduction to the Mediterranean region of Rift Valley fever (Egypt in 1977) is of considerable current concern, with regard both to possible further spread of the virus and to how the virus was introduced into the area.

2. STRUCTURAL COMPONENTS AND THEIR FUNCTIONS

Relatively little physiochemical information is available on the structural components of most bunyaviruses. Only a few viruses have been adapted to tissue culture and cloned. Most of the molecular information that has been obtained has come from studies of the California encephalitis and Bunyamwera serogroups of bunyaviruses and Uukuniemi virus, a bunyaviruslike virus.

2.1. Virus Particle Morphology and Morphogenesis

The published studies on bunyavirus morphology fall into two categories: electron microscopic analyses of purified virus preparations and similar analyses of infected tissues or cell cultures (Figs. 1–4). These latter analyses also relate to the question of viral morphogenesis and so will also be discussed in relation to what is known about the virion morphology.

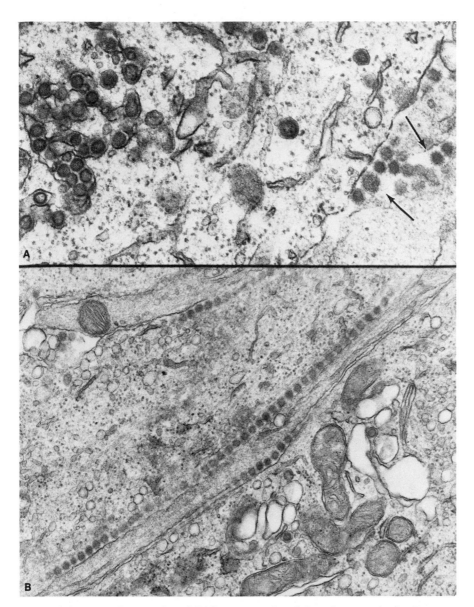

Fig. 1.   Electron micrographs of Bunyamwera virus-infected mouse brain. Bunyamwera virus particles (A) enclosed in complex membrane enclosures within the cytoplasm
of an infected mouse brain neuron. Such masses are commonly observed late in infection. Extracellular virions (arrows) appear round or oval within a ragged surface halo
(mean diameter 98 nm). Magnification ×64,000. Section of Bunyamwera virus-infected
mouse brain tissue (B) in which virus particles are linearly arrayed in intercellular
spaces. Magnification ×34,400. Photographs provided by F. Murphy, CDC, Atlanta.
From Murphy *et al.* (1968*b*). Reduced 20% for reproduction.

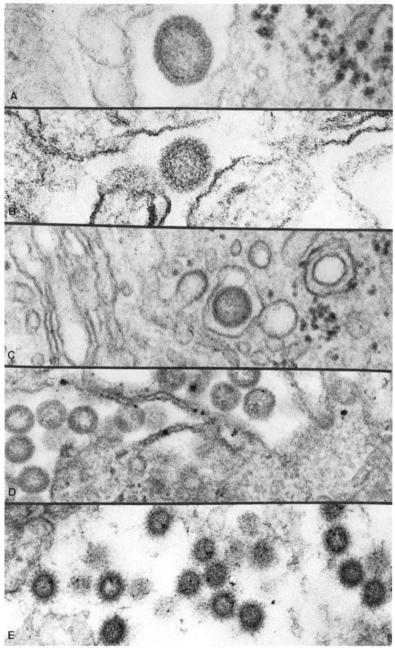

Fig. 2.   Thin-section electron microscopy of bunyaviruslike viruses. A: Hazara virus in suckling mouse brain (×170,000). B: Chagres virus in infected mouse brain (×144,000). C: Congo virus in infected mouse brain (×107,000). D: Rift Valley fever virus in infected mouse brain tissue (×100,000). E: Bhanja virus in mouse brain (×92,000). Photographs provided by F. Murphy, CDC, Atlanta. From Murphy *et al.* (1973). Reduced 9% for reproduction.

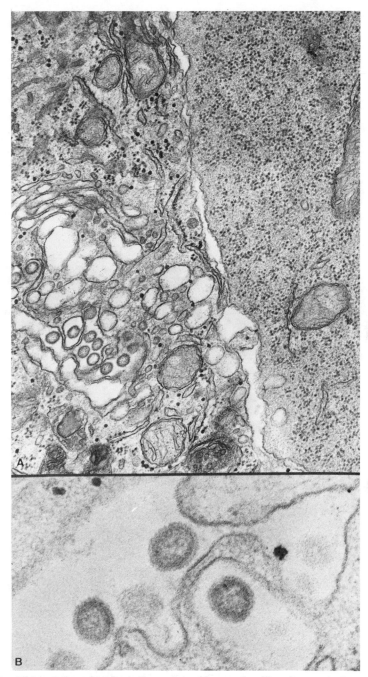

Fig. 3.   Thin-section electron microscopy of bunyaviruslike viruses. A: Lone Star virus in proliferated Golgi vesicules in an infected sucking mouse brain neuron (×38,000). B: Ganjam virus at the plasma membrane of an infected hepatocyte (×114,000). Photographs provided by F. Murphy, CDC, Atlanta. From Murphy *et al.* (1973). Reduced 7% for reproduction.

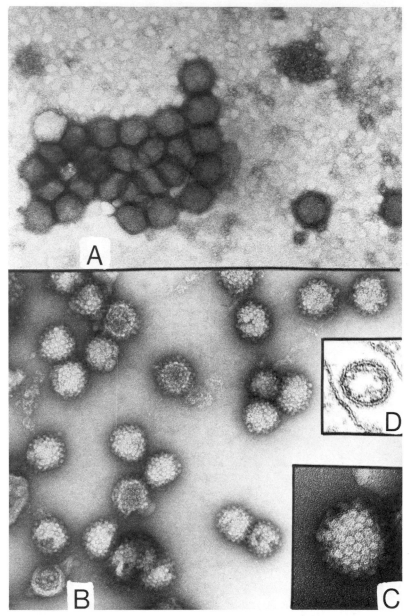

Fig. 4.   Electron micrographs of bunyaviruslike viruses. A: Karimabad virus negatively stained with phosphotungstate (×75,000). B: Uukuniemi virus fixed with 0.7% glutaraldehyde before purification; negatively stained with uranyl acetate. The hexagonal array of subunits and occasional penton groups are evident (×100,000). C: Uukuniemi virion (×180,000). D: Uukuniemi virus-infected chick cells showing internal material in juxtaposition to the viral envelope (×60,000). Uukuniemi photographs provided by C.-H. Bonsdorff, University of Helsinki. From von Bonsdorff and Pettersson (1975). Reduced 11% for reproduction.

2.1.1. Analyses of Infected Tissues and Tissue Culture Cells

Electron microscopic examination of newborn mouse brains infected with five California group viruses (California encephalitis, La Crosse, San Angelo, Keystone, and an isolate NY 658569) by Murphy *et al.* (1968*a*) has revealed that despite the fact that these viruses represent the range of virulence of experimental pathogenicity (Berge, 1975) they induce similar changes on intracerebral inoculation in newborn mice. These changes include perineuronal edema formation, minimal inflammatory cell infiltration, and neuronal degeneration. Similar histological changes in the central nervous system have been observed for several bunyavirus infections of adult mice (and monkeys), except that a slower progression of infection in adult animals leads to an eventual severe inflammation involving neuronophagia, perivascular infiltration, and necrosis (Behbehani *et al.*, 1967; Murphy *et al.*, 1968*a,b*; F. Murphy, personal communication).

Many investigators have reported that bunyavirus infections of animal cell cultures are cytopathic, including those of animal tissue origin such as bovine lymph node cell cultures (March and Hetrick, 1967). However, it has been reported that infection of insect cells produces no gross cytopathic effects (Lyons and Heyduk, 1973).

Morphogenetic studies of bunyavirus-infected tissues, such as thin sections of brain tissues, have shown that virus particles appear in brain neurons coincident with the clinical signs of infection and concurrent with the development of high titers of virus in infected brains (Murphy *et al.*, 1968*a*). Within infected brain or tissue culture cells, virus particles characteristically occur in intracellular cisternae and vacuoles, particularly in association with the Golgi apparatus (Figs. 1–3) (Behbenani *et al.*, 1967; von Bonsdorff and Pettersson, 1975; Holmes, 1971; Lyons and Heyduk, 1973; Murphy *et al.*, 1973). No, or very rare, evidence for plasma membrane budding or nuclear involvement in the infection cycle has been obtained.

The morphogenesis of several bunyaviruses has been studied. Such studies have led to the concept that, despite the hepatotropism of some bunyaviruses (e.g., group C, Nairobi sheep disease, and Guama groups) and neurotropism of others (e.g., Bunyamwera and California encephalitis groups), the process of virus maturation is similar for all the viruses examined in the various tissues that are invaded, and probably characteristic of the intracelllular infection process by all members of the family. Similar results have been obtained for animal and insect tissue culture analyses, as well as from studies of experimentally infected animals. The various viruses in the Bunyavirus genus that have

been examined in one or another system include the following:
Bunyamwera group viruses: Bunyamwera, Maguari, Tensaw (Fig. 1)
(Murphy et al., 1968a, 1973; F. Murphy, personal communication), and
Cache Valley (Holmes, 1971); Anopheles A group viruses: Anopheles A
(Holmes, 1971; Murphy et al., 1973); California encephalitis serogroup
viruses: California encephalitis (Lyons and Heyduk, 1973), California
encephalitis, Keystone, La Crosse, San Angelo, NY 658569 (Murphy et
al., 1968b), and Melao (Holmes, 1971); group C viruses: Gumbo
Limbo, Marituba, Oriboca, and Restan (Holmes, 1971; Murphy et al.,
1973); Simbu group viruses: Oropouche, Manzanilla (Holmes, 1971),
and Mermet (Murphy et al., 1973); Guama group viruses: Catu
(Holmes, 1971); Capim group viruses: Capim and Bushbush (Murphy
et al., 1973); Koongol group viruses: Koongol and Wongal (Stevenson
and Holmes, 1972); unassigned supergroup viruses: Kaeng Khoi
(Murphy et al., 1973).

The bunyaviruslike viruses (other possible members of the
Bunyaviridae family) that have been examined by electron microscopy
include the following: Anopheles B group viruses: Anopheles B
(Murphy et al., 1973); Bakau group viruses: Bakau (Murphy et al.,
1973); Crimean hemorrhagic fever–Congo group viruses: Congo,
Hazara, and Crimean hemorrhagic fever (Fig.2) (Chumakov and
Donets, 1975; Donets and Chumakov, 1975; Donet et al., 1977a;
Jelinkova et al., 1976; Korolev et al., 1975, 1976; Murphy et al., 1973;
Donets, 1975; Donets and Chumakov, 1975; Donet et al., 1977a;
Jelinkova et al., 1976; Korolev et al., 1975, 1976; Murphy et al., 1973;
Popov and Zavodova, 1976); Kaisodi group viruses: Silverwater
(Murphy et al., 1973); Nairobi sheep disease group viruses: Dugbe
(David-West et al., 1972), Ganjam (Fig. 3) (Murphy et al., 1973); Phle-
botomus fever group viruses: Sicilian sandfly fever virus (Behbehani et
al., 1967), Chagres and Punta Toro (Fig. 2) (Murphy et al., 1973); Sak-
halin group viruses: Sakhalin and Avalon (D. Lvov, personal communication); Thogoto group viruses: Thogoto (Murphy et al., 1973); Turlock
group viruses: Turlock (Murphy et al., 1973); Uukuniemi group viruses:
Uukuniemi (von Bonsdorff et al., 1969; Saikku and von Bonsdorff,
1968); unassigned nonsupergroup viruses: Belmont (D. A. McPhee and
E. G. Westaway, personal communication), Rift Valley fever, Witwatersrand, Bhanja, and Lone Star (Figs. 2 and 3) (Levitt et al., 1963;
Murphy et al., 1973), Bhanja, Khasan, Razdan, and Tamdy (D. Lvov,
personal communication).

An overall conclusion drawn from all the reported studies is that
the morphogenesis of bunyaviruses is quite distinct from that of most

other major families of RNA viruses. Both in animal cells and in insect cell lines, the primary site of virus maturation is in smooth endoplasmic membranes, particularly in association with the Golgi apparatus. Apparently late in infection a distension and proliferation of Golgi saccules and vesicles occur (Fig. 3). Virus particles have been observed both budding into vesicules of the smooth endoplasmic reticulum in the region of the Golgi apparatus and accumulating within cisternae of these organelles (Fig. 3). Crescent-shaped segments of thickened membranes observed by Lyons and Heyduk (1973) may represent the initial process of budding into Golgi cisternae. Single virions, small groups, and occasionally large numbers of mature virions have been observed in intracellular vesicles as well as in perinuclear focal groups (Fig. 1). Crystal-like patterns of Crimean hemorrhagic fever virus in infected cells have been reported by Korolev *et al.* (1976).

Virus particles, which are never encompassed by membranous enclosures, have been observed extracellularly where neither evidence of marginal membrane disruption nor loss of cytoplasmic organization was evident (Fig. 1). Late in infection not only do cells often become strikingly vacuolated (Fig. 3), but also peripheral vacuoles containing uniformly dense virus particles have been observed.

These observations, plus the presence of extracellular virus particles in areas of cell breakage, have led to the suggestion that virus release may occur by both cytoplasmic membrane disruption with localized discharge of the cell contents and viral transport to cell margins in organelle cisternae followed by membrane fusion and virus egestion.

No precursor particles have been observed in virus-infected cells, in contrast to the result obtained for alphaviruses (Murphy *et al.*, 1968).

Holmes (1971) has reported an occasional central dense spot (15 nm diameter) in intracellular virions, although most particles that were found in the vacuoles in the vicinity of the Golgi structure appeared to have a central area with fine filamentous material in it. Similar observations have been made by Donets *et al.* (1977) with Crimean hemorrhagic fever–Congo virus. Late in infection Holmes observed peripheral vacuoles in infected cells containing uniformly dense virus particles. Holmes also reported that extracellular virus has a uniformly electron-dense "core" and an electron-lucent envelope. Thus he suggested that there may be a structural transition between newly formed virus particles within a cell and the extracellular virions. Similar conclusions have been reached by Jelinkova *et al.* (1976) for Crimean hemorrhagic fever virus infected monkey cells.

Morphological studies undertaken by Murphy *et al.* (1968*a,b*,1973) did not detect significant differences in intracellular vs. extracellular viruses with regard to particle central density. Virion centers which were smooth, granular, reticular, or filamentous were observed for both types of virus.

However, Murphy *et al.* (1968*a,b*) did notice that the form of the virion surface projection layer was partly related to the location of the virus particles, with intracellular particles having a smoother surface—possibly due to compaction of surface projections. Extracellular particles were seen often to have a more ragged and wide external layer (Fig. 1). Occasionally an ordered array of hexagonal surface projections was observed by Murphy *et al.* (1973), similar to that described for negatively stained purified Uukuniemi (Fig. 4) and Rift Valley fever viruses (von Bonsdorff and Pettersson, 1975; Polson and Stannard, 1970; Saikku and von Bonsdorff, 1968; Saikku *et al.*, 1970).

Analyses of thin sections of Uukuniemi-infected chick embryo fibroblasts have provided some evidence of an association of an irregularly arranged electron-opaque material (probably the viral nucleocapsids) located in a zone beneath the viral membrane (Fig. 4) (von Bonsdorff and Pettersson, 1975).

2.1.2. Virus Particle Morphology

Bunyavirus particles are generally spherical in shape with an external fringe of surface projections (5–10 nm in size) apparently anchored in a lipid bilayer which constitutes the viral envelope. The sizes of extracellular virus particles appear to be the same as those of intracellular particles (Fig. 1). The overall size ranges obtained in analyses involving measurements of a large number of particles vary from 80 to 120 nm, with mean values for particular viruses ranging from 92 to 105 nm (Holmes, 1971; Murphy *et al.*, 1968*a,b*, 1973). Most particles observed by either thin-section electron microscopy of infected tissues or negatively stained purified virus preparation are spherical (Figs. 1–4) or oval in shape, the latter possibly due to compression or collapse during sample preparation (Behbehani *et al.*, 1967; Holmes, 1971; Murphy *et al.*, 1968*a,b*, 1973; Obijeski *et al.*, 1976*a*; Southam *et al.*, 1964). Morphological studies of the viruses listed in Section 2.1.1 indicate that all the bunyaviruses examined are similar in overall shape, size, and internal definition. Similar conclusions have been reached for Mapputta, Trubanaman, and Maprik viruses of the Mapputta group (I.

Holmes, cited in Murphy *et al.*, 1973). Occasionally purified bunyavirus preparations (e.g., Karimabad virus of the Phlebotomus fever group) have aggregates of virus particles (Fig. 4). Slightly larger-sized virus particles have been observed for unfixed Belmont virus (114 nm) when similarly treated Bunyamwera virus preparations give values of 91 nm (D. A. McPhee and E. Westaway, personal communication).

The size estimates obtained by electron microscopic analyses, or controlled pore glass filtration (Donets *et al.*, 1977a), are compatible with the size ranges estimated by membrane ultrafiltration for the different members of the Bunyaviridae family and the bunyaviruslike viruses (Berge, 1975). The values are in contrast to the significantly smaller size estimates of alphaviruses (~55 nm) and flaviviruses (~38 nm).

Occasional aberrant virus forms have been observed in infected tissues, including elongated forms which, however, have a normal width (Murphy *et al.*, 1968a,b, 1973). The significance of such forms is not known.

Studies by Saikku, von Bonsdorff, Oker-Blom, and associates on Uukuniemi virus (von Bonsdorff *et al.*, 1969; von Bonsdorff and Pettersson, 1975; Pettersson *et al.*, 1971; Saikku and von Bonsdorff, 1968; Saikku *et al.*, 1970) indicate that although this virus resembles other bunyaviruses in general morphological properties, hexagonal arrays of surface components can be visualized, particularly after glutaraldehyde fixation (Fig. 4). Such arrays, although occasionally seen for other viruses, have not been seen when La Crosse virus is treated similarly (Obijeski *et al.*, 1976a; F. Murphy, personal communication). The reason is not known. Since the glycoprotein species of Uukuniemi virus are quite different to those of La Crosse virus, it is possible that the apparently unique surface arrangement of Uukuniemi virus reflects these differences (see Section 2.2.7a). The clustered projections observed for Uukuniemi virus (Fig. 4) are in the form of hollow cylindrical morphological units, 8–10 nm long and 10–12 nm in diameter, with a central 5-nm cavity (von Bonsdorff and Pettersson, 1975). Both negative staining and glutaraldehyde fixation plus freeze-etching of Uukuniemi virus prepartions have suggested that the surface units are penton–hexon clusters arranged in a $T = 12$, $P = 3$ icosahedral surface lattice with hexon–hexon distances estimated to be between 12.5 and 16 nm for stained virus particles and 17 nm for the freeze-etched samples. The analyses performed on Uukuniemi virus preparations also indicate that the surface subunits are probably attached to a lipid bilayer which can be freeze-fractured.

2.2.   Composition and Properties of Bunyavirus Particles

2.2.1.   Virus Sedimentation Coefficients and Buoyant Densities

Sedimentation coefficients ($S_{20,w}$) have been reported for various bunyaviruses: Bunyamwera virus (Kascsak and Lyons, 1977), California encephalitis virus (Rosato et al., 1974a), La Crosse virus (McLerran and Arlinghaus, 1973; Obijeski et al., 1976a), Inkoo virus (Brummer-Korvenkontio, 1969), Crimean hemorrhagic fever virus (Donets and Chumakov, 1975; Donets et al., 1977a,b), Rift Valley fever virus (Polson and Levitt, 1963), and Uukuniemi virus (Pettersson et al., 1971). The reported values range from 350 S to 470 S, significantly higher than those obtained for alphaviruses ($\sim$240 S) or flaviviruses ($\sim$200 S). An infectious, slowly sedimenting agent (156 S), obtained as a minor component in Rift Valley fever virus preparations (in addition to an infectious 450 S component), has been reported (Polson and Levitt, 1963). Some evidence that this minor component may be filamentous and lipoidal was obtained, although no electron microscopy of the material was presented.

As with many other lipid-enveloped viruses, the reported buoyant densities of bunyaviruses in sucrose range from 1.17 to 1.19 g/cm³. Such values have been recorded for Bunyamwera virus (Kascsak and Lyons, 1977), California encephalitis virus (Goldman et al., 1977; White, 1975), Lumbo and Tahyna viruses (Bouloy et al., 1973/1974), La Crosse virus (McLerran and Arlinghaus, 1973), Oriboca virus (Rosato et al., 1974b), Crimean hemorrhagic fever virus (Chumakov and Donets, 1975; Donets et al., 1977a,b), and Uukuniemi virus (von Bonsdorff and Pettersson, 1975). Obijeski et al. (1976a) reported that La Crosse virus banded in potassium tartrate at a density of 1.20 g/cm³. A similar value was obtained by Pettersson et al. (1971) for Uukuniemi virus using cesium chloride.

2.2.2.   Particle Weight

The particle weight of La Crosse virus has been determined by McLerran and Arlinghaus (1973), using the formula: particle weight = $N[(4/3)\pi a^3]p$ (Luria and Darnell, 1967), where N is Avogadro's number (6.02×10^{23}), a is the radius of the particle in cm (taken to be 49×10^{-7} cm), π is 3.1416, and p is the buoyant density of the virus (taken to be 1.18 g/cm³). The value McLerran and Arlinghaus obtained for the weight of a La Crosse virus particle was 350×10^6. Similar values have been obtained for Crimean hemorrhagic fever virus (Donets *et al.*, 1977*a,b*) and Inkoo virus (Brummer-Korvenkontio, 1969).

2.2.3. Chemical Composition

The overall chemical composition of Uukuniemi virus has been given as 2% RNA, 58% protein, 33% lipid, and 7% carbohydrate (R. F. Pettersson and O. Renkonen, cited in Obijeski and Murphy, 1977). The chemical composition of other bunyaviruses has not been determined, although RNA-to-protein mass ratios of 1:30 have been reported for La Crosse virus (Obijeski *et al.*, 1976*a*).

2.2.4. Lipid Analyses

The presence of a lipid envelope as an integral part of bunyavirus particles has been deduced from solvent and detergent sensitivity studies performed with most of the known bunyavirus isolates (Berge *et al.*, 1970, 1971; Berge, 1975, Karabatsos, 1978). Treatment of purified virus, or infectious extracts of either animal or arthropod origin, with chloroform, ether, acetone, or sodium deoxycholate has been shown to reduce substantially the infectivity of all bunyaviruses tested.

No data are available on the neutral lipids, sterols, and glycolipids of bunyaviruses. A phospholipid analysis of Uukuniemi virus has been reported by Renkonen *et al.* (1972). Comparisons they made of the BHK-21 total cellular phospholipids with those extracted from purified Uukuniemi virus or the togavirus Semliki Forest virus (both grown in BHK-21 cells) indicated that the phospholipid compositions of the two viruses were strikingly similar, although they both differed in several respects to the total cellular phospholipid composition (Table 17). While Semliki Forest virus buds from the plasma membrane, Uukuniemi virus matures from the smooth endoplasmic reticulum (see Section 2.1).

2.2.5. Carbohydrate Analyses

No carbohydrate analyses of bunyaviruses have been reported.

2.2.6. RNA Genome

The presence of RNA as the genetic information of bunyaviruses has been demonstrated by a variety of procedures including extraction

TABLE 17

Percentage [³²P]Phospholipid Distribution in Uukuniemi Virus, Semliki Forest Virus, and BHK-21 Cells[a]

	Uukuniemi virus	Semiliki Forest virus	BHK-21 cells
Lysobisphosphatidic acid	1.15 ± 0.65	0.41 ± 0.20	1.2
Cardiolipin	0.34 ± 0.33	0.22 ± 0.10	3.3
Phosphatidic acid	1.22 ± 0.48	1.29 ± 0.70	0.6
Phosphatidylethanolamine (plus plasmalogen)	23.4 ± 2.9	23.2 ± 2.3	22.8
Phosphatidylcholine	41.9 ± 5.8	42.4 ± 3.8	49.8
Phosphatidylserine	11.6 ± 1.3	13.4 ± 2.0	6.6
Phosphatidylinositol	3.30 ± 1.24	1.60 ± 0.48	5.7
Sphingomyelin	15.1 ± 3.0	16.0 ± 2.1	6.9
Lysophosphatidylcholine	1.11 ± 0.42	0.47 ± 0.22	0.7

[a] The percentages of phospholipids were determined by Renkonen *et al.* (1972).

of RNA from purified virus preparations and lack of inhibition of virus growth by deoxyribonucleoside analogues (e.g., 5-bromo-2-deoxy-uridine, Whitney *et al.*, 1966) or actinomycin D (Goldman *et al.*, 1977) (see Fig. 15).

Although in early studies up to six virion RNA species were identified for certain bunyaviruses, recent analyses suggest that bunyaviruses only have three viral RNA species (Fig. 5), designated large (L), medium (M), and small (S). Three RNA species have been identified for Lumbo virus (Bouloy *et al.*, 1973/1974), La Crosse virus

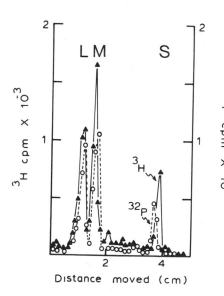

Fig. 5. The three viral RNA species of snowshoe hare and Main Drain viruses. A preparation of [³H]uridine-labeled Main Drain (▲) viral RNA was mixed with ³²P-labeled snowshoe hare (O) viral RNA and resolved by polyacrylamide gel electrophoresis. Three RNA size classes (L, large; M, medium; S, small) were resolved for each sample. From Gentsch *et al.* (1977*a*).

(Obijeski *et al.*, 1976*b*; Clewley *et al.*, 1977), snowshoe hare virus (Gentsch and Bishop, 1976), Uukuniemi virus (Hewlett *et al.*, 1977; Pettersson and Kaariainen, 1973; Pettersson *et al.*, 1977), snowshoe hare, Main Drain, La Crosse and Bunyamwera viruses (Fig. 5) (Gentsch *et al.*, 1977*a*), Guaroa, Lumbo and Tahyna viruses (El Said *et al.*, 1979), Sicilian sandfly fever, Chagres, Punta Toro, and Karimabad viruses (L. El Said, G. Robeson, and D. H. L. Bishop, unpublished observations), and Bunyamwera and Belmont viruses (D. A. McPhee and E. G. Westaway, personal communication).

2.2.6a. Base Ratios and RNA Density

Base-ratio analyses of the L, M, and S RNA species of La Crosse, snowshoe hare, and Uukuniemi viruses have been reported (Table 18). The results obtained indicate that the viral RNA species are single stranded, and this has been confirmed by single-strand specific ribonuclease digestion of the viral RNA species (McLerran and Arlinghaus, 1973).

TABLE 18

Base Ratios of Snowshoe Hare, La Crosse, and Uukuniemi Viral RNA Species[a]

	Base ratio		
RNA species	S	M	L
Snowshoe hare			
CMP	24.1	20.7	19.4
AMP	25.6	27.1	27.3
GMP	19.2	18.0	16.3
UMP	31.1	34.2	36.9
La Crosse			
CMP	22.6	20.3	19.4
AMP	26.6	27.1	27.7
GMP	18.4	17.7	16.1
UMP	32.7	34.9	36.8
Uukuniemi			
CMP	25.0	24.2	24.8
AMP	25.0	25.2	25.0
GMP	24.3	24.0	22.6
UMP	25.7	26.6	28.0

[a] The base ratios of snowshoe hare and La Crosse virus RNA species were determined by Clewley *et al.* (1977), while the base ratios of Uukuniemi viral RNA species were determined by Pettersson and Kaariainen (1973).

A density of 1.66 g/cm³ for La Crosse viral RNA in Cs₂SO₄ has been reported (Dahlberg *et al.*, 1977).

2.2.6b. Analyses of the RNA Termini

The 5'-terminal nucleotide of the viral RNA species of snowshoe hare (Gentsch *et al.*, 1977a), La Crosse (Obijeski *et al.*, 1976b), and Uukuniemi (Pettersson *et al.*, 1977) viruses has been shown to be pppAp. It is neither capped nor methylated. The 3'-terminal nucleotide(s) can be oxidized and reduced by ³H-labeled sodium borohydride (Obijeski *et al.*, 1976b). The identity of the 3'-terminal nucleotide(s) has not been determined. No 3'-polyadenosine tract has been found on the viral RNA species of either Lumbo virus (Bouloy *et al.*, 1973/1974), Uukuniemi virus (Pettersson *et al.*, 1977), snowshoe hare virus, or La Crosse virus (Clewley *et al.*, 1977). End nucleotide to total nucleotide recovery analyses for La Crosse virus (Obijeski *et al.*, 1976b), snowshoe hare virus (Gentsch *et al.*, 1977a), and Uukuniemi virus (Pettersson *et al.*, 1977) have given molecular weight estimates of the viral RNA species similar to those obtained by other methods (Section 2.2.6i).

2.2.6c. Infectivity Analyses

Infectivity associated with RNA extracts of La Crosse virus (McLerran and Arlinghaus, 1973), La Crosse and Restan viruses (Yukhananova *et al.*, 1974), and Catu and Bimiti viruses (Lomonosov and Fadeeva, 1974) has been reported. For the Catu and Bimiti viral extracts, the material was reported to be infectious on suckling mouse brain inoculation, sensitive to ribonuclease digestion, and insensitive to pretreatment with homologous immune ascitic fluids.

In contrast to these observations, no infectious RNA was recovered in extracts of Tahyna virus (Bouloy and Hannoun, 1973), Lumbo virus (Bouloy and Hannoun, 1976a), or La Crosse virus (Obijeski *et al.*, 1976b). In the studies reported by Obijeski *et al.* (1976b), under conditions in which RNA extracts of Sindbis virus gave 8.2×10^4 plaques in BHK-21 cell monolayers, no plaques were obtained with comparable quantities of La Crosse viral RNA. The Sindbis plaques did not develop if the Sindbis RNA-infected cells were treated with anti-Sindbis mouse ascitic fluids. Treatment of the Sindbis RNA extracts with ribonuclease (but not trypsin or deoxyribonuclease) totally reduced its infectivity.

It is currently held that the RNA of bunyaviruses is negative sense, and not infectious *per se*.

2.2.6d. Noncovalently Closed Circular RNA

Following the demonstration that the nucleocapsids of Lumbo (Samso *et al.*, 1975), Uukuniemi (Pettersson and von Bonsdorff, 1975), and La Crosse (Obijeski *et al.*, 1976*b*) viruses are circular (see Section 2.2.8), extracts of bunyavirus nucleic acids have also been shown to contain circular and linear nucleic acid species. This was first demonstrated for Lumbo virus, where in different preparations some 5–50% of the molecules were shown to be circular (Samso, *et al.*, 1976). The observations were confirmed by subsequent analyses of Uukuniemi virus extracts (Fig. 6) (Hewlett *et al.*, 1977).

Dahlberg *et al.* (1977) reported that La Crosse virus extracts contained considerable amounts of double-stranded nucleic acids, mostly DNA. They therefore separated the DNA from the viral RNA (or nucleocapsids) prior to electron microscopic analysis. For RNA samples in 4 M urea and 80% formamide, heated to 53°C for 30 sec, they observed by electron microscopy that their preparations contained mostly linear RNA species, with lengths compatible with the viral RNA sizes estimated by other procedures (see Section 2.2.6i).

The circular and linear structures found in Lumbo extracts by Samso *et al.* (1976), and Uukuniemi extracts by Hewlett *et al.* (1977), were shown to be destroyed by pancreatic ribonuclease treatment but were unaffected by deoxyribonuclease or proteinase K treatment. For the Lumbo viral extracts the circular structures resisted aqueous heat denaturation at 100°C, or denaturation at 55°C in 4 M urea–80% formamide (Samso *et al.*, 1976). For the Uukuniemi virus extracts (Hewlett *et al.*, 1977), the structures were shown to be denatured incompletely by moderate denaturing conditions (50% or 60% formamide). Complete denaturation of the Uukuniemi RNA species was obtained by exposure of the RNA to 99% formamide and 60°C for 15 min. Other denaturing conditions were also shown to lead to loss of the circular Uukuniemi RNA species. Renaturation of denatured Uukuniemi virus RNA preparations was reported to result in the reformation of a substantial percentage of the circular RNA species.

Panhandles of various lengths were seen on some but not all of the circular and linear structures in the Uukuniemi viral RNA extracts (Fig. 6). Their significance is not known.

Taken together with the termini analyses discussed above, the results suggest that the RNA species of bunyaviruses can be isolated as

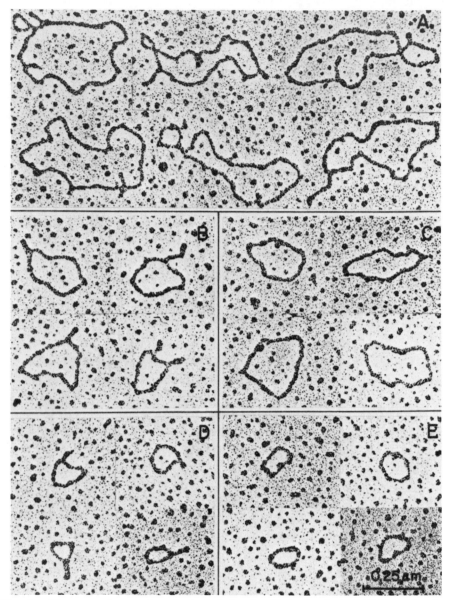

Fig. 6.   Electron micrographs of selected circular Uukuniemi virus RNA molecules. The RNA was spread from 70% formamide onto a 40% hypophase. Shown are the L (A), M (B), and S (D) RNA molecules with distinct panhandles. Many of the M and S molecules were seen without any apparent panhandles (C and E). From Hewlett *et al.* (1977).

noncovalently closed circles. Presumably the circularization involves inverted complementary, "sticky" 5'- and 3'-end sequences. The lengths of the hydrogen-bonded sequences are not known. It is possible that the panhandles seen on certain molecules (Fig. 6) may represent the hydrogen-bonded ends. To what extent, if any, the 5' ends (or 3' ends) of the L, M, and S RNA species are homologous is not known.

2.2.6e. Length Measurements of Bunyavirus RNA Species

Electron microscopic analyses of the circular *or* linear viral RNA species of Uukuniemi virus (Hewlett *et al.*, 1977) indicate that they have similar lengths. Average lengths of the three RNA species were estimated to be (L) 1.59 μm, (M) 0.74 μm, and (S) 0.34 μm. Length measurements from glyoxal-treated samples gave slightly higher values: (L) 1.65 μm, (M) 0.80 μm, and (S) 0.40 μm.

Length estimates of the linear La Crosse RNA species measured by Dahlberg *et al.* (1977) were (L) 3.3 μm, (M) 2.0 μm, and (S) 0.4 μm, while the estimates obtained for Lumbo viral RNA species were (L) 1.40 μm, (M) 0.93 μm, and (S) 0.25 μm (Samso *et al.*, 1976).

The reason for the discrepancies between the results obtained for the different viral RNA samples is not known. By polyacryamide gel electrophoresis the L, M, and S RNA species of Lumbo virus are similar in size to their respective La Crosse counterparts (D. H. L. Bishop, unpublished observations).

2.2.6f. Sedimentation Coefficients of the Viral RNA Species

Sedimentation coefficients have been reported for the three viral RNA species identified for Bunyamwera virus (Kascsak and Lyons, 1977), La Crosse virus (Obijeski *et al.*, 1976*b*), Lumbo virus (Bouloy *et al.*, 1973/1974), and Uukuniemi virus (Pettersson and Kaariainen, 1973). The $s_{20,w}$ values reported by the different investigators for the L (27–32 S), M (22–25 S), and S (12–19 S) RNA species indicate a degree of similarity for the different viruses. Previous reports of two viral RNA species for Uukuniemi virus (27 S and 21 S, Pettersson, *et al.*, 1971) or six RNA species for La Crosse virus (50–60 S, 35 S, 27 S, 20 S, 16 S, and 4 S, McLerran and Arlinghaus, 1973) probably preprent under- and overestimates (respectively) of the number of viral RNA species.

The $s_{20,w}$ values of the three viral RNA species of snowshoe hare, Tahyna, Trivittatus, Guaroa, Main Drain, Sicilian sandfly fever,

Chagres, Punta Toro, and Karimibad viruses are similar to those reported for La Crosse, Lumbo, and Uukuniemi viruses (L. El Said, J. Gentsch, R. Klimas, and D. H. L. Bishop, unpublished observations).

Molecular weight estimates of the Uukuniemi viral RNA species resolved by centrifugation in sucrose gradients containing formaldehyde have given values of (L) 1.9 × 10⁶, (M) 0.9 × 10⁶, and (S) 0.5 × 10⁶ (Pettersson and Kaariainen, 1973).

2.2.6g. Electrophoretic Analyses of the Viral RNA Species

Resolution of bunyavirus RNA species of polyacrylamide gel electrophoresis has identified three RNA species for Lumbo virus (Bouloy *et al.*, 1973/1974), La Crosse virus (Obijeski *et al.*, 1976*b*), snowshoe hare virus (Gentsch and Bishop, 1976), Bunyamwera, Main Drain, snowshoe hare, and La Crosse viruses (Fig. 5) (Gentsch *et al.*, 1977*a*), Trivittatus, Melao, La Crosse, and Lumbo viruses (Clewley *et al.*, 1977). Karimabad and Punta Toro viruses (Fig. 7) (G. Robeson and D. H. L. Bishop, unpublished data), Rift Valley fever virus (G. Eddy and D. Peters, personal communication), and Bunyamwera and Belmont viruses (D. A. McPhee and E. G. Westaway, personal communication). Four RNA species identified in extracts of Uukuniemi virus (Pettersson

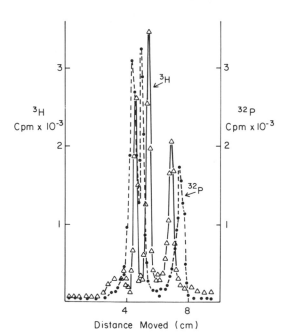

Fig. 7. The viral RNA species of Punta Toro and snowshoe hare viruses. Samples of [³H]uridine-labeled Punta Toro (△) and ³²P-labeled snowshoe hare (●) viruses were resolved by electrophoresis in 2.2% polyacrylamide gels. For each virus three RNA species were resolved.

and Kaariainen, 1973) were not confirmed by later analyses which indicated that Uukuniemi virus has three RNA species (Pettersson *et al.*, 1977). The six RNA species reported by McLerran and Arlinghaus (1973) for La Crosse virus have also not been confirmed by later analyses (Obijeski *et al.*, 1976*b*).

In order to estimate the sizes of La Crosse viral RNA species, labeled RNA preparations have been coelectrophoresed with known marker RNA species (Obijeski *et al.*, 1976*b*), the marker RNA species including VSV Indiana RNA (3.82×10^6, Repik and Bishop, 1973), BHK-21 28 S and 18 S ribosomal RNA species (1.75×10^6 and 0.75×10^6, respectively, Loening, 1968), poliovirus RNA (2.6×10^6, Granboulan and Girard, 1969; Tannock *et al.*, 1970), and tobacco mosaic virus RNA (2×10^6, Szybalski, 1968; Tannock *et al.*, 1970). From their results, Obijeski *et al.* (1976*b*) estimated the molecular weights of the L, M, and S RNA species of La Crosse virus to be 2.9×10^6, 1.8×10^6, and 0.4×10^6, respectively, in essential agreement with the electron microscopic length estimates obtained later by Dahlberg *et al.* (1977).

The molecular weight values for the three viral RNA species of various bunyaviruses, as estimated by gel electrophoresis, are given in Table 19. Variations in the values reported for Uukuniemi viral RNA species may well reflect the systems employed (as indicated in the table footnotes). It is conceivable that the split S peak described by Pettersson and Kaariainen (1973) could represent resolution of circular vs. linear S RNA forms. The 0.8×10^6 dalton RNA obtained by Kascsak and Lyons (1977) may be 18 S ribosomal RNA, since not only is a small peak frequently found in that position in analyses we have undertaken (see Gentsch *et al.*, 1977*a*) but also oligonucleotide fingerprint analyses of M and S RNA preparations sometimes detect unique 18 S BHK-21 ribosomal RNA oligonucleotides contaminating the viral RNA extracts (J. Clewley and D. H. L. Bishop, unpublished observations).

Coelectrophoresis of combinations of ^{3}H-labeled RNA species of La Crosse, or Main Drain (Fig. 5), or Bunyamwera viruses with ^{32}P-labeled snowshoe hare viral RNA species have detected minor but reproducible differences between their respective L, M, and or S RNA species, particularly for the S RNA species (Gentsch *et al.*, 1977*a*). Suggestive evidence that the S RNA may code for the viral N protein was obtained in these studies since a correspondence was observed between the viral S RNA and N protein sizes of the respective viruses. This has been confirmed by analyses of reassortant snowshoe hare–La Crosse viruses (Gentsch *et al.*, 1977*b*; Gentsch and Bishop, 1978).

TABLE 19

Molecular Weights of Bunyavirus RNA Species Estimated by Gel Electrophoresis

Molecular weights ($\times 10^{-6}$)				
L	M	S	Virus	Reference
3.0	1.9	0.34	Bunyamwera[d]	Gentsch et al. (1977)
3.8	2.4	(0.8)0.5	Bunyamwera[a]	Kascsak and Lyons (1977)
2.9	1.8	0.3	Bunyamwera[d]	D. A. McPhee and E. G. Westaway (personal communication)
3.1	2.0	0.4	Main Drain,[d]	Gentsch, et al. (1977)
(6.7)4.1	2.2	0.4	CE BFS-283[a]	Goldman et al. (1977)
2.9	1.8	0.4	La Crosse[a]	Obijeski et al. (1976)
2.9	2.0	0.5	Lumbo[d]	Bouloy et al. (1973/1974)
3.0	1.9	0.45	Snowshoe hare[d]	Gentsch et al. (1977)
2.9	1.9	0.45	Snowshoe hare[d]	Gentsch and Bishop (1976)
2.6	2.2	0.8	Karimabad[d]	G. Robeson and D. H. L. Bishop (unpublished data)
2.8	1.8	0.75	Punta Toro[d]	G. Robeson and D. H. L. Bishop (unpublished data)
4.1	1.0	(0.88)0.78	Uukuniemi[a]	Pettersson and Kaariainen (1973)
2.9	1.3	0.6	Uukuniemi[b]	Pettersson et al. (1977)
2.6	1.2	0.5	Uukuniemi[c]	Pettersson et al. (1977)
3.2	2.4	0.3	Belmont[a]	D. A. McPhee and E. G. Westaway (personal communication)

[a] Polyacrylamide agarose gel electrophoresis.
[b] Formamide gel electrophoresis (Ranki and Pettersson, cited in Pettersson et al., 1977).
[c] 2% polyacrylamide gel (Ranki and Pettersson, cited in Pettersson et al., 1977).
[d] All other electrophoretic systems employed polyacrylamide gels.

Coelectrophoresis of Punta Toro (Phlebotomus fever group) and snowshoe hare viral RNA species indicates that the RNA species of Punta Toro virus are easily distinguished from those of snowshoe hare virus (Fig. 7).

2.2.6h. Oligonucleotide Fingerprint Analyses of Bunyavirus RNA Species

Oligonucleotides derived from the viral L, M, and S RNA species by ribonuclease T1 digestion, resolved by two-dimensional gel electrophoresis according to the procedures described by de Watcher and Fiers (1972), have given characteristic fingerprints for the viral RNA species of snowshoe hare and La Crosse viruses (Fig. 8) (Clewley et al.,

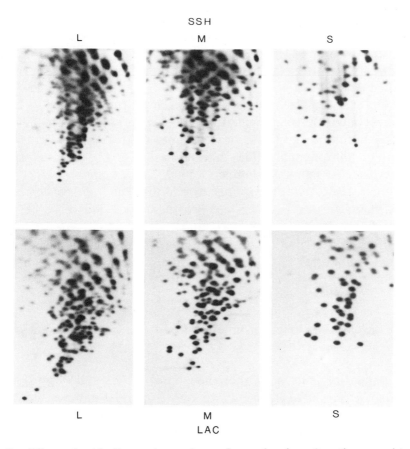

Fig. 8. Oligonucleotide fingerprint analyses of snowshoe hare (top three panels) and La Crosse (bottom three panels) L, M, and S viral RNA species. The fingerprints were obtained as described by Clewly *et al.* (1977).

1977), La Crosse–snowshoe hare reassortant (recombinant) viruses (see later, Gentsch *et al.*, 1977*b*), Uukuniemi virus (Pettersson *et al.*, 1977), and Lumbo, Tahyna, Trivittatus, Guaroa, Karimibad, and Punta Toro viruses (El Said *et al.*, 1979; L. El Said and D. H. L. Bishop, unpublished observations). In all cases the RNA oligonucleotide fingerprints have been shown to be characteristic for a particular virus serotype. Comparison of the L, M, and S RNA fingerprints of a virus indicates that each RNA has a unique nucleotide sequence, suggesting that each codes for separate genetic information.

In a study of La Crosse virus isolates obtained from Wisconsin (courtesy of Dr. W. Thompson and Dr. R. Anslow), Minnesota (courtesy of Dr. W. Thompson), Ohio (courtesy of Dr. C. Calisher), and New York State (courtesy of Dr. M. Grayson), La Crosse virus variants, which differ by a few nucleotide sequences for their respective L, M, and/or S RNA species, and La Crosse virus varieties, which differ by many oligonucleotides for each of their RNA species, have been identified (El Said *et al.*, 1979). The results obtained for some 11 different La Crosse isolates recovered from different regions of the northern United States indicate that in different ecological niches there are distinguishable La Crosse virus variants and varieties present. Comparisons of the oligonuleotide fingerprints of La Crosse virus isolates obtained from human, sentinel rabbit, *Aedes triseriatus*, *Aedes canadensis*, and *Aedes trivittatus* mosquitoes, as well as *Hybomitra lasiophthalmus* horseflies have not provided any evidence for insect or host tropisms. La Crosse virus isolates from various *Aedes triseriatus* mosquitoes were found to be as different from one another as those obtained from other mosquitoes or from human, sentinel rabbit, or other insect sources (El Said *et al.*, 1979).

2.2.6i. Molecular Weight Estimates of Bunyavirus L, M, and S RNA Species

Complexity studies of snowshoe hare L, M, and S viral RNA species (Clewley *et al.*, 1977), involving combined pancreatic ribonuclease and ribonuclease T1 digestion of the individual ^{32}P-labeled viral RNA species, followed by resolution of the resulting oligonucleotides by DEAE column chromotography and computation of the molar recoveries of the hexa- and heptanucleotides, have given molecular weight estimates for the L, M, and S RNA species of $2.8 \pm 0.1 \times 10^6$, $1.6 \pm 0.03 \times 10^6$, and $0.41 \pm 0.02 \times 10^6$, respectively.

Genome complexity studies by Pettersson *et al.* (1977) or Uukuniemi viral RNA species, using pancreatic ribonuclease compositional analyses of the recovered ribonuclease T1 derived viral oligonucleotides, have given molecular weight estimates for the various Uukuniemi viral RNA species of (L) 2.7×10^6, (M) 1.2×10^6, and (S) 0.7×10^6.

For La Crosse and/or snowshoe hare viruses, the molecular weight estimates obtained by electron microscopic analyses, gel electrophoresis, end-to-total nucleotide ratios, and nuclease digestion are in reasonable agreement with each other. The comparable results obtained for Uukuniemi virus, as pointed out by Pettersson *et al.* (1977), are more variable. With the reservation of how the various Uukuniemi viral RNA estimates should be weighted, mean values for Uukuniemi L, M, and S RNA species have been reported to be $2.4 \pm 0.4 \times 10^6$, $1.1 \pm 0.2 \times 10^6$ and $0.5 \pm 0.1 \times 10^6$, respectively.

In conclusion, the sum genetic information of those bunyaviruses that have been analyzed so far is in the region of $4-6 \times 10^6$ daltons of RNA, with three viral RNA species having been identified for viruses belonging to the Bunyavirus genus, as well as certain bunyaviruslike viruses.

2.2.6j. Number of RNA Species per Virus Particle

The molar ratios obtained for the three RNA species of various bunyaviruses, or even different preparations of any one bunyavirus, are highly variable. In some circumstances RNA molar ratios of 1 L, to 1 M, to 1 S RNA species have been observed both by *in vitro* 3'-end labeling of viral RNA preparations and by the incorporation of [^{3}H]nucleoside or [^{32}P]phosphate precursors into RNA (Obijeski *et al.*, 1976*b*). Other RNA ratios have been obtained not only for different bunyaviruses but also for the same virus, depending on the virus preparation (D. H. L. Bishop, unpublished observations). For Uuku-niemi virus, L to M to S RNA ratios 1:4.6:2 have been reported in some virus preparations (Pettersson and Kaariainen, 1973).

It is not known if the number of RNA species per virus particle varies according to host- or viral-determined factors. Although the presence of defective virus particles has not been investigated in any detail, it has been shown that high multiplicity of infection often causes reduced virus yields when compared to the results obtained with lower multiplicities (Obijeski *et al.*, 1976*a*; see Section 5). It is possible that replication of particular viral RNA species may lead to mispackaging of genetic information, if packaging is not a strictly regulated function. Whether this accounts for the variable molar ratios of virus RNA species that are obtained in bunyavirus extracts is not know. For Bunyamwera virus, the four RNA species observed by Kascsak and Lyons (1977) were present (in order of decreasing size) in a 1 (L), to 1 (M), to 1 (18 S), to 3 (S) RNA ratio. They reported, however, that the smallest RNA is found in even larger relative amounts in defective Bunyamwera virus preparations.

2.2.7. Proteins

Three major structural polypeptides, including two external glyco-proteins, G1 and G2, and an internal nucleocapsid protein, N, have

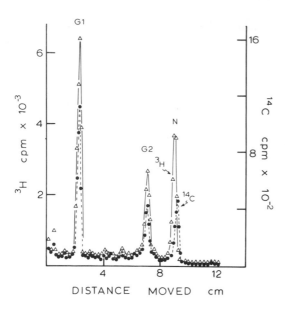

Fig. 9. The viral polypeptides of snowshoe hare and La Crosse viruses. [³H]Amino-acid-labeled La Crosse (LAC), and [¹⁴C] amino-acid-labeled snowshoe hare (SSH) viral polypeptides were resolved by 8% polyacrylamide gel electrophoresis. The viral G1, G2, and N polypeptides are indicated. From Gentsch *et al.* (1977*a*).

been identified for several bunyaviruses (Table 20). A large but minor protein L has also been observed in at least some bunyavirus preparations.

The three major polypeptides have similar size ranges for Bunyamwera, Main Drain, and Guaroa viruses of the Bunyamwera serogroup (Gentsch *et al.*, 1977*a*; Pennington *et al.*, 1977; Rosato *et al.*, 1974*a*; El Said *et al.*, 1979), as well as for California encephalitis, Jamestown Canyon, Keystone, La Crosse, Lumbo, Melao, South River, snowshoe hare, Tahyna, and Trivittatus viruses of the California encephalitis serogroup (Table 20 and Fig. 9) (Bouloy and Hannoun, 1976*b*; El Said *et al.*, 1979; Gentsch and Bishop, 1976; Gentsch *et al.*, 1977*a*; McLerran and Arlinghaus, 1973; Obijeski *et al.*, 1976*a,b*; Rosato *et al.*, 1974*a*). White (1975) identified four major viral polypeptides in California encephalitis virus preparations, three of which correspond in type and size to the proteins identified by others for that virus. The origin of the fourth polypeptide is not known. Studies of Oriboca and Murutucu viruses (Rosato *et al.*, 1974*b*) and Capim, Guama, Oriboca, Patois, and Tete viruses (D. W. Trent, cited in Obijeski and Murphy, 1977) indicate that these viruses also have three major polypeptides similar to those of viruses mentioned above.

The sizes of the G2 polypeptide of Bwamba, Koongol, and Simbu viruses (D. W. Trent, personal communication, cited in Obijeski and Murphy, 1977) are larger than those found for other supergroup viruses such as the California group virus La Crosse. The viral polypeptides of the Phlebotomus fever group viruses (e.g., Karimabad) are also quite different from those of California group viruses (Table 20 and Fig. 10).

Uukuniemi virus is reported to have three major and one minor structural polypeptides (Table 20), although the G1 and G2 proteins are significantly different in size from those of the supergroup or the Phlebotomus fever group viruses (von Bonsdorff and Pettersson, 1975; Pettersson *et al.*, 1971, 1977).

2.2.7a. Viral Glycoproteins G1 and G2

Two viral glycoproteins have been identified in every study of bunyaviruses so far published. Although early studies indicated that the glycoproteins of Bunyamwera, California encephalitis, La Crosse, Lumbo, Murutucu, Oriboca and Tahyna viruses included a G1 polypeptide of size $82–85 \times 10^3$ daltons, and a G2 polypeptide of size $30–45 \times 10^3$ daltons (Bouloy and Hannoun, 1976*b*; McLerran and

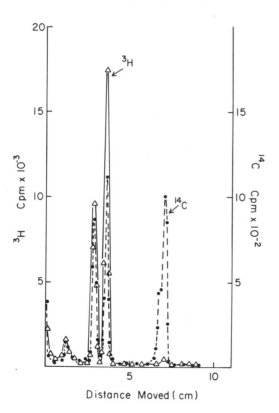

Fig. 10. The viral polypeptides of Karimabad (Phlebotomus fever group) virus. A preparation of [³H]glucosamine- and [¹⁴C]amino-acid-labeled Karimabad virus was resolved by 8% polyacrylamide gel electrophoresis. Two viral glycoproteins (mol. wt. 62 and 50×10^3) and a nonglycosylated polypeptide (mol. wt. 21×10^3) were identified.

TABLE 20

Molecular Weight Estimates of the Virion Polypeptides of Bunyaviruses

Viral polypeptides (mol. wt. ×10³)					Virus	Reference
L[a]	G1[b]	G2	N	Other		
200	115	38	19		Bunyamwera	Gentsch et al. (1977a)
	128	31	23		Bunyamwera	Pennington et al. (1977)
	104	32	22		Bunyamwera	D. A. McPhee and E. G. Westaway (personal communication)
145	85–83	33–30	23–20		Bunyamwera	Rosato et al. (1974a)
	115	38	21		Main Drain	Gentsch et al. (1977a)
	115	32	21		Guaroa	El Said et al. (1979)
	85–83	33–30	23–20		Murutucu	Rosato et al. (1974a)
	85–83	33–30	23–20		Oriboca	Rosato et al. (1974b)
	125	30	22		Oriboca	D. W. Trent (personal communication)
	115	39	21		California encephalitis	El Said et al. (1979)
	82	38	18	30	California encephalitis	White (1975)
	85–83	33–30	23–20		California encephalitis	Rosato et al. (1974a)
	115	38	21		Tahyna	El Said et al. (1979)
	85–83	33–30	23–20		Tahyna	Rosato et al. 1974a
	115	38	22		Lumbo	El Said et al. (1979)
	85	35	25		Lumbo	Bouloy and Hannoun (1976b)

L	G1	G2	N	Virus	Reference
180	120	35	25	La Crosse	Obijeski et al. (1976a)
	110	38	24	La Crosse	Gentsch et al. (1977a)
	85	45	26	La Crosse	McLerran and Arlinghaus (1973)
	115	38	21	Snowshoe hare	Gentsch and Bishop (1976), Gentsch, et al. (1977a)
	117	38	24	Melao	El Said et al. (1979)
	120	38	22	South River	El Said et al. (1979)
	118	38	21	Jamestown Canyon	El Said et al. (1979)
	118	38	23	Trivittalus	El Said et al. (1979)
	118	38	23	Keystone	El Said et al. (1979)
	125	30	22	Capim	D. W. Trent (personal communication)
	125	30	22	Guama	D. W. Trent (personal communication)
	125	30	22	Patois	D. W. Trent (personal communication)
	125	30	22	Tete	D. W. Trent (personal communication)
	62	50	21	Karimabad	G. Robeson and D. H. L. Bishop (unpublished data)
170	75	65	25	Uukuniemi	von Bonsdorff and Pettersson (1975), Pettersson et al. (1971, 1977)
145	104	32[c]	22	Belmont	D. A. McPhee and E. G. Westaway (personal communication)

[a] Inability to detect the L species probably reflects the difficulty of obtaining enough purified virus to unambiguously demonstrate presence of the polypeptide.

[b] Recent studies of the Bunyamwera, group C, and California encephalitis serogroup viruses have not confirmed the lower G1 polypeptide size estimates obtained in earlier studies. Recent studies have, however, confirmed the size estimates of the phlebotomus fever group (Karimabad) and Uukuniemi viral G polypetides.

[c] Not glycosylated.

Arlinghaus, 1973; Rosato *et al.*, 1974*a,b*; White, 1975), subsequent analyses of these viruses, as well as all the Bunyamwera, California encephalitis, group C, Capim, Guama, Patois, and Tete group viruses that have been analyzed, suggest that the G1 polypeptide has a molecular weight between 110 and 130 $\times$ 10³ (El Said *et al.*, 1979; Gentsch and Bishop, 1976; Gentsch *et al.*, 1977*a*; Obijeski *et al.*, 1976*a*; Obijeski and Murphy, 1977). Minor but reproducible differences have been observed between the G1 and/or G2 polypeptides of different California encephalitis (see Fig. 9) and Bunyamwera serogroup viruses (El Said *et al.*, 1979).

There are no published reports on the number of carbohydrate side chains present on the G1 or G2 polypeptides. Glucosamine components in both polypeptides have been inferred from the specific incorporation of ³H-labeled glucosamine into both G1 and G2. Studies on the number of pronase-resistant glycopeptides recovered from La Crosse G1 and G2 polypeptides (after neuraminidase treatment) by V. Vorndam and D. W. Trent (personal communication) indicate that the G1 polypeptide has two oligosaccharide species, each with at least one sialic acid developmental stage, while G2 has only the smaller of these oligosaccharide species and two sialic acid developmental stages. These investigators have obtained evidence that for snowshoe hare virus grown in BHK-21 cells the G1 has four glycosylation sites (Trivittatus virus has only two), while the G2 polypeptide has one major and one minor glycosylation site.

No amino acid or peptide analyses of the two viral glycoproteins have been published. Studies undertaken in the laboratory of one of us (D. H. L. B.) indicate that the peptides of snowshoe hare and La Crosse G2 polypeptides are distinguishable from each other, and from their respective G1 polypeptides.

Uukuniemi virus appears to have two glycoproteins of similar sizes (G1: 75 $\times$ 10³; G2: 65 $\times$ 10³). It is not known whether the Uukuniemi G1 and G2 polypeptides are related to each other (e.g., G2 a cleavage derivation of G1, or G1 an alternate glycosylated form of G2).

The Phlebotomus fever group viruses, Punta Toro and Karimabad, both have two large glycoproteins (Karimabad G1: 62 $\times$ 10³, G2: 50 $\times$ 10³) that can be specifically labeled with [³H]glucosamine (Fig. 10). It is also not known if these two glycoproteins are unique or share common polypeptide sequences. Similar size classes of viral glycoproteins have been reported for Bwamba, Simbu, and Koongol viruses (D. W. Trent, cited in Obijeski and Murphy, 1977).

In contrast to these results with recognized members of the Bunyaviridae family, studies with Belmont virus, a proposed member of the family, indicate that it has a G1-type glycoprotein (107×10^3 daltons) and apparently a nonglycosylated 28×10^3 dalton protein (it does not incorporate [^{3}H]glucosamine) probably located on the external surface of virus particles (D. A. McPhee and E. G. Westaway, personal communication).

The external location of the viral glycoproteins has been inferred from studies involving their specific removal by protease digestion. Such studies have been undertaken for La Crosse, Karimabad, and Uukuniemi viruses. In the analyses reported by Obijeski *et al.* (1976a), La Crosse [^{14}C]amino-acid- and [^{3}H]glucosamine-labeled virus preparations were incubated with bromelain, and the treated material was repurified by sucrose gradient centrifugation. The protease treatment reduced the specific infectivity to about 10^{-5} that of untreated control virus preparations. The bromelain-treated preparations, when examined by electron microscopy, were shown to contain only spikeless particles with intact envelopes. Both the viral N and L proteins remained associated with the spikeless particles. No viral glycoproteins were present. It was shown that in combination glycerol–potassium tartrate gradients, the density of the spikeless particles was 1.16 g/cm³ whereas untreated virus had a density of 1.20 g/cm³.

As an alternate method to demonstrate that the glycoproteins are the only external virion proteins, a preparation of unlabeled La Crosse virus was iodinated with [^{125}I]iodine, lactoperoxidase, and hydrogen peroxide (Obijeski *et al.*, 1976a). After repurification, it was found that only the G1 and G2 polypeptides were iodinated. Iodination of Triton-X-100-disrupted La Crosse virus was shown to label all four structural polypeptides, L, G1, G2, and N.

Earlier analyses of Uukuniemi virus by von Bonsdorff and Pettersson (1975), using the proteolytic enzyme thermolysin showed that enzyme treatment caused the particles to band in sucrose at a density of 1.14 g/cm³, compared to 1.17 g/cm³ for untreated virus. The treated particles were observed to have an RNA to protein label ratio of 1:2.63, as opposed to a ratio of 1:1.73 for untreated virus. Thermolysin treatment of Uukuniemi virus completely removed the G1 and G2 polypeptides and gave a small peptide fragment which migrated in a 15% polyacrylamide gel ahead of the viral N protein. From these results it was concluded that the two viral glycoproteins were external to the viral envelope and that the enyme-resistant fragment might represent a glycoprotein peptide anchor in the lipid bilayer. Electron microscopic studies by von Bonsdorff and Pettersson (1975) also provided evidence that thermolysin treatment removed the visible surface spikes from Uukuniemi virus and produced deformed particles which, unlike the untreated virus, tended to form aggregates. From these observations it was suggested that the viral glycoproteins are largely responsible for the structural stability of the virus particle.

Treatment of Karimabad virus preparations with chymotrypsin has been shown to remove the two viral glycoproteins, leaving spikeless virus particles (G. Robeson and D. H. L. Bishop, unpublished observations).

Whether the viral glycoprotein(s) span the lipid bilayer and make contact with the internal viral nucleocapsid, as suggested for the alphavirus Semliki Forest virus (Garoff and Simons, 1974), is not known.

In summary, two glycoproteins have been identified for all bunyaviruses so far analyzed. The two glycoproteins are either large and small in size (120×10^3 and 38×10^3 daltons), intermediate in size (50–70×10^3 daltons), or possibly large and intermediate in size (120×10^3 and 70×10^3 daltons). The last possibility needs confirmation. The significance of such class ranges at the generic level is not known. The glycoproteins of bunyaviruses form the surface spikes of the virus particles, although part of their polypeptide chain(s) may penetrate and/or span the envelope, possibly making contact with the viral nucleocapsids. The glycoproteins probably are involved in the adsorption process of virus to susceptible cells.

The interrelationship of the two bunyavirus glycoproteins to each other is not known. Which glycoprotein has group- and/or type-specific antigenic determinants is also not known.

2.2.7b. Phosphoproteins and Sulfated Proteins

No evidence for virion phosphoproteins or sulfated proteins was obtained in studies undertaken with La Crosse virus (Obijeski *et al.*, 1976*a*).

2.2.7c. Nucleocapsid Protein N

The major nucleocapsid protein (designated N) of all bunyaviruses so far analyzed has a reported molecular weight of between 19 and 26 $\times 10^3$ (Table 20). Analyses involving both protease digestion of labeled virus preparations and iodination of intact and detergent-dissociated virus samples have established that the N protein is an internal component. Belmont virus, a proposed member of the Bunyaviridae family, also has a 25×10^3 dalton nucleocapsid associated protein (D. A. McPhee and E. G. Westaway, personal communication).

Nonionic detergent treatment of purified preparations of bunya-viruses has shown that particulate nucleocapsids (RNA and protein) can be released from the viruses (Obijeski *et al.*, 1976a; Pettersson *et al.*, 1971; Rosato *et al.*, 1974b; White, 1975). The major protein associated with the nucleocapsids is the small viral polypeptide N, a minor component is the protein L.

Minor but reproducible differences in electrophoretic mobilities have been observed between the N proteins of different bunyaviruses (El Said *et al.*, 1979; Gentsch *et al.*, 1977a). The N protein size differences of Bunyamwera and California group viruses appear to correlate to S RNA size differences, suggesting that the S RNA may code for N protein. Since some $2.5–3.0 \times 10^5$ daltons of RNA would be required to code for N protein, that amount of information is well within the S RNA size ($4–7 \times 10^5$ daltons of RNA) (Table 21).

Tryptic peptide analyses of snowshoe hare and La Crosse viral N

TABLE 21
Structural Components and Genetic Relationships of LAC Virus[a]

Viral polypeptides	Molecular weight	Approximate number of molecules per virion
L	180×10^3	25
G1	120×10^3	650
G2	34×10^3	630
N	23×10^3	2100

Viral RNA species	Molecular weight	Genetic recombination group
L	2.9×10^6	II
M	1.8×10^6	I
S	0.4×10^6	III

Coding relationship	
RNA	Protein
L	?
M	G1, G2
S	N

[a] The information on the identification of the types of LAC virion polypeptides (G1, G2, glycoproteins; N, nucleocapsid protein; L, large protein), their sizes, and number per virion is taken from Obijeski *et al.* (1976a). The LAC RNA size classes are taken from Obijeski *et al.* (1976b). Slightly different values have been observed by others for both the protein and RNA size classes (see Gentsch *et al.*, 1977a; Obijeski and Murphy, 1977). The genetic recombination group segment, RNA segment–protein coding relationships are from Gentsch *et al.* (1977b), Gentsch and Bishop (1978, 1979), and unpublished data.

proteins indicate that these two viruses have N peptide sequences that can easily be distinguished (Fig. 11) (Gentsch and Bishop, 1978).

2.2.7d.   Large Protein L

Minor amounts of a large protein ($170–200 \times 10^3$ daltons) have been observed in preparations of La Crosse virus (Obijeski *et al.*, 1976*a*), snowshoe hare, Bunyamwera, and Main Drain viruses (Gentsch *et al.*, 1977*a*), Bunyamwera virus (Pennington *et al.*, 1977), Bunyamwera and Belmont viruses (D. A. McPhee and E. G. Westaway, personal communication), and Uukuniemi virus (Pettersson *et al.*, 1977). Obijeski *et al.* (1976*a*) determined that the L protein was equivalent to 3–5% of the total virus protein mass and was an internal component associated with the viral nucleocapsids. The function of the viral L protein, its uniqueness, and its associations with other structural components still need to be determined. The possibility that, like the minor L protein of rhabdoviruses, the bunyavirus L protein is a transcriptase component also needs to be investigated.

2.2.7e.   Estimates of the Number of Protein Molecules per Virus Particle

The average numbers of L, G1, G2, and N protein molecules per La Crosse virus particle have been estimated from the viral RNA to protein mass ratio (1:30), the percentage of the total protein present in each protein species (3%, 51%, 14%, and 32%, respectively), the sum molecular weights of the three genome RNA species (5.1×10^6), and assuming that there is only one L, M, and S RNA species per virion (Obijeski *et al.*, 1976*a*). The estimates obtained for the number of molecules per virion (25 L, 650 G1, 629 G2, and 2126 N), while they may be compromised to some extent by the various assumptions, suggest that the two glycoproteins are in equivalent molar proportions. The significance of this observation, and whether it is true for other bunyaviruses, needs to be determined.

2.2.8.   RNA–Protein Coding Relationships

Although not all of the RNA–protein coding assignments are known, it has been shown that the viral S RNA codes for N protein

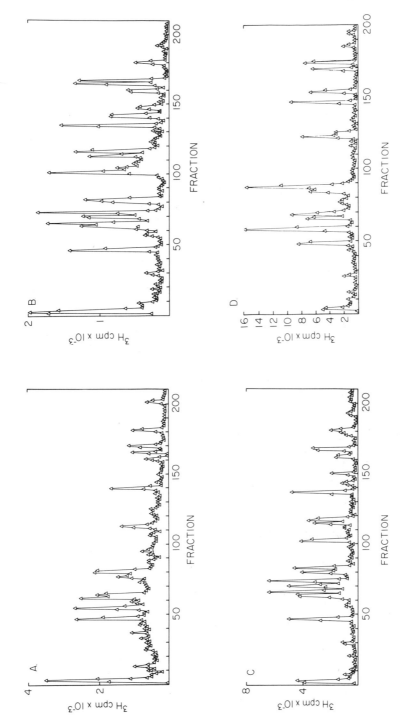

Fig. 11. Tryptic peptide analyses of the nucleocapsid N protein of (A) La Crosse, (LAC), (B) snowshoe hare (SSH), and the recombinant L/M/S (RNA) viruses (C) SSH/LAC/SSH and (D) SSH/LAC/LAC.

(Gentsch and Bishop, 1978). Evidence has been obtained that the M RNA codes for the viral glycoproteins, G1 and G2 and the hemagglutinin (presumed to be the glycoproteins; see later, Gentsch, *et al.*, 1977*b*; Gentsch and Bishop, 1979). The proposed RNA–protein assignments are shown in Table 21.

2.2.9. Viral Nucleocapsids

Nonionic detergent treatment and/or spontaneous lysis of Batai, California encephalitis, Inkoo, La Crosse, Lumbo, Oriboca, and Uukuniemi virus preparations has been shown by electron microscopy to liberate the viral nucleocapsids. They can be recovered by cesium chloride equilibrium gradient centrifugation at a density of 1.31 ± 0.2 g/ml (Obijeski *et al.*, 1976*b*; Pettersson et al., 1971; Rosato *et al.*, 1974*b*; Saikku *et al.*, 1971; Samso *et al.*, 1975; White, 1975). The major protein component of the viral nucleocapsids is the N protein; a minor component is the protein L.

Resolution of the nucleocapsids of La Crosse, Lumbo, and Uukuniemi viruses into three size classes by sucrose gradient centrifugation has been reported (115 S, 90 S, and 65 S for La Crosse virus—Obijeski *et al.*, 1976*b*; 145 S, 112 S, and 88 S for Uukuniemi virus—Pettersson and von Bonsdorff, 1975; and 105 S, 85 S, and 45 S for Lumbo virus—Samso *et al.*, 1975; Bouloy and Hannoun, 1976*b*). Extraction of each size class of nucleocapsid for RNA has yielded primarily L RNA from the largest species, M RNA from the medium-size species, and S RNA from the smallest species. RNA to protein label ratios appear to be the same for each size class of nucleocapsid.

Initial electron microscopic analyses of bunyavirus nucleocapsids reported by von Bonsdorff *et al.*, (1969) and Saikku *et al.*, (1971) with Uukuniemi, Batai, and Inkoo viruses described coiled strands 2–3 nm in diameter and up to 1 μm in length. Supercoiled strands 7–12 nm in diameter were also observed.

For Lumbo virus (Samso *et al.*, 1975), Uukuniemi virus (Pettersson and von Bonsdorff, 1975), and La Crosse virus (Obijeski *et al.*, 1976*b*), supercoiled and/or circular nucleocapsid forms have also been observed.

The modal length distributions of the circular, supercoiled nucleocapsids of La Crosse virus fall into three size classes (0.7 μm, 0.51 μm, and 0.20 μm in length, 10–12 nm wide). Their sizes do not exhibit a simple relationship to the size of their component RNA species (see Section 2.2.6; Obijeski *et al.*, 1976*b*). Some extended nucleocapsid strands have been seen in the La Crosse virus preparations having diameters of 2–3 nm and consisting of "strings of beads" whose total lengths were difficult to measure. The lack of a direct relationship of RNA to nucleocapsid lengths for La Crosse virus has been ascribed to the convoluted, supercoiled configuration of the nucleocapsids.

Whether the supercoiling is due to protein–protein, RNA–protein, or RNA–RNA interactions is not known, nor is it known if these configurations reflect packaging arrangements within the virus particle or artifacts of purification and preparation of the material for electron microscopy.

In contrast to the studies with La Crosse virus, analyses of detergent-treated Uukuniemi virus, resolved into its component nucleocapsids by sucrose gradient centrifugation, identified three distinct size classes of extended nucleocapsids with modal lengths of 2.8 μm, 1.4 μm, and 0.7 μm, and diameters of 2 nm (Pettersson and von Bornsdorff, 1975). The Uukuniemi nucleocapsid lengths were determined to be equivalent to their component L, M, and S RNA sizes (Pettersson *et al.*, 1977). Although no supercoiling was observed for these purified Uukuniemi nucleocapsids, earlier studies of preparations of Uukuniemi, Inkoo, and Batai viruses stored at 4°C (von Bonsdorff *et al.*, 1969) showed that spontaneously ruptured viral envelopes released an inner *coiled* component. For Uukuniemi virus this component apparently consisted of a loosely wound helix, 9 nm in overall width, and composed of one strand approximately 2 nm broad. From these studies it was suggested that the nucleocapsids of the three viruses have a single-stranded, helical symmetry. Helical nucleocapsids have also been reported for Hazara virus (Shestapalova *et al.*, 1975). Uukuniemi nucleocapsids purified from cesium chloride gradients appear by electron microscopy to consist of loosely coiled strands (Pettersson *et al.*, 1971).

Nucleocapsids purified from Inkoo virus, treated with Nonidet P-40, and recovered after cesium chloride centrifugation at a density of 1.31–1.32 g/ml were observed by Saikku *et al.* (1971) to consist of a 2-nm strand having a regular undulation, suggesting an unwound, stretched helix.

In summary, it appears that bunyaviruses have circular nucleocapsids in three distinct size classes. The nucleocapsids may be supercoiled or in a helical configuration (with a 9- to 12-nm span but consisting of a single 2-nm strand), which on release from the virus particles can unwind. While the convoluted or helical configuration may preclude accurate measurements, length measurements have been obtained on the extended nucleocapsids of some viruses, and these

lengths correlate reasonably well with the component RNA size estimates.

Each nucleocapsid contains N protein, L protein, and a single size
class of RNA. It has been estimated for La Crosse virus that there are
1209, 750, and 167 N protein molecules per L, M, and S nucleocapsid,
respectively (Obijeski *et al.*, 1976*b*). While these values indicate that for
each nucleocapsid there is a tenfold mass excess of protein over RNA,
ribonuclease digestion analyses of La Crosse virus nucleocapsids have
shown that the RNA within each nucleocapsid size class is accessible to
digestion by 100 μg pancreatic ribonuclease/ml (37°C, 30 min), in
contrast to the ribonuclease resistance of nucleocapsids of the
rhabdovirus vesicular stomatitis virus (Hefti and Bishop, 1975). For
Uukuniemi virus, it has been reported that 1 μg pancreatic ribonu-
clease/ml (37°C, 30 min) did not solubilize the viral RNA in the
nucleocapsids, while 15 μg pancreatic ribonuclease only made 15% of
the RNA acid soluble (Pettersson *et al.*, 1971).

The reason why the nucleocapsids of bunyaviruses are circular is
not known. Their circular forms can be correlated to the circular RNA
species (Section 2.2.6).

We do not know how the viral RNA species are replicated or how
the viral N protein is related to the RNA replication process. It will be
of interest to know whether the viral N protein addition occurs after
circularization of the viral RNA, or whether the RNA is circularized
only after addition of N protein.

Although in many analyses the internal organization of bunyavirus
particles cannot be easily defined, in thin sections of Uukuniemi-
infected chicken embryo fibroblasts an irregularly arranged electro-
opaque material, presumed to be the viral nucleocapsids, has been
visualized in a zone underneath the viral envelope (Fig. 4) (von Bonsdorff and Pettersson, 1975). How nucleocapsids interrelate with each
other and/or with the viral envelope (and/or glycoproteins) is not
known.

2.2.10.   Virion RNA Polymerase

An RNA-directed RNA polymerase activity has been demonstrated in preparations of Lumbo virus (Bouloy and Hannoun, 1976*a*;
Bouloy *et al.*, 1975) and Uukuniemi virus (Ranki and Pettersson, 1975).
The polymerase activities, assayed *in vitro*, have been shown to be
associated specifically with virus recovered at a bouyant density (in sucrose) of 1.17–1.18 g/cm³. The amount of RNA polymerized is directly

related to the amount of virus protein added to a reaction mixture (at least up to 750 μg/ml for Uukuniemi virus).

The enzymatic activity of both viruses is reported to require all four ribonucleoside triphosphates and to have a broad pH optimum in the range pH 7.0–8.5. For Lumbo virus, magnesium (8 mM) and manganese (2 mM) ions induce higher incorporation of labeled precursors into acid-insoluble products than any other concentration of either manganese or magnesium ions. For Uukuniemi virus, the polymerase activity requires manganese ions (4.5 mM); magnesium ions do not enhance or substitute for this requirement. Monovalent cations (sodium or potassium), or a reducing agent such as mercaptoethanol, although routinely included in reaction mixtures, is not apparently required. The reported temperature optimum for the Lumbo virus polymerase is 38°C, while that of the Uukuniemi virus polymerase is between 37°C and 40°C. Linear incorporation of radioactive ribonucleoside triphosphates into RNA has been obtained for 10–15 hr for Lumbo virus and 1–2 hr for Uukuniemi virus. Ribonuclease, but not deoxyribonuclease, actinomycin D, or rifampin, has been shown to inhibit the synthesis of product RNA by the Uukuniemi virus polymerase.

Analyses of the products of the Lumbo or Uukuniemi virus polymerase reactions have indicated that much of the product after phenol extraction is ribonuclease resistant and cosediments with the viral L, M, and S RNA species. Heat denaturation experiments result in the separation of the product RNA from the viral RNA templates. The separated product is reported to be small (less than 7 S for the Uukuniemi products and less than 18 S for Lumbo product RNA). Reannealing of the heat-denatured reaction products, or annealing to an excess of homologous viral RNA, has been shown to increase the ribonuclease resistance of the product RNA (70–100%). For Lumbo virus, 100% of the product RNA became ribonuclease resistant after annealing to an excess of added viral RNA.

These results indicate that Lumbo and Uukuniemi viruses have a virion RNA-directed RNA polymerase which catalyzes the synthesis of viral complementary RNA and probably is responsible for the *in vivo* synthesis of viral messenger RNA species (see Section 3.2).

2.3. Diagrammatic Represention of Bunyavirus Virions

A schematic representation of a bunyavirus particle is given in Fig. 12. The arrangements of the surface glycoproteins, G1 and G2, the viral nucleocapsids, and their relationships to each other, or to the viral

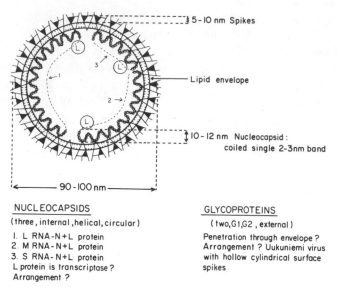

Fig. 12.   A hypothetical bunyavirus particle.

envelope, are hypothetical. The location and function of the L protein are also hypothetical.

3.   REPLICATION OF BUNYAVIRUSES

It is commonly held that the infection of negative-stranded RNA viruses involves the sequence of (1) adsorption, (2) penetration, (3) synthesis of viral complementary messenger RNA (mRNA) by the virion RNA polymerase (primary transcription), (4) translation of the viral mRNA species, (5) replication of the viral RNA when these translation products became available, (6) amplification of the mRNA transcription (secondary transcription), translation, and replication processes, using the new RNA templates generated by the RNA replication processes, and eventually (7) assembly of virus particles by budding.

To what extent bunyavirus replication fits these concepts is not known, because of the lack of information on the replication processes of these viruses. What is known is discussed below using the framework of the sequence of events described in the preceding paragraph.

3.1.   Adsorption and Penetration

No studies on the adsorption process of bunyaviruses have been undertaken. Other than the reduction of infectivity after removal of the external viral glycoproteins by protease (implicating them in the attachment process), it is not known how bunyaviruses initiate an infection or whether there are specific host receptors involved in the adsorption process. It is also not known if penetration involves phagocytosis of complete virus particles and/or viral and cell plasma membrane fusion and deposition of the internal contents of the virus into the cell cytoplasm. Whether one or both viral glycoproteins is primarily responsible for attachment to a susceptible host is not known. If only one glycoprotein species is involved, then it will be of interest to know the function of the other viral glycoprotein.

3.2. Primary Transcription: Early Viral Messenger RNA Synthesis

As discussed in Section 2.2.10, it has been shown by *in vitro* studies that at least some bunyavirus preparations have a virion RNA-dependent RNA polymerase capable of synthesizing viral complementary RNA. *In vivo* studies also support the involvement of a viral polymerase in the synthesis of viral complementary RNA. When snowshoe hare virus is used to infect confluent BHK-21 cell monolayers in the presence of puromycin or cycloheximide (to inhibit protein synthesis), viral complementary RNA is synthesized (Fig. 13). The accumulation of this RNA in the presence of these inhibitors is measured by the amount of the ^{3}H-labeled viral RNA that is rendered ribonuclease resistant when the infected cell nucleic acids are annealed to an excess of ^{3}H-viral RNA (Flamand and Bishop, 1974). This initial RNA synthesis, termed "primary transcription," is soon overtaken by higher rates of RNA synthesis when protein synthesis is allowed to proceed (Fig. 13). It is presumed that the increased synthesis of viral complementary RNA (secondary transcription) is due to the availability of newly synthesized progeny RNA templates in the infected cells. Such progeny templates are believed to originate from the replication of the parental RNA species (see Section 3.4).

Kascsak and Lyons (1977) identified three viral specified RNA species in cycloheximide- and actinomycin D-treated Bunyamwera infected cells having S values of 33 S, 26 S, and 16 S, equivalent to essentially complete transcripts of the viral RNA, although it was not proved that these RNA species were in fact viral complementary.

While host cell factors could be involved in primary transcription, it is probable that the viral complementary RNA synthesis involves the virion polymerase. Although it has been shown that bunyavirus viral complementary RNA can be isolated from infected cell polysomes, it

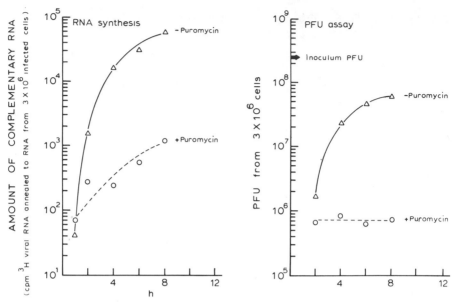

Fig. 13. *In vivo* viral complementary RNA synthesis by snowshoe hare virus. Viral complementary RNA synthesis and released PFU in snowshoe hare infected BHK-21 cells (MOI of 80) in the presence or absence of 100 μg puromycin per milliliter culture fluid were determined as described by Flamand and Bishop (1974). RNA synthesis in the presence of puromycin (primary transcription) is markedly lower than that obtained in its absence (secondary transcription).

remains to be directly shown that this RNA can function as messenger RNA, i.e., RNA that can direct the synthesis of specific viral gene products.

3.3. Viral Protein Synthesis

The synthesis of viral polypeptides in Bunyamwera virus-infected cells has been studied by Pennington *et al.* (1977). Four virus-induced polypeptides were identified in infected BSC-1 cells. These were the viral L, G1, G2, and N polypeptides. Similar results have been obtained by others (personal communications from I. Lazdins and I. H. Holmes, and from D. A. McPhee and E. G. Westaway) for Bunyamwera virus-infected Vero cells. Pulse-chase experiments, short-term labeling experiments, and experiments using amino acid analogues undertaken by Pennington *et al.* (1977) failed to provide any evidence of polypeptide processing involving proteolytic cleavage. These results suggested that L protein is not a precursor of G1, G2, or N and that G2 is not derived from G1. The absence of a precursor for both G1 and G2 may mean either that these proteins are synthesized from separate messenger RNA species or that they are independently initiated from a single messenger RNA (see Section 3.5). The negative evidence for large protein precursors, however, does not preclude a precursor which is processed too quickly for detection.

Analyses we have undertaken with Trivittatus virus-infected cells (Fig. 14), confirm the results reported by Pennington *et al.* (1977) and indicate that at least three viral-specified polypeptides are made in Trivittatus virus-infected cells (G1, G2, and N). No L protein has been detected.

For both Trivittatus and Bunyamwera virus-infected cells, a multiplicity-dependent decrease in the host cell protein synthesis has been observed late in infection (Fig. 14), 5–7 hr after infection for Bunyamwera-infected cells (L. El Said, personal communication; I. Lazdins and I. H. Holmes, personal communication; Pennington *et al.*, 1977).

Analyses of the kinetics of synthesis of Bunyamwera viral polypeptides by Pennington *et al.* (1977) indicated that there were an early phase involving primarily N polypeptide synthesis and a late phase involving primarily G1 and G2 polypeptide syntheses. They observed

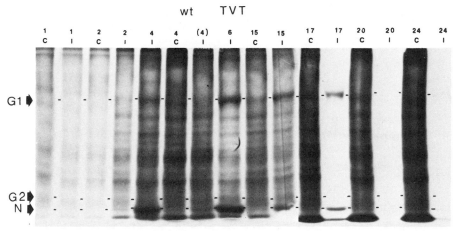

Fig. 14.   Intracellular polypeptides synthesized in Trivittatus (TVT) infected BHK-21 cells. Control cells (C) and TVT-infected cells (I), infected at a MOI of 10 PFU per cell were labeled for 30 min at 1, 2, 4, 6, 15, 17, 20, and 24 hr after infection in the presence of 50 μCi [³H]leucine per milliliter of Eagle's medium. The labeled intracellular proteins were resolved by electrophoresis in 8% polyacrylamide gels. A fluorograph (Bonner and Laskey, 1974) of the polypeptide patterns is presented. The positions of the TVT viral G1, G2, and N polypeptides are indicated. In a center well a 4-hr sample (4) of cells infected at a lower MOI is shown.

that the syntheses of polypeptides N and L peaked and declined earlier than those of G1 and G2. The earliest time new Bunyamwera viral N protein was detected was 2 hr after infection. Similar results have been obtained for Trivittatus virus (Fig. 14).

Taking the L, G1, G2, and N protein molecular weights as 200×10^3, 128×10^3, 31×10^3, and 23×10^3, respectively (sum = 3.82×10^5, Pennington *et al.*, 1977), the amount of RNA genetic information needed to code for these polypeptides is about 4×10^6 daltons. If the Bunyamwera L, M, and S RNA sum molecular weight is 5.24×10^6 (Gentsch *et al.*, 1977*a*), then there is theoretically enough information to code for other viral polypeptide(s). No such polypeptides have been observed in Bunyamwera- or Trivittatus-infected cells. Either there are no other viral-coded polypeptides, or they have molecular weights similar to those of the known viral protein species so that their presence has been overlooked. Alternatively, nonstructural polypeptides may be present in such low quantities that their synthesis has not been detected. This latter possiblity is not unreasonable if L RNA codes for L protein *and* an unidentified protein, since not only does L RNA contain the largest excess of genetic information but also L protein is present in infected cells in the least amounts (Pennington *et al.*, 1977; also see Fig. 14). If the production of multiple L RNA gene products is coordinated, then one might expect difficulty in identifying another protein in view of the difficulty in detecting L protein.

3.4. Virus RNA Replication

The mechanism of virus RNA replication is not known. Intracellular viral nucleocapsids have been detected in Lumbo virus-infected cells (Bouloy and Hannoun, 1976*b*) having the same density and sedimentation coefficients as those isolated from purified virus. The major polypeptide associated with the nucleocapsids has been shown to be the viral N polypeptide. A minor polypeptide associated with the viral nucleocapsids was also reported, similar to a minor component often found in Lumbo virus preparations (Bouloy and Hannoun, 1976*b*); whether it is a virus or a host coded protein is not known.

Hybridization experiments using RNA extracted from the intracellular Lumbo nucleocapsids provided evidence that both positive and negative RNA strands were present, even after removal of nascent transcripts by prior ribonuclease treatment (20 μg/ml, 30 min, 20°C). While it was concluded that the ratio of plus- to minus-strand nucleocapsids (of any size class) was 1:4, the presence of full-length plus strands needs to be demonstrated in order to confirm these results, since others have shown that the RNA in viral nucleocapsids is accessible to ribonuclease digestion.

Despite this, it is reasonable to propose that the replication of bunyavirus RNA species involves plus-strand ribonucleoprotein intermediates. How they are formed or what regulates their synthesis is not known. Inhibition of host cell RNA synthesis in Bunyamwera virus-infected Vero cells has been observed by I. Lazdins and I. H. Holmes (personal communication).

3.5. Secondary Transcription: Amplified Messenger RNA Synthesis

As shown in Fig. 13, amplified viral complementary (putative messenger) RNA synthesis occurs in bunyavirus-infected cells when protein synthesis is allowed to proceed. Such synthesis is responsible for the bulk of the viral complementary RNA that is synthesized in infected cells. The relative proportion of primary to secondary RNA synthesis is about $1:100$ in cells infected at a multiplicity of 80 (Fig. 13). It is not known if higher multiplicities of infection would decrease this ratio. Neither actinomycin D (5 μg/ml), rifampin (100 μg/ml), or α-amanitin (25 μg/ml) effectively inhibited either the overall rate or the accumulation of viral complementary RNA (Fig. 15). Although some effect on the virus yields was observed with one or other of these antibiotics, it is clear that such inhibition was not due to impairment of the processes involved in viral complementary RNA synthesis (Fig. 15). Reduction of California encephalitis virus yields by actinomycin D has also been reported (Goldman *et al.*, 1977).

Lumbo virus-infected cells have been shown to have polysomes containing viral complementary RNA species (Bouloy and Hannoun, 1976a). On extraction, three size classes of viral complementary RNA were identified (32 S, 24 S, and 14 S). Since these sizes are similar to those of the three viral RNA species, it was suggested that the viral messenger RNA species may be essentially complete transcripts of the viral genome segments. If so, then it would indicate that at least one mRNA segment codes for two viral polypeptides since there are four virion polypeptides. However, the evidence for the three mRNA size classes does not preclude the presence of two mRNA species (perhaps derived from different viral RNA segments) within a single size class.

As discussed previously, direct evidence is needed to prove that viral complementary RNA species function as messenger RNA that can program the synthesis of viral polypeptides. If individual messenger

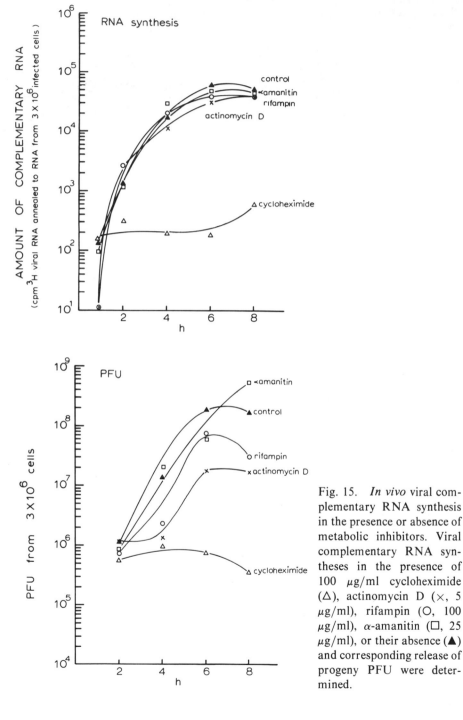

Fig. 15. *In vivo* viral complementary RNA synthesis in the presence or absence of metabolic inhibitors. Viral complementary RNA syntheses in the presence of 100 μg/ml cycloheximide (Δ), actinomycin D (×, 5 μg/ml), rifampin (O, 100 μg/ml), α-amanitin (□, 25 μg/ml), or their absence (▲) and corresponding release of progeny PFU were determined.

RNA species can be isolated in sufficient quantities and sized, then which RNA codes for which protein can be determined. Also, the question can be answered of whether a particular messenger RNA species codes for more than one viral polypeptide. If any messenger RNA codes for two independent polypeptides, then it will be of interest to know how both polypeptides are synthesized and whether their synthesis is initiated independently or whether a polyprotein precursor is involved.

No analyses of the primary nucleotide sequences of messenger RNA species have been published. It is not known if there are 3' polyadenylated sequences and/or 5' capped and methylated termini. How identical the RNA termini are for the various viral messenger RNA species is not known. Whether only three messenger RNA species are found in bunyavirus-infected cells also needs to be confirmed.

Kascsak and Lyons (1977) reported that for Bunyamwera virus-infected cells the peak of actinomycin-D-resistant RNA synthesis occurred 9–11 hr after infection, approximately 6–8 hr prior to the peak of infectious virus release. Pulse-labeling experiments at various times after infection demonstrated that the drug-treated BHK cells, when compared to mock-infected cells, contained three size classes of single-stranded RNA having sedimentation coefficients similar to those of three of the four RNA species these investigators identified in Bunyamwera virus preparations. Some change in the ratio of the three RNA size classes representing a relative decrease in the larger and increase in the smaller was noted as a function of the time of infection. Duplexes of ribonuclease resistant RNA with $s_{20,w}$ values of 27 S, 17.5 S, and 13 S and molecular weights estimated at 7.2×10^6, 4.1×10^6, and 1.7×10^6 were identified. Denaturation of the duplexes apparently yielded 33 S, 26 S, and 16 S single-stranded RNA size classes. No duplex corresponding to the fourth RNA they observed in Bunyamwera virus extracts was identified.

3.6. Virus Assembly and Budding

The morphogenesis of progeny bunyavirus particles probably involves assembly and budding into the Golgi cisternae, as discussed in Section 2.1. How the viral glycoproteins and nucleocapsids translocate and recognize each other, or the Golgi membranes, is not known. Which end or ends of the viral glycoprotein(s) interact with or transect the Golgi membrane lipid bilayer, or make contact with the viral nucleocapsid(s), is not known. An interesting question which also remains unanswered is how packaging of the viral nucleocapsids occurs.

4. GENETICS

Genetic analyses have been undertaken on four bunyaviruses, three belonging to the California encephalitis serogroup, snowshoe hare (SSH), La Crosse (LAC) (Gentsch and Bishop, 1976; Gentsch *et al.*, 1977*b*), and Trivittatus (TVT) viruses (L. El Said and D. H. L. Bishop, unpublished studies), and one belonging to the Bunyamwera serogroup, Guaroa (GRO) virus (R. Klimas and D. H. L. Bishop, unpublished studies).

The genetic analyses have had three objectives: (1) demonstration of the ability of these viruses to form recombinant viruses by segment reassortment, (2) establishment of gene product–RNA coding relationships, and (3) determination of the ability of these viruses to form recombinants from distinguishable virus serotypes.

So far only temperature-sensitive, conditional lethal mutants of the four bunyavirus serotypes have been described. Their isolation, properties, and use in recombination and complementation analyses are described below, together with the limited information that has been accumulated on the heterologous recombination potential of bunyaviruses. The data obtained on establishing the RNA coding assignments (Table 21) will also be discussed below.

4.1. Isolation and Characterization of Temperature-Sensitive, Conditional Lethal Bunyavirus Mutants

The genetic studies so far reported for bunyaviruses have used temperature-sensitive (*ts*), conditional lethal bunyavirus mutants, either derived by mutagen induction or isolated as spontaneous mutants in stocks of wild-type virus. No cold-sensitive, host range, or other mutants have been obtained.

4.1.1. Properties of the Wild-Type Viruses

The growth potential of wild-type La Crosse virus in BHK-21 cells has been studied as a function of multiplicity of infection (MOI) using cloned virus stocks (Obijeski *et al.*, 1976*a*). Even with a virus stock which represents the first passage after picking a plaque plug, lower virus yields were obtained with increasing multiplicities of infection (Obijeski *et al.*, 1976*a*). Thus it was shown that at 33°C by 48 hr after infection with an MOI of 10, the plaque-forming units (PFU) per milliliter (8×10^5) were significantly less than those obtained at a MOI of 1 (8×10^6) or 0.01 (2×10^7), or with virus eluted directly from a plaque plug and used to infect cells at a MOI of 0.002 (8×10^7). Such data suggest that high multiplicities of infection induce interference even on short-term growth with freshly cloned virus stocks. The differences in yields were much less pronounced at 24 hr than at 48 hr after infection (Obijeski *et al.*, 1976*a*). Since recombination assays can be more easily conducted using average multiplicities of infection of greater than 3, the interference observed at a MOI of 10 is of concern.

One-step growth curves at 33°C and 39.8°C have been obtained for snowshoe hare virus using BHK-21 cells. As shown in Fig. 16, with a MOI of 5 PFU per cell, virus production peaked by 24 hr after infection. When compared to the yields at 36 hr for a snowshoe hare virus

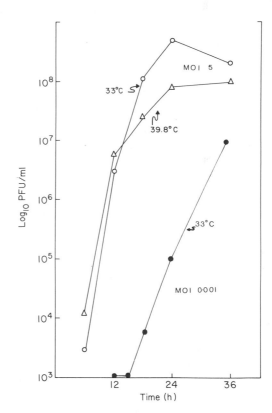

Fig. 16. Growth curves of snowshoe hare virus in BHK-21 cell monolayers. The snowshoe hare progeny PFU/ml from BHK-21 cells infected at input multiplicities of 5 PFU per cell at 39.8°C or 33°C are shown.

infection initiated at a MOI of 0.001 (Fig. 16), in contrast to the La Crosse virus results, no inhibition in virus yields was observed with the higher multiplicity of infection. The yield of snowshoe hare virus at 33°C was somewhat higher than that at 39.8°C, particularly by 18 hr after infection. From these results it was concluded that a single cycle of infection at 33°C or 39.8°C was complete by 24 hr after infection.

The efficiency of plating (EOP) of wild-type snowshoe hare virus (PFU at 39.8°C/PFU at 33°C) is around 1 (see Table 23). For La Crosse and Guaroa viruses, similar EOP values have been obtained, although for Trivittatus virus an EOP of 0.1 was obtained (L. El Said, unpublished results). After six consecutive passages at 39.8°C, the EOP of Trivittatus virus has been shown to increase to 0.5, although to be dependable the plaque assay at 39.8°C requires the use of 80–90% confluent monolayers of BHK-21 cells.

Plaque assays in Vero cells for snowshoe hare, La Crosse, Guaroa, and Trivittatus viruses are less efficient than in BHK-21 cells. Efficiencies range from 10% to 40%. The efficiency of plating these viruses in other cell systems has not been analyzed. Goldman *et al.* (1977) have shown that in BHK, MDBK, HeLa, chick embryo, and XC cells only the last two cell systems supported plaque development (when protamine sulfate or DEAE dextran was used), even though all supported virus growth (with efficiencies varying from 12% to 28% that of the most permissive cell line, XC cells).

4.1.2. Induction of *ts* Mutants Using Mutagens

Using 39.8°C as a nonpermissive temperature, 33°C as a permissive temperature, and BHK-21 cells to select and propagate viruses, temperature-sensitive mutants of snowshoe hare, La Crosse, Trivittatus, and Guaroa viruses have been isolated. The dose–response curves for snowshoe hare virus when grown in the presence of 5-fluorouracil (5-FU) or 5-azacytidine (5-AZA), or after treatment of virus preparations with *N*-methyl-*N*'-nitro-*N*-nitrosoguanidine (NTG), are shown in Fig. 17. Similar dose–response curves have been obtained for La Crosse, Trivittatus, and Guaroa viruses grown in the presence of 5-FU. Of the three mutagens, 5-AZA appears to be the most effective for inhibiting snowshoe hare virus growth.

The frequency of isolation of snowshoe hare *ts* mutants after treatment with various mutagens has been analyzed (Table 22). Although not all concentrations of the mutagens were analyzed, the results indicate that greater percentages of *ts* mutants were obtained from 5-AZA-

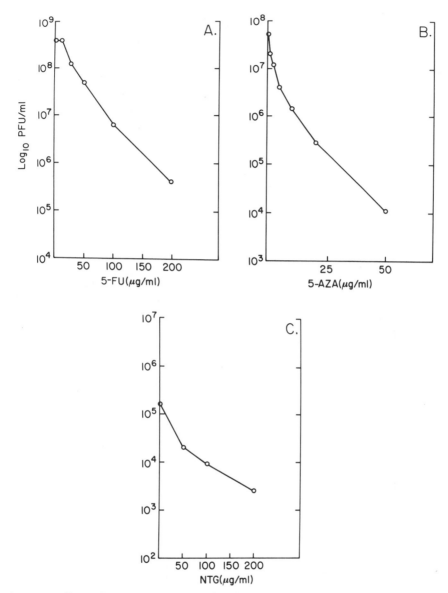

Fig. 17. Effect of mutagens on snowshoe hare progeny virus release. The released PFU/ml snowshoe hare virus from cells treated with various doses of (A) 5-FU, (B) 5-AZA, and (C) NTG was determined.

mutagenized virus than from concentrations of 5-FU- or NTG-mutagenized stocks that gave equivalent inhibitions of infectious virus.

Mutants derived from either 5-FU-, 5-AZA-, or NTG-mutagenized virus stocks have been shown to be capable of recombination. Nonrecombining (presumed multiple) *ts* mutants have been isolated

TABLE 22

Frequency of Isolation of Temperature-Sensitive (*ts*) Mutants of Snowshoe Hare Virus[a]

Method	Concentration (μg/ml)	Number of clones analyzed	%|*ts*	Total number of mutants	Number of mutants kept
5-FU	50	224	14.7	33	26
	100	100	22.0	22	18
5-AZA	5	50	24.0	12	8
	10	100	27.0	27	19
NTG	50	50	6.0	3	3
	200	50	6.0	3	2
Spontaneous	—	475	2.3	11	11
Total	—	1049		111	87

[a] The recovery of spontaneous *ts* mutants in stocks of wild-type SSH virus or following growth of the wild-type virus in the presence of different concentrations of 5-fluorouracil (5-FU), or 5-azacytidine (5-AZA), or treatment of virus suspensions with *N*-methyl-*N'*-nitro-*N*-nitrosoguanidine (NTG) is given. After screening out those *ts* mutants which were too leaky to use in genetic recombination assays, the rest were kept for subsequent analyses.

frequently from mutageneses involving high concentrations of 5-FU (greater than 50 μg/ml).

4.1.3.   Isolation of Spontaneous *ts* Mutants

The frequency of occurrence of spontaneous *ts* mutants in clones of wild-type snowshoe hare virus has been determined to be 2.3% (Table 22). All of the spontaneous *ts* mutants obtained so far appear to be the product of single mutational events, since they all recombine with representative snowshoe hare *ts* mutants of group I or II.

4.1.4.   Properties of the *ts* Mutants

Temperature-sensitive mutants of snowshoe hare (SSH) virus were originally selected on the basis of (1) having EOP values (PFU at 39.8°C/PFU at 33°C) of less than 0.001 and (2) an ability to produce greater than 10^7 PFU/ml when grown at 33°C (Gentsch and Bishop, 1976; Gentsch *et al.*, 1977*b*). Most SSH, LAC, TVT, and GRO mutants have EOP values ranging from 5×10^{-4} to less than 7×10^{-7} (Table 23). Some SSH *ts* mutants are more leaky than others giving plaques at 39.8°C (often smaller than those of wild-type virus), which

TABLE 23

**Virus Yields after Single and Mixed Infections with Snowshoe Hare Virus *ts*
Mutants[a]**

Inoculum viruses	Incubation temperature (°C)	24-hr yield assayed at		CI	%R
		33°C	39.5°C		
ts1	33	4.1×10^7	6×10^3		
	39.5	8×10^3	10^3		
ts2	33	5×10^7	3×10^3		
	39.5	8×10^3	10^3		
ts3	33	6.8×10^7	10^3		
	39.5	10^3	10^3		
ts1 × *ts2*	33	1.1×10^8	2.3×10^6		4
	39.5	4.3×10^5	3.5×10^4	25	
ts1 × *ts3*	33	1.5×10^8	4×10^4		0.05
	39.5	10^3	10^3	0.1	
ts2 × *ts3*	33	7.5×10^7	5.5×10^6		15
	39.5	9.6×10^5	3.4×10^5	78	
Wild type	33	2.3×10^7	2.7×10^7		
	39.5	4.6×10^6	2.7×10^6		

[a] Recombination percentages (%R) and complementation indices (CI) were determined as described in the text (data of Gentsch and Bishop, 1976).

on replating still exhibit a *ts* phenotype. No accurate determination of reversion frequencies to a wild-type phenotype has been made for either SSH, LAC, TVT, or GRO mutants. Reversion frequencies may well be less than 5×10^{-4}.

4.2. High-Frequency Homologous Virus Genetic Recombination

In certain dual SSH mutant virus infections incubated for 24 hr at 33°C, and initiated at an MOI of 5 for each virus, progeny virus are obtained which have higher EOP values than those obtained from the individual SSH mutant virus infections (Table 23) (Gentsch and Bishop, 1976). Clonal analyses of the progeny viruses from the dual mutant infections have indicated that they have a wild-type virus EOP (Gentsch and Bishop, 1976). Similar results have been obtained with other SSH, or LAC, or TVT, or GRO *ts* mutants (Tables 24–27) (Gentsch *et al.*, 1977*b*; L. El Said, R. Klimas, and D. H. L. Bishop, unpublished results). Recombination frequencies (%R) are calculated according to the formula

$$\%R = \frac{[(AB_{33})_{39.8} - (A_{33})_{39.8} - (B_{33})_{39.8}] \times 100 \times 2}{(AB_{33})_{33}}$$

TABLE 24

Recombination Analyses with Snowshoe Hare *ts* Mutants[a]

SSH *ts* mutant	Percentage recombinants with SSH *ts* mutants												
	1	*2*	*3*	*7*	*9*	*12*	*13*	*14*	*15*	*16*	*18*	*20*	*21*
1	.	4	0	7	0	0	0	0	0	0	14	0	21
2	.	.	17	0	18	4	1	0	16	9	0	7	0
3	.	.	.	24	0	0	0	0	0	0	14	0	2
7	.	.	.	.	5	4	3	0	5	5	0	4	0
9	.	.	.	.	.	0	0	0	0	0	5	0	7
12	.	.	.	.	.	.	0	0	0	0	25	0	4
13	.	.	.	.	.	.	.	0	0	0	9	0	6
14	.	.	.	.	.	.	.	.	0	0	0	0	0
15	.	.	.	.	.	.	.	.	.	0	13	0	6
16	.	.	.	.	.	.	.	.	.	.	6	0	2
18	.	.	.	.	.	.	.	.	.	.	.	2	0
20	.	.	.	.	.	.	.	.	.	.	.	.	2

[a] Assignments: Group I: *ts1*, *ts3*, *ts9*, *ts12*, *ts13*, *ts15*, *ts16*, *ts20* (eight mutants).
   Group II: *ts2*, *ts7*, *ts18*, *ts21* (four mutants).
Unassigned: *ts14* (possible double mutant).

Recombination percentages are the average of three separate determinations and were calculated according to the formula given in the text.

In this formula $(AB_{33})_{39.8}$ represents the yield of the mixed mutant virus infection, incubated at 33°C and assayed at 39.8°C, while $(A_{33})_{39.8}$ and $(B_{33})_{39.8}$ represent the yields of the individual A or B (respectively) mutant virus infections, incubated at 33°C and assayed at 39.8°C. The term $(AB_{33})_{33}$ represents the yield of the mixed mutant infection, grown and titered at 33°C. The percentage obtained is multiplied by a factor

TABLE 25

Recombination Analyses with La Crosse *ts* Mutants[a]

LAC *ts* mutant	Percentage recombinants with LAC *ts* mutants																			
	3	*4*	*9*	*13*	*1*	*2*	*5*	*10*	*11*	*12*	*14*	*15*	*16*	*17*	*18*	*19*	*20*	*21*	*22*	*23*
3	—	0	13	11	0	0	0	0	0	0	0	0	10	0	0	8	13	0	0	14
4	.	—	13	5	0	0	0	0	0	0	0	0	12	0	0	7	17	0	0	12
9	.	.	—	0	21	39	10	30	8	33	27	19	0	25	32	0	0	22	7	0
13	.	.	.	—	17	24	4	39	3	7	7	4	0	18	6	0	0	11	2	0

[a] Assignments: Group I: *ts9*, *ts13*, *ts16*, *ts19*, *ts20*, *ts23*.
     Group II: *ts3*, *ts4*, *ts1*, *ts2*, *ts5*, *ts10*, *ts11*, *ts12*, *ts14*, *ts15*, *ts17*, *ts18*, *ts21*, *ts22*.

The recombination percentages were calculated as described in the text.

TABLE 26
Recombination Analyses with Trivittatus Virus *ts* Mutants[a]

TVT *ts* mutant	Percentage recombinants with Trivittatus *ts* mutants											
	1	2	3	4	5	6	7	8	10	11	15	16
1	.	20	11	10	4	5	0	0	0	0	46	0
2	.	.	0	0	0	0	0	4	18	13	0	0
3	.	.	.	0	0	0	0	10	3	13	0	0
4	.	.	.	.	0	0	0	2	10	3	0	0
5	.	.	.	.	.	0	0	30	20	24	0	0
6	.	.	.	.	.	.	0	40	44	28	0	0
7	.	.	.	.	.	.	.	0	0	0	0	0
8	.	.	.	.	.	.	.	.	0	0	40	0
10	.	.	.	.	.	.	.	.	.	0	20	0
11	.	.	.	.	.	.	.	.	.	.	32	0
15	.	.	.	.	.	.	.	.	.	.	.	0

[a] Assignments: Group I: *ts1, ts8, ts10, ts11.*
                  Group II: *ts2, ts3, ts4, ts5, ts6, ts15.*
Unassigned: *ts7, ts16.*

The recombination percentages were calculated as described in the text.

of 2 in order to score for double mutant recombinants which are presumed to be produced at a frequency equal to that of the wild-type recombinants. Although double mutants have been found in virus harvests which give wild-type recombinants, insufficient numbers have been analyzed to prove that they occur at equivalent frequencies.

TABLE 27
Recombination Analyses with Guaroa Virus *ts* Mutants[a]

GRO *ts* mutant	Percentage recombinants with Guaroa *ts* mutants								
	3	4	9	10	11	12	13	14	16
3	.	49	1	0	2	13	0	62	0
4		.	0	0	0	0	32	0	4
9			.	0	0	0	18	0	2
10				.	0	0	0	0	0
11					.	0	3	0	6
12						.	26	0	4
13							.	9	0
14								.	8

[a] Assignments: Group I: *ts3, ts13, ts16.*
                  Group II: *ts4, ts9, ts11, ts12, ts14.*
Unassigned: *ts10.*

The recombination percentages were calculated as described in the text.

Pairwise crosses with 13 SSH *ts* mutants established that the mutants could either be categorized into two nonoverlapping genetic recombination groups (group I, eight mutants; group II, four mutants), or (one mutant) not be so categorized (Table 24) (Gentsch and Bishop, 1976). The mutant which could not be placed in one or other recombination group is probably a multiple mutant having at least both group I and group II type mutations. In these initial (and subsequent) analyses, recombination percentages which were less than 1% were scored as 0 (Tables 24–27). The range of recombination percentages that have been obtained for various snowshoe hare mutant crosses is from 1% to 45%, with most values between 1% and 18%. Replicate crosses can give recombination percentages which vary by as much as 20%, so that the value obtained for particular mutant crosses may reflect only a positive as opposed to a negative result.

Of a total of 65 SSH *ts* mutants we have analyzed, 31 are classified as group I mutants, 24 as group II mutants, and 10 as probable multiple mutants (J. Gentsch and D. H. L. Bishop, unpublished data). We have not isolated any mutants which recombine with both representative group I and representative group II mutants. Evidence to be discussed later (see Section 4.5.3) indicates that SSH group I mutants have M RNA lesions while SSH group II mutants have L RNA lesions (Gentsch *et al.*, 1977*b*). Since the S RNA codes for N protein, and reassorts independently of the M or L RNA (Gentsch *et al.*, 1977*b*), there should be a third group of *ts* mutants (group III). Out of a total of 120 bunyavirus *ts* mutants we have analyzed, we have not detected any that can be unambiguously classified as group III mutants. We have a few SSH mutants which give high recombination percentages with SSH Group II mutants and reproducible, but low, recombination percentages with SSH group I mutants (%*R* of 0.1–1%). However, from heterologous recombination analyses with LAC *ts* mutants (see Section 4.5), these putative group III mutants appear to be leaky group I mutants. Whether this interpretation is correct is uncertain in view of the limitations we have observed on generating all types of SSH-LAC recombinants (see Section 4.5).

The reason why no group III SSH (or LAC, TVT, or GRO) mutants have yet been isolated is not known. The reason is not just that the S RNA represents only 10% of the total RNA target size, since out of 120 *ts* mutants we would expect on that basis to have up to 12 group III mutants. It is possible that mutations in the S RNA gene product are more often lethal than temperature sensitive. Some evidence to support the concept that S RNA resists evolution more than the M or L RNA species has been obtained from LAC oligonucleotide fingerprint analyses (El Said *et al.*, 1979). These analyses indicate that S RNA sequences are more conserved than those of M or L RNA sequences, suggesting that the LAC S RNA resists evolution more than the L or M RNA species.

For reference purposes SSH *ts* mutants are described with both a group and a mutant isolate number. Thus SSH *ts* mutant number 1 is referred to as SSH *tsI-1*, while SSH mutant number 18 is SSH *tsII-18*. A similar convention is used for La Crosse, Trivittatus, and Guaroa *ts* mutants. If snowshoe hare virus mutants are isolated by other investigators, then we propose that a convention including the city of origin be used (e.g., SSH *tsBII-18* for snowshoe hare *ts* mutant 18 isolated in Birmingham). Similar conventions are used for *ts* mutants of viruses belonging to other virus families.

The *ts* mutants of LAC, TVT, and GRO are also each categorized into two recombination groups (groups I and II; Tables 25–27). As discussed above, no group III *ts* mutants have been isolated for either LAC, TVT, or GRO viruses.

The ts^+ recombinants produced from crosses involving different snowshoe hare *ts* mutants have been analyzed in order to determine if they are (1) heterozygotes (containing in their virions duplicate RNA segments, i.e., *ts* and wild type, derived from both viruses), or (2) aggregates of both parental *ts* viruses, or (3) genotypically stable wild-type progeny recombinants. Screening the cloned and recloned ts^+ recombinants generated from particular crosses of snowshoe hare *ts* mutants for *ts* mutant shedding at high frequency has given no indication of *ts* progeny being shed from the recombinants at any frequency higher than that equivalent to the spontaneous rate of *ts* mutant production (Gentsch and Bishop, 1976; Gentsch *et al.*, 1977*b*). These results suggest that the ts^+ recombinants are genotypically stable and probably reassortant wild type viruses (see Section 4.5.1).

4.3. Complementation Analyses

For certain SSH dual mutant virus infections incubated for 24 hr at 39.8°C, and initiated at a MOI of 5 for each virus, enhanced yields of progeny virus have been observed when compared to the sum of the individual virus infections incubated for a similar time at 39.8°C (Tables 23 and 28) (Gentsch and Bishop, 1976). Complementation indices (CI) are calculated according to the formula

$$CI = \frac{(AB_{39.8})_{33} - 2(AB_{39.8})_{39.8}}{(A_{39.8})_{33} + (B_{39.8})_{33}}$$

TABLE 28

Complementation Analyses with SSH *ts* Mutants[a]

SSH *ts* mutant	CI indices with SSH *ts* mutants					
	1	*2*	*3*	*6*	*7*	*9*
1	.	25	0	0	62	0
2	.	.	78	26	0	158
3	.	↕	.	0	7	0
6	.	.	.	.	5	0
7	.	.	.	.	.	6

[a] Complementation indices (CI) were calculated as described in the text.

Assignments: Group I: *ts1, ts3, ts6, ts9.*
                       Group II: *ts2, ts7.*

where $(A_{39.8})_{33}$ and $(B_{39.8})_{33}$ are the yields, titered at 33°C, of the individual mutant virus harvests grown at 39.8°C, and $(AB_{39.8})_{33}$ and $(AB_{39.8})_{39.8}$ are the yields of the dual mutant virus infections at 39.8°C, titered at 33°C or 39.8°C, respectively. The factor of 2 takes into account double mutants that may be generated during the complementation assay. They are presumed to occur as frequently as the wild-type recombinants. Although it has not been proved that such double mutants occur in the same proportion as the wild-type recombinants (see Section 4.2), the equation provides a more rigorous test for complementation than a formula which takes no account of double mutant production.

The complementation indices obtained for dual mutant virus infections involving particular SSH *ts* mutants are given in Tables 23 and 28 (Gentsch and Bishop, 1976). Significant complementation was observed only when recombination occurred (see Tables 23, 24, and 28). The fact that both complementation and recombination occurred was evidenced by the presence of more *ts* progeny in the dual mutant virus yields than wild-type progeny. Complementation indices of less than 2 were scored as zero (Table 28).

An exhaustive search for *ts* mutants which do not recombine with but do complement each other has not yet been undertaken. Some ten SSH recombination group I *ts* mutants and ten SSH recombination group II *ts* mutants show no evidence of intra-recombination group complementation. Since it is likely that at least one of the viral RNA segments codes for more than one gene product (see Section 3.5), intragroup complementation might be expected.

4.4. Group I/II Double Mutants

It has been shown that certain SSH *ts* mutants (e.g., *ts31*) do not recombine with representative SSH group I or group II *ts* mutants (G. Robeson and D. H. L. Bishop, unpublished data). At least some of these mutants are probably double group I/II mutants (e.g., *ts31*). This has been demonstrated by coinfecting BHK cells with wild-type SSH virus and *ts31* at 33°C and screening the progeny for *ts* mutants. Of 32 progeny clones examined, 13 were *ts* (40%); the rest had wild-type EOP values. Recombination analyses with representative SSH group I and group II mutants established that two of the 13 mutants would not recombine with the group I and group II mutants (like *ts31*). Nine of the remaining mutants recombined only with the group I mutants, and the remaining two recombined only with the group II mutants. The high frequency of group I and group II progeny mutants recovered from the *ts31* and wild-type virus cross and lack of any group III mutants indicate that *ts31* is a double group I/II mutant. Although SSH double mutants have been used in screening for SSH group III mutants, no group III SSH mutants have yet been isolated.

4.5. High-Frequency Heterologous Recombination between Certain Bunyaviruses

High-frequency recombination has been obtained between certain *ts* mutants of snowshoe hare and La Crosse viruses (Table 29) (Gentsch *et al.*, 1977*b*). Recombinants were generated from the cross LAC II × SSH I and characterized as reassortant viruses by oligonucleotide fingerprinting. The reciprocal cross, SSH II × LAC I, has not provided

TABLE 29

Recombination betweeen Snowshoe Hare and La Crosse *ts* Mutants[a]

LAC *ts* mutants	Percentage recombinants with SSH *ts* mutants			
	SSH I-1	SSH I-3	SSH II-2	SSH II-18
LAC II-3	3.9	5.4	0	0
LAC II-4	6.5	6.2	0	0
LAC II-5	35.7	16.9	0	0

[a] Recombination percentages were determined as described in the text.

any evidence of recombination. The heterologous crosses involving selected TVT I, TVT II, GRO I, or GRO II mutants with LAC I, LAC II, SSH I, or SSH II mutants have so far also not provided any evidence for heterologous virus recombination (Table 30) (J. Gentsch, R. Klimas, and D. H. L. Bishop, unpublished results).

The lack of recombination between *ts* mutants of GRO or TVT and those of LAC or SSH should be considered in light of the serological relationships of these viruses. Within the California encephalitis serogroup, TVT and MEL are serologically quite distant from LAC and SSH viruses (Table 1), while GRO, on the basis of CF tests, is a member of the Bunyamwera serogroup of bunyaviruses (Table 1). While there is serological evidence to link GRO with various members of the California encephalitis group (HI and neutralization data, Whitman and Shope, 1962), it is quite possible that the constraints for heterologous recombination are rigorous and do not exactly parallel the antigenic relationships. Other explanations for the lack of recombination can also be advanced (e.g., interference). These will need to be investigated further.

The SSH-LAC recombinants that have been obtained are described by the origin of their RNA species. Thus the L/M/S RNA species of the recombinants generated from LAC II × SSH I mutants have the genotypes SSH/LAC/SSH and SSH/LAC/LAC (Gentsch *et al.*, 1977*b*).

Since we do not have SSH or LAC group III mutants, we have no means of directly selecting certain SSH-LAC recombinants. In view of

TABLE 30

Heterologous Recombination Assays between SSH, LAC, TVT, and GRO *ts* Mutants

	SSH I	SSH II	LAC I	LAC II	TVT I	TVT II	GRO I	GRO II
SSH I	0	+	0	+	0	0	0	0
SSH II		0	0	0	0	0	0	0
LAC I			0	+	0	0	0	0
LAC II				0	0	0	0	0
TVT I					0	+	0	0
TVT II						0	0	0
GRO I							0	+
GRO II								0

[a] High-frequency recombination, as detected by the production of wild-type (*ts*⁺) virus in the progeny virus yields from mixed *ts* mutant virus infections, is scored as +, while the lack of recombination is scored by 0.

this, the cloned progeny from coinfections involving wild-type LAC and SSH viruses have been analyzed by oligonucleotide fingerprinting. Of eight progeny analyzed, three were found to have the genotype LAC/LAC/LAC, three were SSH/SSH/SSH, one was SSH/LAC/LAC, and one was SSH/LAC/SSH. Although more clones need to be analyzed, these results suggest that SSH-LAC recombinants may have lower growth potentials than the wild-type LAC or SSH viruses. Backcrosses of a group I *ts* mutant derived from the recombinant SSH/LAC/SSH with a group II *ts* mutant of La Crosse virus have yielded a new recombinant characterized as LAC/LAC/SSH, while backcross analyses of a group I *ts* mutant derived from the SSH/LAC/LAC recombinant with a group II *ts* mutant of snowshoe hare virus yielded SSH/SSH/LAC (J. Gentsch and D. H. L. Bishop, unpublished observations).

If there are restrictions against the formation of certain SSH-LAC recombinants, then the restrictions will have to be considered in relation to the L, M, and S gene products. It is known that the S RNA codes for N protein (Gentsch *et al.*, 1977*b*; Gentsch and Bishop, 1978), while M RNA codes for G1 and G2 (Gentsh and Bishop, 1979), leaving L RNA to code for L protein. If correct, then the fact that the SSH/LAC/LAC and SSH/LAC/SSH viruses have different N polypeptides (Section 4.5.2) suggests that the LAC N polypeptide can function with the snowshoe hare L protein while the SSH L and N proteins can function with the LAC G1 and G2 proteins.

One possibility which needs further investigation is that other SSH-LAC recombinants (e.g., those expected from LAC I × SSH II crosses, LAC/SSH/LAC and LAC/SSH/SSH) are noncytocidal and cannot form plaques, or are not released from infected cells.

4.5.1. Involvement of Segment Reassortment in Bunyavirus Recombination

It has been established by oligonucleotide fingerprinting of the individual RNA segments of the SSH-LAC recombinants (Fig. 18) that they have reassorted genomes derived from the progenitor LAC and SSH viruses (Gentsch *et al.*, 1977*b*). The recombinants derived from the SSH I × LAC II crosses were shown to have the L/M/S genotypes SSH/LAC/LAC and SSH/LAC/SSH. No evidence for heterozygous viruses having L (or M, or S) RNA species derived from *both* LAC and SSH viruses has been obtained, and no evidence has been obtained for

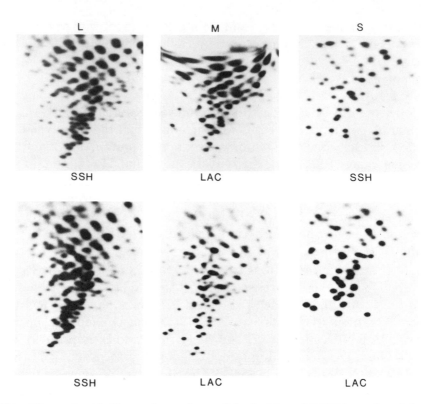

Fig. 18.   Oligonucleotide fingerprint analyses of the L, M, and S RNA species of the recombinant obtained from a LAC *tsII-4* × SSH *tsI-1* cross (upper panels) and a LAC *tsII-5* × SSH *tsI-3* cross (lower panels). The fingerprints were determined as described previously (Clewley *et al.*, 1977; Gentsch *et al.*, 1977*b*).

recombinant viruses having part L (or M, or S) RNA species derived from SSH and part derived from LAC L (or M, or S, respectively) RNA sequences.

4.5.2.   Assignment of Particular Bunyavirus Recombination Groups to Particular RNA Segments

The SSH/LAC/LAC and SSH/LAC/SSH recombinants were both derived from the cross SSH I × LAC II. It can be concluded therefore that the SSH I mutants have a mutation in their M RNA since the only LAC RNA segment common to the two recombinants that corrected the SSH defect was LAC M RNA. Likewise, it can be concluded that the LAC II mutants have a mutation in their L RNA since the only SSH RNA segment common to the two recombinant viruses that corrected the LAC defect was the SSH L RNA.

In view of the fact that both recombinants have a SSH L RNA and a LAC M RNA, it can also be deduced that neither progenitor *ts* mutant had defective S RNA gene products.

If the LAC II and SSH I mutants are single mutants (noted here by an asterisk) in L and M, respectively (i.e., LAC*/LAC/LAC and SSH/SSH*/SSH), then one would expect to generate two wild-type recombinants having the genotypes SSH/LAC/LAC and SSH/LAC/SSH. This is supported by the results obtained.

4.5.3. Proof That the Bunyavirus S RNA Segment Codes for N Protein

Suggestive evidence derived by comparing the S RNA sizes of several bunyaviruses with their respective N protein sizes has been obtained which indicates that the S RNA codes for N protein (Gentsch *et al.*, 1977a). It has been shown that the LAC N protein has a slightly slower electrophoretic mobility than SSH N protein. Since the SSH/LAC/LAC and SSH/LAC/SSH recombinants differ only in their S RNA species, their virion polypeptides were compared in order to determine if they have different N polypeptides. Both electrophoretic analyses of the total virion polypeptides (Fig. 19) and tryptic peptide analyses (Fig. 11) have established that the SSH/LAC/LAC recombinant has a LAC N protein while the SSH/LAC/SSH recombinant has a SSH N protein (Gentsch *et al.*, 1977b; Gentsch and Bishop, 1978).

Fig. 19. Coelectrophoresis of the virion polypeptides of the recombinants SSH/LAC/LAC and SSH/LAC/SSH. [³H]Leucine-labeled SSH/LAC/SSH and [¹⁴C]amino acid-labeled SSH/LAC/LAC virus preparations were dissociated by sodium dodecylsulfate and resolved by electrophoresis in 8% polyacrylamide gels. Data of Gentsch *et al.* (1977b)

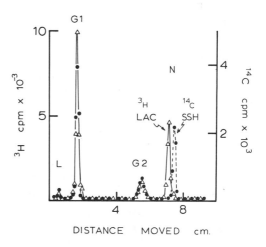

Similar peptide analyses of the recombinant G1 and G2 proteins (Gentsch and Bishop, 1979), when compared to those of SSH and LAC, have allowed us to prove that the M RNA codes for G1 and G2 polypeptides. Whether L RNA codes for L protein remains to be determined.

4.5.4. Pathogenic Potential of SSH-LAC Recombinants

Analyses in suckling mice, hamsters, and guinea pigs of the pathogenic potential of the SSH/LAC/LAC and SSH/LAC/SSH recombinants, when compared to those of the wild-type LAC and SSH viruses, have indicated that the recombinants are no more pathogenic than their wild-type progenitor viruses. Certain but not all recombinants appear to evoke a LAC HI seriological response and a SSH CF response (Gentsch *et al.*, 1977*b*), suggesting that the HI response corresponds to an M RNA gene product (presumed to be the glycoproteins) while the CF response corresponds to an S RNA gene product (N protein).

4.6. Summary of the Bunyavirus Genetic Studies

High-frequency *homologous* virus genetic recombination has been demonstrated for four bunyaviruses: La Crosse, snowshoe hare, Trivittatus, and Guaroa. Limited high-frequency *heterologous* virus genetic recombination has been observed between snowshoe hare and La Crosse viruses (SSH I × LAC II *ts* mutants, but not for SSH II × LAC I *ts* mutants). No heterologous virus recombination has been observed in crosses involving Guaroa or Trivittatus with La Crosse or snowshoe hare virus mutants. The heterologous virus recombination between snowshoe hare and La Crosse viruses has been shown to involve genome segment reassortment. Analyses of SSH-LAC recombinant viruses have shown that the bunyavirus S RNA codes for N protein while the M RNA codes for G1 and G2 glycoproteins.

From two viruses with three segments of genetic information one would expect to obtain for each of them three recombination groups of *ts* mutants, and in heterologous crosses generate $2^3 - 2$ (i.e., six) new genotypes. For snowshoe hare, La Crosse, Trivittatus, and Guaroa viruses only two groups of *ts* mutants have been obtained for each virus serotype, and so far only four SSH-LAC recombinants (SSH/LAC/ LAC, SSH/LAC/SSH, LAC/LAC/SSH, SSH/SSH/LAC) have been generated by mixed mutant virus infections. The reasons for the lack of a third recombination group of mutants and the reasons for restricted recombination need to be studied.

5. DEFECTIVE INTERFERING VIRUS

The possibility of interference in the ability of bunyaviruses to produce infectious virus has been inferred from high multiplicity of infection experiments with La Crosse virus (Obijeski *et al.*, 1976*a*). Whether interference involves the production of progeny with greater than normal amounts of one or another of the viral RNA species (e.g., the S RNA as suggested by Kascsak and Lyons, 1977) and/or the production (and incorporation into virions) of deletion derivatives of one or other of the RNA species remains to be determined. Defective virus with lesser or greater than normal quantities of particular RNA species may be a frequent occurrence based on the variable RNA ratios observed in many preparations of bunyaviruses (see Section 2.2.6j).

6. CONCLUSIONS

The Bunyaviridae are a complex and diverse family of arboviruses. Although morphological, morphogenetic, structural, and certain serological studies indicate that the member viruses are comparable to each other, it is evident both from the diverse nature of the hosts and vectors which can be infected by particular bunyaviruses, and from the limited genetic studies which have been performed, that the various bunyavirus types have evolved in many different directions—presumably by adaptation to particular ecological niches.

Transmission studies suggest that at least certain bunyaviruses could persist in insect populations from year to year without the need for passage in a vertebrate host. Vertebrate hosts may serve (1) for amplification and translocation of the viruses (e.g., as carriers of infected ticks or when viremic by virtue of their habits), or (2) for selection of bunyavirus variants that can productively infect that species of vertebrate, or (3) as a medium in which recombinant viruses are generated. It is possible that the arthropod vector is a preferred medium in which recombinant viruses are formed in view of (1) the limited time of a vertebrate host viremia (for those viruses that have been studied), and (2) the persistent infection in the arthropod species. Whether recombination can be induced in arthropods remains to be determined.

The restriction against recombinant formation that appparently exists needs to be investigated more thoroughly. Both its cause and relationship to gene product functions, and morphogenesis of the viruses, will have to be studied further.

ACKNOWLEDGMENTS

We thank numerous colleagues for consultation and their permission to use unpublished data, and Drs. F. A. Murphy, C.-H. von Bonsdorff, M. S. Hewlett, D. Baltimore, and R. F. Pettersson for electron micrographs used in the text. Studies conducted in our laboratories and reported herein were aided by U.S. Public Health Service Grants A1 13402 and A1 10984, National Science Foundation Grant PCM76-22218, U.S. Army Medical Research and Development Command Contracts DAMD17-78-C-8017 and DADA17-72-C-2170, and the World Health Organization.

Frequent reference is made in the text to the *International Catalogue of Arboviruses* and its supplemental issues (Berge, 1975; Berge *et al.*, 1970, 1971; Karabatsos, 1978; Taylor, 1967) rather than to primary sources. This has been done to minimize the already long list of references and not in any way to slight the many dedicated scientists who have contributed to the study of bunyaviruses. We would like to acknowledge their contributions, many of which have been in the form of personal communications to the *Catalogue*.

7. REFERENCES

Aitken, T. H. G., Woodall, J. P., Andrade, A. H. P., de Bensabath, G., and Shope, R. E., 1975, Pacui virus, phlebotomine flies, and small mammals in Brazil: An epidemiological study, *Am. J. Trop. Med. Hyg.* **24**:358.

Albanese, M., Di Cuonzo, G., Randazzo, G., Srihongse, S., and Tringali, G., 1971. Survey for arbovirus antibodies in domestic animals of western Sicily, *Ann. Sclavo.* **13**:641.

Albanese, M., Bruno-Smiraglia, C., Di Cuonzo, G., Lavagnino, A., and Srihongse, S., 1972, Isolation of Thogoto virus from *Rhipicephalus bursa* ticks in western Sicily, *Acta Virol.* **16**:267.

Alexander, R. A., 1951, Rift Valley Fever in the Union, *J. S. Afr. Vet. Med. Assoc.* **22**:105.

Anderson, C. R., Aitken, T. H. G., Spence, L. P., and Downs, W. G., 1960a, Kairi virus, a new virus from Trinidadian forest mosquitoes, *Am. J. Trop. Med. Hyg.* **9**:70.

Anderson, C. R., Spence, L. P., Downs, W. G., and Aitken, T. H. G., 1960b, Manzanilla virus: A new virus isolated from the blood of a howler monkey in Trinidad, West Indies, *Am. J. Trop. Med. Hyg.* **9**:78.

Anderson, C. R., Spence, L., Downs, W. G., and Aitken, T. H. G., 1961, Oropouche virus: A new human disease agent from Trinidad, West Indies, *Am. J. Trop. Med. Hyg.* **10**:574.

Andrews, W. N., Rowley, W. A., Wong, Y. W., Dorsey, D. C., and Hausler, W. J., 1977, Isolation of Trivittatus virus from larvae and adults reared from field-collected larvae of *Aedes trivittatus* (Diptera: Culicidae), *J. Med. Entomol.* **13**:699.

Anslow, R. O., Thompson, W. H., Thompson, P. H., De Foliart, G. R., Papadopoulos, O., and Hanson, R. P., 1969, Isolation of Bunyamwera-group viruses from Wisconsin mosquitoes, *Am. J. Trop. Med. Hyg.* **18**:599.

Balducci, M., Verani, P., Lopes, M. C., and Gregorig, B., 1973, Isolation in Italy of Bahig and Matruh viruses (Tete group) from migratory birds, *Ann. Microbiol. (Paris)* **124B**:213.

Balfour, H. H. Jr., Edelman, C. K., Cook, F. E., Barton, W. I., Buzicky, A. W., Siem, R. A., and Bauer, H., 1975, Isolates of California encephalitis (La Crosse) virus from field-collected eggs and larvae of *Aedes triseriatus*: Identification of the overwintering site of California encephalitis, *J. Infect. Dis.* **131**:712.

Balfour, H. H. Jr., Edelman, C. K., Bauer, H., and Siem, R. A., 1976, California arbovirus (La Crosse) infections. III. Epidemiology of California encephalitis in Minnesota, *J. Infect. Dis.* **133**:293.

Bardos, V., and Cupkova, E., 1962, The Calovo virus: The second virus isolated from mosquitoes in Czechoslovakia, *J. Hyg. Epidemiol. Microbiol. Immunol.* **6**:186.

Bardos, V., and Danielova, V., 1959, The Tahyna virus—a virus isolated from mosquitoes in Czechoslovakia, *J. Hyg. Epidemiol. Microbiol. Immunol.* **3**:264.

Bardos, V., and Danielova, V., 1961, A study of the relationship between Tahyna virus and *Aedes vexans* in natural conditions, *Cesk. Epidemiol. Mikrobiol. Immunol.* **10**:389.

Bardos, V., Adamcova, J., Sefcovicova, L., and Cervenka, J., 1962, Antibodies neutralizing Tahyna virus in different age-groups of inhabitants of an area with mass prevalence of mosquitoes, *Cesk. Epidemiol. Mikrobiol. Immunol.* **11**:238.

Bardos, V., Ryba, J., and Hubalek, Z., 1975, Isolation of Tahyna virus from field collected *Culiseta annulata* (Schrk) larvae, *Acta Virol.* **19**:446.

Barnard, B. J. H., and Botha, M. J., 1977, An inactivated Rift Valley fever vaccine, *J. S. Afr. Vet. Assoc.* **48**:45.

Barnett, H. C., and Suyemoto, W., 1961, Field studies on Sandfly Fever and Kalaazar in Pakistan, in Iran, and in Baltistan (Little Tibet) Kashmir, *Trans. N.Y. Acad. Sci. Ser. II* **23**:609.

Bartelloni, P. J., and Tesh, R. B., 1976, Clinical and serologic responses of volunteers infected with Phlebotomus fever virus (Sicilian Type), *Am. J. Trop. Med. Hyg.* **25**:456.

Beaty, B. J., and Thompson, W. H., 1975, Emergence of La Crosse virus from endemic foci: Fluorescent antibody studies of overwintered *Aedes triseriatus*, *Am. J. Trop. Med. Hyg.* **24**:685.

Beaty, B. J., and Thompson, W. H., 1976, Delineation of La Crosse virus in developmental stages of transovarially infected *Aedes triseriatus*, *Am. J. Trop. Med. Hyg.* **25**:505.

Beaty, B. J., and Thompson, W. H., 1977, Tropisms of La Crosse virus in *Aedes triseriatus* following infective blood meals, *J. Med. Entomol.* **14**:499.

Begum, F., Wisseman, C. L. Jr., and Casals, J., 1970a, Tick-borne viruses of West Pakistan. II. Hazara virus, a new agent isolated from *Ixodes Redikorzevi* ticks from the Kaghan valley, W. Pakistan, *Am. J. Epidemiol.* **92**:192.

Begum, F., Wisseman, C. L. Jr., and Casals, J., 1970b, Tick-borne viruses of West Pakistan. IV. Viruses similar to, or identical with, Crimean hemorrhagic fever (Congo-Semunya), Wad Medani and Pak Argas 461 isolated from ticks of the Changa Manga forest, Lahore district, and of Hunza, Gilgit Agency, W. Pakistan, 1970, *Am. J. Epidemiol.* **92**:197.

Begum, R., Wisseman, C. L. Jr., and Traub, R., 1970c, Tick-borne viruses of West Pakistan. I. Isolation and general characteristics, *Am. J. Epidemiol.* **92**:180.

Behbehani, A. M., Hiller, M. S., Lenahan, M. F., and Wenner, H. A., 1967, Responses of monkeys to California encephalitis, Sicilian sandfly, and Turlock arboviruses, *Am. J. Trop. Med. Hyg.* **16**:63.

Berge, T. O. (ed.), 1975, *International Catalogue of Arboviruses Including Certain Other Viruses of Vertebrates*, DHEW Publication No. CDC, 75-8301, Washington, D.C.

Berge, T. O., Shope, R. E., and Work, T. H., 1970, The Subcommittee on Information Exchange of the American Committee on Arthropod-borne viruses. Catalogue of arthropod-borne viruses of the world, *Am. J. Trop. Med. Hyg.* **19**:1079.

Berge, T. O., Chamberlain, R. W., Shope, R. E., and Work, T. H., 1971, The Subcommittee on Information Exchange of the American Committee on Arthropod-borne viruses, Catalogue of arthropod-borne and selected vertebrate viruses of the world, *Am. J. Trop. Med. Hyg.* **20**:1018.

Berry, R. L., Lalonde, B. J., Stegmiller, H. W., Parsons, M. A., and Bear, G. T., 1974, Isolation of La Crosse virus (California encephalitis group) from field collected *Aedes triseriatus* (Say) larvae in Ohio (Diptera: Culicidae), *Mosq. News* **34**:454.

Bhatt, P. N., Kulkarni, K. G., Boshell, J., Rajagopalan, P. K., Patil, A. P., Goverdhan, M. K., and Pavri, K. M., 1966, Kaisodi virus, a new agent isolated from *Haemaphysalis spinigera* in Mysore State, South India. I. Isolation of strains, *Am. J. Trop. Med. Hyg.* **15**:958.

Binn, L. N., Randall, R., Harrison, V. R., Gibbs, C. J., Jr., and Aulisio, C. G., 1963, The serological reactions in a case of Rift Valley Fever, *Am. J. Trop. Med. Hyg.* **12**:236.

Blood, D. C., 1956, Arthogryposis and hydraencephaly in newborn calves, *Aust. Vet. J.* **32**:125.

Bond, J. O., Hammon, W. McD., Lewis, A. L., Sather, G. E., and Taylor, D. J., 1966, California group arboviruses in Florida and report of a new strain, Keystone virus, *Public Health Rep.* **81**:607.

Bonner, W. M., and Laskey, R. A., 1974, A film detection method for tritium-labelled proteins and nucleic acids in polyacrylamide gels, *Eur. J. Biochem.* **46**:83.

Boshnell, J., Desai, P. K., Dandawate, C. N., and Goverdhan, M. K., 1970, Isolation of Ganjam virus from ticks *Haemaphysalis intermedia*, *Indian J. Med. Res.* **58**:561.

Bouloy, M., and Hannoun, C., 1973, Effet de l'actinomycine D sur la multiplication du virus Tahyna, *Ann. Microbiol. (Inst. Pasteur)* **124b**:547.

Bouloy, M., and Hannoun, C., 1976a, Studies on Lumbo virus replication. I. RNA-dependent RNA polymerase associated with virions, *Virology* **69**:258.

Bouloy, M., and Hannoun, C., 1976b, Studies on Lumbo virus replication. II. Properties of viral ribonucleoproteins and characterization of messenger RNAs, *Virology* **71**:363.

Bouloy, M., Krams-Ozden, S., Horodniceanu, F., and Hannoun, C., 1973/1974, Three segment RNA genome of Lumbo virus (bunyavirus), *Intervirology* **2**:173.

Bouloy, M., Colbere, F., Krams-Ozden, S., Vialat, P., Garapin, A. C., and Hannoun, C., 1975, Activité RNA polymerasique associée à un Bunyavirus (Lumbo), *C. R. Acad. Sci. Paris* **280**:213.

Bres, P., Williams, M. C., and Chambon, L., 1966, Isolation of a new arbo-virus prototype the "Tataguine" strain (IPD/A 252) in Senegal, *Ann. Inst. Pasteur* **111**:585.

Brummer-Korvenkontio, M., 1969, in: Arboviruses of the California complex and the Bunyamwera group, *Proc. Smolenice Symp. Slovak Acad. Sci. Bratislava*, p. 131.

Brummer-Korvenkontio, M., 1973*a*, Arboviruses in Finalnd. V. Serological survey of antibodies against Inkoo virus (California group) in human, cow, reindeer, and wild life sera, *Am. J. Trop. Med. Hyg.* **22**:654.

Brummer-Korvenkontio, M., 1973*b*, Batai (Calovo) arbovirus neutralising antibodies in Finland, *Ann. Med. Exp. Biol. Fenn.* **51**:158.

Brummer-Korvenkontio, M., Saikku, P., Korheonen, P., Ulmanen, I., Reunala, T., and Karvonen, J., 1973, Arboviruses in Finland. IV. Isolation and characterization of Inkoo virus, a Finnish representative of the California group, *Am. J. Trop. Med. Hyg.* **22**:404.

Buckley, S. M., 1974, Cross plaque neutralization tests with cloned Crimean hemorrhagic fever-Congo (CHF-C) and Hazara viruses, *Proc. Soc. Exp. Biol. Med.* **146**:594.

Burgdorfer, W., Newhouse, V. F., and Thomas, L. A., 1961, Isolation of a California encephalitis virus from the blood of a snowshoe hare (*Lepus americanus*) in western Montana, *Am. J. Hyg.* **73**:344.

Calisher, C. H., and Goodpasture, H. C., 1975, Human infection with Bhanja virus, *Amer. J. Trop. Med. Hyg.* **24**:1040.

Calisher, C. H., Kokernot, R. H., de Moore, J. F., Boyd, K. R., Hayes, J., and Chappell, W. A., 1969, Arbovirus studies in the Ohio-Mississippi Basin, 1964–1967. VI. Mermet: A Simbu-group arbovirus, *Am. J. Trop. Med. Hyg.* **18**:779.

Calisher, C. H., Chappell, W. A., Maness, K. S. C., Lord, R. D., and Sudia, W. D., 1971, Isolations of Nepuyo virus strains from Honduras, 1967, *Am. J. Trop. Med. Hyg.* **20**:331.

Calisher, C. H., Sasso, D. R., Maness, K. S. C., Gheorghiu, V. N., and Shope, R. E., 1973, Relationships of *Anopheles A* group arboviruses, *Proc. Soc. Exp. Biol. Med.* **143**:465.

Calisher, C. H., Lindsey, H. S., Ritter, D. G., and Sommerman, K. M., 1974, Northway virus: A new Bunyamwera group arbovirus from Alaska, *Can. J. Microbiol.* **20**:219.

Calisher, C. H., McLean, R. G., Smith, G. C., Szmyd, D. M., Muth, D. J., and Lazuick, J. S., 1977, Rio Grande—A new Phlebotomus fever group virus from south Texas, *Am. J. Trop. Med. Hyg.* **26**:997.

Carey, D. E., Reuben, R., Myers, R. M., and George, S., 1968, Japanese encephalitis studies in Vellore, South India. IV. Search for virological evidence of infection in animals other than man, *Indian J. Med. Res.* **56**:1340.

Casals, J., 1963, New developments in the classification of arthropod-borne animal viruses. *Ann. Microbiol.* **11**:13.

Casals, J., 1968, Filtration of arboviruses through 'Millipore' membranes, *Nature (London)* **217**:648.

Casals, J., 1969, Antigenic similarity between the virus causing Crimean hemorrhagic fever and Congo virus (33847), *Proc. Soc. Exp. Biol. Med.* **131**:233.

Casals, J., 1971, Arboviruses: Incorporation in a general system of virus classification, in: *Comparative Virology* (K. Maramorosch and E. Kurstak, eds.), p. 307, Academic Press, New York.

Casals, J., 1972, Serological and physio-chemical considerations, in: *International Symposium on Tick-borne Viruses* (*Excluding Group B*), p.13, Publishing House of the Slovak Academy of Sciences, Bratislava.

Casals, J., 1978, Crimean-Congo hemorrhagic fever, in: *Proceedings of the International Colloquium on Ebola-virus Infection and Other Hemorrhagic Fevers* (S. R. Pattyn, ed.), Prince Leopold Institute of Tropical Medicine, Antwerp, Belgium.

Casals, J., and Brown, L. V., 1954. Hemagglutination with arthropod-borne viruses, *J. Exp. Med.* **99**:429.

Casals, J., and Tignor, G. H., 1974, Neutralization and hemagglutination-inhibition tests with Crimean hemorrhagic fever–Congo virus, *Proc. Soc. Exp. Biol. Med.* **145**:960.

Casals, J., and Whitman, L., 1960, A new antigenic group of arthropod-borne viruses, the Bunyamwera group, *Am. J. Trop. Med. Hyg.* **9**:73.

Casals, J., and Whitman, L., 1961, Group C, a new serological group of hitherto undescribed arthropod-borne viruses. Immunological studies, *Am. J. Trop. Med. Hyg.* **10**:250.

Casals, J., Hoogstraal, H., Johnson, D. M., Shelokov, A., Wiebenga, N. H., and Work, T. H., 1966, A current appraisal of hemorrhagic fevers in the USSR, *Am. J. Trop. Med. Hyg.* **15**:751.

Causey, O. R., and Shope, R. E., 1965, Icoaraci, a new virus related to Naples phlebotomus fever virus, *Proc. Soc. Exp. Biol. Med.* **118**:420.

Causey, O. R., Causey, C. E., Maroja, O. M., and Macedo, D. G., 1961, The isolation of arthropod-borne viruses, including members of two hitherto undescribed serological groups, in the Amazon region of Brazil, *Am. J. Trop. Med. Hyg.* **10**:227.

Causey, O. R., Shope, R. E., and Rodrigues, A., 1962, The isolation of Guaroa virus by liver biopsy from a patient suffering from paralysis, *Rev. Serv. Espec. Saude Publica* **12**:55.

Causey, O. R., Kemp, G. E. Madbouly, M. H., and Lee, V. H., 1969, Arbovirus surveillance in Nigeria, 1964–1967, *Bull. Soc. Pathol. Exot.* **62**:249.

Causey, O. R., Kemp, G. E., Madbouly, M. H., and David-West, T. S., 1970, Congo virus from domestic livestock, African hedgegog, and arthropods in Nigeria, *Am. J. Trop. Med.* **19**:846.

Causey, O. R., Kemp, G. E., Casals, J., Williams, R. W., and Madbouly, M. H., 1971, Dugbe virus, a new arbovirus from Nigeria, *Niger. J. Sci.* **5**:41.

Causey, O. R., Kemp, G. E., Causey, C. E., and Lee, V. H., 1972, Isolations of Simbu-group viruses in Ibadan, Nigeria 1964–69, including the new types Sango, Shamonda, Sabo, and Shuni, *Ann. Trop. Med. Parasitol.* **66**:357.

Chamberlain, R. W., 1963, Anophelines as arbovirus vectors of Tensaw virus in southeastern USA, *Ann. Microbiol.* **11**:89.

Chamberlain, R. W., Sudia, W. D., and Coleman, P. H., 1969, Isolations of an arbovirus of the Bunyamwera group (Tensaw Virus) from mosquitoes in the southeastern United States, *Am. J. Trop. Med. Hyg.* **18**:92.

Chumakov, M. P., 1946, in: *Crimean Hemorrhagic Fever*, p. 26, Krymizdat, Simpheropol.

Chumakov, M. P., 1947, A new virus disease, Crimean hemorrhagic fever, *News Med. Virus Dis.* **4**:9.

Chumakov, M. P., 1963, Studies of virus haemorrhagic fevers, *J. Hyg. Epidemiol. Microbiol. Immunol.* **7**:125.

Chumakov, M. P. (ed.), 1969a, in: *Etiology, Epidemiology and Clinical Manifestations of Crimean Hemorrhagic Fever and West Nile Fever*, Acad. Med. Sci., U.S.S.R., Astrakhan Dist., San. Epidemiol. Serv.

Chumakov, M. P., 1969b, *Vth Symposium on the Study of the Role of Migrating Birds in the Distribution of Arboviruses*, Novosibersk 1969, Acad. Sci. U.S.S.R., Siberian Branch.

Chumakov, M. P., 1973, On the results of investigations of the etiology and epidemiology of Crimean hemorrhagic fever in the USSR. *9th Int. Congr. Trop. Med. Malaria*, Vol. 1: *Abstracts of Invited Papers*, p. 33, Athens.

Chumakov, M. P., and Donets, M. A., 1975, Virion and subvirion constituents of Crimean hemorrhagic fever virus, *Int. Virol.* **3**:193.

Chumakov, M. P., Smirnova, S. E., and Tkachenko, E. A., 1969, Antigenic relationships between Soviet strains of Crimean hemorrhagic fever virus and Afro-Asian strains of Congo virus (in Russian), in: *Materials 16th Sci. Conf. USSR AMS Inst. Poliomyelitis Virus Encephalitides*, Vol. 2, pp. 152–154, Moscow.

Chumakov, M. P., Smirnova, S. E., and Tkachenko, E. A., 1970, Antigenic relationships between strains of Crimean heamorrhagic fever and Congo viruses, *Acta Virol.* **14**:82.

Clewley, J., Gentsch, J., and Bishop, D. H. L., 1977, Three unique viral RNA species of snowshoe hare and La Crosse bunyaviruses, *J. Virol.* **22**:459.

Coetzer, J. A. W., and Barnard, B. J. H., 1977, Hydrops amnii in sheep associated with hydranencephaly and arthrogryposis with Wesselbron disease and Rift Valley fever viruses as aetiological agents, *Onderstepoort J. Vet. Res.* **44**:119.

Coleman, P. H., 1969, Tensaw virus, a new member of the Bunyamwera arbovirus group from the southern United States, *Am. J. Trop. Med. Hyg.* **18**:81.

Coleman, P. H., Ryder, S., and Work, T. H., 1969, Mahogany Hammock virus, a new Guama group arbovirus from the Florida Everglades, *Am. J. Epidemiol.* **89**:217.

Converse, J. D., Hoogstraal, H., Moussa, M. I., and Bafort, J. M., 1974a, Isolation of Dugbe virus from *Amblyomma variegatum* ticks in Cameroun, *Tr. R. Soc. Trop. Med. Hyg.* **68**:411.

Converse, J. D., Hoogstraal, H., Moussa, M. I., Stek, M. Jr., and Kaiser, M. N., 1974b, Bahig virus (Tete group) in naturally and transovarially infected *Hyalomma marginatum* ticks from Egypt and Italy, *Arch. Gesamte Virusforsch.* **46**:29.

Coverdale, O. R., Cybinski, D. H., and St. George, T. D., 1978, Congenital abnormalities in calves associated with Akabane virus and Aino virus, *Aust. Vet. J.* **54**:151.

Cramblett, H. G., Stegmiller, H., and Spencer, C., 1966, California encephalitis virus infections in children: Clinical and laboratory studies, *J. Am. Med. Assoc.* **198**:108.

Crane, G. T., Elbel, R. E., and Calisher, C. H., 1977, Transovarial transmission of California encephalitis virus in the mosquito *Aedes dorsalis* at Blue Lake, Utah, *Mosq. News* **37**:479.

Cupkova, E., 1971, Comparative serological studies of some strains of Tahyna virus, Part I, *J. Hyg. Epidemiol. Microbiol. Immunol.* **15**:66.

Dahlberg, J. E., Obijeski, J. F., and Korb, J., 1977, Electron microscopy of the segmented RNA genome of La Crosse virus: Absence of circular molecules, *J. Virol.* **22**:203.

Dandawate, C. N., and Shah, K. V., 1969, Ganjam virus: A new arbovirus isolated from ticks *Haemaphysalis intermedia* Warburton and Nuttall, 1909 in Orissa, India, *Indian J. Med. Res.* **57**:799.

Dandawate, C. N., Rajagopalan, P. K., Pavri, K. M., and Work, T. H., 1969, Virus isolations from mosquitoes collected in North Arcot district, Madras State, and Chittoor district, Andhra Pradesh between November 1955 and October 1957, *Indian J. Med. Res.* **57**:1420.

Daubney, R., Hudson, J. R., and Garnham, P. C., 1931, Enzootic hepatitis or Rift Valley fever. An undescribed virus disease of sheep, cattle, and man from East Africa, *J. Pathol. Bacteriol.* **34**:545.

David-West, T. S., 1974, Polyacrylamide gel electrophoresis of Dunbe virus infected cells, *Micribios* **11**:21.

David-West, T. S., Labzoffsky, N. A., and Hamvas, J. J., 1972, Electron microscopy of virus IB AR 1972 (Dugbe), *W. Afr. Med. J.* **21**:10.

David-West, T. S., Cooke, A. R., and David-West, A. S., 1974, Seroepidemiology of Congo virus (related to the virus of Crimean haemorrhagic fever) in Nigeria, *Bull. WHO* **51**:543.

Davies, F. G., 1975, Observations on the epidemiology of Rift Valley Fever in Kenya, *J. Hyg.* **75**:219.

De Foliart, G. R., Anslow, R. O., Hanson, R. P., Morris, C. D., Papadopoulos, O., and Sather, G. E., 1969, Isolations of Jamestown Canyon serotype of California encephalitis virus from naturally infected *Aedes* mosquitoes and Tabanids, *Am. J. Trop. Med. Hyg.* **18**:440.

De Paola, D., 1963, Pathology of the arboviruses (mouse, man), in: Proceedings of the Seventh International Congress on Tropical Medicine and Malaria, Rio de Janerio, *An. Microbiol.* **11**:187.

De Rodaniche, E., De Andrade, A. P., and Galindo, P., 1964, Isolation of two antigenically distinct arthropod-borne viruses of group C in Panama, *Am. J. Trop. Med. Hyg.* **13**:839.

De Wachter, R., and Fiers, W., 1972, Preparative two-dimensional polyacrylamide gel electrophoresis of ^{32}P-labeled RNA, *Anal. Biochem.* **49**:184.

Digoutte, J. P., Bres, P., Nguyen Trung Luong, and Durand, B., 1969, Isolement du virus Tataguine à partir de deux cas de fièvres exanthematiques, *Bull. Soc. Pathol. Exot.* **62**:72.

Digoutte, J. P., Pajot, F. X., Henderson, B. E., Bres, P., and Nguyen Trung Luong, P., 1970, Le virus M'Poko (BA365). Nouveau prototype d'arbovirus isolé en Centrafrique, *Ann. Inst. Pasteur*, **119**:512.

Doerr, R. and Russ, V. K., 1909, Weitere Untersuchungen über das Pappataci Fieber, *Arch. Schiffs. Trop. Hyg.* **13**:693.

Doerr, R., Franz, K., and Taussig, S., 1909, *Das Pappataci Fieber*, Deuticke, Leipzig.

Doherty, R. L., Carley, J. G., Mackerras, M. J., and Marks, E. N., 1963, Studies of arthropod-borne virus infections in Queensland. III. Isolation and characterization of virus strains from wild-caught mosquitoes in north Queensland, *Aust. J. Exp. Biol. Med. Sci.* **41**:17.

Doherty, R. L., Whitehead, R. H., Wetters, E. J., and Gorman, B. M., 1968, Studies of the epidemiology of arthropod-borne virus infections at Mitchell River Mission, Cape York Peninsula, North Queensland. II. Arbovirus infections of mosquitoes, man and domestic fowls, 1963–1966, *Tr. R. Soc. Trop. Med. Hyg.* **62**:430.

Doherty, R. L., Whitehead, R. H., Wetters, E. J., Gorman, B. M., and Carley, J. G., 1970, A survey of antibody to 10 arboviruses (Koongol group, Mapputta group and ungrouped) isolated in Queensland, *Tr. R. Soc. Trop. Med. Hyg.* **64**:748.

Doherty, R. L., Carley, J. G., Standfast, H. A., Dyce, A. L., and Snowdon, W. A., 1972, Virus strains isolated from arthropods during an epizootic of bovine ephemeral fever in Queensland, *Aust. Vet. J.* **48**:81.

Doherty, R. L., Carley, J. G., Murray, M. D., Main, A. J., Kay, S. H., and Domrow, R., 1975, Isolation of arboviruses (Kemerovo group, Sakhalin group) from *Ixodes uriae* collected at Macquarie Island, Southern Ocean, *Am. J. Trop. Med. Hyg.* **24**:521.

Donchev, D., Kebedzhiev, G., and Rusakiev, M., 1974, *Misc. Publ.* **9**:194.

Donets, M. A., and Chumakov, M. P., 1975, Several characteristics of the virions of the viruses Crimean hemorrhagic fever and Congo, in: *Voprosi Medical Virology* (Transactions of the Institute of Poliomyelitis and Viral Encephalitis), p. 287, Moscow.

Donets, M. A., Chumakov, M. P., Korolev, M. B., and Rubin, S. G., 1977a, Physicochemical characteristics, morphology and morphogenesis of virions of the causative agent of Crimean hemorrhagic fever, *Intervirology* **8**:294.

Donets, M. A., Korolev, M. B., and Chumakov, M. P., 1977b, Study of physicochemical properties, morphology and morphogenesis of arboviruses of the CHF (Crimean hemorrhagic fever) Congo group to determine the taxonomic position of these agents in the modern classification system, *Vestn. Akad. Med. Nauk. SSSR* **5**:28.

Edelsten, R. M., 1975, The distribution and prevalence of Nairobi sheep disease and other tick-borne infections of sheep and goats in northern Somalia, *Trop. Anim. Health Prod.* **7**:29.

El Said, L. H., Vorndam, V., Gentsch, J. R., Clewley, J. P., Calisher, C. H., Klimas, R. A., Thompson, W. H., Grayson, M., Trent, D. W., and Bishop, D. H. L., 1979, A comparison of La Crosse virus isolates obtained from different ecological niches and an analysis of the structural components of California encephalitis serogroup viruses and other bunyaviruses, *Am. J. Trop. Med. Hyg.* **28**:364.

Embil, J. A., Embree, J. E., Artsob, H., Spence, L., and Rozee, K. R., 1978, Antibodies to snowshoe hare virus of the California group in the snowshoe hare (*Lepus americanus*) population of Nova Scotia, *Am. J. Trop. Med. Hyg.* **27**:843.

Fagbami, A. H., Monath, T. P., Tomori, O., Lee, V. H., and Fabiyi, A., 1972, Studies on Tataguine infection in Nigeria, *Trop. Geogr. Med.* **24**:298.

Fagbami, A. H., Tomori, O., Fabiyi, A., and Isoun, T. T., 1975, Experimental Rift Valley fever in West African dwarf sheep, *Res. Vet. Sci.* **18**:334.

Fenner, F., 1976a, Classification and nomenclature of viruses, *Intervirology* **7**:1.

Fenner, F., 1976b, The classification and nomenclature of viruses. Summary of results of meetings of the International Committee on Taxonomy of Viruses in Madrid, September 1975, *Virology* **71**:371.

Fenner, F., Pereira, H. G., Porterfield, J. S., Joklik, W. K., and Downie, A. W., 1974, Family and generic names for viruses approved by the International Committee on Taxonomy of Viruses, June 1974, *Intervirology* **3**:193.

Fields, B. N., Henderson, B. E., Coleman, P. H., and Work, T. H., 1969, Pahayokee and Shark River, two new arboviruses related to Patois and Zegla from the Florida Everglades, *Am. J. Epidemiol.* **89**:222.

Flamand, A., and Bishop, D. H. L., 1974, *In vivo* synthesis of RNA by vesicular stomatitis virus and its mutants, *J. Mol. Biol.* **87**:31.

Gaidamovich, S. Y., Nikiforov, L. P., Gromashevsky, V. L., Obukhova, V. F., Klisenko, G. A., Chervonsky, V. I., and Melnikova, E. E., 1971*a*, Isolation and study of Sumakh virus, a member of the Uukuniemi group, in the U.S.S.R., *Acta Virol.* **15**:155.

Gaidamovich, S. Y., Vinograd, I. A., and Obukhova, V. R., 1971*b*, Isolation in Southwest Ukraine of viruses of the Uukuniemi group, *Acta Virol.* **15**:333.

Gaidamovich, S. Y., Kiryushchenko, T. V., Peikre, E. Y., and Vasilenko, V. A., 1973, Detection of antibodies to Sumakh-Uukunemi virus in birds in the complement fixation inhibition test, *Acta Virol.* **17**:69.

Gaidamovich, S. Y., Kurakhmedova, S. A., and Melnikova, E. E., 1974, Aetiology of Phlebotomus fever in Ashkabad studied in retrospect, *Acta Virol.* **18**:508.

Galindo, P., and Srihongse, S., 1967, Transmission of arboviruses to hamsters by the bite of naturally infected *Culex* (*Melanoconicon*) mosquitoes, *Am. J. Trop. Med. Hyg.* **16**:525.

Gard, G., Marshall, I.D., and Woodroofe, G. B., 1973, Annual recurrent epidemic polyarthritis and Ross River virus activity in a coastal area of New South Wales. II. Mosquitoes, viruses and wildlife, *Am. J. Trop. Med. Hyg.* **22**:551.

Garoff, H., and Simons, K., 1974, Location of the spike glycoproteins in the Semliki Forest virus membrane, *Proc. Natl. Acad. Sci. USA* **71**:3988.

Gauld, L. W., Hanson, R. P., Thompson, W. H., and Sinha, S. K., 1974, Observations of a natural cycle of La Crosse virus (California group) in south western Wisconsin, *Am. J. Trop. Med. Hyg.* **23**:983.

Gauld, L. W., Yuill, T. M., Hanson, R. P., and Sinha, S. K., 1975, Isolation of La Crosse virus (California encephalitis group) from the chipmunk (*Tamias striatus*), an amplifier host, *Am. J. Trop. Med. Hyg.* **24**:999.

Gear, J., de Meillon, B., Measroch, V., and Davis, D. H. S., 1955, Rift Valley fever in South Africa. 2. The occurrence of human cases in the Orange-free State, the Northwestern Cape Province, the Western and Southern Transvaal. B. Field and laboratory investigations, *S. Afr. Med. J.* **25**:908.

Gentsch, J., and Bishop, D. H. L., 1976, Recombination and complementation between temperature sensitive mutants of the bunyavirus, snowshoe hare virus, *J. Virol.* **20**:351.

Gentsch, J., and Bishop, D. H. L., 1978, The small viral RNA segment of bunyaviruses codes for the viral nucleocapsid (N) protein, *J. Virol.* **28**:417.

Gentsch, J., and Bishop, D. H. L., 1979, The M RNA segment of bunyaviruses codes for two glycoproteins, G1 and G2, *J. Virol.* **30**:767.

Gentsch, J., Bishop, D. H. L., and Obijeski, J. F., 1977*a*, The virus particle nucleic acids and proteins of four bunyaviruses, *J. Gen. Virol.* **34**:257.

Gentsch, J., Wynne, L. R., Clewley, J. P., Shope, R. E., and Bishop, D. H. L., 1977*b*, Formation of recombinants between snowshoe hare and La Crosse bunyaviruses, *J. Virol.* **24**:893.

George, J. E., 1971, Isolation of Phlebotomus fever virus from *Phlebotomus papatasi* and determination of the host ranges of sandflies (*Diptera: Psychodidae*) in West Pakistan, *J. Med. Entomol.* **7**:670.

Goldman, N., Presser, I., and Sreevalsan, T., 1977, California encephalitis virus: Some biological and biochemical properties, *Virology* **76**:352.

Goverdhan, M. K., Dhanda, V., Modi, G. B., Bhatt, P. N., Bhagwat, R. B., Dandawate, C. N., and Pavri, K. M., 1976, Isolation of *Phlebotomus* (sand fly) fever from sandflies and humans during the same season in Aurangabad district, Maharashtra State, India, *Indian J. Med. Res.* **64**:57.

Granboulan, N., and Girard, M., 1969, Molecular weight of poliovirus ribonucleic acid, *J. Virol.* **4**:475.

Grimes, J. E., Garza, E. H., and Irons, J. V., 1962, *Abstr. Annu. Meet. Am. Soc. Trop. Med. Hyg.*

Grimstad, P., Craig, G. B., Ross, Q. E., and Yuill, T. M., 1977, *Aedes triseriatus* and La Crosse virus: Geographic variation in vector susceptibility and ability to transmit, *Am. J. Trop. Med. Hyg.* **26**:990.

Groot, H., Oya, A., Bernal, C., and Barreto-Reyes, P., 1959, Guaroa virus, a new agent isolated in Colombia, South America, *Am. J. Trop. Med. Hyg.* **8**:604.

Haig, D. A., Woodall, J. P., and Danskin, D., 1965, Thogoto virus: A hitherto undescribed agent isolated from ticks in Kenya, *J. Gen. Microbiol.* **38**:389.

Hammon, W. McD., and Reeves, W. C., 1952, California encephalitis virus, a newly described agent. I. Evidence of natural infection in man and other animals, *Calif. Med.* **77**:303.

Hammon, W. McD., and Sather, G., 1966, History and recent reappearance of viruses in the California encephalitis group, *Am. J. Trop. Med. Hyg.* **15**:199.

Hammon, W. McD., Reeves, W. C., and Sather, G., 1952, California encephalitis virus, a newly described agent. II. Isolations and attempts to identify and characterize the agent. *J. Immunol.* **69**:493.

Hannoun, C., Corniou, B., and Rageou, J., 1970, Isolation in Southern France and characterization of new tick-borne viruses related to Uukuniemi: Grand Arabaud and Ponteves, *Acta Virol.* **14**:167.

Hardy, J. L., Scrivani, R. P., Lyness, R. N., Nelson, R. L., and Roberts, D. R., 1970, Ecologic studies on buttonwillow virus in Kern County, California, *Am. J. Trop. Med. Hyg.* **19**:552.

Hartley, W. J., Wanner, R. A., Della-Porta, A. J., and Snowdon, W. A., 1975, Serological evidence for the association of Akabane virus with epizootic bovine congenital arthrogryposis and hydranencephaly syndromes in New South Wales, *Aust. Vet. J.* **51**:103.

Hayes, R. O., La Motte, L. C., and Holden, P., 1967, Ecology of arboviruses in Hale County, Texas during 1965, *Am. J. Trop. Med. Hyg.* **16**:675.

Hefti, E., and Bishop, D. H. L., 1975, The 5′ sequence of VSV viral RNA and its *in vitro* transcription product RNA, *Biochem. Biophys. Res. Commun.* **66**:785.

Henderson, B. E., and Coleman, P. H., 1971, The growing importance of California arboviruses in the etiology of human disease, *Prog. Med. Virol.* **13**:404.

Henderson, B. E., Calisher, C. H., Coleman, P. H., Fields, B. N., and Work, T. H., 1969, Gumbo Limbo, a new group C arbovirus from the Florida Everglades, *Am. J. Epidemiol.* **89**:227.

Henderson, B. E., McCrae, A. W. R., Kirva, B. G., Ssenkubuge, Y., and Sempala, S. D. K., 1972, Arbovirus epizootics involving man, mosquitoes, and vertebrates at Lunyo, Uganda, 1968, *Ann. Trop. Med. Parasitol.* **66**:343.

Hewlett, M. J., Pettersson, R. F., and Baltimore, D., 1977, Circular forms of Uukuniemi virion RNA: An electron microscopic study, *J. Virol.* **21**:1085.

Hilty, M. D., Haynes, R. E., Azimi, P. H., and Cramblett, H. G., 1972, California encephalitis in children, *Am. J. Dis. Child.* **124**:530.

Hoff, G. L., Anslow, R. O., Spalatin, J., and Hanson, R. P., 1971*a*, Isolation of Montana snowshoe hare serotype of California encephalitis virus group from a snowshoe hare and *Aedes* mosquitoes, *J. Wildl. Dis.* **7**:28.

Hoff, G. L., Iversen, J. O., Yuill, T. M., Anslow, R. O., Jackson, J. O., and Hanson, R. P., 1971*b*, Isolation of Silverwater virus from naturally infected snowshoe hares and *Haemaphysalis* ticks from Alberta and Wisconsin, *Am. J. Trop. Med. Hyg.* **20**:320.

Hoff, G. L., Yuill, T. M., Iversen, J. O., and Hanson, R. P., 1971*c*, Silverwater virus serology in snowshoe hares and other vertebrates, *Am. J. Trop. Med. Hyg.* **20**:326.

Holden, P., and Hess, A. D., 1959, Cache valley virus, a previously undescribed mosquito-borne agent, *Science* **130**:1187.

Holmes, I. H., 1971, Morphological similarity of Bunyamwera supergroup viruses, *Virology* **43**:708.

Horvath, L. B., 1975, Incidence of antibodies to Crimean haemorrhagic fever in animals, *Acta Microbiol. Acad. Sci. Hung.* **22**:61.

Horvath, L. B., 1976, Precipitating antibodies to Crimean haemorrhagic fever virus in human sera collected in Hungary, *Acta Microbiol. Acad. Sci. Hung.* **23**:331.

Hunt, A. R., and Calisher, C. H., 1979, Relationships of Bunyamwera group viruses by neutralization, *Am. J. Trop. Med. Hyg.* **28**:740.

Inaba, Y., Kurogi, H., and Omori, T., 1975, Akabane disease: Epizootic abortion, premature birth, stillbirth and congenital arthrogryposis-hydranencephaly in cattle, sheep and goats caused by Akabane virus, *Aust. Vet. J.* **51**:584.

Institut Pasteur de Bangui, *Annual Report*, 1971.

Institut Pasteur de Dakar, *Annual Report*, 1971.

Institut Pasteur de Dakar, *Annual Report*, 1972.

Issel, C. J., 1973, Isolation of Jamestown Canyon virus (a California group arbovirus) from a white-tailed deer, *Am. J. Trop. Med. Hyg.* **22**:414.

Issel, C. J., Trainer, D. O., and Thompson, W. H., 1972, Experimental studies with white-tailed deer and four California group arboviruses (La Crosse, Trivittatus, snowshoe hare, and Jamestown Canyon), *Am. J. Trop. Med. Hyg.* **21**:979.

Issel, C. J., Hoff, G. L., and Trainer, D. O., 1973, Serologic evidence of infection of white-tailed deer in Texas with three California group arboviruses (Jamestown Canyon, San Angelo and Keystone), *J. Wildl. Dis.* **9**:245.

Iversen, J., Hanson, R. P., Papadopoulos, O., Morris, C. V., and De Foliart, G. R., 1969, Isolations of virus of the California encephalitis virus group from boreal *Aedes* mosquitoes, *Am. J. Trop. Med. Hyg.* **18**:735.

Iversen, J. O., Wagner, R. J., Dejong, C., and McLintock, J., 1973, California encephalitis virus in Saskatchewan: Isolation from boreal *Aedes* mosquitoes, *Can. J. Public Health* **64**:590.

Jelinkova, A., Brenda, R., and Novak, M., 1976, Electron microscopic demonstration of Crimean hemorrhagic fever virus in CV-1 (monkey) cells, *Acta Virol. (Prague)* **19**:369.

Jennings, W. L., Lewis, A. L., Sather, G. E., Hammon, W. McD., and Bond, J. O., 1968, California-encephalitis-group viruses in Florida rabbits, *Am. J. Trop. Med. Hyg.* **17**:781.

Johnson, B. K., Chanas, A. C., Tayeb, E. E., Abel-Wahab, K. S. E., Sheheta, F. A., and Mohamed, A. E., 1978, Rift Valley fever in Egypt 1978, *Lancet* **8092**:745.

Jonkers, A. H., Metselaar, D., Paes De Andrade, A. H., and Tikasingh, E. S., 1967, Restan virus, a new group C arbovirus from Trinidad and Surinam, *Am. J. Trop. Med. Hyg.* **16**:74.

Jonkers, A. H., Spence, L., Downs, W. G., Aitken, T. H. G., and Tikasingh, E. S., 1968, Arbovirus studies in Bush Bush Forest, Trinidad, W. I., September 1959–December 1964. V. Virus Isolations, *Am. J. Trop. Med. Hyg.* **17**:276.

Kaiser, M. N., Hoogstraal, H., and Watson, G. E., 1974, Ticks (*Ixodoidea*) on migrating birds in Cyprus, Fall 1967 and Spring 1968, and epidemiological considerations, *Bull Entomol. Res.* **64**:97.

Kalmar, E., Peleg, B. A., and Sayir, D., 1975, Arthrogryposis-hydranencephaly syndrome in newborn cattle, sheep, and goats: Serological survey for antibodies against the Akabane virus, *Refu. Vet.* **32**:47.

Karabatsos, N. (ed.), 1978, Supplement to International Catalogue of Arboviruses including certain other viruses of vertebrates, *Am. J. Trop. Med. Hyg.* **27**:372.

Karabatsos, N., and Henderson, J. R., 1969, Cross-neutralization studies with group C arboviruses, *Acta Virol.* **13**:544.

Kascsak, R. J., and Lyons, M. J., 1977, Bunyamwera virus: I. The molecular complexity of the virion RNA, *Virology* **82**:37.

Kascsak, R. J., Shope, R. E., Donnenfeld, H., and Bartfeld, H., 1978, Antibody response to arboviruses—Absence of increased response in amyotrophic lateral sclerosis and multiple sclerosis, *Arch. Neurol.* **35**:440.

Kemp, G. E., Causey, O. R., and Causey, C. E., 1971, Virus isolations from trade cattle, sheep, goats and swine at Ibadan, Nigeria, *Bull. Epizoot Dis. Afr.* **19**:131.

Klisenko, G. A., Gaidamovich, S. Y., Obukhova, V. R., Agafanov, V. I., and Nikolaev, V. P., 1973, Identification of a virus from the Uukuniemi group isolated in the Far East, *Vopr. Virusol.* **18**:594.

Kokernot, R. H., Smithburn, K. C., and Weinbren, M. P., 1956, Neutralizing antibodies to arthropod-borne viruses in human beings and animals in the Union of South Africa, *J. Immunol.* **77**:313.

Kokernot, R. H., Smithburn, K. C., Weinbren, M. P., and De Mellon, B., 1957a, Studies on arthropod-borne viruses of Tongaland. VI. Isolation of Pongola virus from *Aedes* (*Banksinella*) *circumlyteolus theo*, *S. Afr. J. Med. Sci.* **22**:81.

Kokernot, R. H., Heymann, C. S., Muspratt, J., and Wolstenholme, B., 1957b, Studies on arthropod-borne viruses of Tongaland. V. Isolation of Bunyamwera and Rift Valley fever viruses from mosquitoes, *S. Afr. J. Med. Sci.* **22**:71.

Kokernot, R. H., Smithburn, K. C., De Meillon, B., and Paterson, H. R., 1958, Isolation of Bunyamwera virus from a naturally infected human being and further isolations from *Aedes* (*Banksinella*) *circumluteolus Theo*, *Am. J. Trop. Med. Hyg.* **7**:579.

Kokernot, R. H., Smithburn, K. C., Paterson, H. E., and McIntosh, B. M., 1960, Isolation of Germiston virus, a hitherto unknown agent, from culicine mosquitoes, and a report of infection in two laboratory workers, *Am. J. Trop. Med. Hyg.* **9**:62.

Kokernot, R. H., McIntosh, B. M., Worth, C. B., DeMorais, T., and Weinbren, M. P., 1962, Isolation of viruses from mosquitoes collected at Lumbo, Mozambique. I. Lumbo virus, a new virus isolated from *Aedes* (*skusea*) *pembaensis* Theobald, *Am. J. Trop. Med. Hyg.* **11**:678.

Kokernot, R. H., Calisher, C. H., Stannard, L. J., and Hayes, J., 1969, Arbovirus studies in the Ohio-Mississippi Basin 1964–1967. VII. Lone Star Virus. A hitherto unknown agent isolated from the tick *Amblyomma americanum* (Linn), *Am. J. Trop. Med. Hyg.* **18**:789.

Kolman, J. M., and Husova, M., 1971, Virus carrying ticks *Ixodes ricinus* in the mixed natural focus of the Central European Tick-Borne Encephalitis virus (CETE) and Uukuniemi virus (UK), *Folia. Parasitol. (Prague)* **18**:329.

Kolman, J. M., Malkova, D., and Smetana, A., 1966, Isolation of a presumable new virus from unengorged *Ixodes ricinus* ticks, *Acta Virol.* **10**:171.

Kondratenko, V. F., 1976, The role of ixodid ticks in the transmission and preservation of Crimean hemorrhagic fever in infection foci, *Parazitologiya* **10**:297.

Korolev, M. B., Donets, M. A., and Chumakov, M. P., 1975, Electron microscope study of Crimean hemorrhagic fever virus in brains of infected mice and in pig kidney cell cultures (in Russian). (Conf. Abstracts USSR AMS Inst. of Poliomyelitis and Virus Encephalitides), *Vopr. Med. Virusol.* p. 302.

Korolev, M. B., Donets, M. A., Rubin, S. G., and Chumakov, M. P., 1976, Morphology and morphogenesis of Crimean hemorrhagic fever virus, brief report, *Arch. Virol.* **50**:169.

Kozuch, O., Gresikova, M., Nosek, J., and Chmela, J., 1970a, Uukuniemi virus in western Slovakia and northern Moravia, *Folia Parasitol. (Prague)* **17**:337.

Kozuch, O., Rajacni, J., Sekeyova, M., and Nosek, J., 1970b, Uukuniemi virus in small rodents, *Acta Virol.* **14**:163.

Ksiazek, T. G., and Yuill, T. M., 1977, Viremia and antibody response to La Crosse virus in sentinel gray squirrels (*Sciurus carolinesis*) and chipmunks (*Tamias striatus*), *Am. J. Trop. Med. Hyg.* **26**:815.

Kunz, C., and Aspock, H., 1967, Rapid identification of Tahyna virus by means of the immunofluorescent method, *Zentralbl. Bakteriol. Parasitenkd. Infektionskr. Hyg. Abt. Orig.* **203**:25.

Kunz, C., Buckley, S. M., and Casals, J., 1964, Antibodies in man against Tahyna and Lumbo viruses determined by hemagglutination-inhibition and tissue culture neutralization tests, *Am. J. Trop. Med. Hyg.* **13**:738.

Kurogi, H., Inaba, Y., Goto, Y., Miura, Y., Takahashi, H., Sato, K., Omori, T., and Matumoto, M., 1975, Serologic evidence for etiologic role of Akabane virus in epizootic abortion–arthrogryposis–hydranencephaly in cattle in Japan, 1972–1974, *Arch. Virol.* **47**:71.

Kurogi, H., Inaba, Y., Takahashi, E., Sato, K., Omori, T., Miura, Y., Goto, Y., Fujiwara, Y., and Hatano, Y., 1976, Epizootic congenital arthrogryposis–hydranencephaly syndrome in cattle: Isolation of Akabane virus from affected fetuses, *Arch. Virol.* **51**:67.

Kurogi, H., Inaba, Y., Takahashi, E., Sato, K., Satoda, K., Goto, Y., Omori, T., and Matumoto, M., 1977, Congenital abnormalities in newborn calves after inoculation of pregnant cows with Akabane virus, *Infect. Immun.* **17**:338.

Le Duc, J. W., Suyemeto, W., Eldridge, B. F., Russell, P. K., and Barr, A. R., 1975a, Ecology of California encephalitis viruses on the Del Mar Va Penninsula. II. Demonstration of transovarial transmission, *Am. J. Trop. Med. Hyg.* **24**:124.

Le Duc, J. R., Suyemoto, W., Keife, T. J., Burger, J. F., Eldridge, B. F., and Russell, P. K., 1975b, Ecology of California encephalitis viruses on the Del Mar Va Peninsula. I. Virus isolations, *Am. J. Trop. Med. Hyg.* **24**:118.

Lennette, E. H., Ota, M. I., Fujimoto, F. Y., Wiener, A., and Loomis, E. C., 1957, Turlock virus: A presumably new arthropod-borne virus. Isolation and identification, *Am. J. Trop. Med. Hyg.* **6**:1024.

Levitt, J., Naude, W. du T., and Polson, A., 1963, Purification and electron microscopy of pantropic Rift Valley fever virus, *Virology* **20**:520.

Likar, M., and Casals, J., 1963, Isolation from man in Slovenia of a virus belonging to the California Complex of arthropod-borne viruses, *Nature* (*London*) **197**:1131.

Lindsey, H. S., Calisher, C. H., and Mathews, J. H., 1976, Serum dilution neutralization test for California group virus identification and serology, *J. Clin. Microbiol.* **4**:503.

Lindsey, H. S., Klimas, R. A., and Obijeski, J. F., 1977, La Crosse virus soluble cell culture antigen, *J. Clin. Microbiol.* **6**:618.

Loening, U. E., 1968, Molecular weights of ribosomal RNA in relation to evolution, *J. Mol. Biol.* **38**:355.

Lomonosov, N. N., and Fadeeva, L. L., 1974, Isolation of infectious RNA from the Guama group of arboviruses, *Vopr. Virusol.* **6**:719.

Lopes, O. De S., Foratinni, O. P., Fonseca, I. E. M., Lacerda, J. P. G., Sacchetta, L. A., and Rabello, E. X., 1966, Boraceia virus. A new virus related to *Anopheles* B virus, *Proc. Soc. Exp. Biol. Med.* **123**:502.

Lopes, O. de S., and Sacchetta, L. de A., 1974, Epidemiology of Boraceia virus in a forested area in Sao Paulo, Brazil, *Am. J. Epidemiol.* **100**:410.

Lopes, O. de S., Sacchetta, L. de A., Fonesca, I. E. M., and Lacerda, J. P. G., 1975, Bertioga (Guama group) and Anhembi (Bunyamwera group), two new arboviruses isolated in Sao Paulo, Brazil, *Am. J. Trop. Med. Hyg.* **24**:131.

Luria, S. E., and Darnell, J. E., 1967, *General Virology*, Wiley, New York.

Lvov, D. K., Timofeeva, V. L., Gromashevski, V. I., Chervonsky, A. I., Gromov, A. I., Tsyrkin, Y. M., Pogrebenko, A. G., and Kostyrko, I. N., 1972, Sakhalin virus: A new arbovirus isolated from *Ixodes* (*Ceratixodes*) *putus* Pick.-Camb. 1878 collected on Tuleniy Island, Sea of Okhotsk, *Arch. Gesamte Virusforsch.* **38**:133.

Lvov, D. K., Smirnov, V. A., Gromashevskii, V. L., Veselovskaya, V., and Lavrova, N. A., 1973a, Isolation of the arbovirus of Patience Bay from *Ixodes* (*Ceratixodes*) *putus Pick-Cambr.* 1878 ticks in the Murmansk oblast, *Med. Parazitol. Parazit. Bolezni.* **42**:728.

Lvov, D. K., Timopheeva, A. A., Gromashevski, V. L., Gostinshchikova, G. V., Veselovskaya, O. V., Chervonski, V. I., Fomina, K. B., Gromov, A. I., Pogrebenko, A. G., and Zhezmer, V. Yu., 1973b, "Zaliv Terpeniya" virus, a new Uukuniemi group arbovirus isolated from *Ixodes* (*Ceratixodes*) *putus Pick. Camb. 1878* on Tyuleniy Island (Sakhalin Region) and Commodore Islands (Kamchatsk Region), *Arch. Gesamte Virusforsch.* **41**:165.

Lvov, D. K., Timofeeva, A. A., Gromashevski, V. L., Tsyrkin, Yu. M., Sazonov, A. A., Togredenko, A. G., Sidorova, G. A., Gostinshcikova, G. V., Khytoretskaya, N. V., Gusha, V. I., Fomina, K. B., Chervonski, V. I., Aristova, V. A., Leonova, G. N., Zhezmer, V. Yu., Shibaev, Yu. B., Yudakov, A. J., Philatov, Ph. P., and Chumakov, V. M., 1974, The ecology of Sakhalin virus in the north of the Far East of the U.S.S.R., *J. Hyg. Epidemiol. Microbiol. Immunol.* **18**:87.

Lyons, M. J., and Heyduk, J., 1973, Aspects of the developmental morphology of California encephalitis virus in cultured vertebrate and arthropod cells and in mouse brain, *Virology* **54**:37.

Main, A. J., Downs, W. G., Shope, R. E., and Wallis, R. C., 1976, Avalon and Clo Mor: Two new Sakhalin group viruses from the North Atlantic, *J. Med. Entomol.* **13**:309.

Malkova, D., Danielova, V., Minar, J., Rosicky, B., and Casals, J., 1972, Isolations of Yaba-1 arbovirus in Czechoslovakia, *Acta Virol.* **16**:93.

Malkova, D., and Reddy, N., 1975, Influence of early passages on the character of freshly isolated strains of Tahyna virus, *Acta Virol.* **19**:333.

March, R. W., and Hetrick, F. M., 1967, Studies on Guaroa virus. I. Virus characteristics, *Am. J. Trop. Med. Hyg.* **16**:191.

Masterson, R. A., Stegmiller, H. W., Parsons, M. A., Croft, C. C., and Spencer, C. B., 1971, California encephalitis: An endemic puzzle in Ohio, *Health Lab. Sci.* **8**:89.

Matevosyan, K. S., Semashko, I. V., and Chumakov, M. P., 1974, Isolation of Bhanja virus from ticks *Dermacentor marginatus* in the Armenian SSR, *Zh. Eksp. Klin. Med.* **14**:9.

McIntosh, B. M., Kokernot, R. H., and Paterson, H. E., 1960, Witwatersrand virus: An apparently new virus isolated from culicine mosquitoes, *S. Afr. J. Med. Sci.* **25**:33.

McIntosh, B. M., McGillivray, G. M., and Dickinson, D. B., 1965, Ingwavuma virus: an arbovirus isolated in South Africa, *S. Afr. J. Med. Sci.* **30**:67.

McIntosh, B. M., Anderson, D., Jupp, P. G., Dickinson, D. B., Bromfeld, J. A., Dos Santos, I., Gutteling, M. B., Meenhan, G. M., and Tew, M. G., 1972, *Annual Report for the Year 1972*, South African Institute for Medical Research, Johannesburg, p. 181.

McIntosh, B. M., Jupp, P. G., Anderson, D., and Dickinson, D. B., 1973, Rift Valley fever: 2. Attempts to transmit virus with seven species of mosquito, *J. S. Afr. Vet. Assoc.* **44**:57.

McIntosh, B. M., Dos Santos, I. S. L., and Meenehan, G. M., 1976, *Culex (Eumelanomyia) rubinotus* Theobald as vector of Banzi, Germiston, and Witwatersrand viruses: III. Transmission of virus to hamsters by wild-caught infected *C. rubinotus, J. Med. Entomol.* **12**:645.

McKiel, J. A., Hall, R. R., and Newhouse, V. F., 1966, Viruses of the California encephalitis complex in indicator rabbits, *Am. J. Trop. Med. Hyg.* **15**:98.

McLean, D. M., 1961, Silverwater virus: Characterization of virus isolated from ticks collected in Eastern Canada, *Fed. Proc.* **20**:443.

McLean, D. M., Crawford, M. A., Ladyman, S. R., Peers, R. R., and Purvin-Good, K. W., 1970, California encephalitis and Powassan virus activity in British Columbia, 1969, *Am. J. Epidemiol.* **92**:266.

McLean, D. M., Goddard, E. J., Graham, E. A., Hardy, G. J., and Purvin-Good, K. W., 1972, California encephalitis virus isolations from Yukon mosquitoes, 1971, *Am. J. Epidemiol.* **95**:347.

McLean, D. M., Bergman, S. K. A., Gould, A. P., Gross, P. N., Miller, M. A., and Spratt, E. E., 1975*a*, California encephalitis virus prevalence throughout the Yukon Territory, 1971–74, *Am. J. Trop. Med. Hyg.* **24**:676.

McLean, D. M., Gubash, S. M., Grass, P. N., Miller, M. A., Petric, M., and Walters, T. E., 1975*b*, California encephalitis virus development in mosquitoes as revealed by transmission studies, immunoperoxidase staining and electron microscopy, *Can. J. Microbiol.* **21**:453.

McLerran, C. J., and Arlinghaus, R. B., 1973, Structural components of a virus of the California encephalitis complex: La Crosse virus, *Virology* **53**:247.

McLintock, J., Curry, P. S., Wagner, R. J., Leung, M. K., and Iversen, J. O., 1976, Isolation of snowshoe hare virus form *Aedes implicatus* larvae in Saskatchewan, *Mosq. News* **36**:233.

Metselaar, D., 1966, Isolation of arboviruses of group A and group C in Surinam, *Trop. Geogr. Med.* **18**:137.

Metselaar, D., and Robin, Y., 1976, Akabane virus isolated in Kenya, *Vet. Rec.* **99**:86.

Miller, B. R., De Foliart, G. R., and Yuill, T. M., 1977, Vertical transmision of La Crosse virus (California encephalitis group): Transovarial and filial infection rates in *Aedes triseriatus* (Diptera: Culcidae), *J. Med. Entomol.* **14**:437.

Monath, T. P. C., Nuckolls, J. G., Berall, J., Bauer, H., Chappell, W. A., and Coleman, P. H., 1970, Studies on California encephalitis in Minnesota, *Am. J. Epidemiol.* **92**:40.

Monath, T. P. C., Henderson, B. E., and Kirya, G. B., 1972, Characterization of viruses (Witwatersrand and Germiston) isolated from mosquitoes and rodents collected near Lunyo Forest, Uganda in 1968, *Arch. Gesamte Virusforsch.* **38**:125.

Montgomery, R. E., 1917, On a tick-borne gastro-enteritis of sheep and goats occurring in British East Africa, *J. Comp. Pathol. Ther.* **30**:28.

Moulton, D. W., and Thompson, W. H., 1971, California group virus infections in small, forest-dwelling mammals of Wisconsin: Some ecological considerations, *Am. J. Trop. Med. Hyg.* **20**:474.

Moussa, M. I., Imam, I. Z., Converse, J. D., and El-Karamany, R. M., 1974, Isolation of Matruh virus from *Hyalomma marginatum* ticks in Egypt, *J. Egypt. Public Health Assoc.* **49**:341.

Muria, Y., Hayashi, S., Ishihara, T., Inaba, Y., Omori, T., and Matumoto, M., 1974, Neutralizing antibody against akabane virus in precolostral sera from calves with congenital arthrogyrposis–hydranencephaly syndrome, *Arch. Gesamte Virusforsch.* **46**:377.

Murphy, F. A., and Coleman, P. H., 1967, California group arboviruses: Immunodiffusion studies, *J. Immunol.* **99**:276.

Murphy, F. A., Whitfield, S. G., Coleman, P. H., Calisher, C. H., Rabin, E. R., Jenson, A. B., Melnick, J. L., Edwards, M. R., and Whitney, E., 1968a, California group arboviruses: Electron microscopic studies, *Exp. Mol. Pathol.* **9**:44.

Murphy, F. A., Harrison, A. K., and Tzianabos, T., 1968b, Electron microscopic observations of mouse brain infected with Bunyamwera group arboviruses, *J. Virol.* **2**:1315.

Murphy, F. A., Harrison, A. K., and Whitfield, S. G., 1973, Bunyaviridae: Morphologic and morphogenetic similarities of Bunyamwera serologic supergroup viruses and several other arthropod-borne viruses, *Intervirology* **1**:297.

Nelson, R. L., and Scrivani, R. P., 1972, Isolation of arboviruses from parous midges of the *Culicoides variipennis* complex, and parous rates in biting populations, *J. Med. Entomol.* **9**:277.

Newhouse, V. F., Burgdorfer, W., McKiel, J. A., and Gregson, J. D., 1963, California encephalitis virus. Serologic survey of small wild mammals in northern United States and southern Canada and isolation of additional strains, *Am. J. Hyg.* **78**:123.

Newhouse, V. F., Burgdorfer, W., and Corwin, D., 1971, Field and laboratory studies on the hosts and vectors of the snowshoe hare strain of California virus, *Mosq. News* **31**:401.

Obijeski, J. F., and Murphy, F. A., 1977, Bunyaviridae: Recent biochemical developments, *J. Gen. Virol.* **37**:1.

Obijeski, J. G., Bishop, D. H. L., Murphy, F. A., and Palmer, E. L., 1976a, Structural proteins of La Crosse virus, *J. Virol.* **19**:985.

Obijeski, J. G., Bishop, D. H. L., Palmer, E. L., and Murphy, F. A., 1976*b*, Segmented genome and nucleocapsid of La Crosse virus, *J. Virol.* **20**:664.

Ogunbi, O., 1968, Ukauwa virus proliferation in mosquitoes, *Can. J. Microbiol.* **14**:125.

Oker-Blom, N., Salminin, A., Brummer-Korvenkontio, M., 1964, Isolation of some viruses other than typical tick-borne encephalitis viruses from *Ixodes ricinus* ticks in Finland, *Ann. Med. Exp. Biol. Fenn.* **42**:109.

Okuno, T., 1961, Immunological studies relating two recently isolated viruses, Germiston virus from South Africa and Ilesha virus from West Africa, to the Bunyamwera group, *Am. J. Trop. Med. Hyg.* **10**:223.

Ota, W. K., Watkins, H. M. S., Neri, P., Schmidt, M. L., and Schmidt, J. R., 1976, Arbovirus recoveries from mosquitoes collected in Gambela, Illubabor province, Ethiopia, 1970, *J. Med. Entomol.* **13**:173.

Oya, A., Ogata, T., Kobayashi, I., and Matsuyama, T., 1961, Akabane, a new arbovirus isolated in Japan, *Jpn. J. Med. Sci. Biol.* **14**:101.

Pak, T. P., 1972, Division into epidemiological districts of Crimean haemorrhagic fever (CHF) in the Tadzhik S.S.R., *Zh. Mikrobiol. Epidemiol. Immunobiol.* **12**:112.

Pantuwatana, S., Thompson, W. H., Watts, D. M., and Hanson, R. P., 1972, Experimental infection of chipmunks and squirrels with La Crosse and trivittatus viruses and biological transmission of La Crosse by *Aedes triseriatus*, *Am. J. Trop. Med. Hyg.* **21**:476.

Pantuwatana, S., Thompson, W. H., Watts, D. M., Yuill, T. M., and Hanson, R. P., 1974, Isolation of La Crosse virus from field collected *Aedes triseriatus* larvae, *Am. J. Trop. Med. Hyg.* **23**:246.

Parkin, E. E., Hammon, W. M., and Sather, G. E., 1972, Review of current epidemiological literature on viruses of the California arbovirus group, *Am. J. Trop. Med. Hyg.* **21**:964.

Parsonson, I. M., Della-Porta, A. J., and Snowdon, W. A., 1975, Congenital abnormalities in foetal lambs after inoculation of pregnant ewes with Akabane virus, *Aust. Vet. J.* **51**:585.

Parsonson, I. M., Della-Porta, A. J., and Snowdon, W. A., 1977, Congenital abnormalities in newborn lambs after infection of pregnant sheep with Akabane virus, *Infect. Immun.* **15**:254.

Paterson, H. E., Kokernot, R. H., and David, D. H. S., 1957, Studies of arthropodborne viruses of Tongaland. IV. The birds of Tongaland and their possible role in virus disease, *S. Afr. J. Med. Sci.* **22**:63.

Pavri, K. M., and Casals, J., 1966, Kaisodi virus, a new agent isolated from *Haemaphysalis spinigera* in Mysore State, South India. II. Characterization and identification, *Am. J. Trop. Med. Hyg.* **15**:961.

Pennington, T. H., Pringle, C. R., and McCrae, M. A., 1977, Bunyamwera virus-induced polypeptide synthesis, *J. Virol.* **24**:397.

Peralta, P. H., Shelokov, A., and Brody, J. A., 1965, Chargres virus: A new human isolate from Panama, *Am. J. Trop. Med. Hyg.* **14**:146.

Perelatov, V. D., Vostokova, K. K., Butenko, A. M., and Donets, M. A., 1972, Epidemiology of Crimean haemorrhagic fever (CHF). Communication II. Features of the epidemiology of CHF in the Belokalitvensk district of the Rostov on Don region, *Med. Parazitol.* **41**:718.

Pettersson, R., and Kaariainen, L., 1973, The ribonucleic acids of Uukuniemi virus, a noncubical tickborne arbovirus, *Virology* **56**:608.

Pettersson, R., and von Bonsdorff, C.-H., 1975, Ribonucleoproteins of Uukuniemi virus are circular, *J. Virol.* **15**:386.

Pettersson, R., Kaarianen, L, von Bonsdorff, C.-H., and Oker-Blom, N., 1971, Structural components of Uukuniemi virus, a non-cubical tick-borne arbovirus, *Virology* **46**:721.

Pettersson, R. F., Hewlett, M. J., Baltimore, D., and Coffin, J. M., 1977, The genome of Uukuniemi virus consists of three unique RNA segments, *Cell* **11**:51.

Pinheiro, F., Pinheiro, M., Bensabath, G., Causey, O. R., and Shope, R., 1962, Epidemic of Oropouche virus in Belem, *Rev. Serv. Espec. Saude Publica* **12**:15.

Pinheiro, F. P., Travassos Da Rosa, A. P. A., Travassos Da Rosa, J. F., and Bensabath, G., 1976, An outbreak of Oropouche virus disease in the vicinity of Santarem, Para, Brazil, *Tropenmed. Parasitol.* **27**:213.

Polson, A., and Levitt, J., 1963, A slowly sedimenting infectious component of Rift Valley fever virus, *J. Yg.* **61**:451.

Polson, A., and Stannard, L., 1970, Concentration of viruses at low rotor velocities, *Virology* **40**:781.

Popov, G. V., and Zavodova, T. I., 1976, Morphology of the virus of Crimean hemorrhagic fever, International Virology 3, p. 257, *Proc. 3rd Int. Congr. Virol.*, Madrid 1975, Karger, Basel.

Porterfield, J. S., Casals, J., Chumakov, M. P., Gaidamovich, S. Y., Hannoun, C., Holmes, I. H., Horzinek, M. C., Mussgay, M., and Russell, P. K., 1973/1974, Bunyaviruses and Bunyaviridae, *Intervirology* **2**:270.

Porterfield, J. S., Casals, J., Chumakov, M. P., Gaidamovich, S. Y., Hannoun, C., Holmes, I. H., Horzinek, M. C., Mussgay, M., Okerk-Blom, N., and Russell, P. K., 1975/1976, Bunyaviruses and Bunyaviridae, *Intervirology* **6**:13.

Pringer, R. R., Rowley, W. A., Wong, Y. W., and Dorsey, D. C., 1975, Trivittatus infections in wild mammals and sentinel rabbits in central Iowa, *Am. J. Trop. Med. Hyg.* **24**:1006.

Quick, D. T., Smith, A. G., Lewis, A. L., Sather, G. E., and Hammon, W. McD., 1965, California encephalitis virus infection: A case report, *Am. J. Trop. Med. Hyg.* **14**:456.

Radev, M., and Bakardjiev, T., 1975, Comparative clinico-anatomical study of Crimean haemorrhagic fever, *Problemi Zaraznite Paraznite Bolesti* **3**:135.

Rajagopalan, P. K., Sreenivasan, M. A., and Sharda, D. P., 1970, Isolation of Ganjam virus from the bird tick *Haemaphysalis wellingtoni* Nuttall and Warburton 1907, *Indian J. Med. Res.* **58**:1195.

Randall, R., Gibbs, C. J., Jr., Aulisio, C. G., Binn, L. N., and Harrison, V. R., 1962, The development of a formalin-killed Rift Valley fever virus vaccine for use in man, *J. Immunol.* **89**:660.

Ranki, M., and Pettersson, R., 1975, Uukuniemi virus contains an RNA polymerase, *J. Virol.* **16**:1420.

Reeves, W. C., and Hammon, W. McD., 1952, California virus, a newly described agent. III. Mosquito infection and transmission, *J. Immunol.* **69**:511.

Reeves, W. C., Scrivani, R. P., Hardy, J. L., Roberts, D. R., and Nelson, R. L., 1970, Buttonwillow virus, a new arbovirus isolated from mammals and *Culicoides* midges in Kern County, California, *Am. J. Trop. Med. Hyg.* **19**:544.

Renkonen, O., Kaarianen, L., Pettersson, R., and Oker-Blom, N., 1972, The phospholipid composition of Uukuniemi virus, a non-cubical tick-borne arbovirus, *Virology* **50**:899.

Repik, P., and Bishop, D. H. L., 1973, Determination of the molecular weight of animal RNA virus genomes by nuclease digestions. I. Vesicular stomatitis virus and its defective T particle, *J. Virol.* **12**:969.

Rickenbach, A., Le Gonidec, G., and Ravisse, P., 1976, Arboviruses isolated from mosquitoes in south Cameroun forest country, Yaounde area, *Bull. Soc. Pathol. Exot.* **69**:372.

Ritter, D. G., and Feltz, E. T., 1974, On the natural occurrence of California encephalitis virus and other arboviruses in Alaska, *Can. J. Microbiol.* **20**:1359.

Roca-Garcia, M., 1944, The isolation of three neurotropic viruses from forest mosquitoes in eastern Colombia, *J. Infect. Dis.* **75**:160.

Rodriques, F. M., and Dandawate, C. N., 1977, Arthropod-borne viruses in northeastern India: A serological survey of Arunachal Pradesh and northern Assam, *Indian J. Med. Res.* **65**:453.

Rosato, R. R., Dalrymple, J. M., Brandt, W. E., Cardiff, R. D., and Russell, P. K., 1974*a*, Biophysical separation of major arbovirus serogroups, *Acta Virol.* **18**:25.

Rosato, R. R., Robbins, M. L., and Eddy, G. A., 1974*b*, Structural components of Oriboca virus, *J. Virol.* **13**:780.

Sabin, A. B., 1951, Experimental studies on Phlebotomus (Pappataci, Sandfly) fever during World War II, *Arch. Gesamte Virusforsch.* **4**:367.

Sabin, A. B., 1955, Recent advances in our knowledge of Dengue and Sandfly fever, *Am. J. Trop. Med. Hyg.* **4**:198.

Sacca, G., Mastrilli, M. L., Balducci, M., Verani, P., and Lopes, M. C., 1969, Studies on the vectors of arthropod-borne viruses in central Italy: Investigations on ticks, *Ann. Ist. Super. Sanita* **5**:21.

Saidi, S., Casals, J., and Faghih, M. A., 1975, Crimean hemorrhagic fever Congo (CHF-C) virus antibodies in man, and in domestic and small mammals, in Iran, *Am. J. Trop. Med. Hyg.* **24**:353.

Saikku, P., 1973, Arboviruses in Finland. III. Uukuniemi virus antibodies in human, cattle, and reindeer sera, *Am. J. Trop. Med. Hyg.* **22**:400.

Saikku, P., 1974, Passerine birds in the ecology of Uukuniemi virus, *Med. Biol.* **52**:98.

Saikku, P., and von Bonsdorff, C.-H., 1968, Electron microscopy of the Uukuniemi virus, an ungrouped arbovirus, *Virology* **34**:804.

Saikku, P., and Brummer-Korvenkontio, M., 1973, Arboviruses in Finland. II. Isolation and characterization of Uukuniemi virus, a virus associated with ticks and birds, *Am. J. Trop. Med. Hyg.* **22**:390.

Saikku, P., von Bonsdorff, C.-H., and Oker-Blom, N., 1970, The structure of Uukuniemi virus, *Acta Virol.* **14**:103.

Saikku, P., von Bonsdorff, C.-H., Brummer-Korvenkontio, M., and Vaheri, A., 1971, Isolation of non-cubical ribonucleoprotein from Inkoo virus, a Bunyamwera supergroup arbovirus, *J. Gen. Virol.* **13**:335.

Samso, A., Bouloy, M., and Hannoun, C., 1975, Presence de ribonucleoproteins circulaires dans le virus Lumbo (Bunyavirus), *C. R. Acad. Sci., Paris* **D280**:779.

Samso, A., Bouloy, M., and Hannoun, C., 1976, Mise en evidence de molécules d'acide ribonucleique circulaire dans le virus Lumbo (Bunyavirus), *C. R. Acad. Sci., Paris* **D282**:1653.

Sather, G. E., and Hammon, W. McD., 1967, Antigenic patterns within the California-encephalitis-virus group, *Am. J. Trop. Med. Hyg.* **16**:548.

Schaffer, P. A., and Scherer, W. F., 1972, Growth of a candidate arbovirus (Tsuruse) in *Aedes aegypti* mosquitoes following intrathoracic inoculation, *Proc. Soc. Exp. Biol. Med.* **139**:1298.

Scherer, W. F., Campillo-Sainz, C., Dickerman, R. W., Diaz-Najera, A., and Madalengoitia, J., 1967, Isolation of Tlacotalpan virus, a new Bunyamwera-group virus from Mexican mosquitoes, *Am. J. Trop. Med. Hyg.* **16**:79.

Scherer, W. F., Anderson, K., Dickerman, R. W., and Ordonez, J. V., 1972, Studies of Patois group arboviruses in Mexico, Guatemala, Honduras, and British Honduras, *Am. J. Trop. Med. Hyg.* **21**:194.

Scherer, W. F., Dickerman, R. W., Ordonez, J. V., Seymour, III., C., Kramer, L. D., Jahrling, P. B., and Powers, C. D., 1967a, Ecologic studies of Venezuelan encephalitis virus and isolations of Nepuyo and Patois viruses during 1968–1973 at a marsh habitat near the epicenter of the 1969 outbreak in Guatemala, *Am. J. Trop. Med. Hyg.* **25**:151.

Scherer, W. F., Ordonez, J. V., Dickerman, R. W., and Navarro, J. E., 1976*b*, Search for persistent epizootic Venezuelan encephalitis virus in Guatemale, El Salvador and Nicaragua during 1970–1975, *Am. J. Epidemiol.* **104**:60.

Schmidt, J. R., Schmidt, M. L., and McWilliams, J. G., 1960, Isolation of phlebotomus fever virus from *Phlebotomus papatasi*, *Trop. Med. Hyg.* **9**:450.

Schmidt, J. R., Williams, M. C., Lule, M., Mivule, A., and Mujomba, E., 1966, Viruses isolated from mosquitoes collected in the southern Sudan and western Ethiopia, *East Afr. Virus Res. Inst. Rep.* **18**:31.

Schmidt, J. R., Schmidt, M. L., and Said, M. I., 1970, Phlebotomus fever in Egypt. Isolation of Phlebotomus fever viruses from *Phlebotomus papatasi*, *Am. J. Trop. Med. Hyg.* **20**:483.

Scott, G. R., 1963, Pigs and Rift Valley fever, *Nature (London)* **200**:920.

Scott, G. R., Coackley, W., Roach, R. W., and Cowdy, N. R., 1963, Rift Valley fever in camels, *J. Pathol. Bacteriol.* **86**:229.

Sekoyova, M., Gresikova, M., and Stupalova, S., 1970, Serological study on distribution of Uukuniemi virus in man, *Folia Parasitol.* **17**:341.

Shah, K. V., and Work, T. H., 1969, Bhanja virus: A new arbovirus from ticks *Haemaphysalis intermedia* Warburton and Nuttall, 1909, in Orissa, India, *Indian J. Med. Res.* **57**:793.

Shanmugam, J., Smirnova, S. E., and Chumakov, M. P., 1976, Presence of antibody to arboviruses of the Crimean haemorrhagic fever-Congo (CHF-Congo) group in human beings and domestic animals in India, *Indian J. Med. Res.* **64**:1403.

Shestopalova, N. M., Reingold, V. N., Averina, S. M., and Smirnova, S. E., 1975, Electron microscope study of Hazara virus in white mouse brains, *U.S.S.R. Acad. Med. Sciences, Proc. Conf. Vop. Med. Virus (Moscow)*, pp. 374–375.

Shope, R. E., 1965, Antigenic variation among arboviruses, *Cienc. Cult.* **17**:30.

Shope, R. E., and Causey, O. R., 1962, Further studies on the serological relationships of group C arthropod-borne viruses and the application of these relationships to rapid identification of types, *Am. J. Trop. Med. Hyg.* **11**:283.

Shope, R. E., and Whitman, L., 1966, Nepuyo virus, a new group C agent isolated in Trinidad and Brazil. II. Seriological studies, *Am. J. Trop. Med. Hgy.* **15**:772.

Shope, R. E., Causey, C. E., and Causey, O. R., 1961, Itaqui virus, a new member of arthropod-borne group C, *Am. J. Trop. Med. Hyg.* **10**:264.

Shope, R. E., Andrade, A. H. P. de, Bensabath, G., Causey, O. R., and Humphrey, P. S., 1966, The epidemiology of EEE, WEE, SLE and Turlock viruses, with special reference to birds, in a tropical rain forest near Belem, Brazil, *Am. J. Epidemiol.* **84**:467.

Simpson, D. I. H., Knight, E. M., Courtois, G., Williams, M. C., Weinbren, M. P., and Kibukamusoke, J. W., 1967, Congo Virus: A hitherto undescribed virus occurring in Africa. Part I. Human isolations-clinical notes, *East Afr. Med. J.* **44**:87.

Smithburn, K. C., 1954, Neutralizing antibodies against arthropod-borne viruses in the sera of long time residents of Malaya and Borneo, *Am. J. Hyg.* **59**:157.

Smithburn, K. C., Mahaffy, A. F., and Paul, J. H., 1941, Bwamba fever and its causative virus, *Am. J. Trop. Med.* **21**:75.

Smithburn, K. C., Haddow, A. J., and Mahaffy, A. F., 1946, A neurotropic virus isolated from *Aedes* mosquitoes caught in the Semliki forest, *Am. J. Trop. Med.* **26**:189.

Smithburn, K. C., Haddow, A. J., and Lumsden, W. H. R., 1949, Rift Valley fever: Transmission of the virus by mosquitoes, *Br. J. Exp. Pathol.* **30**:35.

Sommerman, K. M., 1977, Biting fly: Arbovirus probe in interior Alaska (Culicidae) (Similiidae): (SSH: California complex) (Northway: Bunyamwera group), *Mosq. News* **37**:90.

Southam, C. M., Shipkey, F. H., Babcock, V. I., Bailey, R., and Erlandson, R. A., 1964, Virus biographies. I. Growth of West Nile and Guaroa viruses in tissue culture, *J. Bacteriol.* **88**:187.

Spence, L., Anderson, C. R., Aitken, T. H. G., and Downs, W. G., 1962*a*, Bimiti virus, a new agent isolated from Trinidadian mosquitoes, *Am. J. Trop. Med. Hyg.* **11**:414.

Spence, L., Anderson, C. R., Aitken, T. H. G., and Downs, W. G., 1962*b*, Melao virus, a new agent isolated from Trinidadian mosquitoes, *Am. J. Trop. Med. Hyg.* **11**:687.

Spence, L., Anderson, C. R., Aitken, T. H. G., and Downs, W. G., 1966, Nepuyo virus, a new group C agent isolated in Trinidad and Brazil. I. Isolation and properties of the Trinidadian strain, *Am. J. Trop. Med. Hyg.* **15**:71.

Spence, L., Anderson, C. R., Aitken, T. H., and Downs, W. G., 1967, Bushbush, Ieri and Lukuni viruses, three unrelated new agents isolated from Trinidadian forest mosquitoes, *Proc. Soc. Exp. Biol. Med.* **125**:45.

Sprance, H. E., and Shope, R. E., 1977, Single inoculation immume hamster sera for typing California group arboviruses by the complement-fixation test, *Am. J. Trop. Med. Hyg.* **26**:544.

Srihongse, S., and Johnson, C. M., 1965, Wyeomyia subgroups of arbovirus: Isolation from man, *Science* **149**:863.

Srihongse, S., and Johnson, C. M., 1974, Human infections with Chagres virus in Panama, *Am. J. Trop. Med. Hyg.* **23**:690.

Srihongse, S., and Shope, R. E., 1968, The Patois group of arboviruses, *Acta Virol.* **12**:453.

Srihongse, S., Galindo, P., and Grayson, M. A., 1966, Isolation of group C arboviruses in Panama including two new members, Patois and Zegla, *Am. J. Trop. Med. Hyg.* **15**:379.

Srihongse, S., Albanese, M., and Casals, J., 1974, Characterization of Thogoto virus isolated from ticks (*Rhipicephalus bursa*) in Western Sicily, Italy, *Am. J. Trop. Med. Hyg.* **23**:1161.

Stevenson, A. E., and Holmes, I. H., 1972, Electron microscopy of Koongol group arboviruses, *Aust. J. Biol. Sci.* **25**:53.

Sudia, W. D., Newhouse, V. F., Calisher, C. H., and Chamberlain, R. W., 1971, California group arboviruses: Isolations from mosquitoes in North America, *Mosq. News* **31**:576.

Sudia, W. D., Fernandez, Z., Newhouse, V. F., Sanz, B. R., and Calisher, C. H., 1975, Arbovirus vector ecology studies in Mexico during the 1972 Venezuelan equine encephalitis outbreak, *Am. J. Epidemiol.* **101**:51.

Sureau, P., Ravisse, P., Germain, M., Rickenbach, A., Cornet, J. P., Fabre, J., Jan, C., and Robin, Y., 1976, Isolation of Thogoto virus from *Amblyomma* and *Boophilus* ticks in Central Africa, *Bull. Soc. Pathol. Exot.* **69**:207.

Swanepoel, R., 1976, Studies on the epidemiology of Rift Valley fever, *J. S. Afr. Vet. Assoc.* **47**:93.

Szybalski, W., 1968, Use of cesium sulfate for equilibrium density gradient centrifugation, *Methods Enzymol.* **B12**:330.

Takahashi, K., Oya, A., Okada, T., Matsuo, R., Kuma, M., and Noguchi, H., 1968, Aino virus, a new member of Simbu group of arbovirus from mosquitoes in Japan, *Jpn. J. Med. Sci. Biol.* **21**:95.

Tan, D. S. K., Smith, C. E. G., McMahon, D. A., and Bowen, E. T. W., 1967, Lanjan virus, a new agent isolated from *Dermacentor auratus* in Malaya, *Nature (London)* **214**:1154.

Tannock, G. A., Gibbs, A. J., and Cooper, P. D., 1970, A re-examination of the molecular weight of polio-virus RNA, *Biochem. Biophys. Res. Commun.* **38**:298.

Taylor, R. M., 1967, *Catalogue of Arthropod-borne Viruses of the world*, Public Health Service Pub. No. 1760, USGPO, Washington, D.C.

Tesh, R. B., and Gubler, D. J., 1975, Laboratory studies of transovarial transmission of La Crosse and other arboviruses by *Aedes albopictus* and *Culex fatigans*, *Am. J. Trop. Med. Hyg.* **24**:876.

Tesh, R. B., and Papaevangelou, G., 1977, Effect of insecticide spraying for malaria control on the incidence of sandfly fever in Athens, Greece, *Am. J. Trop. Med. Hyg.* **26**:163.

Tesh, R. E., Chaniotis, B. N., Peralta, P. H., and Johnson, K. M., 1974, Ecology of viruses isolated from Panamanian phlebotomine sandflies, *Am. J. Trop. Med. Hyg.* **23**:258.

Tesh, R. B., Peralta, P. H., Shope, R. E., Chaniotis, B. N., and Johnson, K. M., 1975, Antigenic relationships among Phlebotomus fever group arboviruses and their implication for the epidemiology of sandfly fever, *Am. J. Trop. Med. Hyg.* **24**:135.

Tesh, R. B., Saidi, S., Gajdamovic, S. J., Rodhain, F., and Vesenjak-Hirjan, J., 1976, Serological studies on the epidemiology of sandfly fever in the Old World, *Bull. WHO* **54**:663.

Theiler, M., and Downs, W. G., 1973, *The Arthropod-Borne Viruses of Vertebrates*, Yale University Press, New Haven.

Thomas, L. A., Clifford, C. M., and Yunker, C. E., 1973, Tick-borne viruses in western North America. I. Viruses isolated from *Ixodes uriae* in coastal Oregon in 1970, *J. Med. Entomol.* **10**:165.

Thompson, W. H., 1977, Transovarial transmission of California arbovirus group, *Second International Symposium on Arctic Arboviruses*, May 26–28, Mont Gabriel, Quebec, Canada.

Thompson, W. H., and Beaty, B. J., 1978, Veneral transmission of La Crosse virus from male to female *Aedes triseriatus*, *Am. J. Trop. Med. Hyg.* **27**:187.

Thompson, W. H., and Evans, A. O., 1965, California encephalitis virus studies in Wisconsin, *Am. J. Epidemiol.* **81**:230.

Thompson, W. H., Kalfayan, B., and Anslow, R. O., 1965, Isolation of California encephalitis group virus from a fatal human illness, *Am. J. Epidemiol.* **81**:245.

Thompson, W. H., Engeseth, D. J., Jackson, J. O., De Foliart, G. R., and Hanson, R. P., 1967, California encephalitis-group virus infections in small mammals and insects in a deciduous forest area of southwestern Wisconsin, *Bull. Wildl. Dis. Assoc.* **3**:92.

Thompson, W. H., Anslow, R. O., Hanson, R. P., and De Foliart, G. R,. 1972, La Crosse virus isolations from mosquitoes in Wisconsin, 1964–68, *Am. J. Trop. Med. Hyg.* **21**:90.

Tikasingh, E. S., Ardoin, P., and Williams, M. C., 1974, First isolation of Catu virus from a human in Trinidad, *Trop. Geogr. Med.* **26**:414.

Top, F. H., Jr., Kraivapan, C., Grossman, R. A., Rozimarek, H., Edelman, R., and Gould, D. J., 1974, Ingwavuma virus in Thailand: Infection of domestic pigs, *Am. J. Trop. Med. Hyg.* **22**:251.

Traavik, T., Mehl, R., and Petterson, E. M., 1974, The isolation of an agent related to Uukuniemi virus from Norwegian *Ixodes ricinus* ticks, *Acta Pathol. Microbiol. Scand. Sect. B* **82**:297.

Trapp, E. E., Andrade, A. H. R. de, and Shope, R. E., 1965, Itaporanga, a newly recognized arbovirus from Sao Paulo State, Brazil, *Proc. Soc. Exp. Biol. Med.* **118**:421.

Van Velden, D. J. J., Meyer, J. D., Oliver, J., Gear, J. H. S., and McIntosh, B., 1977, Rift Valley fever affecting humans in South Africa, *S. Afr. Med. J.* **51**:867.

Verani, P., Balducci, M., and Lopes, M. C., 1970, Isolation of Bhanja virus in Italy and serologic evidence of its distribution in man and animals of different Italian regions, *Folia Parasitol.* **17**:367.

Vianna, N., Whitney, E., Bast, T., Deibel, R., Doll, J., and Culver, J., 1971, California encephalitis in New York State, *Am. J. Epidemiol.* **94**:50.

Vinograd, I. A., Krasovskaia, I. A., and Sidorova, G. A., 1975, Isolation of Bhanja arbovirus from *Boophilus decoloratus* ticks in Cameroun, *Vopr. Virusol.* **1**:63.

von Bonsdorff, C.-H., and Pettersson, R., 1975, Surface structure of Uukeniemi virus, *J. Virol.* **16**:1296.

von Bonsdorff, C.-H., Saikku, P., and Oker-Blom, N., 1969, The inner structure of Uukuniemi virus and two Bunyamwera supergroup arboviruses, *Virology* **39**:342.

Wagner, R. J., De Jong, D., Leung, M. K., McLintock, J., and Iversen, J. O., 1975, Isolations of California encephalitis virus from tundra mosquitoes, *Can. J. Microbiol.* **21**:574.

Walker, J. S., Stephen, E. L., Remmele, N. S., Carter, R. C. Mitten, J. Q., Schuh, L. G., and Klein, G., 1970, The clinical aspects of Rift Valley fever virus in household pets. II. Susceptibility of the cat, *J. Infect. Dis.* **121**:19.

Watts, D. M., Morris, C. D., Wright, R. E., DeFoliart, G. R., and Hanson, R. P., 1972, Transmission of La Crosse virus (California encephalitis group) by the mosquito *Aedes triseriatus*, *J. Med. Entomol.* **9**:125.

Watts, D. M., Pantuwatana, S., De Foliart, G. R., Yuill, T. M., and Thompson, W. H., 1973, Transovarial transmission of La Crosse virus (California encephalitis group) in the mosquito, *Aedes triseriatus*, *Science* **182**:1140.

Watts, D. M., Thompson, W. H., Yuill, T. M., De Foliart, G. R., and Hanson, R. P., 1974, Over-wintering of La Crosse virus in *Aedes triseriatus*, *Am. J. Trop. Med. Hyg.* **23**:694.

Watts, D. M., Grimstad, P. R., De Foliart, G. R., and Yuill, T. M., 1975, *Aedes hendersoni:* Failure of laboratory-infected mosquitoes to transmit La Crosse virus (California encephalitis group), *J. Med. Entomol.* **12**:451.

Watts, D. M., De Foliart, G. R., and Yuill, T. M., 1976, Experimental transmission of Trivittatus virus (California virus group) by *Aedes trivittatus*, *Am. J. Trop. Med. Hyg.* **25**:173.

Weinbren, M. P., Heymann, C. S. Kokernot, R. H., and Paterson, H. E., 1957*a*,

Studies on arthropod-borne viruses of Tongaland. VII. Simbu virus, a hitherto unknown agent isolated from *Aedes* (Banksinella) *circumluteolus Theo*, *S. Afr. J. Med. Sci.* **22**:93.

Weinbren, M. P., Williams, M. C., and Haddow, A. J., 1957*b*, A variant of Rift Valley fever virus, *S. Afr. Med. J.* **31**:951.

Weinbren, M. P., Gourlay, R. N., Lumsden, W. H. R., and Weinbren, B. M., 1958, An epizootic of Nairobi sheep disease in Uganda, *J. Comp. Pathol. Ther.* **68**:174.

Weiss, K. E., 1962, Studies on Rift valley fever. Passive and active immunity in lambs, *Onderstepoort J. Vet. Res.* **29**:3.

Wellings, F. M., 1969, Doctoral Thesis, University of Pittsburgh Graduate School of Public Health.

Wellings, F. M., Lewis, A. L., and Pierce, L. V., 1972, Agents encountered during arboviral ecological studies: Tampa Bay area, Florida, 1963 to 1970, *Am. J. Trop. Med. Hyg.* **21**:201.

White, A. B., 1975, Structural polypeptides of California encephalitis virus: BFS-283, *Arch. Virol.* **49**:281.

Whitman, L., and Casals, J., 1961, The Guama group: A new serological group of hitherto undescribed viruses. Immunological studies, *Am. J. Trop. Med. Hyg.* **10**:259.

Whitman, L., and Shope, R. E., 1962, The California complex of arthropod-borne viruses and its relationship to the Bunyamwera group through Guaroa virus, *Am. J. Trop. Med. Hyg.* **11**:691.

Whitney, E., Jamnback, H., Means, R. G., Roz, A. P., and Rayner, G. A., 1969, California virus in New York state. Isolation and characterization of California encephalitis virus from *Aedes cinereus*, *Am. J. Trop. Med. Hyg.* **18**:123.

Whittingham, H. E., 1924, The etiology of phlebotomus fever, *J. State Med.* **32**:461.

Williams, J. E., Imlarp, S., Top, F. H. Jr., Cavanaugh, D. C., and Russel, P. K., 1976, Kaeng Khoi virus from naturally infected bedbugs (*Cimicidae*) and immature freetailed bats, *Bull. WHO.* **53**:365.

Wong, Y. W., Rowe, J. A., Dorsey, D. C., Humphreys, M. J., and Hausler, W. J., 1971. Arboviruses isolated from mosquitoes collected in southeastern Iowa in 1966, *Am. J. Trop. Med. Hyg.* **20**:726.

Wong, Y. W., Rowley, W. A., Rowe, J. A. Dorsey, D. C., Humphreys, M. J., and Hausler, W. J. Jr., 1973, California encephalitis studies in Iowa during 1969, 1970, and 1971, *Health Lab. Sci.* **10**:88.

Woodall, J. P., 1967, Virus Research in Amazonia, *Atas Simpos. Biota Amazon* **6**:31.

Woodall, J. P., Williams, M. C., and Simpson, D. I. H., 1967, Congo virus: A hitherto undescribed virus occurring in Africa. Part 2. Identification studies, *East Afr. Med. J.* **44**:93.

Wright, R. E., Anslow, R. O., Thompson, W. H., De Foliart, G. R., Seawright, G., and Hanson, R. P., 1971, Isolations of La Crosse virus from *Tabanidae* in Wisconsin, *Mosq. News* **30**:600.

Wroblewska-Mularczykowa, Z., Sadowski, W., and Zukowski, K., 1970, Isolation of arbovirus strains of Uukuniemi type in Poland, *Folia Parasitol.* **17**:375.

Yaba Annual Report, 1957, *West African Council for Medical Research*, p. 123, Yaba, Lagos, Nigeria.

Young, D. J., 1966, California encephalitis virus. Report of three cases and review of the literature, *Ann. Intern. Med.* **65**:419.

Yuill, T. M., and Buescher, E. L., 1970, Cache Valley virus in the Del Mar Va peninsula. II. Identity of virus recovered from mosquitoes, *Am. J. Trop. Med. Hyg.* **19**:503.

Yuill, T. M., Iversen, J. O., and Hanson, R. P., 1969, Evidence for arbovirus infections in a population of snowshoe hares: A possible mortality factor, *Bull. Wild. Dis. Assoc.* **5**:248.

Yukhananova, S. A., Nikolayeva, O. V., Fadeyeva, L. L., and Parfanovich, M. I., 1974, Isolation of infectious RNA from arboviruses of the California and C groups, *Acta Virol.* **18**:88.

Yunker, C. E., 1975, Tick-borne viruses associated with seabirds in North America and related islands, *Med. Biol.* **53**:302.

Yunker, C. E., Clifford, C. M. Thomas, L. A., Kierans, J. E., Casals, J., George, J. E., and Parker, J. C., 1977, Sunday Canyon virus, a new ungrouped agent from the tick *Argas* (A.) *cooleyi* in Texas, *Acta Virol.* **21**:36.

Zarate, M. L., Geiger, R. H., Shope, R. E., and Scherer, W. F., 1968, Intergroup antigenic relationships among arboviruses manifested by a Mexican strain of Patois virus and viruses of the Bunyamwera, C, California, Capim, and Guama groups, *Am. J. Epidemiol.* **88**:273.

Zeitlenok, N. A., Vanag, K. A., and Pilie, E. R., 1957, Cases of illness of the Crimean haemorrhagic fever type observed in the Astrakhan oblast, *Probl. Virol.* **2**:90.

CHAPTER 2

Arenaviruses

William E. Rawls and Wai-Choi Leung*

Department of Pathology
McMaster University
Hamilton, Ontario, Canada

1. INTRODUCTION

There have been two principal stimuli behind efforts to gain a better understanding of the arenaviruses. Four members of this group cause severe and sometimes fatal diseases in man; thus efforts have been made to acquire knowledge which could be used to aid in the prevention and/or treatment of these human ailments. These diseases, i.e., lymphocytic choriomeningitis, Argentine hemorrhagic fever, Bolivian hemorrhagic fever, and Lassa fever, represent zoonosis, and all except lymphocytic choriomeningitis occur in well-circumscribed geographic areas. Because of the limited geographic distribution of these diseases, research efforts devoted to this virus group have not been so intense as those devoted to other groups of viruses which produce disease worldwide.

The second stimulus for study has been to understand the mechanisms and possible sequelae of persistent virus infections. The arenaviruses characteristically produce persistent infections in their natural hosts. Lymphocytic choriomeningitis virus has been a major tool in studies examining the virus–host interaction of virus persistence associated with neonatal infection. The immune-induced pathology

* Wai-Choi Leung is a Research Scholar of the Medical Research Council of Canada. Studies in the authors' laboratory were supported by grants from the Medical Research Council of Canada.

157

which is associated with acute meningoencephalitis of adult mice infected with lymphocytic choriomeningitis virus and the antigen–antibody complexes found in the glomeruli of chronically infected animals have provided concepts applicable to the pathogenesis of other virus diseases. More recently, the role of the histocompatibility complex in immune recognition for lymphocyte destruction of target cells became evident in studies using the murine-lymphocytic choriomeningitis virus system. No attempt will be made in this chapter to review comprehensively the information available about the human diseases caused by agents of the group (for review, see Casals, 1975). Neither will the biological and immunological aspects of virus–host interaction be described in depth. Instead, we will review the biochemical composition of the arenaviruses and detail some of the information available on the mode of virus replication.

2. HISTORICAL CONSIDERATIONS

Lymphocytic choriomeningitis virus (LCM), the prototype of the arenavirus group, was initially isolated in 1933 from a monkey used for the passage of St. Louis encephalitis virus (Armstrong and Lillie, 1934). Soon thereafter, the virus was isolated from a human case of aseptic meningitis (Rivers and Scott, 1935), and subsequent studies established the house mouse as the principal reservoir of the agent (Lepine et al., 1937; Armstrong and Sweet, 1939). The unusual feature of virus persistence associated with congenital and neonatal infection of mice was recognized not long after the virus was first isolated (Traub, 1936), and this virus–host interaction has been extensively studied over the years (see reviews by Lehmann-Grube, 1971; Hotchin, 1971; Cole and Nathanson, 1974).

About two and one-half decades elapsed before Junin and Tacaribe viruses were isolated. Tacaribe virus was isolated from tissues of fruit-eating bats (Downs et al., 1963), while Junin virus was isolated from human cases of Argentine hemorrhagic fever (Parodi et al., 1958). These two viruses were unrelated to any known arboviruses but were found to be serologically related to each other. When Machupo virus, the etiological agent of Bolivian hemorrhagic fever, was found by serological means to be related to Tacaribe virus and Junin virus (Johnson et al., 1965a), it was clear that a new virus group could be defined. These agents were thus aggregated into what became known as the Tacaribe complex. Subsequently, the complex was expanded with the isolation and identification of Amapari virus (Pinheiro et al., 1966),

Parana virus (Webb *et al.*, 1970), Tamiami virus (Calisher *et al.*, 1970) Pichinde virus (Trapido and Sanmartin, 1971), and Latino virus (Johnson *et al.*, 1973).

The first suggestions that the viruses of the Tacaribe complex might be related to LCM came from observed similarities in the virus–host interaction; the patterns of infection of Machupo virus in hamsters and in *Calomys callosus*, the natural host of Machupo virus, were similar to those of LCM in mice (Johnson *et al.*, 1965b; Webb, 1965). Murphy *et al.* (1969) noted a morphological similarity of Machupo virus to that reported for LCM by Dalton *et al.* (1968). All members of the Tacaribe complex were found to share the morphological features of Machupo virus and LCM (Murphy *et al.*, 1970). The demonstration of a one-way cross reaction between antigens of LCM and antisera to viruses of the Tacaribe complex (Rowe *et al.*, 1970a) provided further evidence of the relatedness of these viruses and led to the acceptance of the viruses as a new taxonomic group (Rowe *et al.*, 1970b; Pfau *et al.*, 1974).

The arenaviruses and the principal vertebrate host of each virus are listed in Table 1. Expansion of the group beyond LCM and members of the Tacaribe complex came with the isolation of Lassa virus, the etiological agent of a severe febrile illness which occurs in West Africa (Buckley and Casals, 1970). Additional viruses which appear to be

TABLE 1

Members of the Arenavirus Group

Virus	Principal vertabrate host	References
Lymphocytic choriomeningitis	*Mus musculus*	Armstrong and Lillie (1934)
Junin	*Calomys laucha* *Calomys musculinus* *Akodon azarae*	Parodi *et al.* (1958)
Tacaribe	*Antibesis liturates* *Antibesis jamaicensis*	Downs *et al.* (1963)
Machupo	*Calomys callosus*	Johnson *et al.* (1965b)
Amapari	*Oryzomys goeldi* *Neacomys guianae*	Pinheiro *et al.* (1966)
Parana	*Oryzomys buccinatus*	Webb *et al.* (1970)
Tamiami	*Sigmodon hispideis*	Calisher *et al.* (1970)
Lassa	*Mastomys natalensis*	Monath *et al.* (1974)
Pichinde	*Oryzomys albigularis*	Trapido and Sanmartin (1971)
Latino	*Calomys callosus*	Johnson *et al.* (1973)

members of the group have recently been isolated in Brazil (F. P. Pinheiro, personal communication) and in Mozambique (Wulff *et al.*, 1978). It seems likely that the arenavirus group will expand when more studies of rodent populations of various areas of the world are undertaken.

3. PATHOBIOLOGY

While the arenaviruses are capable of infecting a variety of mammals under experimental conditions, the agents have a remarkably restricted host range in nature; most of the viruses have one principal rodent host (Johnson *et al.*, 1973). An explanation for the high degree of specificity may be that the agents are capable of producing persistent infection only in the appropriate host, and the virus is maintained in nature by persistently infected animals. Persistent infections have been documented for LCM in *Mus musculus* (Traub, 1936), Machupo virus in *Calomys callosus* (Johnson *et al.*, 1965*b*), Junin virus in *Calomys musculinus* (Sabattini and Maiztequi, 1970), Pichinde virus in *Oryzomys albigularis* (Trapido and Sanmartin, 1971), and Lassa virus in *Mastomys natalensis* (Monath *et al.*, 1974; Walker *et al.*, 1975*a*). A persistent infection of the Syrian hamster, *Mesocricetus auratus*, with LCM can also occur (Parker *et al.*, 1976). Where examined, the conditions for producing viral persistence appear to be similar to those detailed for LCM virus. The major determinant is the age at infection. Infections acquired either congenitally or in the newborn period frequently become chronic, while infections acquired in adult life do not normally result in continued virus excretion. Thus animals infected early in life excrete virus in the urine and saliva throughout life, and these animals serve as a reservoir for infection of the species progeny (Johnson *et al.*, 1973; Webb *et al.*, 1975).

The arenavirus infections are systemic in nature, and evidence of virus replication can be detected in multiple tissues. The lymphoreticuloendothelial system has been identified as a major tropic site for several of the viruses (Murphy *et al.*, 1976, 1977). However, course of infection, pathological changes induced by the viruses, and clinical manifestations of the virus–host interaction vary considerably. The spectrum of virus–host interactions thus far observed can be divided into four types. Adults of strains of laboratory mice injected intracerebrally with neurotropic strains of LCM or intraperitoneally with viscerotropic strains of virus exemplify the most severe type of interaction. Virus replicates in the leptomeninges or in the liver, kidney, and spleen, and the pathological changes which develop as a consequence of the virus produce death. Peripheral inoculation of temperate strains of virus results in a second type of infection in which there is limited virus replication in vital organs, an effective immune response against the virus, minimal or no virus shedding, and no clinical disease. A third type of interaction is that seen when immunologically hyporesponsive animals are infected. In the natural setting the hyporesponsive period of early life is the period when infections of this type occur. These congenital or newborn infections may establish a persistent infection in which there appears to be a lifelong functional tolerance to the virus. The animals continually shed virus but develop no clinical manifestations of the infection. A fourth variation is observed when there is persistence but the carrier state is gradually modified by a low level of immune reactivity (Oldstone and Dixon, 1967). Animals with this type of infection may manifest late-onset diseases (Oldstone and Dixon, 1969). The particular type of infection which develops depends on a number of factors such as the age and genetic constitution of the host and the strain, and dose and route of inoculation of the virus.

An apparent contrast in arenavirus infections is evident when comparing the influence of age on the outcome of infections by LCM and members of the Tacaribe complex. The most extensively studied response has been the lethal infection of adult mice by LCM. Intracerebral inoculation of the virus results in the development of pathological changes in the central nervous system which can be explained by cell-mediated immune responses to the virus. In contrast, inoculation of newborn mice by a similar route does not produce disease; this has been attributed to an immunological hyporesponsiveness of the newborn animals (see reviews by Lehmann-Grube, 1971; Hotchin, 1971; Cole and Nathanson, 1974). A reverse pattern has been found for members of the Tacaribe complex which produce lethal disease when injected into newborn mice or hamsters but do not kill adult animals. In these cases, the immune response appears to have two detectable effects: one effect is to limit the virus replication and spread (Mims and Blanden, 1972), while the other is to induce an inflammatory reaction in tissues which contain virus antigen. Thus in adult animals the immune response prevents the accumulation of sufficient numbers of infected cells to lead to overt disease. The relative nonresponsiveness of newborn animals allows virus spread, and when an immune response does develop the cell destruction is widespread (Borden and Nathanson, 1974; Nathanson *et al.*, 1975). The central role of cell-mediated immune processes in experimental arenavirus disease has been repeatedly demonstrated;

however, exceptions have been described (Besuschio *et al.*, 1973; Buch-meier and Rawls, 1977; Murphy *et al.*, 1977).

In the principal host reservoir, the arenaviruses usually replicate well in both newborn and adult animals, but acute disease is seldom observed (Johnson *et al.*, 1973). The adult infections are limited in duration, while the newborn infections often persist. Although acute disease is not observed, the infections that persist may not be totally harmless. Neonatal infection of certain strains of mice with LCM has been found to retard growth and to reduce fertility (Hotchin, 1962; Mims, 1970). Retarded growth and relative infertility were also observed among *C. callosus* infected as newborns with Machupo virus (Webb *et al.*, 1975). In addition, the weights of captured *M. natalensis* which were excreting Lassa virus were less than uninfected animals captured in the same area (Walker *et al.*, 1975*a*). Certain strains of mice chronically infected with LCM develop a late-onset disease (Hotchin, 1962) which includes a form of chronic glomerulonephritis, and it has been demonstrated that the glomerular disease is mediated by the deposition of antigen–antibody complexes (Oldstone and Dixon, 1967, 1969; Buchmeier and Oldstone, 1978). More recently, changes in behavior have also been associated with persistent LCM infections of mice (Hotchin and Seegal, 1977).

A further appreciation of the varied responses to the arenaviruses can be derived from a review of the pathological changes observed during acute infections. Intracerebral inoculation of LCM in adult mice produces an inflammatory reaction of the leptomeninges, choroid plexus, and ependyma (Walker *et al.*, 1975*b*). The inflammatory exudate is composed primarily of lymphocytes and monocytes. In addition, perivascular infiltration of mononuclear cells is observed in the adjacent brain tissue. Weanling mice injected intracerebrally with Lassa virus develop similar histological abnormalities (Henderson *et al.*, 1972). Like mice injected intracerebrally with LCM, the mice injected with Lassa virus have minimal changes in other organs of the body, although the viruses can be detected in a number of tissues. The newborn mice which develop fatal disease after intracerebral injection of the Tacaribe complex viruses also develop lesions of the central nervous system consisting of the infiltration of lymphocytes and monocytes. As in the adult mice injected with LCM, the lesions in the newborn mice are thought to be mediated through thymus-derived lymphocytes (Besuschio *et al.*, 1973; Borden and Nathanson, 1974).

In addition to the well-described pathological changes which follow intracerebral injection, lesions may develop in other tissues when arenaviruses are injected intraperitoneally or intravenously. The type and extent of changes vary with the host and with virus strains. For example, intravenous injection of the WEHI strain of mice with LCM was found to produce focal areas of necrosis in the spleen, with depletions of lymphoid elements from the spleen follicles (Mims and Tosolini, 1969). Focal areas of necrosis of hepatocytes were also found in these animals (Tosolini, 1970). Somewhat similar lesions of the spleen and liver were noted in the MHA strain of hamsters injected intraperitoneally with Pichinde virus. Tubular necrosis of the outer zone of the renal medulla was also found in the animals infected with Pichinde virus (Murphy et al., 1977). The investigators of the mouse model felt that cell-mediated immune responses played a role in the tissue damage they observed, while direct destruction of cells by the virus was thought to account for the damages observed in the hamsters.

Guinea pigs are susceptible to some of the arenaviruses, and the pathological changes of the disease produced in these animals appear to be unique from those described above. Junin virus produces a fatal illness associated with hemorrhagic lesions of multiple tissues, necrosis of bone marrow elements, and depletion of the lymphocyte populations in spleen, in lymph nodes, and in the lymphoid elements of the lungs and bowel (Wiessenbacher et al., 1975). The illnesses induced in guinea pigs by LCM and Lassa virus have been characterized by extensive involvement of the lungs; respiratory insufficiency has been attributed to pulmonary edema and hyaline membranes in alveoli. Myocarditis was also noted in the Lassa virus-infected animals (Walker et al., 1975a). No experimental evidence exists regarding the role of the immune response in the development of the lesions found in the guinea pigs.

Some of the pathological features noted in experimentally induced diseases were also found in tissues of patients suffering from fatal arenavirus infections. The generalized hemorrhages noted in guinea pigs infected with Junin virus were found in patients with Argentine hemorrhagic fever (Elsner et al., 1973). In addition, the patients had evidence of myocarditis, foci of necrotic hepatocytes, and reticulum cell hypersplasia in lymph nodes. [A form of reticuloendothelial hyperplasia has been associated with some forms of arenavirus infections in rodents (Murphy et al., 1976).] Congestion and hemorrhage in multiple tissues have similarly been found in patients with Bolivian hemorrhagic fever, and focal liver necrosis, hyperplasia of reticulum cells, and interstitial pneumonia were also observed (Child et al., 1967). Few patients with LCM die of their disease; however, pneumonitis and hemorrhagic lesions were described in one of two reported cases, while pneumonitis was the major feature of the second case (Smadel *et al.*, 1942). Extensive necrosis of liver cells not unlike that found in hamsters infected with Pichinde virus was a prominent feature in fatal cases of Lassa fever. In addition, congestion, focal interstitial pneumonitis, focal necrosis of renal tubules, and splenic lesions have been described (Winn and Walker, 1975). Immune complexes do not appear to play a role in the pathological changes of Argentine hemorrhagic fever (deBraco *et al.*, 1978), and the genesis of the lesions produced in humans by the arenaviruses is poorly understood.

4. MORPHOLOGIC AND PHYSICAL PROPERTIES

All members of the arenavirus group appear similar when viewed by electron microscopy (Dalton *et al.*, 1968; Lascano and Berria, 1974; Mannweiler and Lehmann-Grube, 1973; Murphy *et al.*, 1969, 1970, 1973; Murphy and Whitfield, 1975; Spier *et al.*, 1970). The general features of the viruses seen on examination of ultrathin sections are shown in Fig. 1. The particles are usually round or oval, but pleomorphic particles are sometimes seen. The particles range in diameter from 50 to 300 nm, with a mean diameter of approximately 110–130 nm. Surface projects extend from the unit membrane of the virus, and the interior of the particles contain variable numbers of 20- to 25-nm electron-dense granules. No discrete nucleocapsid structures commonly found in other viruses are found in arenaviruses. The internal granules are morphologically indistinguishable from ribosomes; however, the structures are not organized in tight, orderly configurations as in polyribosomes (Murphy and Whitfield, 1975). In some virus particles, the ribosomelike structures appear to be attached at varying intervals to a filamentous structure which is less than 20 nm in diameter (Fig. 2). The ribosomelike structures may not necessarily be distributed at random within the virus particles since the distribution in larger particles appears to be arranged in circular fashion beneath the envelope of the virus. The surface projections are about 10 nm in length and are club shaped. When examined in cross-section perpendicular to the long axis, these projections appear hollow by negative-contrast microscopy (Murphy and Whitfield, 1975).

While the above-described particles have been repeatedly identified in cultures of cells infected with arenaviruses, doubt has been raised regarding their infectivity. A smaller particle (50–65 nm) with a more dense internal structure was also observed in cell cultures infected with LCM virus (Mannweiler and Lehmann-Grube, 1973). These investiga-

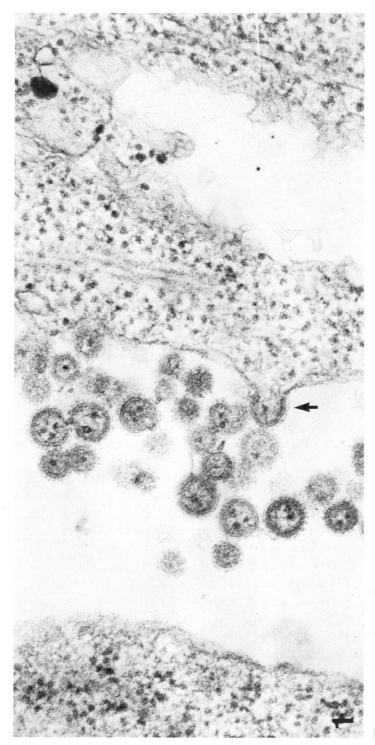

Fig. 1. Machupo virus replicated in Vero cells. The virus particles are characterized by a layer of surface projections, a distinct envelope, and an interior containing variable numbers of granules. A particle which appears to be budding from the plasma membranes of the cell is shown (arrow). ×114,000.

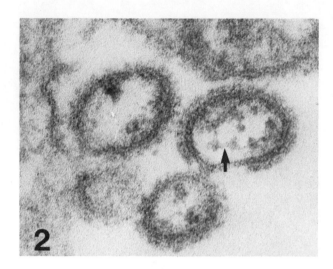

Fig. 2.   Lassa virus. The granules within one of the virus particles shown are arranged along a filamentous structure (arrow). ×173,000.

tors and others have suggested that the majority of infectivity resides with the smaller particles, while the larger particles containing the granules are not infectious. The findings of Blechschmidt and Thomssen (1976) do not support this hypothesis. The smaller particles have not been reported routinely in ultrastructural studies of other arenaviruses; however, somewhat similar structures were noted in the tissues of a patient with Argentine hemorrhagic fever (Maiztegui *et al.*, 1975).

As can be seen in Fig. 1, the arenaviruses appear to mature by budding in a fashion similar to that of a number of other enveloped RNA viruses. Budding takes place at the plasma membrane, and membrane changes detectable by electron microscopy occur at the site of virus formation. Early in infection, these changes are limited to the site of budding; however, late in infection, there are large areas of the membrane that become dense, and a thick layer of an amorphous material may be found in patches (Mannweiler and Lehmann-Grube, 1973; Murphy and Whitfield, 1975). LCM may assimilate host cell components onto the virus envelope as shown by the host cell-dependent inactivation of virus by human complement (Walsh, 1977); however, mouse H-2 antigens are not incorporated into virus grown in L cells (Blechschmidt and Thomssen, 1976). The process of maturation seems to be similar for virus replicating in cell cultures and in the animal host.

In addition to the membrane changes, alterations in the distribution of the intracytoplasmic ribosomes have been repeatedly reported (Abelson *et al.*, 1969; Murphy *et al.*, 1970: Mannweiler and Lehmann-Grube, 1973; Murphy and Whitfield, 1975). These changes are illustrated in Fig. 3. Aggregates of ribosomelike structures have been noted dispersed throughout the cytoplasm of L cells infected with LCM; these aggregates are larger than polysomelike structures seen in uninfected cells (Mannweiler and Lehmann-Grube, 1973). More impressive are the intracytoplasmic inclusion bodies which have been found both in cells from cultures and in cells from infected animals. These inclusions appear to be composed of masses of ribosomes embedded in a matrix of virus-specified proteins (Abelson *et al.*, 1969). The inclusion formation seems to begin with the diffuse aggregation of ribosomes into small units, and, with time, these aggregates condense into a large inclusion body. Inclusions with a loose matrix or a filamentous matrix have been observed, and it is believed that these forms may precede the tightly packed structure (Murphy and Whitfield, 1975).

The stability and physical properties of the arenaviruses have been detailed elsewhere (Pfau *et al.*, 1974; Rawls and Buchmeier, 1975). As

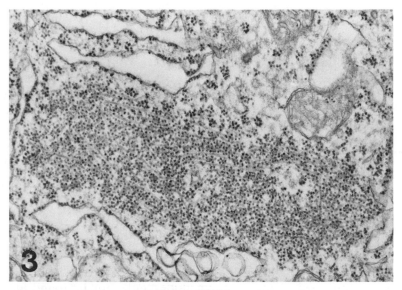

Fig. 3. Inclusion within a cell infected with Tamiami virus. The inclusion consists of an aggregate of ribosomes in a matrix of viral protein. An unusual clustering of ribosomes scattered throughout the cytoplasm is also a feature noted in arenavirus-infected cells. ×55,000.

expected for enveloped viruses, the arenaviruses are sensitive to lipid solvents such as sodium deoxycholate, chloroform, and ether. Virus infectivity was found to be lost at pH values below 5.5 and above 8.5. Arenaviruses replicated in the cell cultures have been shown to be relatively sensitive to heat; this sensitivity could be reduced by the addition of protein to the medium. The buoyant densities of the viruses were recorded as 1.17–1.18 g/cm^3 in sucrose gradients, 1.18–1.20 g/cm^3 in CsCl gradients, and 1.14 g/cm^3 in amido triazole gradients (Gschwender et al., 1975). The reported sedimentation velocities have varied from 76 S to 470–500 S for LCM, and a value of 300–325 S was found for Pichinde virus.

5. PROTEINS

The structural proteins of the virion can be defined according to functional, antigenic, or physical characteristics. Three antigens have been described in cells infected with arenaviruses, and some efforts have been made to correlate these with polypeptides identified by electrophoresis of SDS-disrupted virus in polyacrylamide gels. Several enzymatic activities, including RNA transcriptase activity have also been described. However, the relation of the enzymatic activities to the polypeptides or antigens has not yet been determined.

5.1. Polypeptides

The structural polypeptides of five members of the arenavirus group have been examined. The findings are summarized in Table 2. The major polypeptide (designated as NP, VP1, N, or 3) is not glycosylated and has a molecular weight of about 63,000–72,000. A second consistent finding is a glycosylated polypeptide with a molecular weight of about 34,000–44,000; this polypeptide has been designated GP2, VP3, G2, 5, or G. Another glycopeptide migrating close to the major polypeptide was clearly demonstrated in LCM (GP1) and Pichinde viruses (VP2 or G1), and a glycopeptide with similar relative migration characteristics, i.e., a molecular weight of 58,000, was identified in preparations of Junin virus. However, it was present in lesser amounts, and a similar polypeptide could not be found at all in Tacaribe virus or Tamiami virus.

The location of the virus polypeptides in the virion has been examined by solubilizing the viruses with nonionic detergent and

TABLE 2

Structural Polypeptides[a]

Virus	Nucleoproteins		Envelope proteins		Minor proteins		References
	Name	Molecular weight	Name	Molecular weight	Name	Molecular weight	
LCM	NP	63,000	GP1	54,000	—	—	Buchmeier et al.
			GP2	35,000			(1978)
Pichinde	VP1	72,000	VP2	72,000	VP4	12,000	Ramos et al. (1972)
			VP3	34,000			
Pichinde	N	66,000	G1	64,000		77,000	Vezza et al. (1977)
			G2	38,000		12,000	
Junin	3	64,000			1	91,000 (g)	Martinez-Segovia
			5	38,000	2	71,000 (g)	and de Mitri (1977)
					4	58,000 (g)	
					6	25,000	
Tacaribe	N	68,000	G	42,000		79,000	Gard et al. (1977)
Tamiami	N	66,000	G	44,000		77,000	Gard et al. (1977)

[a] g, Glycopeptides.

separating the components by velocity sedimentation in sucrose gradients or by equilibrium centrifugation in CsCl or metrizimide gradients. The major nonglycosylated polypeptide was found to be tightly associated with the ribonucleic acid; thus this polypeptide is thought to be part of the ribonucleoprotein complex. Furthermore, polyethylene glycol–dextran phase extraction of detergent-disrupted virus demonstrated that the polypeptide separated with the dextran phase, which is a property common to ribonucleoprotein complexes of other viruses (see Table 2). The major polypeptide is the most abundant of the polypeptide species, and estimates of 1530 molecules of N, 390 molecules of G1, and 440 molecules of G2 for each virion have been derived from studies of Pichinde virus (Vezza et al., 1977).

Of the two glycopeptides found in Pichinde virus, the one of low molecular weight (VP3) could be easily removed from the virion by treatment with Nonidet P-40 in low salt conditions. However, under the same conditions, the high molecular weight glycopeptide (VP2) remained with the ribonucleoprotein complex (Ramos et al., 1972). Subsequent studies suggest that both glycopeptides are primarily structures of the envelope. When the virus was solubilized with nonionic detergent in high salt, both glycopeptides were freed from the ribonucleoprotein complex (Vezza et al., 1977). It was also found that treatment of purified Pichinde virus (Vezza et al., 1977) or LCM (Buchmeier et al., 1978) with protease resulted in the removal of the

[³H]glucosamine label of the glycopeptides. Both glycopeptides can be labeled with ¹²⁵I by surface-labeling techniques utilizing lactoperoxidase (SenGupta and Rawls, unpublished observations), indicating that at least part of the glycopeptides are exposed on the surface of the viral envelope. Since removal of the glycopeptides by protease coincided with the disappearance of the surface spike structures on the virus envelope, the glycopeptides probably reside on the spikes (Vezza *et al.*, 1977).

The three major polypeptides of LCM were found to be distinct when the externally labeled polypeptides were submitted to digestion with trypsin and the tryptic fragments analyzed (Buchmeier *et al.*, 1978). Similar techniques applied to Pichinde virus have led to the same conclusion (Vezza *et al.*, 1978; SenGupta and Rawls, unpublished observations).

A fourth nonglycosylated polypeptide was found in Pichinde virus (Ramos *et al.*, 1972). Less abundant species of both glycosylated and nonglycosylated polypeptides were also present in preparations of other arenaviruses examined (see Table 2). The nature and significance of these minor polypeptides are unknown. No significant amount of phosphate or sulfate was present in the structural polypeptides of Pichinde, Tacribe, and Tamiami viruses (Vezza *et al.*, 1977; Gard *et al.*, 1977).

Information concerning the synthesis of the viral polypeptides is limited. In cells infected with Pichinde virus and incubated in the presence of [³⁵S]methionine or [³H]glucosamine, VP1, VP2, and VP3 can be identified by polyacrylamide gel electrophoresis (Leung and Rawls, unpublished observations). The NP polypeptide of LCM has been identified in lysates of infected cells; this polypeptide could be initially detected 6 hr after infection, which corresponds to the beginning of the exponential phase of virus replication. By immune precipitation, a glycopeptide was also found in lysates of cells infected with LCM. This glycopeptide, designated GPC, has a molecular weight of about 75,000 and is antigenically distinct from the NP polypeptide (Buchmeier *et al.*, 1978). Based on peptide mapping studies which showed structural homology between GPC and GP1, GPC has been postulated as a precursor protein for GP1 (Buchmeier, personal communication). Similar large molecular weight polypeptides have also been observed in Tacaribe (Vezza *et al.*, 1978c) and Pichinde virus-infected cells.

5.2. Antigens

Antigens detectable by several assay techniques have been described for the arenaviruses. Broadly, the antigens can be grouped as those which are virus type specific and those which are cross-reacting. Antigens detected in neutralization tests are generally considered type specific and are used to define the distinctness of the members of the virus group. However, varying degrees of cross-reactivity are often observed when the virus preparations are assayed by complement-fixation or immunofluorescence tests (Rowe *et al.*, 1970*a*; Casals *et al.*, 1975; Wulff *et al.*, 1978). The antigens have also been identified by immunodiffusion (Bro-Jorgensen, 1971; Gschwender *et al.*, 1976; Buchmeier *et al.*, 1977) and by indirect hemagglutination (Gajdamovic *et al.*, 1975); the techniques detect cross-reacting antigens. The reaction of antibodies to the surface of viable cells (Cole *et al.*, 1973; Hotchin *et al.*, 1975; Gschwender *et al.*, 1976; Rawls *et al.*, 1976) detect envelope-associated antigens which appear to be similar to those present on the surface of the virion.

A soluble substance produced in cells infected with LCM and reactive in a complement-fixation assay was found to be separable from infectious viruses (Smadel *et al.*, 1939, 1940; Smadel and Wall, 1940). The soluble preparation, called CF antigen, was subsequently examined in some detail and was found to contain two antigens detectable by immunodiffusion (Bro-Jorgensen, 1971). One of the antigens was thermolabile and was not characterized in detail. The other antigen was thermostable, had a sedimentation coefficient of about 3.5 S, and was resistant to prolonged digestion with protease. Antigens with similar properties were found in BHK-21 cells infected with Pichinde virus (Buchmeier *et al.*, 1977); partially purified preparations contained two antigens detectable by immunodiffusion, and one was heat stable while the other was labile. The thermostable antigen was present in abundance and was resistant to pronase digestion. Polyacrylamide gel electrophoresis of purified preparations of this antigen yielded two low-molecular-weight polypeptides which did not comigrate with any of the viral structural polypeptides. However, CF antigenic activity could be demonstrated in purified preparations of the LCM and Pichinde virus by disrupting the viruses (Gschwender *et al.*, 1976; Rawls and Buchmeier, 1975). Antiserum prepared against the ribonucleoprotein complex of Pichinde virus was found to react with the heat-resistant, soluble antigen (Buchmeier *et al.*, 1977), and antiserum prepared against purified soluble antigen was found to precipitate the major polypeptide of the ribonucleoprotein of the virus (Buchmeier and Oldstone, 1978*a*). Thus the major antigenic determinant for this antigen appears to reside in the nucleoprotein. The discrepancy in the properties of the antigen with respect to migration in polyacrylamide gels has been attibuted to the breakdown, probably by proteolysis, of the large structural polypeptide into a soluble pronase-resistant fragment which contains the antigenic component (Buchmeier *et al.*, 1977).

When examined by immunofluorescence, the distribution of antigen in fixed cells is primarily cytoplasmic. The antigens are detectable by 6–8 hr after infection and increase thereafter. Two elements of the staining patterns are distinguishable, a fine diffuse staining and aggregates or granules of fluorescence. The heat-stable, pronase-resistant antigen accounts for the granular fluorescence (Gschwender *et al.*, 1976), and it is likely that this is the same antigen found in the inclusions containing aggregates of ribosomelike structures (Abelson *et al.*, 1969). No information is available on the nature of the antigen giving rise to the fine, diffuse fluorescence.

The serological interrelationship of members of the arenavirus group has been examined by complement fixation and by immunofluorescence (Casals *et al.*, 1975; Wulff *et al.*, 1978). The cross-reactions between members of the Tacaribe complex are more extensive than between members of this complex and Lassa virus or LCM. Lassa virus and LCM do not cross-react strongly, but these two viruses appear to be more closely related to each other than to the other viruses. The cross-reactions between members of the Tacaribe complex are not uniform; Junin, Machupo, Amapari, and Tacaribe viruses tend to cluster together, while Tamiami and Pichinde viruses appear more closely related to each other than to the other members of the group. The ribonucleoprotein of the virion has been shown to contain cross-reacting antigens (Buchmeier and Oldstone, 1978*a*). When antisera to Pichinde, Amapari, Junin, and Tacaribe viruses were used to immunoprecipitate radiolabeled components of disrupted Pichinde virus, only the large polypeptide (NP or VP1) was precipitated by the heterologous antiserum. The percentages of the protein precipitated were 85.9, 30.0, 12.9, and 8.9 by antisera to Pichinde virus, Amapari virus, Tacaribe virus, and Junin virus, respectively. While the antisera were not characterized adequately enough to conclude that the amounts precipitated represented relatedness, the ordering is not dissimilar from that suggested when other assay systems were used.

6. NUCLEIC ACIDS

Five species of RNA have been repeatedly isolated from different members of the arenavirus group. These observatons are summarized in Table 3. The 31–33 S RNA and the 22–25 S RNA are thought to represent genomic RNA of the viruses, while the 28 S, 18 S, and 4–6 S

TABLE 3

RNA Species Isolated from Arenaviruses

Viruses	Genomic RNA	Ribosomal RNA	Small RNA	References
LCM	31 S $(2.1 \times 10^6)^a$	28 S (1.7×10^6)	4 S	Pedersen (1971,
	23 S (1.1×10^6)	18 S (0.7×10^6)	5 S	1973)
			5.5 S	
Pichinde virus L	31 S (2.1×10^6)	28 S (1.7×10^6)	4–6 S	Carter et al.
S	22 S (1.1×10^6)	18 S (0.7×10^6)		(1973)
L	(3.2×10^6)	28 S		Vezza et al.
S	(1.6×10^6)	18 S		(1977, 1978a)
Junin virus	33 S (2.4×10^6)	28 S	4 S	Anon et al.
	25 S (1.34×10^6)	18 S	5 S	(1976)
Parana virus	37 S	28 S		Dutko et al.
	24 S	18 S		(1978)

[a] Molecular weight.

RNA species are thought to be of host cell origin. In addition, a 15 S RNA species has been reported to be present in some preparations of Pichinde virus (Farber and Rawls, 1975; Dutko et al., 1976). The RNA appears to be primarily single stranded.

The evidence for the host cell origin of the 28 S and 18 S RNA comes from the ability to isolate these RNA species from 60 S and 40 S ribosomal subunits, respectively, released from purified virus (Farber and Rawls, 1975; Pedersen and Konigshofer, 1976). In addition, the *in vivo* incorporation of radiolabel into the 28 S and 18 S RNA of LCM and Pichinde virus was inhibited by a low concentration of actinomycin D, which prevents the synthesis of ribosomal RNA (Pedersen, 1971; Carter et al., 1973a). However, under similar conditions, the 28 S and 18 S RNA in Junin virus (Anon et al., 1976) and Parana virus (Dutko, Helfand, and Pfau, personal communication) were relatively insensitive to this concentration of actinomycin D. The base composition and methylation ratio (Carter et al., 1973a) and oligonucleotide fingerprint patterns (Vezza et al., 1978a) of the 28 S and 18 S RNA in Pichinde virus were similar to those of cellular ribosomal RNA. These studies all indicate that the 28 S and 18 S RNA in arenaviruses are derived from host cell ribosomes.

The 4–6 S RNA of LCM was further resolved into 4 S, 5 S, and 5.5 S RNA (Pedersen, 1973). Base composition data suggested that the 4–6 S was not the breakdown product of one of the larger RNA species. Moreover, the size and methylation ratio of the 4–6 S RNA were similar to those of the host cell transfer RNA. The relative amounts of 28 S and 18 S RNA in certain virus preparations have accounted for up to 50% of the total [³H]uridine incorporated into the viruses (Pedersen, 1971; Carter *et al.*, 1973*a*). However, in a heat-resistant clone of Pichinde virus initially selected for studies of temperature-sensitive mutants, relatively small amounts of 28 S RNA and trace amounts of 18 S RNA were found (Vezza *et al.*, 1978*a*). The 4–6 S RNA constituted about 6% of the total radiolabeled RNA in LCM (Pedersen, 1973) and about 7% of the RNA in Junin virus (Anon *et al.*, 1976).

The genetic information of arenaviruses appears to reside in the L (31–33 S) and S (22–25 S) RNA species (see Table 3). A somewhat larger molecular weight of L and S RNA has been estimated from one strain of Pichinde virus (Vezza *et al.*, 1977). The L and S RNA species of Pichinde virus do not contain methylated residues (Carter *et al.*, 1973*a*). Structural characteristics of messenger RNA such as the presence of capped and methylated structures and 3′-polyadenylated sequences were not found in the L and S RNA of Pichinde virus. Nor was the viral RNA able to translate into viral structural polypeptides in an *in vitro* protein-synthesizing system. These studies suggested that a messenger function is not associated with the virion RNA (Leung *et al.*, 1977; Leung, 1978*a*). A molar ratio of 1.3 : 1 has been accorded to the L and S RNA in Junin virus (Anon *et al.*, 1976). The oligonucleotide fingerprint patterns of the L and S RNA of Pichinde virus were found to be distinct (Vezza *et al.*, 1978*a*). No cross-hybridization was observed when the two RNAs were examined by reannealing with complementary DNAs synthesized *in vitro* from individual L and S RNA (Leung *et al.*, 1979*b*). Thus the two RNA species do not appear to be related. These observations, if taken to indicate that the L and S RNA species each have unique genetic information, is in agreement with the high-frequency genetic recombination with temperature-sensitive Pichinde virus mutants (Vezza and Bishop, 1977).

No abnormal resistance to ionizing radiation has been described, and a single-hit kinetics of inactivation by ultraviolet light was observed with Pichinde virus. This latter observation was interpreted as evidence for a single genome copy per particle (Carter *et al.*, 1973*b*). The inactivation kinetics by γ-irradiation of Pichinde virus indicated that the radiosensitive genome of Pichinde virus was about 6–8 × 10⁶ daltons (Carter *et al.*, 1973*b*), which was larger than those estimated by biochemical analysis (i.e., polyacrylamide gel electrophoresis in aqueous solution). However, the molecular weight of RNA with considerable secondary structures cannot be accurately estimated by this method. Since closed circular molecules as well as linear and hairpin forms have been observed in Tacaribe and Tamiami viral RNA, and since considerable RNase-resistant structures were also present in Pichinde, Tacaribe, and Tamiami viral RNAs (Vezza *et al.*, 1978), the absolute value of the molecular weight of arenavirus genomic RNA remains uncertain.

7. INTERNAL COMPONENTS OF THE VIRUS

Knowledge regarding the packaging of the genome and functional proteins within arenaviruses is limited in comparison to our understanding of members of certain other virus groups. Unique features of arenaviruses are the apparent unstructured interior and the presence of variable numbers of ribosomes.

7.1. Virus-Associated Ribosomes

Electron microscopic examination of ultrathin sections of arenavirus-infected cells revealed that, for all arenaviruses surveyed, the virion had an unstructured interior with variable numbers of electron-dense granules which were indistinguishable from cell ribosomes. As indicated above, RNA extracted from purified virus contained 28 S, 18 S, and 4–6 S species in addition to the L and S genomic RNA. Ribosomal structures with sedimentation coefficients of 80 S, 60 S, and 40 S were isolated from disrupted Pichinde virus (Farber and Rawls, 1975). 60 S and 40 S structures were also isolated from LCM which had been treated with nonionic detergent in the presence of high salt (Pedersen and Konigshofer, 1976). As with ribosomes, the integrity of these structures was lost in the presence of EDTA. The buoyant density of the structures isolated from Pichinde virus was the same as that of ribosomes isolated from BHK-21 cells; after formaldehyde fixation, they banded at 1.61 g/cm³ in CsCl. The 40 S subunit isolated from LCM banded at 1.52 g/cm³ and the 60 S subunit banded at 1.60 g/cm³ in CsCl. 28 S and 18 S RNA with characteristics of ribosomal RNA could be isolated from the 60 S and 40 S structures, respectively.

Although the evidence obtained from morphological and biochemical studies indicates that host cell ribosomes are present within the arenaviruses, the significance of this finding is unclear. The relative amounts of ribosomal RNAs and ratio of 28 S to 18 S RNA extracted from different virus preparations are not constant. A possible role of ribosomes in the initial phases of replication was examined using clones of a cell mutant. The cell mutant was temperature sensitive, with thermolabile 60 S ribosomal subunits, and at the nonpermissive temperature protein synthesis did not occur. Pichinde virus replicated in the mutant cells at the permissive temperature were found to incorporate the temperature-sensitive ribosomal subunit. The virus carrying the temperature-sensitive ribosomal subunit was able to replicate as well as virus carrying wild-type ribosomes at the nonpermissive temperature. This result suggests that the protein-synthesizing function and integrity of the ribosomes associated with the viruses are not required for the initial phase of virus replication (Leung and Rawls, 1977).

7.2. Ribonucleoprotein Core

An electron-dense nucleocapsid structure has not been readily demonstrated in thin section or negative-contrast staining of arenaviruses. Only in one instance in which uranyl acetate could penetrate the virion was an electron-dense center of supercoiled strands of indeterminant length seen (Palmer *et al.*, 1977). However, when virus disrupted by nonionic detergent was centrifuged to equilibrium in CsCl, a ribonucleoproteinlike structure banded at 1.31–1.37 g/cm^3 (see Table 4). Examination of the ribonucleoprotein of Pichinde virus under the electron microscope indicated the presence of convoluted, filamentous strands 9–15 nm in diameter (Vezza *et al.*, 1978). Convoluted strands of 30–40 Å in diameter were also observed in Tacaribe virus preparations, while in Tamiami virus preparations strands were observed which were beaded structures that were spaced at a periodicity of 45 Å. A careful examination of Tacaribe virus ribonucleoprotein structures by Palmer *et al.* 1977) revealed supercoiled structures which appeared as strings of beads. The strands did not appear as typical helixes and could be traced as closed circles. The length of the circles fell into two predominant size classes, 640 nm and 1300 nm; length of the circles did not bear a simple relationship to the size of virus genomic RNA. Some large aggregates of coiled filament with free ends were also observed.

When Pichinde virus was disrupted with detergent and sedimented in sucrose gradients, a fast-sedimenting ribonucleoprotein structure was demonstrated (Farber and Rawls, 1975; Buchmeier *et al.*, 1977). Pedersen and Konigshofer (1976) treated LCM with detergent in high salt and, on certrifugation in sucrose gradient, three size classes of ribonucleoprotein were seen: V1 (148 S), V2 (123 S), and V3 (83 S). V1 and V2 contained both 31 S and 23 S RNA, while only 23 S RNA was present in V3. The authors suggested that the V1 and V2 might be an

TABLE 4

Density of Ribonucleoproteinlike Structures

Virus	CsCl	Sucrose	Metrizamide	Reference
LCM	1.37 g/cm³	—	—	Pedersen and Konigshofer (1976)
	—	—	1.16–1.17 g/cm³	Buchmeier et al. (1978)
Pichinde	1.32–1.34 g/cm³	—	—	Ramos et al. (1972)
	1.37 g/cm³	—	—	Farber and Rawls (1975)
	1.31 g/cm³	—	—	Vezza et al. (1977)
		> 1.24 g/cm³	—	Buchmeier et al. (1977)
Tacaribe	1.31 g/cm³	—	—	Palmer et al. (1977)
	1.36 g/cm³	—	—	Gard et al. (1977)
Tamiami	1.36 g/cm³	—	—	Gard et al. (1977)

aggregate of V3 and another ribonucleoprotein containing only 31 S RNA.

The ribonucleoproteins in arenavirus were found to be sensitive to RNase. The predominant protein species contained in this structure is a 66,000-dalton polypeptide in Pichinde virus (Buchmeier et al., 1977) and a 63,000-dalton polypeptide in LCM (Buchmeier et al., 1978). A minor polypeptide of 79,000 daltons, along with the major polypeptide of 68,000 daltons, was found in the ribonucleoprotein structures of Tacaribe and Tamiami viruses (Gard et al., 1977). An RNA transcriptase activity has been found to be associated with the ribonucleoprotein structure of Pichinde virus (Leung, 1978a; Leung et al., 1979a).

7.3. Virus-Associated Enzymes

An RNA-dependent RNA polymerase was found to be associated with purified Pichinde virus preparations (Carter et al., 1974). Disruption of the virus by nonionic detergent was required to detect the enzyme activity, which also needed both Mg^{2+} and Mn^{2+} for maximal activity. The in vitro polymerization product formed an RNase-resistant product when hybridized with RNA extracted from the virus. This RNA–RNA hybrid sedimented in sucrose gradients at a broad peak of about 16 S. On more careful analysis of the polymerase activity associated with Pichinde virus, three types of activities have been delineated (Leung, 1977; Leung et al., 1979a). By subjecting the detergent-disrupted virus to velocity sedimentation in sucrose gradients, an RNA transcriptase activity was found to be associated with the fast-sedimenting ribonucleoprotein complex, while poly(U) and poly(A) polymerase activities were found to be associated with the ribosomes. The transcriptase activities synthesized long strands of heteropolymeric RNA in the *in vitro* reaction. Multiple RNA species of varied sizes were observed when the product was analyzed by polyacrylamide gel electrophoresis. The product was also found to hybridize with the virion RNA but not with ribosomal RNA or transfer RNA.

The ribosome-associated RNA-polymerizing activities exhibited properties similar to the poly(U) and poly(A) polymerases associated with the polyribosome fractions prepared from uninfected BHK-21 cells. The poly(U) polymerase required Mg^{2+} while Mn^{2+} alone was sufficient to catalyze the polymerizing activity of poly(A) polymerase. *In vitro*, both activities synthesized short segments of RNA, and most of the synthesized products of both enzymes existed in the reaction mixture as free RNA segments. Portions of the synthesized products, however, were attached to the 28 S and 18 S rRNA of the virus, probably by terminal addition. The poly(A) polymerase was found to have an additional property in that it could accept, as a primer, exogenous viral complementary RNA which had been synthesized *in vitro* by the viral transcriptase. This observation raises the possibility that the poly(A) polymerase may function *in vivo* to add poly-adenylated sequences to complementary RNA synthesized by the virion-associated transcriptase. No comparable role could be postulated for the poly(U) polymerase. However, as with the virion-associated ribosomes, the incorporation of these polymerases into the virion may inadvertently occur during morphogenesis and may have no required role in virus replication.

8. REPLICATION IN CULTURED CELLS

The arenaviruses replicate in a variety of mammalian cells; however, most information about virus replication has been derived from studies carried out in L cells and BHK-21 cells. The adsorption of LCM, Pichinde virus, and Machupo virus has been examined, and maximum adsorption occurred within 1.5–2 hr. Examination of the kinetics of penetration of LCM demonstrated that this process was complete after 45 min at 37°C; uncoating of the penetrated virus was thought to be complete within 2 hr (review by Pfau, 1974). Virus progeny can be detected between 7 and 8 hr after infection, and, during the exponential phase of growth, more virus is cell associated than is free in the culture medium. Maximum titers of virus are detected 24–36 hr after infection of cultures with a multiplicity of 1 infectious unit per cell or greater (Mifune *et al.*, 1971; Von Boekmer *et al.*, 1974; Lehmann-Grube *et al.*, 1975).

There are several aspects of the interaction between cells and arenaviruses which deserve consideration. Unlike as with a number of other viruses, infection by the arenaviruses is not usually associated with marked alterations of host cell macromolecular synthesis. Variable effects of the viruses on the cells have been reported. In certain instances, the cells appear to undergo cytopathogenic changes rather soon after infection, while in other circumstances the cytopathogenic changes do not develop until some time after maximum infectious virus is produced. However, the virus is not lethal to many cells, and carrier cultures have been readily established (Wagner and Synder, 1962; Traub and Kesting, 1963; Lehmann-Grube *et al.*, 1969; Boxaca, 1970; Staneck *et al.*, 1972). Cells in the chronically infected cultures are morphologically similar to uninfected cells and have similar growth characteristics. Alterations in the production of specific enzymes of differentiated cells were noted in cultures of murine neuroblastoma cells infected with LCM whereas the vital functions of the cell were not affected (Oldstone *et al.*, 1977). This observation on the ability of the cell to synthesize or degrade acetylcholine, the major neurotransmitter substance, may be related to the recently reported behavioral aberration observed in the LCM carrier mouse (Hotchin and Seegal, 1977).

Where examined, carrier cultures appeared to have the characteristics of the carrier state defined by Walker (1964) as a regulated infection. Such cultures were characterized by the presence of viral antigens in a large fraction of the cells, and clones of infected cells could be readily obtained. If uninfected cells were cloned from the carrier cultures, the cells were susceptible to infection by the virus, while chronically infected cells were resistant to homologous virus. These cultures also did not require antibodies for the maintenance of the carrier state nor were the cultures readily freed of virus by the addition of antiviral antibody to the medium. Thus the expression of the genome of the arenavirus-infected cells appeared to be regulated in the cells, and both virus and cell could coexist.

The factors which regulate the expression of the virus genome in the carrier state are poorly understood. Studies of L cells infected with LCM virus have provided evidence suggesting that cells are transiently infected with the virus (Hotchin, 1973). This evidence has been reviewed by Hotchin (1974), who postulates that the virus may go through a replicative cycle without producing cell death. Furthermore, the data are compatible with the cell's ultimately losing the genetic information of the virus and becoming susceptible to reinfection. Persistence in cell cultures or in animals could thus result from repeat cyclic infections of cells.

Strains with different plaquing and organ tropism can be derived from stocks of LCM virus; however, the strains, although differing in their characteristics in carrier cultures, are all capable of existing in a carrier state (Hotchin *et al.*, 1975). The production of nonreplicating defective particles which interfere with productive virus replication has also been suggested as a mechanism for maintenance of the carrier state (Welsh *et al.*, 1972).

Another possible mechanism of persistence of the arenaviruses in through a DNA transcript of the virus genome. Attempts to detect virion-associated reverse transcriptase activity were unsuccessful (Carter *et al.*, 1974; Welsh *et al.*, 1975). DNA extracted from LCM virus carrier cultures was found by Holland *et al.* (1976) not to transfer LCM in transfection experiments. Contrary to these observations, Gaidamovich *et al.* (1978) reported transfer of LCM genetic information from a carrier culture of Detroit-6 cells to a mouse lymphoid cell line using extracted DNA. While the bulk of evidence indicates a DNA provirus form as an unlikely mechanism for persistence of the virus genome, this possibility cannot be completely excluded.

Virus antigens which are detectable by immunofluorescence appear in the cytoplasm and on the surface of virus-infected cells. The major antigen detectable in the cytoplasm is represented in the core of the virion, while the antigens detectable at the surface of the cell are thought to be represented at the surface of the virion (Lehmann-Grube *et al.*, 1975; Gschwender *et al.*, 1976; Buchmeier *et al.*, 1977). During acute infection, intracytoplasmic antigen becomes detectable about the time new virus production begins (Lehmann-Grube *et al.*, 1975), and the same is true for cell-surface antigens. The appearance of these antigens in carrier cultures has been found, at times, to be discordant; a greater percentage of cells normally contain detectable intracytoplasmic antigen than cell-surface antigen. In the cultures, there may be a cycling of the proportion of cells expressing the antigens at the two sites, and the intracytoplasmic antigen and cell-surface antigen expression need not cycle synchronously. These observations suggest that replication and/or expression of genes for the different antigens might be independent of each other in the carrier state (Hotchin *et al.*, 1975).

Inhibitors of DNA synthesis such as 5-bromodeoxyuridine and 5-

iododeoxyuridine do not inhibit the replication of arenaviruses (see Pfau, 1974). This observation and the absence of a virion-associated RNA-dependent DNA polymerase (Carter *et al.*, 1974) suggest that the virus RNA does not replicate through a DNA intermediate. As indicated above, a RNA transcriptase has been found in association with Pichinde virus, and the virus RNA was found to lack characteristics of messenger RNA. Polysomal RNA isolated from cells infected with Pichinde virus was found to hybridize to RNA extracted from purified virus. The polysomal RNA used in the hybridization studies had messenger function as determined by the presence of polyadenylated sequences and the ability of the polysomal RNA to translate into virus structural proteins in an *in vitro* protein-synthesizing system (Leung *et al.*, 1977; Leung, 1978*a*). Thus the RNA of the arenaviruses appears to be negative stranded. While no information is available on the replication of RNA of the arenaviruses within infected cells, it can be expected to be similar to that observed for other negative-stranded RNA viruses.

The expression of virus genome appears to be influenced in part by host cell factors. For example, the yield of infectious LCM and Pichinde virus was found to be about tenfold greater from BHK-21 cells when the cells were in the exponential phase of growth than when the cells were in stationary phase (Pfau *et al.*, 1973; Rawls *et al.*, 1976). As observed with Japanese encephalitis virus and influenza virus, no antigens of Pichinde virus were synthesized in cells which had been enucleated with cytochalasin B (Banerjee *et al.*, 1976). Nuclear functions were required for initiation of antigen production, and studies with actinomycin D suggest that a cell function is required for maturation. Actinomycin D at concentrations which inhibit cellular RNA synthesis inhibited the production of infectious virus (Buck and Pfau, 1969; Mifune *et al.*, 1971; Stanwick and Kirk, 1971). The drug did not inhibit antigen synthesis but did appear to block a late step in the replicative cycle of Pichinde virus (Rawls *et al.*, 1976) and LCM virus (Buchmeier and Welsh, personal communication). An exception to this effect of actinomycin D has been observed by Coto and Vomberger (1969), who found that Junin virus was not inhibited by the drug. α-Amanitin, at concentrations which blocked cellular mRNA synthesis, also inhibited the synthesis of Pichinde virus. The inhibitory effect of α-amanitin was not observed in α-amanitin-resistant cells with a genetic lesion in the cellular DNA-dependent RNA polymerase II. This indicates that a cellular function expressed by the RNA polymerase II is required for virus replication (Leung, 1978*b*).

In addition to actinomycin D and α-amanitin, other compounds have been shown to inhibit the replication of arenaviruses in tissue cultures (Pfau, 1975). High concentration of glucosamine (16 mM) was found to inhibit the synthesis of viral antigens which appear on the cell surface and infectious virus production but not antigens located in the cytoplasm of the cell (L. A. Martinez-Peralta, personal communication). Amantadine hydrochloride was found to inhibit the replication of LCM and members of the Tacaribe complex (Coto *et al.*, 1969; Pfau *et al.*, 1972). The experimental data suggested that the drug delayed or prevented the penetration step in LCM replication and also inhibited a late function of the replicative cycle such as virus maturation or release.

9. INTERFERENCE AND DEFECTIVE INTERFERING PARTICLES

The phenomenon of homologous interference was first described by Traub (1938), who was studying mice persistently infected with LCM. It was subsequently shown that cells grown *in vitro* and persistently infected with LCM were resistant to superinfection by the virus but were susceptible to unrelated viruses (Lehmann-Grube *et al.*, 1969; Staneck *et al.*, 1972). Interestingly, cells infected with one arenavirus are resistant to the replication of another arenavirus (Staneck and Pfau, 1974). A number of studies have provided evidence that defective interfering particles are produced which reduce the yields of infectious virus and prevent CPE in lytic virus–cell combinations (Welsh and Pfau, 1972; Welsh *et al.*, 1972, 1975; Staneck *et al.*, 1972; Staneck and Pfau, 1974; Dutko *et al.*, 1976; Popescu *et al.*, 1976; Dutko and Pfau, 1978).

The characterization of the interfering particle was achieved by a quantitative assay based on the interference with infectious center formation by standard virus (Welsh and Pfau, 1972). A more sensitive and accurate assay has recently been described which is based on the ability of the defective interfering (DI) particle to protect L cells against the cytolytic effect of concomitantly added standard LCM virus; the protected cells are visible as foci or colonies of surviving cells (Popescu *et al.*, 1976). The DI particles of LCM virus have been studied in some detail. Prior infection of cells with DI particles blocks the expression of the genome of the standard virus; the synthesis of polypeptides NP and GPC is inhibited, and viral antigen and infectious virus are not produced (Welsh and Oldstone, 1977; Welsh and Buchmeier, personal communication). The interference by LCM DI particles can be neutralized by antiserum to LCM, and DI particles prevent cell death in cells which are normally destroyed by standard virus (Dutko and Pfau, 1978).

Particles with antigenicity of LCM virus were found in the culture medium of persistently infected cultures, although infectious virus could not be detected (Lehmann-Grube *et al.*, 1969). The antigenic particle could represent a low-pathogenicity variant of the virus which plaqued poorly (Hotchin and Sikova, 1973) or DI particles. In other studies, LCM DI particles were detected in abundance after the initial peak of infectious virus production, and they appear to represent the major particulate product in carrier cultures.

Characterization of DI particles has been somewhat hampered by the difficulty of separating DI particles from standard virus by physical means. Initial efforts to characterize biochemically the DI particles utilized material obtained from culture medium collected from persistently infected cells; the production of infectious virus is minimal under these conditions.

The interfering activity of LCM and Parana DI particles was found to be more resistant to UV irradiation than that of standard virus, which has been interpreted as a smaller nucleic acid target size for interference than for infectivity (Welsh *et al.*, 1972; Staneck and Pfau, 1974). Biochemical analysis of Pichinde virus DI particles revealed alterations in the nucleic acid composition of particles harvested at different passage times; initially no 22 S RNA and 15 S RNA were found. On subsequent passages there was a loss of 31 S RNA, while on 175 or more passages of the persistently infected cells a new 20 S RNA species appeared (Dutko *et al.*, 1976). In Parana virus DI particles, the 24 S RNA disappeared while the 37 S RNA remained unchanged (Dutko *et al.*, 1978). Although the LCM DI particle has buoyancy density slightly lower than that of the standard virus in Renograffin 76, no differences in RNA profiles or protein composition were found between DI particles and infectious LCM (Welsh *et al.*, 1975; Welsh and Buchmeier, personal communication). The reasons for these discrepancies are not apparent.

The role of DI particles in infections by arenaviruses in animals is not clear. LCM DI particles injected concomitantly with standard virus were found to reduce the synthesis of infectious virus and the production of virus antigen, and prevented the development of virus-induced cerebellar disease in rats (Welsh *et al.*, 1977). This effect was not observed if the DI particles were injected prior to standard virus. An analysis of the production of infectious virus and DI particles in mice acutely and persistently infected with LCM was carried out by Popescu

and Lehmann-Grube (1977). Initially, both standard virus and DI particles multiplied to high titers, after which the concentrations of both
declined until relatively constant levels were reached when the animals
were 1–2 months of age. The quantities of both entities as well as their
ratios varied between organs and also changed with time. The relative
quantities of a turbid-plaque variant were also found to increase with
time. While these studies indicate that DI particles may be produced *in
vivo*, the role of these particles in the pathogenesis of the infection
remains uncertain.

10. CONCLUDING REMARKS

The persistence of the arenaviruses in their reservoir host is a
central issue of interest. The persistently infected rodents are the major
source of virus which infects man and gives rise to the hemorrhagic
fevers, aseptic meningitis, and Lassa fever. Despite our understanding
of the epidemiology of these diseases, the illnesses continue to occur,
and in some areas the incidence of the diseases is increasing (Maiztequi,
1975). In addition, it is becoming apparent that persistent virus infections may be responsible for certain chronic diseases in humans (Fuccillo *et al.*, 1974). Thus the stimuli to understand the persistence of
arenaviruses both from the point of view of the diseases they produce
and as a model for studying the persistence of other viruses have
intensified.

The information available indicates that the arenaviruses are
enveloped, negative-stranded RNA viruses with segmented genomes.
They are unique with respect to the presence of ribosomes within the
virion and apparently unstructured core. No function has yet been
assigned to the ribosomes. The viruses have a major polypeptide that is
associated with the genome, and one or two glycopeptides which are
located on the virus envelope. This descriptive information yields no
clues as to the molecular basis for persistence.

Our knowledge of the intracellular events which occur during
replication is very rudimentary. One would anticipate that knowledge in
this area would be most fruitful in unraveling the secret of persistence.
Indirect evidence suggests that the virus can complete a replicative
cycle without producing cell death. However, to appreciate the significance of this possibility, the mechanism controlling virus gene
expression and the means whereby the virus genome is lost need to be
delineated. Equally attractive is the hypothesis of defective interfering
virus as an explanation of regulation of virus replication. The existence

of interfering particles is reasonably well established, but the difficulty in easily separating these particles from infectious virus by physical means leaves some doubt as to their actual composition. Information on the molecular events giving rise to such particles and the means by which the particles interfere with the production of infectious virus is also needed to reveal the significance of the interfering particles in persistence. It is clear that more information than presently exists is needed before we will be able to appreciate the molecular events involved in arenavirus persistence.

ACKNOWLEDGMENTS

The photomicrographs were kindly provided by Dr. F. A. Murphy. Studies in the authors' laboratory were supported by grants from the Medical Research Council of Canada.

11. REFERENCES

Abelson, H. T., Smith, G. H., Hoffman, H. A., and Rowe, W. P., 1969, Use of enzyme-labeled antibody for electron microscopic localization of lymphocytic choriomeningitis virus antigen in infected cell cultures, *J. Natl. Cancer Inst.* **42**:497.

Anon, M. C., Grau, O., Martinez-Segovia, Z., and Franze-Fernandez, M. T., 1976, RNA Composition of Junin virus, *J. Virol.* **18**:833.

Armstrong, C., and Lillie, R. D., 1934, Experimental lymphocytic choriomeningitis of monkeys and mice produced by a virus encountered in studies of the 1933 St. Louis encephalitis epidemic, *Public Health Rep.* **49**:1019.

Armstrong, C., and Sweet, L. K., 1939, Lymphocytic choriomeningitis report of two cases with recovery of the virus from gray mice (*Mus musculus*) trapped in the two infected households, *Public Health Rep.* **54**:673.

Banerjee, S. N., Buchmeier, M., and Rawls, W. E., 1976, Requirement of cell nucleus for the replication of an arenavirus, *Intervirology* **6**:190.

Besuschio, S. C., Weissenbacher, M. C., and Schmunis, G. A., 1973, Different histopathological responses to arenovirus infection of thymectomized mice, *Arch. Gesamte Virusforsch.* **40**:21.

Blechschmidt, M., and Thomssen, R., 1976, Electron-microscopic identification of infectious particles of lymphocytic choriomeningitis, *Med. Microbiol. Immunol.* **162**:193.

Borden, E. C., and Nathanson, N., 1974, Tacaribe virus infection of the mouse: An immunopathologic disease model, *Lab. Invest.* **30**:465.

Boxaca, M., 1970, Estabecimiento y caracteristicas de civa Sublinea de celulas Vero persistentemente infectadas con virus Junin, *Medicina* (Buenos Aires) **30**:50.

Bro-Jorgensen, K., 1971, Characterization of virus-specific antigen in cell cultures infected with lymphocytic choriomeningitis virus, *Acta Pathol. Microbiol. Scand. Sect. B* **79**:466.

Buchmeier, M. J., and Oldstone, M. B. A., 1978*a*, Identity of the viral protein responsible for serologic cross reactivity among the Tacaribe complex arenavirus, in: *Negative Strand Viruses and the Host Cell* (B. W. J. Mahy and R. D. Barry, eds.), pp. 91–97, Academic Press, New York.

Buchmeier, M. J., and Oldstone, M. B. A., 1978*b*, Virus induced immune complex disease: Identification of specific viral antigens and antibodies deposited in complexes during chronic lymphocytic choriomeningitis virus infection, *J. Immunol.* **120**:1297.

Buchmeier, M. J., and Rawls, W. E., 1977, Variation between strains of hamsters in the lethality of Pichinde virus infections, *Infect. Immun.* **16**:413.

Buchmeier, M. J., Gee, S. R., and Rawls, W. E., 1977, The antigens of Pichinde virus. I. The relationship of soluble antigens derived from infected BHK_{21} cells with the structural components of the virion, *J. Virol.* **22**:175.

Buchmeier, M. J., Elder, J. H., and Oldstone, M. B. A., 1978, Protein structure of lymphocytic choriomeningitis virus: Identification of the virus structural and cell associated polypeptides, *Virology* **89**:133.

Buck, L. L., and Pfau, C. J., 1969, Inhibition of lymphocytic choriomeningitis virus replication by actinomycin D and 6 azauridine, *Virology* **37**:698.

Buckley, S. M., and Casals, J., 1970, Lassa fever, a new virus disease of man from West Africa. III. Isolation and characterization of the virus, *Am. J. Trop. Med. Hyg.* **19**:680.

Calisher, C. H., Tzianabos, T., Lord, R. D., and Coleman, P. H., 1970, Tamiami virus, a new member of the Tacaribe group, *Am. J. Trop. Med. Hyg.* **19**:520.

Carter, M. F., Biswal, N., and Rawls, W. E., 1973*a*, Characterization of nucleic acids of Pichinde virus, *J. Virol.* **11**:61.

Carter, M. F., Murphy, F. A., Brunschweg, J. P., Noonan, C., and Rawls, W. E., 1973*b*, Effects of actinomycin D and ultra-violet and ionizing radiation on Pichinde virus, *J. Virol.* **12**:33.

Carter, M. F., Biswal, N., and Rawls, W. E., 1974, Polymerase activity of Pichinde virus, *J. Virol.* **13**:577.

Casals, J., 1975, Arenaviruses, *Yale J. Biol. Med.* **48**:115.

Casals, J., Buckley, S. M., and Cedeno, R., 1975, Antigenic properties of the arenaviruses, *Bull. WHO* **52**:421.

Child, P. L., MacKenzie, R. B., Valverde, L., and Johnson, K. M., 1967, Bolivian hemorrhagic fever. A pathological description, *Arch. Pathol.* **83**:434.

Cole, G. A., and Nathanson, N., 1974, Lymphocytic choriomeningitis pathogenesis, *Prog. Med. Virol.* **18**:94.

Cole, G. A., Predergast, P. A., and Henney, C. S., 1973, *In vitro* correlates of LCM virion-induced immune responses, in: *Lymphocytic Choriomeningitis Virus and Other Arenaviruses*, (F. Lehmann-Grube, ed.), pp. 60–71, Springer, Berlin.

Coto, C. E., and Vomberger, M. D., 1969, The effect of 5-iododeoxyuridine and actinomycin D on the multiplication of Junin virus, *Arch. Gesamte Virusforsch.* **27**:307.

Coto, C. E., Calello, M. A., and Parodi, A. S., 1969, Efecto de la amantadana HCl sobre la infectividad del virus de Junin (F. H. A.) *in vitro* y *in vivo*, *Rev. Asoc. Argent. Microbiol.* **1**:3.

Dalton, A. J., Rowe, W. P., Smith, G. H., Wilsnack, R. E., and Pugh, W. E., 1968, Morphological and cytochemical studies on lymphocytic choriomeningitis virus, *J. Virol* **2**:1465.

de Bracco, M. M. E., Rimoldi, M. T., Cossio, P. M., Rabinovich, A., Maiztequi, J. I., Carballal, G., and Arana, R. M., 1978, Argentine hemorrhagic fever, alterations of the complement system and anti-Junin-virus humoral response, *New Engl. J. Med.* **299**:216.

Downs, W. G., Andersen, C. R., Spence, L., Aitken, T. H. G., and Greenhall, A. H., 1963, Tacaribe virus, a new agent isolated from antibesis bats and mosquitoes in Trinidad, West Indies, *Am. J. Trop. Med. Hyg.* **12**:640.

Dutko, F. J., and Pfau, C. J., 1978, Arenaviruses defective interfering particles mask the cell-killing potential of standard virus, *J. Gen. Virol.* **38**:195.

Dutko, F. J., Wright, E. A., and Pfau, C. J., 1976, The RNA's of defective interfering Pichinde virus, *J. Gen. Virol.* **31**:417.

Dutko, F. J., Helfand, J., and Pfau, C. J., 1978, The RNAs of standard and defective interfering Parana virus, Abstracts for Annual Meeting of American Society for Microbiology.

Elsner, B., Schwarz, E., Mondo, O. G., Maiztequi, J., and Vitches, A., 1973, Pathology of 12 fatal cases of Argentine hemorrhagic fever, *Am. J. Trop. Med. Hyg.* **22**:229.

Farber, F. E., and Rawls, W. E., 1975, Isolation of ribosome-like structure from Pichinde virus, *J. Gen. Virol.* **26**:21.

Fuccillo, D. A., Kurent, J. E., and Sever, J. L., 1974, Slow virus diseases, *Am. Rev. Microbiol.*, 231.

Gaidamovich, S. Ya., Cherednichenko, Y. N., and Rdanov, V. M., 1978, On the mechanism of the persistence of lymphocytic choriomeningitis virus in the continuous cell line Detroit-6, *Intervirology* **9**:156.

Gajdamovic, S. J., Klisenko, G. A., Kocerovskaja, M. J., and Sanojan, N. K., 1975, Antigenic relationships of lymphocytic choriomeningitis virus and Tacaribe virus in the indirect haemagglutination test, *Bull. WHO* **52**:437.

Gard, G. P., Vezza, A. C., Bishop, D. H. L., and Compans, R. W., 1977, Structural proteins of Tacaribe and Tamiami virions, *Virology* **83**:84.

Gschwender, H. H., Brummund, M., and Lehmann-Grube, F., 1975, Lymphocytic choriomeningitis virus. I. Concentration and purification of the infectious virus, *J. Virol.* **15**:1317.

Gschwender, H. H., Rutter, G., and Lehmann-Grube, F., 1976, Lymphocytic choriomeningitis virus. II. Characterization of extractable complement-fixing activity, *Med. Microbiol. Immunol.* **162**:119.

Henderson, B. E., Guay, G. W., Jr., Kissling, R. E., Fraenes, J. D., and Carey, D. E., 1972, Lassa fever, virological and serological studies, *Trans. R. Soc. Trop. Med. Hyg.* **66**:409.

Holland, J. J., Villarreal, L. P., Welsh, R. M., Oldstone, M. B. A., Kohne, D., Lazzarini, R., and Scolnicks, E., 1976, Long term persistent vesicular stomatitis virus and rabies virus infection of cells *in vitro*, *J. Gen. Virol.* **33**:193.

Hotchin, J., 1962, The biology of lymphocytic choriomeningitis infection. Virus-induced immune disease, *Cold Spring Harbor Symp. Quant. Biol.* **27**:479.

Hotchin, J., 1971, Persistent and slow virus infections, Monographs in Virology 3, S. Karger, Basel.

Hotchin, J., 1973, Transient virus infection: Spontaneous recovery mechanism of lymphocytic choriomeningitis virus-infected cells, *Nature (London) New Biol.* **241**:270.

Hotchin, J., 1974, The role of transient infection in arenavirus persistence, *Prog. Med. Virol.* **18**:81.

Hotchin, J., and Seegal, R., 1977, Virus-induced behavioral alterations of mice, *Science* **196**:671.

Hotchin, J., and Sikora, E., 1973, Low-pathogenicity variant of lymphocytic chorio-meningitis virus, *Infect. Immun.* **7**:825.

Hotchin, J., Kinch, W., Benson, L., and Sikora, E., 1975, Role of substrains in persistent lymphocytic choriomeningitis virus infection, *Bull. WHO* **52**:457.

Johnson, K. M., 1965, Epidemiology of Machupo virus infection. III. Significance of virological observations in man and animals, *Am. J. Trop. Med. Hyg.* **14**:816.

Johnson, K. M., Wiebenga, U. H., MacKenzie, R. B., Kuns, M. L., Tauraso, N. M., Sholokov, A., Webb, P. A., Justines, G., and Beye, H. K., 1965a, Virus isolations from human cases of hemorrhagic fever in Bolivia, *Proc. Soc. Exp. Biol. Med.* **118**:113.

Johnson, K. M., MacKenzie, R. B., Webb, P. A., and Kuns, M. L., 1965b, Chronic infection of rodents by Machupo virus, *Science* **150**:1618.

Johnson, K. M., Webb, P. A., and Justines, G., 1973, Biology of Tacaribe-complex viruses, in: *Lymphocytic Choriomeningitis Virus and Other Arenaviruses* (F. Lehmann-Grube, ed.), pp. 241–258, Springer, Berlin.

Lascano, E. F., and Berria, M. I., 1974, Ultrastructure of Junin in mouse whole brain and mouse brain tissue culture, *J. Virol.* **14**:965.

Lehmann-Grube, F., 1971, *Lymphocytic Choriomeningitis Virus*, Virology Monographs 10, Springer-Verlag, New York.

Lehmann-Grube, F., Slenezka, W., and Tees, R., 1969, A persistent and inapparent infection of L cells with the virus of lymphocytic choriomeningitis, *J. Gen. Virol.* **5**:63.

Lehmann-Grube, F., Popescu, M., Schaefer, H., and Gschwender, H. H., 1975, LCM virus infection of cells *in vitro*, *Bull WHO* **52**:443.

Lepine, P., Molldret, P., and Kreis, B., 1937, Receptivite de l'homme au virus murin de la choriomeningite lymphocytaire. Reproduction experimentale de la meningite lymphocytaire benigne, *C. R. Acad. Sci.* **240**:1846.

Leung, W.-C., 1978a, Considerations of the replication of Pichinde virus—An arenavirus, in: *Negative Strand Viruses and the Host Cell* (B. W. J. Mahy and R. D. Barry, eds.), pp. 415–426, Academic Press, New York.

Leung, W.-C., 1978b, Involvement of cellular DNA-dependent RNA polymerase II in the replication of Pichinde virus, in: *Proceedings of the Fourth International Congress for Virology*, Hague, the Netherlands.

Leung, W.-C., and Rawls, W. E., 1977, Virion-associated ribosomes are not required for the replication of Pichinde virus, *Virology* **81**:174.

Leung, W.-C., Ghosh, H. P., and Rawls, W. E., 1977, Strandedness of Pichinde virus RNA, *J. Virol.* **22**:235.

Leung, E.-C., Leung, M. F. K. L., and Rawls, W. E., 1979a, Distinctive RNA transcriptase, polyadenylic acid polymerase, and polyuridylic acid polymerase activities associated with Pichinde virus. *J. Virol.* **30**:98.

Leung, W.-C., Dimock, K., Petrovich, J., Leung, M. F. K. L., Guerra, M. R., and Rawls, W. E., 1979b, *In vitro* synthesis of complementary DNA to Pichinde virus RNA, Abstracts for 1979 Annual meeting of American Society for Microbiology.

Maiztegui, J. I., 1975, Clinical and epidemiological patterns of Argentine haemorrhagic fever, *Bull. WHO* **52**:567.

Maiztegui, J. I., Laquens, R. P., Cassio, P. M., Cassanova, M. B., de la Vega, M. T., Ritacco, V., Segal, A., Fernandez, N. J., and Arana, R. M., 1975, Ultrastructural and immunohistochemical studies in five cases of Argentine hemorrhagic fever, *J. Infect. Dis.* **132**:35.

Mannweiler, K., and Lehmann-Grube, F., 1973, Electron microscopy of LCM virus-infected L cells, in: *Lymphocytic Choriomeningitis Virus and Other Arenaviruses* (F. Lehmann-Grube, ed.), pp. 37–48, Springer, Berlin.

Martinez-Segovia, Z., and de Mitri, M. I., 1977, Junin virus structural proteins, *J. Virol.* **21**:579.

Mifune, K., Carter, M., and Rawls, W. E., 1971, Characterization studies of the Pichinde virus—a member of the arenavirus group, *Proc. Soc. Exp. Biol. Med.* **136**:637.

Mims, C. A., 1970, Observations on mice infected congenitally or neonatally with lymphocytic choriomeningitis (LCM) virus, *Arch. Gesamte Virusforsch.* **30**:67.

Mims, C. A., and Blanden, R. V., 1972, Antiviral action of immune lymphocytes in mice infected with lymphocytic choriomeningitis virus, *Infect. Immun.* **6**:695.

Mims, C. A., and Tosolini, F. A., 1969, Pathogenesis of lesions in lymphoid tissue of mice infected with lymphocytic choriomeningitis (LCM) virus, *Br. J. Exp. Pathol.* **50**:584.

Monath, T. P., Newhouse, V. F., Kemp, G. E., Setzer, H. W., and Cacciapicoti, A., 1974, Lassa virus isolation from *Mastomys natalensis* rodents during an epidemic in Sierra Leone, *Science* **185**:263.

Murphy, F. A., and Whitfield, S. G., 1975, Morphology and morphogenesis of arenaviruses, *Bull. WHO* **52**:409.

Murphy, F. A., Webb, P. A., Johnson, K. M., and Whitfield, S. G., 1969, Morphological comparison of Machupo with lymphocytic choriomeningitis virus: Basis for a new taxonomic group, *J. Virol.* **4**:535.

Murphy, F. A., Webb, P. A., Johnson, K. M., Whitfield, S. G., and Chappell, W. A., 1970, Arenaviruses in Vero cells: Ultrastructural studies, *J. Virol.* **6**:507.

Murphy, F. A., Whitfield, S. G., Webb, P. A., and Johnson, K. M., 1973, Ultrastructural studies of arenaviruses, in: *Lymphocytic Choriomeningitis Virus and Other Arenaviruses* (F. Lehmann-Grube, ed.), pp. 273–285, Springer, Berlin.

Murphy, F. A., Winn, W. C., Jr., Walker, P. H., Flemister, M. R., and Whitfield, S. G., 1976, Early lymphoreticular viral tropism and antigen persistence: Tamiami virus infection in the cotton rat, *Lab. Invest.* **34**:125.

Murphy, F. A., Buchmeier, M. J., and Rawls, W. E., 1977, The reticuloendothelium as the target in a virus infection: Pichinde virus pathogenesis in two strains of hamsters, *Lab. Invest.* **37**:502.

Nathanson, N., Monjan, A. H., Panitch, H. S., Johnsen, E. D., Peturssen, G., and Cole, G. A., 1975, Virus-induced cell-mediated immunopathological disease, in: *Viral Immunology and Immunopathology* (A. L. Notkins, ed.), pp. 357–391, Academic Press, New York.

Oldstone, M. B. A., and Dixon, F. S., 1967, Lymphocytic choriomeningitis; production of antibody by "tolerant" infected mice, *Science* **158**:1193.

Oldstone, M. B. A., and Dixon, F. J., 1969, Pathogenesis of chronic disease associated with persistent lymphocytic choriomeningitis viral infection. I. Relationship of antibody production to disease in neonatally infected mice, *J. Exp. Med.* **129**:483.

Oldstone, M. B. A., Holmstoen, J., and Welsh, R. M., Jr., 1977, Alterations of acetylcholine enzymes in neuroblastoma cells persistently infected with lymphocytic choriomeningitis virus, *J. Cell. Physiol.* **91**:459.

Palmer, E. L., Obijeski, J. F., Webb, P. A., and Johnson, K. M., 1977, The circular segmented nucleocapsid of an arenavirus—Tacaribe virus, *J. Gen. Virol.* **36**:541.

Parker, J. C., Igel, H. J., Reynolds, R. K., Lewis, A. M., Jr., and Rowe, W. P., 1976, Lymphocytic choriomeningitis virus infection in fetal newborn and young adult Syrian hamsters (*Mesocricetus auratus*), *Infect. Immun.* **13**:967.

Parodi, A. J., Greenway, D. J., Rugiero, H. R., Rivers, S., Figerio, M., De la Barrera, J. M., Mattler, N., Garzon, F., Boxaca, M., de Guerrero, L., and Nota, N., 1958, Sobre la etiologia del brote epidermico de Junin, *Dia Med.* **30**:2300.

Pedersen, I. R., 1971, Lymphocytic choriomeningitis virus RNAs, *Nature (London)* **234**:112.

Pedersen, I. R., 1973, Different classes of ribonucleic acid isolated from lymphocytic choriomeningitis virus, *J. Virol.* **11**:416.

Pedersen, I. R., and Konigshofer, E. R., 1976, Characterization of ribonucleoproteins and ribosomes isolated from lymphocytic choriomeningitis virus, *J. Virol.* **20**:14.

Pfau, C. J., 1974, Biochemical and biophysical properties of the arenaviruses, *Prog. Med. Virol.* **18**:64.

Pfau, C. J., 1975, Arenavirus chemotherapy—Retrospect and prospect, *Bull WHO* **52**:737.

Pfau, C. J., Trowbridge, R. S., Welsh, R. M., Staneck, L. D., and O'Connell, C. M., 1972, Arenaviruses: Inhibition by amantadine hydrochloride, *J. Gen. Virol.* **14**:209.

Pfau, C. J., Welsh, R. M., and Trowbridge, R. S., 1973, Plaque assays and current concepts of regulation in arenavirus infections, in: *Lymphocytic Choriomeningitis Virus and Other Arenaviruses* (F. Lehmann-Grube, ed.), pp. 101–111, Springer, Berlin.

Pfau, C. J., Bergold, G. H., Casals, J., Johnson, K. M., Murphy, F. A., Pedersen, I. R., Rawls, W. E., Rowe, W. P., Webb, P. A., and Weissenbacher, M. C., 1974, Arenaviruses, *Intervirology* **4**:207.

Pinheiro, F. P., Shope, R. E., de Androde, A. H. P., Bensabeth, G., Cacios, G. V., and Casals, J., 1966, Amapari, a new virus of the Tacaribe group from rodents and mites of Amapa territory, Brazil, *Proc. Soc. Exp. Biol. Med.* **122**:531.

Popescu, M., and Lehmann-Grube, F., 1977, Defective interfering particles in mice infected with lymphocytic choriomeningitis virus, *Virology* **77**:78.

Popescu, M., Schaefer, H., and Lehmann-Grube, F., 1976, Homologous interference of lymphocytic choriomeningitis virus: Detection and measurement of interference focus-forming units, *J. Virol.* **20**:1.

Ramos, B. A., Courtney, R. J., and Rawls, W. E., 1972, The structural proteins of Pichinde virus, *J. Virol.* **10**:661.

Rawls, W. E., and Buchmeier, M., 1975, Arenaviruses: Purification and physicochemical nature, *Bull. WHO* **52**:393.

Rawls, W. E., Banerjee, S. N., McMillan, C. A., and Buchmeier, M. J., 1976, Inhibition of Pichinde virus replication by actinomycin D, *J. Gen. Virol.* **33**:421.

Rivers, T. M., and Scott, T. F. M., 1935, Meningitis in man caused by a filterable virus, *Science* **81**:439.

Rowe, W. P., Pugh, W. F., Webb, P. A., and Peters, C. J., 1970a, Serological relationships of the Tacaribe complex of viruses to lymphocytic choriomeningitis virus, *J. Virol.* **5**:289.

Rowe, W. P., Murphy, F. A., Bergold, G. H., Casals, J., Hotchin, J., Johnson, K. M., Lehmann-Grube, F., Mims, C. A., Traub, E., and Webb, P. A., 1970b, Arenoviruses: Proposed name for a newly defined virus group, *J. Virol.* **5**:651.

Sabattini, M. S., and Maiztequi, I. I., 1970, Fiebra hemorrhagica Argentina, *Medicina* (Buenos Aires) **30**:8.

Smadel, J. E., and Wall, M. J. 1940, A soluble antigen of lymphocytic choriomeningitis. III. Independence of anti-soluble substances antibodies and neutralizing antibodies and the role of soluble antigen and inactive viruses in immunity to infection, *J. Exp. Med.* **72**:389.

Smadel, J. E., Baird, R. D., and Wall, M. J., 1939, A soluble antigen of lymphocytic choriomeningitis. I. Separation of soluble antigen from virus, *J. Exp. Med.* **70**:53.

Smadel, J. E., Wall, M. J., and Baird, R. D., 1940, A soluble antigen of lymphocytic choriomeningitis. II. Characteristics of the antigen and its use in precipitin reactions, *J. Exp. Med.* **71**:43.

Smadel, J. E., Green, R. H., Paltauf, R. M., and Gonzales, T. A., 1942, Lymphocytic choriomeningitis; two human fatalities following an unusual febrile illness, *Proc. Soc. Exp. Biol. Med.* **49**:683.

Spier, R. W., Wood, O., Liebheber, H., and Buckley, S. M., 1970, Lassa fever, a new virus disease of man from West Africa. IV. Electron microscopy of Vero cell cultures infected with Lassa virus, *Am. J. Trop. Med. Hyg.* **19**:692.

Staneck, L. D., and Pfau, C. J., 1974, Interfering particles from a culture persistantly infected with parana virus, *J. Gen. Virol.* **22**:437.

Staneck, L. D., Trowbridge, R. S., Welsh, R. M., Wright, E. A., and Pfau, C. J., 1972, Arenaviruses. Cellular responses to long term *in vitro* infection with Parana and LCM, *Infect. Immun.* **6**:444.

Stanwick, T. L., and Kirk, B. F., 1971, Effect of actinomycin D on the yield of lymphocytic choriomeningitis virus in baby hamster kidney cells, *Infect. Immun.* **4**:511.

Tosolini, F. A., 1970, The response of mice to the intravenous infection of lymphocytic choriomeningitis virus, *Aust. J. Exp. Biol. Med. Sci.* **48**:445.

Trapido, H., and Sanmartin, C., 1971, Pichinde virus: A new virus of the Tacaribe group from Colombia, *Am. J. Trop. Med. Hyg.* **20**:631.

Traub, E., 1936, Persistence of lymphocytic choriomeningitis virus in immune animals and its relation to immunity, *J. Exp. Med.* **63**:847.

Traub, E., 1938, Factors influencing the persistence of choriomeningitis virus in the blood of mice after clinical recovery, *J. Exp. Med.* **68**:229.

Traub, E., and Kesting, F., 1963, Experiments in heterologous and homologous interference in LCM-infected cultures of murine lymph node cells, *Arch. Gesamte Virusforsch.* **14**:55.

Vezza, A. C., and Bishop, D. H. L., 1977, Recombination between temperature sensitive mutants of the arenavirus, Pichinde, *J. Virol.* **24**:712.

Vezza, A. C., Gard, G. P., Compans, R. W., and Bishop, D. H. L., 1977, Structural components of the arenavirus Pichinde, *J. Virol.* **23**:776.

Vezza, A. C., Clewley, J. P., Gard, G. P., Abraham, N. Z., Compans, R. W., and Bishop, D. H. L., 1978*a*, The virion RNA species of the arenaviruses Pichinde, Tacaribe and Tamiami, *J. Virol.* **26**:485.

Vezza, A. C., Gard, G. P., Compans, R. W., and Bishop, D. H. L., 1978*b*, Genetic and molecular studies of arenaviruses, in: *Negative Strand Viruses and the Host Cell* (B. W. J. Mahy and R. D. Barry, eds.), pp. 71–90, Academic Press, New York.

Vezza, A., Clewley, J. P., Gard, G. P., Saleh, F., Compans, R. W., and Bishop, D. H. L., 1978*c*, Comparative studies of arenavirus RNA and polypeptides, Abstracts of the Fourth International Congress for Virology, Hague, the Netherlands.

Von Boekmer, H., Lehman-Grube, F., Flower, R., and Heuwinkel, R., 1974, Multiplication of lymphocytic choriomeningitis virus in cultivated foetal inbred mouse cells and in neonatally infected inbred carrier mice, *J. Gen. Virol.* **25**:219.

Wagner, R. R., and Snyder, R. M., 1962, Viral interference induced in mice by acute or persistent infection with the virus of lymphocytic choriomeningitis, *Nature (London)* **196**:393.

Walker, D. H., Wulff, H., Lange, J. V., and Murphy, F. A., 1975a, Comparative pathology of Lassa virus infection in monkeys, guinea-pigs and *Mastomys natalensis*, *Bull. WHO* **52**:523.

Walker, D. H., Murphy, F. A., Whitfield, S. G., and Bauer, S. P., 1975b, Lymphocytic choriomeningitis: Ultrastructural pathology, *Exp. Mol. Pathol.* **23**:245.

Walker, D. L., 1964, The viral carrier state in animal cell cultures, *Prog. Med. Virol.* **6**:111.

Webb, P. A., 1965, Properties of Machupo virus, *Am. J. Trop. Med. Hyg.* **14**:799.

Webb, P. A., Johnson, K. M., Hibbs, J. B., and Kuns, M. L., 1970, Parana, a new Tacaribe complex virus from Paraguay, *Arch. Gesamte Virusforsch.* **32**:379.

Webb, P. A., Justines, G., and Johnson, K. M., 1975, Infection of wild and laboratory animals with Machupo and Latino viruses, *Bull WHO* **52**:493.

Welsh, R. M., 1977, Host cell modification of lymphocytic choriomeningitis virus and Newcastle disease virus altering viral inactivation by human complement, *J. Immunol.* **118**:348.

Welsh, R. M., and Oldstone, M. B. A., 1977, Inhibition of immunologic injury of cultered cells infected with lymphocytic choriomeningitis virus: Role of defective interfering virus in regulating viral antigen expression, *J. Exp. Med.* **145**:1449.

Welsh, R. M., and Pfau, C. J., 1972, Determinants of lymphocytic choriomeningitis interference, *J. Gen. Virol.* **14**:177.

Welsh, R. M., Trowbridge, R. S., Kowalski, J. B., O'Connell, C. M., and Pfau, C. J., 1971, Amantadine hydrochloride inhibition of early and late stages of lymphocytic choriomeningitis virus cell interactions, *Virology* **45**:679.

Welsh, R. M., O'Connell, C. M., and Pfau, C. J., 1972, Properties of defective lymphocytic choriomeningitis virus, *J. Gen. Virol.* **17**:355.

Welsh, R. M., Burner, P. A., Holland, J. J., Oldstone, M. B. A., Thompson, H. A., and Villarreal, L. P., 1975, A comparison of biochemical and biological properties of standard and defective lymphocytic choriomeningitis viruses, *Bull. WHO* **52**:403.

Welsh, R. M., Lampert, P. W., and Oldstone, M. B., 1977, Prevention of virus-induced cerebellar disease by defective-interfering lymphocytic choriomeningitis virus, *J. Infect. Dis.* **136**:391.

Wiessenbacher, M. C., de Guerrero, L. B., and Boxaca, M. D., 1975, Experimental biology and pathogenesis of Junin virus infection in animals and man, *Bull. WHO* **52**:507.

Winn, W. C., Jr., and Walker, D. H., 1975, The pathology of human Lassa fever, *Bull. WHO* **52**:535.

Wulff, H., Lange, J. V., and Webb, P. A., 1978, Interrelationships among arenaviruses measured by indirect immunofluorescences, *Intervirology* **9**:344.

CHAPTER 3

Coronaviridae

James A. Robb and Clifford W. Bond*

Department of Pathology
University of California, San Diego
La Jolla, California 92093

1. INTRODUCTION

1.1. Summary

Coronaviruses are widespread in nature, but relatively little attention has been given to them. They are pathogenic, enveloped RNA viruses whose large, single-stranded, nonsegmented genome is of a positive polarity. They cause a broad spectrum of disease in their natural hosts, including man, primarily by a cytocidal virus–cell interaction. The structure of the virion, the molecular mechanisms of their multiplication strategy, and their pathogenesis are just beginning to receive the attention they deserve.

Our goals in this chapter are three: (1) to define the criteria for membership and the present members of the coronavirus family; (2) to define the structure of the virion and the multiplication strategy for this family; and (3) to describe the spectrum and pathogenesis of disease produced by this family of important pathogenic viruses in their natural hosts. The preprints and unpublished data supplied by many of our colleagues are appreciated. Our emphasis will be, whenever possible, on the molecular description of the multiplication strategy of these viruses

* Present addresses: J. A. R., Department of Pathology, The Green Hospital of Scripps Clinic, La Jolla, California 92037. C. W. B., Department of Microbiology, Montana State University, Bozeman, Montana 59717.

and on the molecular mechanisms involved in the pathogenesis of the disease produced by these viruses. There are at present large gaps in the description of the molecular virology of this family. In an attempt to bridge some of these gaps and make the review as up to date as possible, prudent speculation will be used and identified as such.

1.2   Definition and Members of the Coronavirus Family

1.2.1.   Criteria for Membership and Tentative Members

Until recently, enveloped, RNA-containing viruses that budded solely from the endoplasmic reticular membranes, that had a spherical shape with a 60–220 nm diameter, and that had a "corona" of widely spaced, bulbous peplomers 12–24 nm in length were defined as coronaviruses (McIntosh, 1974). Acceptable biochemical criteria were not available. Such biochemical criteria are now available using avian infectious bronchitis virus (IBV) as the prototype virus for this family (Schochetman *et al.*, 1977; Lomniczi, 1977; Lomniczi and Kennedy, 1977). The virion genome of enveloped viruses of the above morphology must be a large (6–8 $\times$ 10^6 daltons) single piece of single-stranded infectious RNA of messenger (positive) polarity. In addition to IBV, the virions of mouse hepatitis virus (MHV), human coronavirus (HCV), and porcine transmissible gastroenteritis virus (TGEV) probably contain a genome of positive polarity as described in Section 2.2.2. In addition, several other viruses have satisfied the electron microscopic criteria for membership in this family and are listed in Table 1. Additional biochemical criteria will soon be forthcoming because the investigation of the molecular virology of the coronavirus family is rapidly gaining momentum.

1.2.2.   Serological Relatedness of Members

The intraspecies and interspecies serological relatedness of the various viruses are complex and not yet fully understood (Table 1). The production of useful vaccines against coronavirus diseases, many of which are economically important in agriculture and probably in the human economy as well, will require a more detailed understanding of the serological relatedness of these viruses than is currently available. The major problem in acquiring these data, as well as in understanding

TABLE 1
Tentative Members of the Coronavirus Family and Their Serological Relatedness

Virus[a]	Natural host	Serotypes[c]	Serologically related to[c]
Avian infectious bronchitis (IBV)	Chicken	Many[1]	? TGEV[2]
Canine coronavirus (CCV)	Dog	? One[3]	TGEV[2,4]
Feline coronavirus (FCV) (infectious peritonitis)	Cat	? One[3]	TGEV, but not HEV[5]
Human coronavirus (HCV)	Man	Several[2,3,6]	HEV, MHV[2,7]
Human enteric coronavirus (HECV)	Man	? One	TGEV[2]
Murine hepatitis virus (MHV)	Mouse	Many[2]	RCV, SDAV, HCV, ?HEV[2,7]
Neonatral calf diarrhea corona-virus[b] (NCDCV)	Bovine	Several[8]	
Porcine transmissible gastro-enteritis virus (TGEV)	Pig	One[2,3,9]	CCV[4], FCV[5], ?HEV[2], ?IBV[2]
Porcine hemagglutinating encephalitis virus (HEV)	Pig	? One[3]	
Rat coronavirus (RCV)	Rat	? One[3]	MHV[2]
Rat sialodacryoadenitis virus (SDAV)	Rat	? One[3]	MHV[2]
Runde tick coronavirus (RTCV)	? Tick ? Sea bird	? One[10]	Not to IBV or MHV[10]
Turkey bluecomb disease virus (TCDV)	Turkey	? One[3]	

[a] These names and abbreviations conform to those suggested by Tyrrell *et al.* (personal communication) in a revision to the previous recommendations (Tyrrell *et al.*, 1975).
[b] Mucosal disease virus (border disease, Plant *et al.*, 1976) of sheep may belong in this group (Snowdon *et al.*, 1975).
[c] References: 1, Cowen and Hitchner (1975); 2, McIntosh (1974); 3, Kapikian (1975); 4, Binn *et al.* (1974); 5, Reynolds *et al.* (1977); 6, Monto (1974); 7, Kaye *et al.* (1977); 8, Hafez *et al.* (1976); 9, Kemeny (1976); 10, Traavik *et al.* (1977).

the molecular virology, is the relative difficulty in isolating and growing these viruses in cell culture. This problem is discussed in Section 3.

2. VIRIONS

2.1. Morphology

Coronavirus virions are pleomorphic spherical particles of 80–160 nm diameter with characteristic large, widely spaced, 12- to 24-nm-long spikes or peplomers that form a corona around the particle and provide the name for this virus family. Figures 1 and 2 show the novel mor-

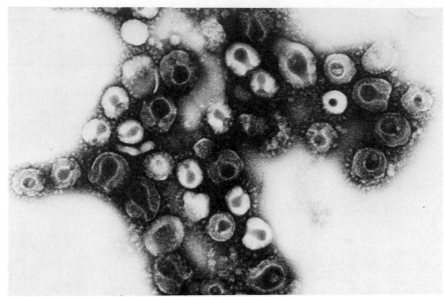

Fig. 1. A group of IBV virions treated with formaldehyde before staining with phosphotungstic acid. Almost all reveal the internal component. The majority display the tongue or flask orientation, but others show a circular structure or even two concentric rings. Figure 2 shows that all of these patterns are compatible with an internal membranous sac continuous with the outer membrane. Magnification ×135,000 (reduced 20% for reproduction). From Bingham and Almeida (1977); used by permission.

phology of the infectious bronchitis virion (Bingham and Almeida, 1977). Whether this is the only internal morphology available to a coronavirus virion remains to be determined. The topology of the ribonucleocapsid within a virion is not yet known. The nucleocapsid is composed of a 9-nm-wide ribonucleoprotein that forms a helical structure (Kennedy and Johnson-Lussenburg, 1975/1976; Pocock and Garwes, 1977) and probably corresponds to the flasklike structure within the virion (Fig. 2). Using transmission electron microscopy, we have observed in mouse hepatitis virus (JHMV and A59V) infected 17CL-16 cells and BALB/c brains that the apparent nucleocapsids in cytoplasmic factories and in early stages of budding have horseshoe or flasklike configurations (Robb *et al.*, 1979a,b). Purification of nucleocapsids from virions and infected cells will be necessary to clarify the internal structure of the coronavirus virion.

The mass of a human coronavirus (OC43) is $390 \pm 5 \times 10^6$ daltons as determined by analytical ultracentrifugation (Hierholzer *et al.*, 1972). Similar experiments with another human coronavirus (229E) did not give reliable data because the virus particles disintegrated too rapidly. The mass of other coronaviruses has not been determined.

2.2. Composition

2.2.1. Overall Chemical Composition

The virions of coronaviruses contain RNA, protein, carbohydrate, and lipid. The buoyant density of the virion in sucrose or potassium tartrate is in the range of 1.17–1.19 g/cm^3 [IBV: MacNaughton and Madge, 1977a; NCDCV: La Porte, personal communication; HCV (299E): Hierholzer, 1976; FCV: Horzinek et al., 1977; MHV (A59V, JHMV): Lai and Stohlman, 1978; Stohlman, personal communication; Leibowitz, Bond, and Robb, manuscript in preparation].

2.2.2. RNA

The genome of coronaviruses has been amply demonstrated to be single-stranded RNA. Lomniczi (1977) and Schochetman et al. (1977) have shown that the genome of infectious bronchitis virus (IBV) is

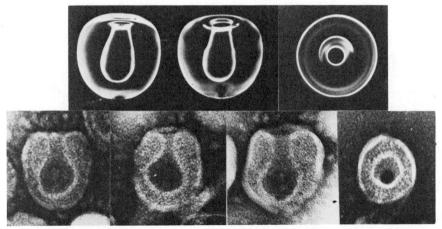

Fig. 2. Three different transilluminated orientations of a glass model are compared to four individual virus particles printed at ×330,000 (reduced 20% for reproduction). Although both refraction and reflection will occur with the glass model, the overall correlation is good. From Almeida (1977); used by permission.

infectious, and Lomniczi (personal communication) has shown that the genome of transmissible gastroenteritis virus (TGEV) is infectious.

The molecular size of the virion RNA of IBV has been variously reported to be 0.5–3.0 million daltons (4–40 S) by Tannock (1973), 9.0 million daltons (50 S) by Watkins *et al.* (1975), 8 million daltons (64 S) by Lomniczi and Kennedy (1977), 8 million daltons (58 S) by MacNaughton and Madge (1977*b*), and 5.5–5.7 million daltons (48 S) by Schochetman *et al.*, (1977).

These variable data reflect the fact that the genome of corona-viruses is the largest viral RNA genome known and, as a result, no standards exist to size the RNA by traditional techniques. Lomniczi and Kennedy (1977) used the elegant method of RNase T1 oligonu-cleotide fingerprinting to confirm the molecular size of 8.1 ± 0.2 million daltons which had been determined on methyl mercury gels and isokinetic sucrose gradients.

Tannock and Hierholzer (1977) have shown that the RNA of a human coronavirus (HCV-OC43) is 6.1 million daltons (70 S). The genome RNAs of two mouse hepatitis viruses (MHV-A59V and JHMV) were found to be identical and to have a molecular size of about 5.4 million daltons (60 S) (Lai and Stohlman, 1978). The genome RNAs of coronavirus have covalently attached poly(A) (IBV: Lomniczi, 1977; Schochetman *et al.*, 1977; MacNaughton and Madge, 1977b; MHV: (A59V and JHMV), Lai and Stohlman, 1978; Leibowitz, Chun-Akana, Bond, and Robb, unpublished observations; Yogo *et al.*, 1977; HCV (OC43): Tannock and Hierholzer, 1978). Most of the reports indicate that only a portion (25–50%) of labeled RNA was bound by oligo(dT) cellulose, suggesting (1) that the length of the poly(A) tract may be short, (2) that the RNA in the purified prepara-tions may be degraded, or (3) that a percentage of the molecules have their poly(A) tract in a conformation that prevents binding to the oligo(dT) cellulose. However, Leibowitz, Chun-Akana, Bond, and Robb (unpublished observation) have demonstrated that nearly 100% of MHV RNA (A59V) from purified virions binds to poly(U) sepharose, which binds poly(A) tracts of less than 40–60 nucleotides. These data suggest that the poly(A) sequence may be less than 40 nucleotides in length (Hunter and Garrels, 1977). The poly(A) tract is presumably 3′ terminal, but this must be demonstrated.

Treatment of the genomic RNA with heat, chaotropic agent, or high salt does not significantly alter the size or migration in gels or suc-rose gradients of several coronavirus RNAs [IBV: Lomniczi and Ken-nedy, 1977; Schochetman *et al.*, 1977; MacNaughton and Madge,

1977*b*; MHV (A59V and JHMV); Lai and Stohlman, 1978; Leibowitz, Bond, and Robb, unpublished observation]. In the cases where heat or chaotropic agents do alter the size or migration of the RNA (TGEV/HEV: Garwes *et al.*, 1975; HCV-OC43: Tannock and Hierholzer, 1977), the reason may be contamination by the RNA of an activated retrovirus or the presence of an internal ribonuclease (Schochetman *et al.*, 1977; Lai and Stohlman, 1978), or the nicking of the large RNA during isolation.

A RNA-dependent RNA polymerase has not been detected in the virions of IBV (Schochetman *et al.*, 1977) or HCV (OC43) (Tannock and Hierholzer, 1978). A RNA-dependent DNA polymerase (reverse transcriptase) was not detected in the virion of IBV (H. Temin, personal communication). These findings support the contention that the coronavirus genome is of positive polarity and separate coronaviruses from retroviruses which are also enveloped RNA viruses containing a genome of positive polarity.

2.2.3. Proteins

The structural proteins that compose the virion of several coronaviruses have been analyzed in detail by several laboratories (Table 2). The variety in the number and size of the structural proteins indicates some degree of complexity in the structure of the coronavirus virion. Much of the variability in the data can be accounted for by the different methods used in virion purification and detection of separated proteins on polyacrylamide gels. It is difficult to synthesize the data in Table 2 into a general description of the protein content of coronavirus virions. The number of different proteins in a virion, however, appears to be about four to six, of which two or more are glycoslyated. All of the reports indicate the presence of a major nonglycosylated protein in the range of 45,000–65,000 daltons, probably the nucleocapsid protein. A glycolipoprotein has also been identified in the virions of human coronaviruses (OC43: Hierholzer *et al.*, 1972; 229E: Hierholzer, 1976).

2.2.4. Lipids

The lipid content of transmissible gastroenteritis virions grown in either primary pig kidney cells or secondary adult pig thyroid cells has been compared to the lipid content of whole cells (Pike and Garwes,

TABLE 2
Structural Proteins of Coronaviruses

IBV			MHV (A59V)		MHV (JHMV)	HCV (229E)	HCV (OC43)	TGEV	HEV	NCDCV
(1)[a]	(2)	(3)	(4)	(5)	(5)	(6)	(7)	(8)	(9)	(10)
130[b] (GP)[c]	52 (GP)	180 (GP)	180 (GP)	150 (GP)	150 (GP)	196 (GP)	191 (GP)	200 (GP)	180 (GP)	125
105 (GP)	45	120	90	89	100	165 (GP)	104 (GP)	50	125 (GP)	65
97	34	106	50	60	63	105 (GP)	60 (GP)	30 (GP)	100 (GP)	50
81 (GP)	32 (GP)	93 (GP)	23 (GP)	20	18	66 (GP)	47	28 (GP)	56	45
74 (GP)	+10 minor species	70				47	30	+2 minor species	26 (GP)	36
		58				31 (GP)	15 (GP)			
51		53				17				34
33		49								28
		43								
		40								
		37 (GP)								
		32								
		29								
		24								
		16								
		14 (GP)								
Stain[d]	Stain	Stain	Isotope	Isotope	Isotope	Stain and Isotope	Stain	Isotope	Isotope	Stain

[a] References: 1, MacNaughton and Madge (1977a); 2, Collins et al. (1976); 3, Bingham (1975); 4, Sturman (1977); 5, Leibowitz, Bond, and Robb (unpublished observations); 6, Hierholzer (1976); 7, Hierholzer et al. (1972); 8, Garwes and Pocock (1975); 9, Pocock and Garwes (1977); 10, La Porte (personal communication).

[b] Molecular weight of protein $\times 10^{-3}$.

[c] (GP) indicates identification of the protein as a glycoprotein.

[d] Method of detection of protein.

1977). The lipid content of the TGEV virion reflected the lipid content of the host cell in which it was grown, suggesting that the lipids of the virion are derived from the lipids of the host cell. As noted above, the virions of human coronaviruses (OC43 and 229E) contain lipoglycoprotein.

2.2.5. Carbohydrates

Glycoproteins are important in the structure of the coronavirus virion, especially in the formation of peplomers. Sturman and Holmes (1977) isotopically labeled cells infected by mouse hepatitis virus (A59V) with glucosamine and fucose and found that the GP180 and GP90 proteins were highly labeled with both sugars, while GP23 was labeled only with glucosamine. The analogous intracellular GP150 and GP90 proteins of mouse hepatitis virus (JHMV), however, are highly labeled with both glucosamine and fucose (Robb, unpublished observation). Differential labeling of carbohydrates in the virions of other coronaviruses has not been reported.

2.3.   Fine Structure and Arrangement of Virion Components

2.3.1.   Peplomers

The peplomers, or spikes, or coronavirus virions contain a major large glycoprotein. They are readily removed by treatment with bromelin or other proteases, a treatment that reduces the density of the virion. For example, the virion of human coronavirus (OC43) has a density of 1.18 g/cm^3, and the "despiked" particle has a density of 1.15 g/cm^3 (Hierholzer *et al.*, 1972). The results of treating the virions of six different coronaviruses with bromelin are shown in Table 3. Again, the results are variable but indicate that there are only one or two proteins in coronavirus peplomers.

The hemagglutinating activity in the coronaviruses that possess this property probably resides in the peplomers for the following reasons. Treatment of the neonatal calf diarrhea coronavirus virion with bromelin removes the peplomers and abolishes hemagglutinating activity (Laporte, personal communication). Concanavalin A does not bind to bromelin-treated hemagglutinating encephalomyelitis virions (HEV) that have lost their peplomers (Greig and Bouillant, 1977). The binding of concanavalin A to untreated HEV virions with intact

TABLE 3
Localization of Structural Proteins in the Virions of Coronavirus

	IBV		MHV (A59V)	HCV (229E)	HCV (OC43)	TGEV	HEV	NCDCV
	(1)[a]	(2)	(3, 4)	(5)	(6)	(7, 8)	(9)	(10)
Spikes (Peplomers)	180[b] (GP)[c] 130 106 83 (GP) 70	130 (GP) 105 (GP) 74	180 (GP) 90 (GP)	105 (GP) 17 (GP)	104 (GP) 15 (GP)	200 (GP)	180 (GP) 125 (GP) 100 (GP)	125 65
Envelope		97 81 (GP) 33	23 (GP)			30 (GP) 28 (GP)	26 (GP)	
Nucleocapsid		51	50			50	56	
Detection method		Stain	Isotope	Stain and isotope	Stain	Isotope	Isotope	Stain

[a] References: 1, Bingham (1975); 2, MacNaughton et al. (1977a); 3, Sturman (1977); 4, Sturman and Holmes (1977); 5, Hierholzer (1976); 6, Hierholzer et al. (1972); 7, Garwes et al. (1976); 8, Garwes and Pocock (1975); 9, Pocock and Garwes (1977); 10, La Porte (personal communication).

[b] Molecular weight of protein $\times 10^{-3}$.

[c] (GP) indicates identification of the protein as a glycoprotein.

[d] Method of detection of protein.

peplomers produces a loss in the hemagglutinating activity of the virions.

2.3.2. Envelope

The coronavirus virion envelope probably contains two to three proteins, at least one of which is glycosylated. Treatment of coronavirus virions with the detergent NP40 results in the release of a ribonucleoprotein complex from the virion (Kennedy and Johnson-Lussenburg, 1975/1976; MacNaughton et al., 1977). Through the use of this method and bromelin digestion, MacNaughton et al. (1977) suggested that the proteins VP97, GP81, and VP33 are located in the viral envelope of infectious bronchitis virus. In like manner, GP30 and GP28 are probably components of the envelope of transmissible gastroenteritis virus (Garwes and Pocock, 1975; Garwes et al., 1976). When virions of mouse hepatitis virus (A59V) are digested with pronase or bromelin, GP23 is digested to a nonglycosylated protein, P*18, suggesting that GP23 is on the surface of the envelope with a tail of about 18,000 daltons embedded in the envelope (Sturman, 1977; Sturman and Holmes, 1977).

2.3.3. Nucleocapsid

2.3.3a. Structure

The ribonucleoprotein that forms the coronavirus nucleocapsid is probably a 9-nm-wide, helical structure that has a buoyant density of 1.27–1.30 g/cm^3 and can be released from the virion by treatment with the detergent NP40 (Kennedy and Johnson-Lussenburg, 1975/1976; Garwes et al., 1976; MacNaughton et al., 1977). The topography of the helical nucleocapsid within the virion remains to be defined but may be the flask-shaped structure shown in Figs. 1 and 2.

2.3.3b. Protein Subunit

The 50,000–63,000 dalton nonglycosylated, arginine-rich virion protein is present in the nucleocapsid of mouse hepatitis virus (A59V: Sturman, 1977), transmissible gastroenteritis virus (TGEV: Garwes et al., 1976) and infectious bronchitis virus (MacNaughton and Madge,

1977*a*). In support of this suggestion is the finding that the internal RNA-associated protein of retroviruses is also rich in arginine (Fleissner, 1971). A minor glycoprotein(s) may also be associated with the nucleocapsid of TGEV (Garwes *et al.*, 1976) and hemagglutinating encephalomyelitis virus (Pocock and Garwes, 1977).

3. GROWTH PROPERTIES IN CELL AND ORGAN CULTURE

3.1. Infectivity Assays

The major impediment to investigating both the pathogenesis and molecular virology of coronaviruses has been the difficulty in isolating and growing to sufficient titer many of the coronaviruses (McIntosh, 1974). The following *in vitro* systems have been used for coronavirus isolation, growth, and adaption. *Infectious bronchitis virus:* embryonated chicken eggs, chicken tracheal ring organ culture, and primary chicken kidney cells (Darbyshire *et al.*, 1975, 1976; Dutta, 1974; Cook *et al.*, 1976; Egan and Tannock, 1978). *Canine coronavirus:* primary dog kidney cells (Takeuchi *et al.*, 1976). *Feline coronavirus:* primary kitten peritoneal cells (Pedersen, 1976). *Human coronavirus:* secondary human embryonic kidney cells, WI38 cells, HeLa cells, human embryonic trachael organ culture, L132 cells, and human embryonic lung cells (McIntosh, 1974; Kennedy and Johnson-Lussenberg, 1975/1976; Hierholzer, 1976). *Mouse hepatitis virus:* primary mouse macrophage cells, mouse DBT cells, and mouse 17CL-1 cells (McIntosh, 1974; Hirano *et al.*, 1974, 1976; Takayama and Kirn, 1976; Sturman and Takemoto, 1972; Robb *et al.*, 1979*a*). Mouse NCTC-1469 liver cells are heavily infected with a murine retrovirus (McIntosh, 1974), and we have found this line to be unacceptable for the growth of MHV because of very poor experimental reproducibility (Robb *et al.*, 1979*a*). *Neonatal calf diarrhea coronavirus:* rhesus monkey kidney cells and fetal bovine kidney cells (King and Harkness, 1975; Inaba *et al.*, 1976; Sharpee *et al.*, 1976; Matsuno *et al.*, 1977). *Transmissible gastroenteritis virus/hemagglutinating encephalomyelitis virus:* primary pig kidney, spleen, and thyroid cells and pig testis cells (McIntosh, 1974; Kemeny *et al.*, 1974; Stark *et al.*, 1974; Thomas and Dulac, 1976; Werdin *et al.*, 1976). *Rat coronavirus:* primary rat kidney cells (McIntosh, 1974).

Plaque, cytopathic effect, and virus-specific immunofluorescence assays can be used in most of these systems. We have developed cytopathic effect and immunofluorescence microassays for mouse hepatitis virus that should be applicable to many other coronavirus systems (Robb *et al.*, 1979*a*). These microassays are comparable to plaque assays, but are more rapid, precise, and economical. See Section 7.3.4 for additional references.

3.2. Growth Curves and Multiplication Kinetics

In general, most coronavirus infections have a 2- to 4-hr eclipse phase and a maximum progeny yield at 12–16 hr after infection at 37°C (McIntosh, 1974). The multiplication of infectious bronchitis virus (IBV) in chicken tracheal ring organ culture, embryonated chicken eggs, or primary chicken kidney cells is dependent on the IBV isolate (Cook *et al.*, 1976). We have found that the maximum yield of progeny mouse hepatitis virus (JHMV and A59V) in mouse 17CL-16 cells, a subclone of BALB/3T3 cells, occurs by 11 hr after infection at 38.5°C and is *independent* of the multiplicity of infection between 0.01 and 10 (Robb *et al.*, 1978*a*). The maximum yield of progeny JHMV in the brain of 4-week-old BALB/c mice after intracerebral inoculation is also independent of the multiplicity of infection between 1 and 10^4 IU/animal (Robb *et al.*, 1979*b*). Furthermore, the production of progeny JHMV and A59V in 17CL-16 cells and mouse brain is independent of intercellular fusion and formation of syncytia (Fig. 3) (Robb *et al.*, 1979*a*). These interesting properties have yet to be explained, but may represent general properties of coronavirus infection *in vitro* and *in vivo*. The only data we found concerning the number of coronavirus particles required to initiate an infection are our own for mouse hepatitis virus: JHMV and A59V have one-hit kinetics in 17CL-16 cells (Robb *et al.*, 1979*a*).

Cytoplasmic coronavirus-specific antigen begins to appear at the end of the 2- to 4-hr eclipse phase. In addition, we have found MHV-specific (JHMV and A59V) granular intranuclear (Fig. 4) and patchy plasma membrane-associated antigens (Fig. 5) in infected 17CL-16 cells (Robb *et al.*, 1979*a*). The intranuclear antigen appears before the cytoplasmic and surface antigens (Fig. 6), while the appearance of the surface antigen coincides with the appearance of the cytoplasmic antigen. All cells that contain the intranuclear antigen during the low-multiplicity infection (less than 0.5 IU/cell) go on to make cytoplasmic and surface antigens. In addition, some clones of 17CL-1 cells persistently infected with JHMV or A59V contain intranuclear antigen in the

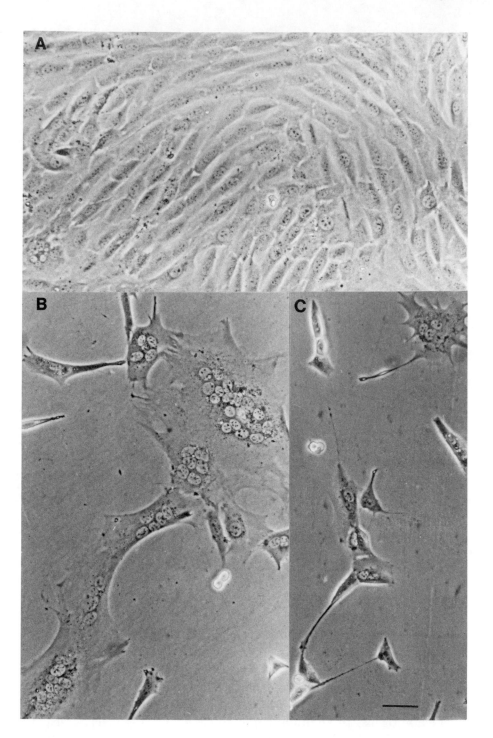

absence of cytoplasmic or surface antigen (Leibowitz, Bond, and Robb, manuscript in preparation). No other report of coronavirus-specific intranuclear or surface antigen was found in our search of the literature.

3.3. Modification of Infectivity

Any agent that disrupts plasma membranes will disrupt the envelope of coronavirus virions and decrease or abolish infectivity (McIntosh, 1974). The infectivity of most coronaviruses is stable to repeated freeze-thaw, heating, and acid environment (McIntosh, 1974; Robb *et al.*, 1979*a*), but each isolate has to be studied for optimum storage conditions. Any alteration of the peplomer structure may decrease virion infectivity (L. Sturman, personal communication).

4. MULTIPLICATION OF VIRUS

4.1. Adsorption

Little is presently known about the molecular events in coronavirus adsorption. Their very narrow host range and organ tropism strongly suggest the presence of specific cell surface receptors. As described in Section 2.3, the peplomers of the virion are probably glycoprotein(s) and represent the most likely site for adsorptive specificity. Adsorption of canine coronavirus and neonatal calf diarrhea coronavirus takes place on the plasma membrane of microvilli, crypts, and invaginations of intestinal absorptive epithelial cells or enterocytes (Doughri *et al.*, 1976; Takeuchi *et al.*, 1976).

Fig. 3. Cytopathic effect of mouse hepatitis virus (JHMV and A59V) infection in 17CL-16 mouse cells. A: Fibroblastoid morphology of the mock-infected 17CL-16 subclone. B,C: Characteristic coronaviral syncytial formation of JHMV and A59V, respectively. The nuclei in JHMV-induced syncytia are usually two- to threefold more numerous than those produced by A59V. A syncytium will stay attached to the substrate for about 2 hr at 38.5°C and 3–4 hr at 33°C after its initial development. The unattached syncytia are apparently "dead," because they are freely permeable to trypan blue. Infected single cells can continue mitosis through telophase. See Robb *et al.* (1979*a*) for details. Scale bar in C is 30 μm.

4.2. Penetration and Uncoating

Little is presently known about the penetration and uncoating phase of coronavirus replication. Viropexis and envelope-membrane fusion have both been described as mechanisms of coronavirus penetration. One mechanism may predominate for one virus isolate or stock, while both mechanisms may be used by other isolates. Fusion of virion envelope to plasma membrane has been described for the penetration

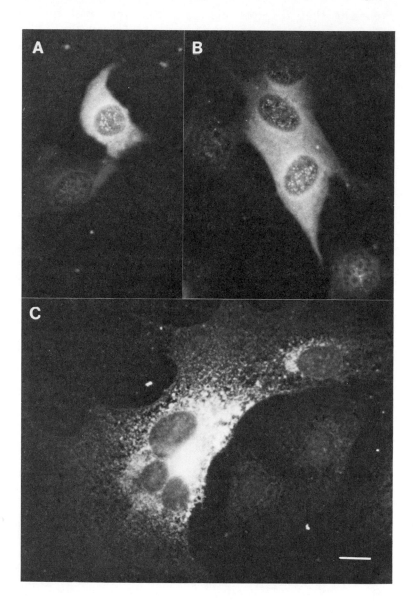

mechanism of neonatal calf diarrhea coronavirus into enterocytes of the bovine small intestine (Doughri *et al.*, 1976). Viropexis, on the other hand, appears to be the predominant penetration mechanism of infectious bronchitis virus (IBV) into chicken chorioallantoic membrane and primary chicken kidney cells (Chasey and Alexander, 1976; Patterson and Bingham, 1976). IBV attachment, but not viropexis, occurs at 4°C (Chasey and Alexander, 1976). The following finding suggests that the penetration of IBV is fairly rapid. The addition of neutralizing antiserum at 90 min after IBV infection at 4°C decreases the number of attached plaque-forming virions, while treatment after 90 min at 37°C does not decrease the number of attached plaque-forming virions (Chasey and Alexander, 1976). The mechanism of uncoating of any coronavirus is not known. The IBV-containing cytoplasmic vesicles formed by viropexis apparently do not fuse with lysosomes as a mechanism of uncoating (Chasey and Alexander, 1976).

4.3. Biosynthesis of Viral Macromolecules

4.3.1. Proof of Messenger Function of RNA

The genomic RNA of coronaviruses is of positive polarity. Lomniczi (1977), Schochetman *et al.* (1977) and Norman *et al.* (1968) have shown that purified infectious virion RNA from bronchitis (IBV) and transmissible gastroenteritis virus, respectively, is infectious. Lomniczi (personal communication) has demonstrated in preliminary experiments that the genomic RNA of IBV can be translated into IBV-

←――

Fig. 4. Intranuclear and cytoplasmic mouse hepatitis virus (JHMV and A59V) specific antigens in 17CL-16 mouse cells. Cells were infected with a MOI of 0.1 and incubated at 38.5°C for 4 hr. They were either fixed with methanol (A,B) or formaldehyde-triton (C) before staining with polyspecific mouse anti-JHMV or anti-A59V. The photographs are of JHMV-infected cells. The immunofluorescent staining patterns are similar for both JHMV and A59V using virus-specific antiserum and in reciprocally stained preparations. The pattern is the same at 33°C. The sequence of syncytial formation is cell–cell contact (A), intercellular fusion (B), and continued recruitment of uninfected cells (C). The intranuclear antigen appears to be predominantly in the perinucleolar regions. The intranuclear and ground-glass cytoplasmic antigens are diminished after formaldehyde–triton treatment. The fluorescence remaining after formaldehyde–triton treatment appears to be in the Golgi apparatus and endoplasmic reticulum, the site of virus budding. Golgi apparatuses appear to coalesce during syncytial formation (C). See Robb *et al.* (1979*a*) for details. The scale bar in C is 10 μm.

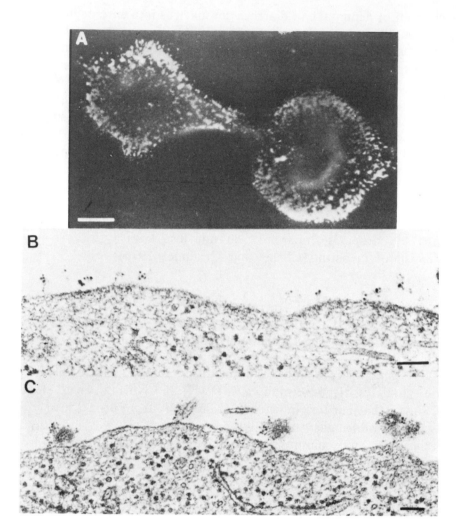

Fig. 5.   Presence of JHMV-specific antigen on the surface of living infected 17CL-16 cells. Cells were infected with a MOI of 0.1 and incubated at 38.5°C for 4 hr. A: Patchy distribution of the JHMV-specific surface antigen on attached living cells. B: Patchy distribution of the JHMV-specific surface antigen at 3 hours after infection. Viral ribonucleoprotein has not been identified by transmission electron microscopy anywhere beneath the plasma membrane, including the regions containing surface antigen C: Specificity of the anti-JHMV serum as ferritin-labeled antibody attaches only to the infecting JHMV particles and not to adjacent plasma membrane. Scale bar in A is 10 μm and in B and C is 100 nm. Similar results are obtained using mouse anti-A59V serum and A59V-infected cells. JHMV- and A59V-infected cells give similar results with reciprocal antisera. Immune electron microscopy kindly performed by R. Garrett. See Robb *et al.* (1979*a*) for details.

specific proteins in a cell-free protein synthesis system. The genomic RNA also contains a covalently linked tract of polyadenylic acid, presumably at the 3′ terminus (IBV: Lomniczi, 1977; Schochetman *et al.*, 1977; MacNaughton and Madge, 1977*b*; mouse hepatitis virus: Lai and Stohlman, 1978; Leibowitz, Chun-Akana, Bond, and Robb, unpublished observations; human coronavirus: Tannock and Hierholzer, 1978).

4.3.2. Species of Coronavirus RNAs in Infected Cells

Although very little information is available, there are probably four major groups of coronavirus-specific RNA species in infected cells: (1) genomic RNA, (2) double-stranded replicative intermediates, (3) mutliple discrete species of mRNA, and (4) defective or deleted RNA species. The synthesis of all these groups of intracellular viral RNA is resistent to treatment with actinomycin D. Mishra and Ryan (1973) demonstrated coronavirus-specific intracellular RNA in pig kidney cells

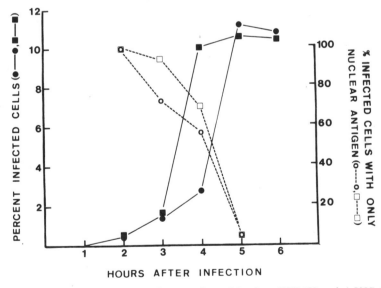

Figure 6. Temporal appearance of mouse hepatitis virus (JHMV and A59V) infected 17CL-16 cells at 38.5°C as detected by virus-specific immunofluorescence. Cells were infected with a MOI of 0.10 in 32-mm Petri dishes and fixed at the indicated times with methanol before immunofluorescent staining with mouse anti-JHMV or anti-A59V. JHMV (O) and A59V (□) infected cells have only intranuclear fluorescence; total number of JHMV (●) or A59V (■) infected cells, i.e., both nuclear-positive and cytoplasmic/nuclear-positive cells, were counted.

treated with actinomycin D and infected with transmissible gastroenteritis virus. During a 1-hr pulse, [³H]uridine was incorporated primarily into 18 S and 4 S RNA, and to a lesser extent into 28 S RNA.
During a 10-min pulse, label was similarly incorporated into 28 S, 18 S,
and 4 S regions. Ribonuclease-resistant RNA in the 18–28 S size range
was synthesized during the 10-min pulse.

Robb *et al.* (1979*a*) have demonstrated major species of 18 S to 28
S and 50 S RNAs in 17CL-16 cells treated with actinomycin D and
infected with mouse hepatitis virus (JHMV and A59V). Virus-specific
cytoplasmic ribonucleoproteins were analyzed by sucrose gradients in
the presence or absence of EDTA. The species of virus-specific
ribonucleoprotein that shifted from higher to lower S values in the
presence of EDTA were presumed to contain mRNA species (Figs. 7
and 8). Several discrete species of mRNA ranging in size from 4 S to
28 S, and possibly 50 S, were detected by agarose gel electrophoresis. A
species of ribonucleoprotein that sedimented at 200 S (A59V) or 230 S
(JHMV) did not shift its S value in the presence of EDTA (Fig. 7). This
large ribonucleoprotein species contains 50 S RNA, and is likely to be
an intermediate in progeny virus formation, probably the nucleocapsid.
No data are available on the mechanism of replication or polyadenyla-
tion of the viral RNA species found in infected cells. Both the single-

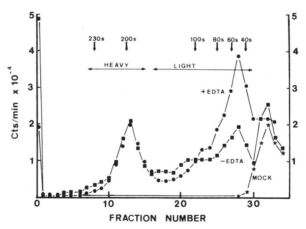

Fig. 7.   Analysis of A59V-specific intracellular provirion (nucleocapsid) and messenger
ribonucleoprotein (RNP). Cytoplasmic ribonucleoprotein (RNP) synthesized and
labeled with [³H]uridine in the presence of 1 μg/ml actinomycin D was extracted with
1% NP40 from mock- and A59V-infected 17CL-16 cells. This extracted RNP was
analyzed on 10–30% equal mass sterile sucrose–RSB gradient. Half of the extracted
RNP was treated with 10 mM EDTA (●——●) before centrifugation. See Robb *et al.*
(1979*a*) for details.

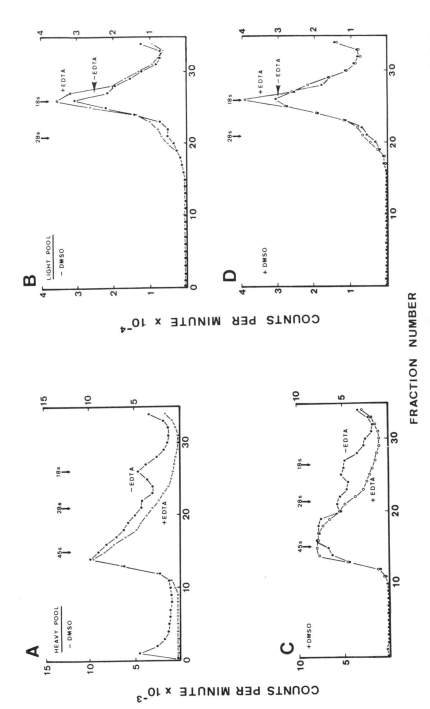

FRACTION NUMBER

Fig. 8. Analysis of A59V-specific intracellular nucleocapsid and messenger RNA. The "heavy" (A) and "light" (B) pools derived from the gradients shown in Fig. 7 were deproteinized by proteinase K–cold phenol extraction and analyzed on 10–30% equal mass sucrose 0.1% SDS gradients. Half of each sample of RNA was denatured with DMSO (C,D) before centrifugation. See Robb *et al.* (1979a) for details.

stranded RNA species (mRNA and deleted defective RNA) and the double-stranded RNA species (replicative intermediates) need to be purified by suitable gel electrophoresis, fingerprinted, and mapped onto the genomic RNA. The putative mRNA species have to be analyzed for the presence of 3'-terminal poly(A) tracts and for their ability to direct the cell-free synthesis of coronaviral proteins. These putative coronaviral proteins will have to be rigorously identified by radioimmune precipitation, high-resolution two-dimensional gel electrophoresis, and peptide analysis.

As noted above, actinomycin D is a useful drug for inhibiting cellular, but not coronaviral, RNA synthesis during infection. Although coronaviral RNA synthesis is not affected by the drug, the multiplication of progeny virus is inhibited during human coronavirus infection (229E, C. M. Johnson-Lussenburg, personal communication). The multiplication of mouse hepatitis virus (JHMV) is also inhibited by the drug, whereas the multiplication of MHV-A59V is not inhibited (S. Stohlman, personal communication; Leibowitz, Bond, and Robb, unpublished observations). Although the mechanism of the inhibition of JHMV multiplication is not yet known, it may involve the intranuclear antigen and putative nuclear phase of this virus (see Section 4.5). Other coronaviruses need to be investigated for the sensitivity of their replication and multiplication to actinomycin D.

4.3.3. Proteins

Bond and Robb (1978) have demonstrated nine viral-specific proteins in cells infected by mouse hepatitis virus (JHMV and A59V). The molecular weights of the viral-specific proteins synthesized in cells infected by JHMV are slightly different from those in cells infected by A59V and are in the range of 18,000–150,000. The viral-specific intracellular proteins are first detectable at 4 hr after infection at 38.5°C and at 7 hr after infection at 33°C. The functions of the proteins, other than some being structural virion proteins (Table 2), are not known. In all probability, one or more of the proteins is a RNA-dependent RNA polymerase responsible for messenger and genomic RNA synthesis, because such an enzyme is not present in the virion. No other data concerning the synthesis of intracellular coronaviral proteins have been reported.

Twelve to 16 proteins of 50,000 daltons each can be encoded in the coronaviral genomic RNA, depending on its size. For example, the mouse hepatitis viral genome is about 6×10^6 daltons, encoding about

600,000 daltons of protein, while the infectious bronchitis viral genome is about 8×10^6 daltons, encoding about 800,000 daltons of protein. The virion proteins of both viruses account for about 250,000–350,000 daltons, leaving about half to two-thirds of the genome available for regulatory activity and encoding of nonstructural proteins. It is difficult to determine how many independent polypeptides are encoded in the coronaviral genome because we have detected the posttranslational processing of at least two of the nine intracellular mouse hepatitis virus proteins. The identification of the protein(s) synthesized by each of the separate mRNA species and the genomic RNA in cell-free translation systems is essential for a complete definition of the coding capacity of the coronaviral genome.

4.4. Assembly

The following sequence of events is probably the most likely mode of coronavirus assembly (McIntosh, 1974). Nucleocapsids are assembled in cytoplasmic viral factories and associate with the cisternal membranes of the endoplasmic reticulum and Golgi apparatus. As the nucleocapsid begins envelopment or budding, peplomers are added to some emerging particles. Not all budding particles receive peplomers, a fact that may account for the low burst size of about 10–100 IU/cell for coronaviruses (Patterson and Bingham, 1976; Robb *et al.*, 1979*a*). Release of virus particles occurs by lysis of the plasma and/or endoreticular membranes and occasionally by fusion of virus-containing cytoplasmic vacuoles with the plasma membrane (Doughri *et al.*, 1976). Both of these mechanisms may be mediated by the membrane-associated coronavirus protein (Chun-Akana, Bond, and Robb, manuscript in preparation).

4.5. General Comments

The following "most likely" scenario is based on the above facts and the known multiplication strategies of two other single-strand RNA viruses whose genomes are of positive polarity and whose virions do not contain a RNA-dependent RNA polymerase: the Picornaviridae and Togaviridae. Picornaviruses utilize their genomic RNA as a polycistronic mRNA to translate a very large polypeptide that is specifically cleaved to produce the terminal proteins. No other mRNA species is found in picornavirus-infected cells. Togaviruses, on the other hand, have two species of mRNA. Their genomic RNA is polycistronic and encodes the nonstructural viral proteins, while a smaller mRNA species is also polycistronic and encodes the virion structural proteins. Coronaviruses are different from both of these families in their multiplication strategy because they use several species of mRNA, one or more of which may be polycistronic. Only additional data will improve the accuracy of the following coronavirus multiplication sequence.

A coronavirus virion adsorbs to a susceptible cell through the interaction of an envelope glycoprotein (peplomer) with a specific glycoprotein receptor on the plasma membrane. Penetration requires energy and a fluid membrane and is accomplished by viropexis and/or envelope-membrane fusion. Uncoating occurs within the cytoplasm, and cytoplasmic "factories" arc established for the synthesis of coronavirus RNA and protein. A nuclear function is probably involved in this phase of replication because of the presence of the early intranuclear antigen found in mouse hepatitis virus infection (Robb et al., 1979a). The infecting genomic RNA is of a positive polarity (mRNA) and, after being uncoated and activated, directs the synthesis of a virus-specific RNA polymerase (replicase) which replicates a complementary negative RNA strand. Multiple discrete mRNA species are then transcribed from the negative-strand RNA by a transcriptase, a function possibly residing in the replicase molecule. Viral protein synthesis occurs on both membrane-associated polysomes (glycoproteins) and on non-membrane-associated polysomes (nonglycosylated proteins). The nucleocapsids assemble in the cytoplasmic factories and mature by budding through the membrane of the cisternae of the endoplasmic reticulum and Golgi apparatus. Peplomers are added at the time of budding. Nucleocapsids do not migrate to positions beneath the plasma membrane, and budding does not occur from the plasma membrane, although a virus-specific plasma membrane-associated antigen is present. Both infectious (containing peplomers) and noninfectious (without peplomers) virus are released by cell lysis. Cell death may be mediated by altered membrane function induced by the presence of virus protein in the cellular membrane. The formation of syncytia (intercellular fusion) is not necessary for the production of progeny virions, nor does it amplify the yield of progeny virions (Robb et al., 1979a).

5. ALTERATION IN HOST CELL METABOLISM

Almost no work has been performed on the alteration of host cell metabolism during coronavirus infection. Information concerning the regulation of nucleic acid, protein, carbohydrate, and lipid synthesis during infection is lacking. We have observed that general cellular protein synthesis is not affected until very late in the infectious cycle for mouse hepatitis virus. JHMV and A59V (Bond and Robb, 1978). We have observed, however, that synthesis of specific cellular proteins can be stimulated or abolished during JHMV and A59V infection in 17CL-16 cells when radiolabeled proteins are analyzed by high-resolution, two-dimensional gel electrophoresis (Bond and Robb, 1978). As described below, the investigation of cells persistently infected by coronaviruses may be helpful in understanding the regulation of specific cellular protein synthesis during infection (Leibowitz, Bond, and Robb, manuscript in preparation).

6. DEFECTIVE VIRUS AND VIRAL INTERFERENCE

6.1. Defective Virus

Evidence of defective virus has been obtained in 17CL-16 cells infected at a multiplicity of 0.1 IU/cell by mouse hepatitis virus, JHMV and A59V (Bond, Leibowitz, and Robb, unpublished observations). The defective virus has a density of 1.16 g/cm³, as compared to a density of 1.18 g/cm³ for intact virions. These defective particles have the same structural proteins as do virions. The RNA in the defective virus, however, is only 18 S in size.

6.2. Interference by Defective Virus

The only available data regarding the production of defective coronavirus particles are those briefly described for mouse hepatitis virus (JHMV and A59V) in Section 6.1. Whether these defective particles have any interfering potential in homologous or heterologous infections *in vitro* and *in vivo* remains to be investigated. These defective particles may not have an interference potential because we have serially passaged both JHMV and A59V 20 times in 17CL-16 cells using multiplicities of infection of 10^{-4}, 0.1, and 20–100 (undiluted) IU/cell. No decrease in the yield of progeny virions occurred. An additional 20 serial undiluted passages of both JHMV and A59V had no effect on the yield of progeny virions.

6.3. Other Forms of Interference

We have found that the dose–response curve for mouse hepatitis virus (JHMV and A59V) is linear for multiplicities between 0.01 and 0.5 IU/cell in 17CL-16 cells (Robb *et al.*, 1979*a*) when the percentage of infected cells is scored by immunofluorescence. The experimental percentages of infected cells are similar to those predicted by the Poisson distribution. Above 0.5 IU/cell, the percentage of infected cells falls significantly below the values predicted by the Poisson distribution. The maximum yield of progeny virions, however, is independent of the multiplicity between 0.01 and 10 IU/cell. In addition, many infected cells at the higher multiplicities contain only the intranuclear MHV-specific antigen and do not develop the cytoplasmic antigen. The mechanism of this apparent interference during virus replication is not known. A possible role for defective particles is being examined. Reports concerning homologous interference in other coronavirus infections were not discovered in our search of the literature.

7. PATHOGENESIS OF CORONAVIRUS DISEASE

7.1. Spectrum of Disease

Three important facts should be borne in mind when the pathogenesis of coronavirus disease is discussed. First, many organs are infected and affected by natural coronavirus infections in animals when the infected animal is carefully examined. Second, variant viruses can be isolated from natural or experimental animal infections that have a more-or-less organ-specific tropism rather than the polyorgan tropism of the original infecting virus. Third, the spectrum of disease is very dependent on the age of the animal, the genetic background of the animal, and the route of inoculation. Although these three factors produce a very complex pathogenesis, they also provide a fertile ground for the molecular investigation of the pathogenesis of organ-specific virus-caused disease. The serological relatedness of some of the mammalian viruses (Table 1) allows some extrapolation of data from one animal to another. This type of extrapolation is important for human coronavirus disease because the pathogenesis of the human disease cannot be adequately investigated in infected humans. The murine model is probably the most suitable model for extrapolation to human disease because of the serological relatedness between the human and murine coronaviruses.

Table 4 lists the spectrum of disease produced by members of the coronavirus family. Of particular interest is the multiorgan involvement produced by the mammalian viruses. The data strongly suggest that evidence for an etiological role for human coronaviruses should be actively sought in human meningoencephalitis (as in the mouse, Fig. 9), primary demyelination of the central nervous system (as in the mouse, Figs. 10 and 11), hepatitis, interstitial nephritis, interstitial pneumonitis, and impaired immune responsiveness. If an etiological role in one or more of these diseases can be proven for these viruses, the development of suitable vaccines would be a reasonable objective, because limited studies on human populations indicate very high infection rates: 50% of 3-year-old children and 69% of adults are seropositive for OC43, one strain of human coronavirus (Monto, 1976). The infection rate could be shown to be much higher if infection with all of the human coronavirus serotypes were adequately investigated in the same population.

Nothing is presently known about the molecular mechanisms underlying the organ tropism of the coronaviruses. Our speculation is that one of the envelope glycoproteins plays a significant receptor function in recognizing appropriate plasma membrane receptors on susceptible cells. The identification of the virion molecule(s) and/or virus–cell interaction(s) (Robb, 1977) that is responsible for the organ tropism should be possible by correlating the altered organ tropism produced by variant virions with altered virion protein(s) or multiplication strategy. The murine model presently offers the greatest potential in this regard.

7.2. Route of Infection

The type of disease produced by a coronavirus is markedly influenced by the route of inoculation, the age of the animal, the genetic background of the animal, and the virus isolate. Intravenous, intranasal, oral, intraocular, intraperitoneal, intramuscular, subcutaneous, and intramammary routes have been used with various viruses and animals.

Natural infections are primarily transmitted by oral ingestion of virus-contaminated fluid and/or particulate matter and by intranasal inoculation with aerosols and/or droplets. The remarkable stability of these enveloped viruses in acid environments, pH 2–3, ensures their passage through the stomach into the small intestine, which is the primary replication site for the viruses that produce significant enteritis.

TABLE 4

Spectrum of Disease Produced by Members of the Coronavirus Family

Virus[a]	Host	Encephalitis demyelination	Enteritis	Hepatitis	Lymphoid adenitis	Nephritis	Pancreatitis	Peritonitis	Upper respiratory pneumonitis	Miscellaneous
IBV	Chicken					1, 2, 3, 4[f]			4	Gonaditis 5
CCV	Dog		5							
FCV	Cat	6	7	7, 8		7		7, 8	7	Eye infection 7 / Ependymitis 6
HCV	Man	(+)[b] + in mice[9]							10, 11	
HECV	Man		12, 13	(+)[c]		(+)[d,2]				
MHV[e]	Mouse	14, 15, 16, 17	15, 18	15	15	2, 15	19	15	14, 15	
NCDCV	Bovine		20, 21							
TGEV	Pig		22			2			23, 24	
HEV	Pig	25, 26, 27	27						27	
RCV	Rat								5, 28	
SDAV	Rat									Salivary adenitis 29, 30, 31
RTCV	Tick	Pathogenesis not yet investigated								
	Bird									
TBDV	Turkey		32						32	

[a] These abreviations follow those suggested by the Coronavirus Study Group, chaired by Dr. D. A. J. Tyrrell, in a revision (Tyrrell, personal communication) of the previous recommendations (Tyrrell et al., 1975). RTCV is a newly described virus whose abbreviation may be modified.
[b] The production of meningoencephalitis in humans is a speculation based on several observations: the headache accompanying many coronavirus colds is not relieved by nonnarcotic analgesics, suggesting at least meningeal involvement; the human coronavirus OC43 produces lethal panencephalitis after I.C. inoculation into suckling mice (9); OC43 is serologically related to the hemagglutinating encephalomyelitis virus of swine (9); essentially all members of the coronavirus family produce meningoencephalitis when neuropathogenesis is examined.

[c] Many human cases of hepatitis are not caused by the hepatitis A or B viruses (Zuckerman, 1978). We speculate that the human coronaviruses are prime suspects in at least some of these non-A, non-B cases, because most of the mammalian coronaviruses produce hepatitis in their natural hosts.

[d] Apostolov et al. (1977a) have made a strong argument that a porcine coronavirus is capable of infecting humans in close contact with pigs. An acute nephronitis occurs that slowly progresses into a chronic active interstitial nephritis, the endemic (Balkan) nephropathy. It therefore seems reasonable to speculate that at least some cases of nonbacterial interstitial nephritis in humans may be caused by a persistent infection with a human coronavirus. Indeed, when such a pathogenesis has been sought, many of the coronaviruses do cause interstitial nephritis in their natural hosts (see table above).

[e] Piazza (1969) describes the pathogenesis of this group of murine viruses in depth. The references given in the table are more recent investigations.

[f] References: 1, Alexander et al. (1978); 2, Apostolov et al. (1977a); 3, Apostolov et al. (1977b); 4, Purcell et al. (1976); 5, Takeuchi et al. (1976); 6, Krum et al. (1975); 7, Timoney (1976); 8, Horzinek et al. (1977); 9, Kaye et al. (1977); 10, Gump et al. (1976); 11, McIntosh et al. (1974); 12, Caul and Egglestone (1977); 13, Moore et al. (1977); 14, Goto et al. (1977); 15, Ward et al. (1973); 16, Lampert et al. (1973); 17, Weiner (1973); 18, Broderson et al. (1976); 19, Fujiwara et al. (1975); 20, Chasey and Lucas (1977); 21, Morin et al. (1976); 22, Morin et al. (1973); 23, Kemeny et al. (1974); 24, Underdahl et al. (1974); 25, Greig et al. (1971); 26, Mengeling and Cutlip (1976); 27, Werdin et al. (1976); Bhatt and Jacoby (1977); 29, Jacoby et al. (1975); 30, Lai et al. (1976); 31, Weisbroth and Peress (1977); 32, Naqi et al. (1975).

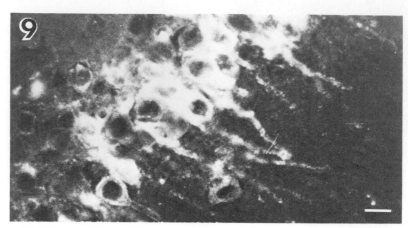

Figure 9.   Demonstration of mouse hepatitis virus-caused acute encephalomyelitis in a 4-week-old BALB/c mouse given 100 infectious units of JHMV intranasally and sacrificed 4 days later. JHMV-specific infection of neurons and glial cells in the hippocampus is demonstrated by immunofluorescence using sections of ethanol-fixed, paraffin-embedded brain. See Robb *et al.* (1979*b*) for details. Scale bar is 10 μm.

The subsequent viremia produces disease in other organs such as the liver, brain, kidneys, and lungs. After intranasal inoculation, however, coronaviruses can infect the brain by direct extension from the nasal mucosa without the assistance of a viremia, as shown for mouse hepatitis virus (MHV) by Goto *et al.* (1977) and for rat sialodacryoadenitis by Jacoby *et al.* (1975). Another possible route in natural infections is the aerosol/droplet infection of the eye as shown for infectious bronchitis virus by Cowen *et al.* (1971). Venereal transfer for MHV infection has been suggested by Nelson (1952).

Finally, a most intriguing possible natural route of infection, that of mechanical and/or biological transfer by infected insects, has been suggested. Ishii *et al.* (1974) showed that MHV produced virus-specific fluorescence in intestinal cells of the mosquito *Aedes aegypti* for at least 14 days after ingestion of blood from infected mice. Furthermore, the blood in these engorged mosquitoes was infectious when inoculated into mice. Recently, a coronavirus has been demonstrated by transmission electron microscopy in ticks, *Ixodes uriae*, that feed on sea birds in Runde, Norway (Traavik *et al.*, 1977). The sea birds were seropositive for the virus.

The following references provide a more detailed examination of the effect of route of inoculation and age of animal on the pathogenesis of coronavirus disease. IBV: Alexander *et al.* (1978); CCV: Binn *et al.* (1974); FCV: Timoney (1976); HCV: Monto (1976); HECV: Caul and

Egglestone (1977); MHV: Bailey *et al.* (1949), Piazza (1969), Sebesteny and Hill (1974), Hirano *et al.* (1975*b*), Taguchi *et al.* (1977); Fox *et al.* (1977); TGEV: Kemeny and Woods (1977); HEV: Mengeling and Cutlip (1976), Werdin *et al.* (1976); TBDV: Naqi *et al.* (1975), Gonder *et al.* (1976).

A very important area of coronavirus-caused disease that has received very little attention is that of intrauterine infection. A beginning has been made into the pathogenesis of neonatal calf diarrhea coronavirus intrauterine infection because of its economic impact on the production of dairy and beef cattle. This virus is also called mucosal

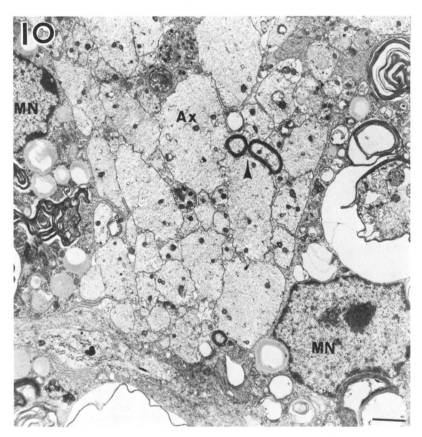

Fig. 10. Demyelination in the brain of a 4-week-old BALB/c mouse that was given 100 infectious units of JHMV by the intranasal route 21 days before examination by transmission electron microscopy. Two small, normally myelinated axons (arrow) are present within a large group of demyelinated axons (Ax) in the spinal cord. MN indicates the nuclei within two macrophages that have removed the damaged myelin from the demyelinated axons. See Robb *et al.* (1979*b*) for details. Scale bar is 1 μm.

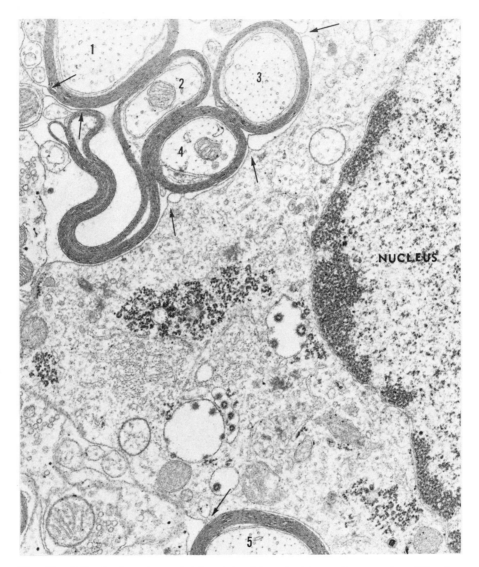

Fig. 11. Oligodendrocyte containing intracisternal virions of mouse hepatitis virus (JHMV). Aggregates of electron-dense particles, filaments, and vacuoles are prominent in the hypertrophic cytoplasm. Plasma membrane connections to myelin lamellae (arrows) are seen around axons 1–3. A redundant myelin loop is connected with an oligodendroglial process (axon 2). ×50,000 (reduced 38% for reproduction). Reproduced from Powell and Lampert (1975).

disease virus of sheep and bovine diarrhea virus. Although limited numbers of animals were investigated, a maternal viremia probably produces abortion and fetal death during early pregnancy, congenital anomalies during middle pregnancy, and little effect during late pregnancy (Brown *et al.*, 1974; Snowdon *et al.*, 1975: Gard *et al.*, 1976; Plant *et al.*, 1976; Allen, 1977). The significant congenital anomalies were in the central nervous system and consisted of cerebellar degeneration, cavitation, and hypoplasia. These anomalies were attributed to the cytocidal effect of the virus and the subsequent cerebellar edema. One indication of fetal reaction to the viral infection was the production of interferon in the fetal tissues from 4 to 21 days after infection and in the fetal serum from 13 to 21 days after infection (Rinaldo *et al.*, 1976).

Turkey poults hatched from eggs infected with turkey bluecomb disease virus 24 days after being laid have a disease syndrome that is similar to that occurring in poults inoculated at 1 day after hatching (Deshmukh *et al.*, 1976). Clearly, a great deal more attention has to be given to this area. The murine model offers the greatest potential for interested investigators.

7.3. Animal Response to Infection

7.3.1. Virus–Cell Interaction

The primary virus–cell interaction in coronavirus-caused disease is a cytocidal interaction (Robb, 1977). As described in more detail in Section 4, the virus adsorbs to a susceptible cell, penetrates the cell, replicates its RNA and protein species primarily in the cytoplasm, assembles by budding into cisternae of the endoplasmic reticulum and Golgi appartus, and kills the cell by a presently unknown mechanism. One possible cytocidal mechanism is the alteration of membrane function by the incorporation of a viral protein into the membrane. We have found that a newly synthesized virus-specific protein is associated early after infection with the plasma membrane of mouse hepatitis virus-infected cells (Fig. 5) (Robb *et al.*, 1979*a*). Shortly after the appearance of this protein in the plasma membrane, the cells become permeable to trypan blue, suggesting that coronavirus infection may rapidly alter the function of the plasma membrane.

The association of a viral protein with the plasma membrane may also account for the loss of glucose-stimulated sodium transport in the plasma membrane of jejunal mucosal enterocytes infected with transmissible gastroenteritis virus (TGEV) (McClung *et al.*, 1976; Kerzner *et al.*, 1977). This altered transport is probably responsible for the TGEV-caused diarrhea. This alteration is not simply the result of a general malfunction of plasma membrane transport, because adenyl cyclase-dependent sodium transport remains intact. The diarrhea produced by TGEV is, therefore, different from the diarrhea produced by the *E. coli* and *C. vibrio* entertoxins, which alter the adenylyl cyclase-dependent sodium transport and leave the glucose-stimulated sodium transport intact.

Lymphoid and reticuloendothelial cells, endothelial cells, and parenchymal cells such as neurons, glia, hepatocytes, renal podocytes, and nasointestinal epithelial cells are all subject to cytocidal attack by members of the coronavirus family. This cytocidal interaction has been demonstrated by light microscopy, virus-specific immunofluorescence, and/or transmission electron microscopy in infected animals and/or organ culture. The formation of typical coronavirus syncytia in organs, probably mediated by the plasma membrane-associated viral protein, is dependent on the virus isolate used for the infection. The following references provide pertinent details. IBV: Cowen *et al.* (1971), Purcell *et al.* (1976), Alexander and Gough (1977), Apostolov *et al.* (1977*a*); CCV: Keenan *et al.* (1976), Takeuchi *et al.* (1976); FCV: Krum *et al.* (1975); HCV: Apostolov *et al.* (1977*a*); HECV: Caul and Clarke (1975), Caul and Egglestone (1977); MHV: Bailey *et al.* (1949), Sebesteny and Hill (1974), Fujiwara *et al.* (1975), Smith *et al.* (1975/1976), Broderson *et al.* (1976), Taguchi *et al.* (1976), Goto *et al.* (1977), Namiki *et al.* (1977), Ward *et al.* (1977); NCDCV: Morin *et al.* (1976), Doughri and Storz (1977); TGEV: Morin *et al.* (1973), Underdahl *et al.* (1974), Kemeny *et al.* (1974), Sprino *et al.* (1976); HEV: Mengeling and Cutlip (1976), Sprino *et al.* (1976), Werdin *et al.* (1976); SDAV: Jacoby *et al.* (1975); TBDV: Deshmukh *et al.* (1976), Gonder *et al.* (1976).

7.3.2. Resistance to Infection

The mechanism of resistance to coronavirus infection in animals is very complex. A comprehensive understanding of the molecular/cellular mechanisms underlying this resistance has not yet emerged, although significant insights have been obtained. As detailed below, resistance is dependent on the interaction of at least four factors in the murine model: (1) ability of virus to produce progeny virus in cells of the reticuloendothelial system (macrophages), (2) production of lymphokines by lymphoid cells, (3) production of interferon, and (4) development of virus-specific cellular immunity. The role of humoral immunity appears to be relatively unimportant in this resistance.

Weiser, Bang, and their co-workers have shown that the resistance to mouse hepatitis virus (MHV) infection in mice is due both to a genetically transmitted "resistance gene(s)" that inhibits MHV replication in macrophages and to a "susceptibility factor(s)" that is produced by lymphoid cells, possibly a lymphokine. The susceptibility factor makes genetically resistant macrophages susceptible to MHV replication (Weiser and Bang, 1976, 1977; Weiser *et al.*, 1976). Stohlman and Frelinger (1978) have found that the resistance of SJL mice to central nervous system infection by JHMV is mediated by two genes, one dominant and one recessive.

Virelizier and his co-workers have found that type I interferon (virus induced) has an important role in providing resistance to acute, but not chronic, MHV disease in resistant strains of mice (Virelizier *et al.*, 1976, Virelizier and Gresser, 1978). Although type II interferon (non-virus-induced) inhibits MHV replication in macrophages *in vitro*, it may have little effect in providing resistance to MHV infection *in vivo* (Taguchi *et al.*, 1976; Virelizier *et al.*, 1976). Additional detailed studies are needed to establish the role, if any, of the various interferons in animal resistance to coronavirus infection.

The murine resistance gene described by Weiser and Bang may involve the *H-2* region of the murine genome because *H-2^{ff}* and *H-2^{bf}* strains of mice are resistant to the chronic phase of MHV-caused disease, while *H-2^{ss}*, *H-2^{aa}*, and *H-2^{bb}* strains are susceptible (Oth *et al.*, 1976). The acute phase of the disease occurs in all the *H-2* strains. Additional detailed studies are needed to determine whether an immune response gene is involved in this model of resistance.

Cellular immunity does have an important but poorly understood role in the resistance of mice to MHV disease. Nude (*nu/nu*) mice develop lethal acute and chronic hepatitis and encephalitis after MHV infection, while the infection in their *nu/+* heterozygote littermates has no clinical effect (Sebesteny and Hill, 1974; Tamura *et al.*, 1976; Ward *et al.*, 1977). Furthermore, *nu/nu* mice can be immunized with inactive MHV only after they have been inoculated with *nu/+* spleen cells (Fujiwara *et al.*, 1976). Cortisone treatment renders *nu/+* heterozygotes susceptible to MHV disease with a pathogenesis similar to that in their *nu/nu* homozygous littermates without cortisone treatment (Hirano *et al.*, 1975*b*). Cortisone or cyclophosphamide treatment also increases the susceptibility of non-nude mice to MHV disease (Hirano *et al.*, 1975*a,b*; Taguchi *et al.*, 1977). Radiation or antilymphocyte serum treatment makes normally resistant mice susceptible to MHV disease (Dupuy *et al.*, 1975; LePrevost *et al.*, 1975*a*). Cell-mediated immunity is also important in transmissible gastroenteritis virus (TGEV) infections (Frederick and Bohl, 1976; Woods, 1977).

Coronavirus infection stimulates a normal humoral immune response in the natural host. The early appearance of IgM is followed by an increasing amount of IgG. Antiviral IgA is readily produced. The antibody levels stay high for months to years after a single exposure. Different temporal and quantitative responses in neutralizing, complement-fixing, immunofluorescent, and hcmagglutination-inhibiting antibodies occur during infection and vary between individuals. The role of humoral immunity in the resistance of mice to MHV infection is less clear. Although neutralizing antibody is transferred to suckling mice via the milk, these mice are still susceptible to MHV disease (Kiuchi *et al.*, 1974). Furthermore, passive immunity with anti-MHV neutralizing serum or transplacental anti-MHV neutralizing antibodies does not make susceptible mice resistant (LePrevost *et al.*, 1975*a*; Dupuy *et al.*, 1975; Taguchi *et al.*, 1976). The inoculation of thymectomized, irradiated mice with T-cell-deficient embryonic liver cells does not protect them from MHV disease (Dupuy *et al.*, 1975; LePrevost *et al.*, 1975*a*). However, orally given anti-TGEV IgG, IgM, or IgA protects neonatal pigs from lethal TGEV infection (Stone *et al.*, 1977).

Immune complex disease may occur during coronavirus infection, especially during the chronic phase of disease. Chicks that develop chronic interstitial nephritis after infectious bronchitis virus (IBV) infection have higher anti-IBV HI titers than do chicks that do not develop chronic interstitial nephritis (Alexander and Gough, 1978). Apostolov has found granular deposits in the glomerular basement membrane and subendothelial space in kidneys from humans with endemic Balkan nephropathy. These deposits contain IgG and C3 by immunofluorescence (Apostolov *et al.*, 1977*a*). This disease is believed to be produced by a chronic TGEV infection in people closely associated with pigs. This observation warrants confirmation and expansion.

The production and use of vaccines for coronaviruses is beyond the scope of this chapter, but the following references will facilitate an introduction to the literature. IBV: Cowen and Hitchner (1975), Thornton and Muskett (1975), Alexander *et al.* (1976), Alexander and Chettle (1977), Alexander and Gough (1978), HCV: Monto (1976); MHV: Dupuy *et al.* (1975), Hirano *et al.* (1975*b*), LePrévost *et al.*

(1975*a*), Fujiwara *et al.* (1976); NCDCV: Hafez *et al.* (1976), Shope *et al.* (1976), Whitmore and Archbald (1977); TGEV: Kemeny (1976), Sprino *et al.* (1976), Stone *et al.* (1976), Kemeny and Woods (1977); SDAV: Jacoby *et al.* (1975); TBDV: Gonder *et al.* (1976).

7.3.3. Mixed Infections of Coronavirus with Other Agents

Few pertinent reports were found concerning mixed infections between a coronavirus and other agent(s). Giambrone *et al.* (1977) showed that 1-day-old chicks infected with infectious bursal disease virus and challenged at 35 days of age with infectious bronchitis virus (IBV) developed lower anti-IBV neutralizing antibody titers and had an increased incidence and severity of disease than did 35-day-old control chicks that had not been previously infected with infectious bursal disease virus (Giambrone *et al.*, 1977). Morin *et al.* (1976) investigated 55 cases of spontaneous calf diarrhea and found 11 of them to involve neonatal calf diarrhea coronavirus and one or more other etiologically significant agents. A review of the viruses, including human enteric coronavirus found in human diarrhea, is given by Flewett and Boxall (1976).

7.3.4. Diagnostic Techniques

Various diagnostic techniques for coronavirus identification and serotyping have been applied to infected animals, tissues, organ cultures, and cell cultures. These techniques include cytopathic effect, virus-specific immunofluorescence, hemagglutination inhibition, neutralization, complement fixation, hemadsorption, immune electron microscopy, negative-contrast electron microscopy, and single radial hemolysis. The following references will provide access to this literature. IBV: Lucio and Hitchner (1970), Cowen and Hitchner (1975), Alexander *et al.* (1976), Hidalgo and Raggi (1976), Alexander and Chettle (1977), Wooley and Brown (1977), Egan and Tannock (1978); CCV: Takeuchi *et al.* (1976); FCV: Pedersen (1976); HCV: Flewett and Boxall (1976); Hierholzer and Tannock (1977), Monto and Rhodes (1977), Riski *et al.* (1977); MHV: Robb (1979*a,b*), Hirano *et al.* (1975*a*), Namiki *et al.* (1977); NCDCV: England *et al.* (1975), Morin *et al.* (1976), Sharpee *et al.* (1976); TGEV: Thomas and Dulac (1976), Werdin *et al.* (1976), Saif *et al.*, 1977; TBDV: Patel *et al.* (1976, 1977);

RTCV: Traavik *et al.* (1977). Also see the additional references listed in Sections 3.1 and 7.1.

7.4.   Summary of Pathogenesis

The spectrum of disease in the natural hosts of coronaviruses depends on the age, genetic background, route of infection, and virus dose. The primary natural routes of coronaviral infection are aerosol/droplet infection of the nasopharynx and oral ingestion of infected particulate matter. More unusual routes have been described such as veneral, intraocular, and biological and/or mechanical transfer from insects (mosquitoes and ticks).

The primary mechanism of disease production during acute, and probably chronic, coronavirus infection is a direct cytocidal attack on susceptible cells. These viruses can destroy epithelial, endothelial, and lymphoid cells. When parenchymal cells are killed, diseases such as hepatitis, encephalomyelitis, enteritis, nasopharyngitis, pneumonitis, and nephritis are produced. The acute lymphadenitis may produce transient or prolonged depression of both humoral and cellular immunity. The destruction of endothelial cells may produce localized or generalized vasculitis. Direct infection of susceptible cells, and extension without a requirement for viremia, can produce enteritis, nasopharyngitis, pneumonitis, lymphadenitis, and, after nasopharyngeal infection, encephalomyelitis. A secondary viremia produces hepatitis, nephritis, and, after oral ingestion, encephalomyelitis and pneumonitis as well.

Resistance to acute infection depends on the ability of the infecting virus to multiply in reticuloendothelial cells, a property that is genetically controlled. In addition, virus-induced interferon production and cell-mediated immunity are important in limiting the extent of infection, while humoral immunity is relatively unimportant. The molecular mechanisms of resistance to coronavirus infection have yet to be fully elucidated.

Chronic coronavirus disease, in the form of demyelination, hepatitis, and/or immune deficiency, is produced primarily by a smoldering cytocidal infection by cell-to-cell spread of the virus. Although coronaviruses produce a plasma membrane-associated antigen in acutely and persistently infected cells, there is at present no evidence that an immune-mediated cytocidal attack on persistently infected cells in chronically infected animals is an important mechanism in the pathogenesis of chronic coronavirus disease. Immune-mediated chronic disease does, however, remain a likely possibility in conjunction with the slowly progressive cell-to-cell spread of the virus.

The murine models available for both acute and chronic coronavirus infections should enhance our presently meager understanding of acute and chronic coronavirus disease in humans. An elucidation of the molecular virology of murine coronaviruses, however, is necessary before the murine models of disease will be fully informative.

8. PERSISTENT INFECTIONS

The persistent infections established by some coronaviruses in their natural hosts should provide very good experimental models for elucidating the pathogenic mechanisms of some important human diseases. The murine models of chronic hepatitis and persistent demyelination of the central nervous system are receiving significant attention. Table 5 lists the pertinent work in these areas. It must be noted that several biologically different variants are listed under one name as if they were all the same virus when they are not, i.e., mouse hepatitis virus: JHMV.

The persistent infections with JHMV that produce a smoldering demyelination (Figures 10 and 11) (Herndon et al., 1975; LePrévost et al., 1975b; Virelizier et al., 1975) may be relevant to human multiple sclerosis because coronaviruslike particles have been observed in the brain of a patient with multiple sclerosis by transmission electron microscopy (Tanaka et al., 1976), and coronaviruses have been isolated from the brains of two patients dying from multiple sclerosis (J. Burks, University of Colorado Medical Center, personal communication). Both findings await confirmation and expansion. The hepatitis models may be analogous to some of the non-A, non-B forms of chronic human hepatitis (Zuckerman, 1978).

The disease produced by a persistent coronavirus infection may be due to a smoldering cytocidal attack on susceptible cells rather than to an immune attack specifically directed against coronavirus-modified cells. Lampert (1978) has reviewed these mechanisms in human demyelinating diseases. A cell-to-cell spread of the virus could be one mechanism that would produce continued cytocidal activity in the presence of high levels of neutralizing antibody. Tentatively, cell-to-cell spread of mouse hepatitis virus (MHV) in 17CL-16 cells infected with an A59V recovered from persistently infected 17CL-1 cells has been

TABLE 5

Persistent MHV Infection in Mice

Virus	Source of virus	Infection parameters				Type of acute disease[c]	Chronic disease >2 mo p.i.[d]	Evidence of persistence	Reference[g]
		Strain	Age	Route[a]	Dose[b]				
JHMV	C57/B1 liver	Swiss	3 wk	i.c.	$100\ LD_{50}$	EM	Porencephaly	None	1
JHMV	Mouse brain	BALB/c	4 wk	i.c.	$50\%\ LD_{50}$	EM	None	Active demyelination 16 mo p.i.	2
MHV3	DBA/2 brain	C3H	10 wk	i.p.	$10^3\ LD_{50}$	EM and H	Paralysis Hepatitis Immune deficiency	Virus isolation from liver, brain and lymph nodes 3 mo p.i.	3
MHV_3	C57/B1 liver	A2G C3H	7 wk 6mo	i.p. i.p.	$10^2\ LD_{50}$ $10^2\ LD_{50}$	None None	Paralysis Vasculitis Immune deficiency	FA+ ependymal cells, virus isolated FA+ endothelial cells, virus isolated	4
NuU (MHV2)	nu/mu, BALB/c on DBT cells	nu/nu BALB/c	7 wk	i.n. i.p. i.v.	$10^2\ PFU$ $10^4\ PFU$	EM and H Lymph node adenitis	Hepatitis Encephalitis LN adenopathy	Virus isolation	5
JHMV-R[e]	17CL-16 cells	BALB/c	4 wk	i.c. i.n.	$10^2\ IU$ $10^3\ IU$	Demyelination (not lethal)	None	Remyelination, ? demyelination with light mononuclear cell infiltrate at 3 months p.i.	6
A59VC[f]	17CL-16 cells	BALB/c	4 wk	i.c. i.n.	$10^3\ IU$ $10^3\ IU$	Demyelination (not lethal)	None	Remyelination, ? demyelintion with light mononuclear cell infiltrate at 3 months p.i.	6
A59VC-R[f]	17CL-16 cells	BALB/c	4 wk	i.c. i.n.	$10^3\ IU$ $10^3\ IU$	Demyelination (increased lethality)	None	Remyelination, ? demyelination with light mononuclear cell infiltrate at 3 months p.i.	6

						Demyelination (not lethal)			
JHMV-ts 8, 11	17CL-16 cells	BALB/c	4 wk	i.c.	10^4 PFU	Demyelination (not lethal)	None	Remyelination, ? demyelination with light mononuclear cell infiltrate at 3 months p.i.	7
JHMV	Swiss brain	C57/BL	12 wk	i.c.	25 SLD_{50}	EM	None	Continuing demyelination with macrophage infiltrate, FA^+, no virus rescued: 3 and 6 mo p.i.	8

[a] i.c., Intracerebral; i.p., intraperitoneal; i.n., intranasal; i.v., intravenous.

[b] LD_{50}, Amount of virus that will kill 50% of infected mice; PFU, plaque-forming units; IU, infectious units.

[c] EM, Acute lethal encephalomyelitis; H, acute hepatitis.

[d] Chronic disease occurring greater than 2 months after infection defined by clinical symptoms.

[e] Revertant of JHMV selected by repeat passage in 17CL-16 cells; markedly deceased tropism for neurons.

[f] A59C, 17CL-1 adapted A59V; A59VC-R, revertant selected for increased neurotropism and lethality by repeated passages in mouse brains. 1976); 6, J. Robb and P. Lampert (unpublished data); 7, M. Haspel (personal communication); 8, S. Stohlman and L. Weiner (personal communication).

[g] References: 1, Bailey et al. (1949); 2, Herndon et al. (1975); 3, LePrévost, et al. (1975b); 4, Virelizier et al. (1975); 5, Tamura et al. (1976); 6, J. Robb and P. Lampert (unpublished data); 7, M. Haspel (personal communication); 8, S. Stohlman and L. Weiner (personal communication).

observed (Robb, unpublished observation). A specific immune attack cannot be ruled out as a mechanism of persistent coronavirus disease, however, because of the presence of a coronavirus antigen associated with the plasma membrane (Robb *et al.*, 1979*a*) and the involvement of cellular immunity in the resistance and susceptibility to coronavirus disease (see Section 7.3.2). Both mechanisms may be important in chronic disease.

One approach to understanding the molecular mechanisms underlying persistent coronavirus infection in animals has been to establish and biochemically investigate persistent coronavirus infections in cell culture. To date, persistent infections *in vitro* using only murine coronaviruses have been reported. Table 6 lists the available data concerning cells persistently infected with MHV. Several comments can be made from the preliminary data. First, persistent infections are very easily established using low or high multiplicities of infection in growing or confluent cultures (Leibowitz, Bond, and Robb, manuscript in preparation). Second, the virus recovered from the persistently infected cells can have biological characteristics similar to or different from those of the pool of virus used in the original infection. Third, neutralizing antibodies may decrease the yield of virus from the cells but do not eradicate the persistent infection (Stohlman and Weiner, 1978). Fourth, cell clones derived from persistently infected cells may vary in the percentage of cells expressing cytoplasmic and surface antigens and releasing infectious virus (infectious centers) while maintaining intranuclear antigen in 100% of the cells (Leibowitz, Bond, and Robb, manuscript in preparation). Several mechanisms of persistence (Huang and Baltimore, 1977) may therefore be available to coronaviruses in establishing and maintaining persistent infections *in vitro* and *in vivo*.

Other members of the coronavirus family are probably able to establish persistent infections in their host animals although very few data are available. Infectious bronchitis virus (IBV) can be recovered for several weeks after infection from organs of infected pullets and for several months in their feces (Fabricant and Levine, 1951; Alexander and Gough, 1977). IBV can also produce a chronic nephritis in chickens (Alexander and Gough, 1978). In human infections, human coronavirus (HCV) can be isolated from nasal washings for up to 18 days (Monto, 1976) and human enteric coronavirus (HCEV) can be isolated from feces for several months (Moore *et al.*, 1977). The inability to temporally assay human tissues for HCV and HECV after acute infection has made the investigation of persistent human coronavirus infection very difficult. The sheep counterpart of NCDCV, mucosal disease virus, can be isolated for months after birth in tissues of lambs infected

TABLE 6

Persistent MHV Infection in Cell Culture

Virus	Cell line	Properties of persistent virus				Superinfection[e]		Mechanism of persistence[f]			Reference[i]
		Temp. sens.[a]	Plq. morph.[b]	Syn.[-c]	Path.[d]	Homologous	Heterologous	IF	Extracell	DI	
A59VC	NCTC-1469 (mouse)	?	?	?	WT	?	?	?	?	?	1
A59VC	17CL-1 (mouse)	?	+	?	?	?	?	?	?	?	2
JHMV	Neuro 2A (mouse)	No	No	No	WT	No	VSV(MOI = 1)	No	±Yes	?No	3
JHMV	17CL-1 (mouse)	No	?	Yes	?	No	±[g]	?	?No	?	4
A59V	17CL-1 (mouse)	No	?	Yes	?	No	±[g]	?	?No	?	4
JHMV	Neuro 2A (mouse)	No	?	Yes	?	?	Yes[h]	?	?No	?	4
JHMV	Glial RN2 (rat)	No	No	No	WT	?	VSV(MOI = 0.1)	?	?	?	5

[a] Temp. sens., virus isolate was inhibited either in its ability to be titered or in progeny virus production at restrictive temperature (38–39°C).

[b] Plq. morph., virus isolate produced plaques that were different from the original infecting virus.

[c] Syn.⁻, virus isolate was unable to induce intracellular fusion (syncytial formation) during infection of susceptible cells.

[d] Path., type of pathogenesis occurring after animal infection with the virus isolate; WT, the infections with the wild-type virus (original infecting virus) and the virus isolate were similar.

[e] Superinfection of the persistently infected lines with the original infecting virus (homologous) or a different strain of MHV or virus group (heterologous). VSV (MOI = 1) means that the superinfection of cells with VSV using a multiplicity of 1 was inhibited.

[f] Three common mechanisms of persistence are the production of interferon (IF), the continued spread of extracellular virus in a carrier state (Extracell.), and the production of interfering defective virus particles (DI).

[g] Depends on the clone of persistently infected cells. For example, five clones from each line were tested for heterologous superinfection with vesicular stomatitis virus (VSV) and mengovirus using multiplicities of infection of 0.1, 1.0, and 10 IU/cell. All ten clones were sensitive to mengovirus infection. Sensitivity to VSV superinfection was clone dependent: some were fully sensitive, some were sensitive only at higher multiplicity, and some were fully resistant.

[h] Sensitive to VSV and mengovirus at multiplicities of 0.1, 1.0, and 10 IV/cell.

[i] References: 1, Sabesin (1972); 2, Holmes and Allen (1977); 3, Stohlman and Weiner (1978); 4, Leibowitz, Bond, and Robb (manuscript in preparation); 5, Lucas et al. (1977).

in utero (Gard *et al.*, 1976). Transmissible gastroenteritis virus (TGEV) and hemagglutinating encephalomyelitis virus (HEV) produce chronic disease in pigs. TGEV could be isolated from lungs and intestine for up to 104 days after infection (Underdahl *et al.*, 1975), while HEV could not be isolated from tissues of pigs dying of chronic disease up to 123 days after infection (Mengeling and Cutlip, 1976). Sialodacryoadenitis virus produces chronic disease in the eye, but virus cannot be recovered (Lai *et al.*, 1976).

In summary, coronaviruses can easily establish and maintain persistent infections in cell culture and probably in host animals. Such persistent infections in man could be etiologically significant in some cases of chronic hepatitis, nephritis, demyelination, pneumonitis, enteritis, and altered immune responsiveness. The mechanisms underlying coronavirus persistence are not known, but they are probably multiple, varied, and interacting. The elucidation of these mechanisms requires (1) the definition of the species of virus-specific intracellular mRNA and protein, and the regulation of the synthesis of these species within persistently infected cells and animals; (2) the definition of the role, if any, of interfering defective homologous virus in coronavirus persistence; and (3) a more precise definition of the immune response in acute and chronic coronavirus infection.

9.   GENETICS

There are no published reports concerning the genetics of coronavirus as of February 1978. Preliminary information is available for some murine coronaviruses. We have isolated 34 independent temperature-sensitive mutants of mouse hepatitis virus (JHMV) (Robb *et al.*, 1979*b*). Complementation assays monitoring the production of immunofluorescent antigens, syncytia, and yield of infectious virus at restrictive temperature have not yet provided separable complementation groups for these 34 mutants. The situation may be analogous to that of another enveloped positive-strand RNA virus, Semliki Forest virus, an alpha togavirus (Atkins *et al.*, 1974). Sindbis virus, another alpha togavirus, has yielded to complementation analysis (Pfefferkorn and Shapiro, 1974). Our collection of mutants contains varied members representing RNA^+/RNA^-, syn^+/syn^-, and FA^+/FA^- combinations. Grouping by affected protein is now under way to bypass the problem with complementation analysis. Another collection of temperature-sensitive mutants of JHMV has not yet been biochemically characterized (M. Haspel, personal communication). Plaque morphology mutants of mouse hepatitis virus (A59V) have been isolated but not biochemically characterized (Holmes and Allen, 1977).

10. CONCLUSION

The following properties presently define the coronavirus family. Virion maturation, or budding, occurs only from the cisternal membranes of the endoplasmic reticulum and Golgi apparatus. The cell is killed during virus multiplication, possibly by the alteration of membrane function secondary to the insertion of a viral protein in the endoreticular and plasma membranes. Nucleocapsids and/or maturing virus particles are not associated with the plasma membrane. The infectious virion contains a nonsegmented, single-strand RNA of 6–8 $\times$ 10^6 daltons that is infectious and therefore of a positive (messenger) polarity. The genome RNA contains a polyadenylic acid tract, presumably at the 3' terminal. There are four to six virion structural proteins. A major glycoprotein in the virion is the predominant protein in the large widely spaced peplomers that provide the corona of the virion and the name for this virus family. The major nonglycosylated virion protein is associated with the nucleocapsid. The virion does not contain a RNA-dependent RNA or DNA polymerase.

Coronaviruses are an important group of pathogenic viruses in all of their natural hosts, which range from fowl to man. They produce disease in many organs in susceptible animals. The primary mechanism of pathogenesis is a direct cytocidal attack on the cell. Genetic background, interferon production, and cell-mediated immunity are important factors in limiting the extent of acute coronavirus disease. Chronic or persistent disease can occur after an acute infection. This persistent disease is mediated primarily by a slow cell-to-cell spread of virus that produces cell death by a direct cytocidal action and possibly by a cell-mediated immune attack on infected cells. The molecular mechanisms underlying the pathogenesis of coronavirus disease cannot be well understood until the molecular virology of this virus family has been elucidated. At present, the murine models of coronavirus infection provide the best opportunity for such an elucidation.

11. REFERENCES

Alexander, D. J., and Chettle, N. J., 1977, Procedures for the haemagglutination and the haemagglutination inhibition tests for avian infectious bronchitis virus, *Avian Pathol.* **6**:9.

Alexander, D. J., and Gough, R. E., 1977, Isolation of avian infectious bronchitis virus from experimentally infected chickens, *Res. Vet. Sci.* **23**:344.

Alexander, D. J., Gough, R. E., and Pattison, M., 1978, A long-term study of the pathogenesis of infection of chickens with three strains of avian infectious bronchitis virus, *Res. Vet. Sci.* **24**(2):228.

Alexander, D. J., Bracewell, C. D., and Gough, R. E., 1976, Preliminary evaluation of the haemagglutination and haemagglutination inhibition tests for avaian infectious bronchitis virus, *Avian Pathol.* **5**:125.

Allen, J. G., 1977, Congenital cerebellar hypoplasia in jersey calves, *Aust. Vet. J.* **53**:173.

Apostolov, K., Spasic, P., and Bojanic, N., 1977*a*, Comparative ultrastructural studies on endemic (Balkan) nephropathy and chicken embryo nephritis caused by infectious bronchitis virus. I. Endemic (Balkan) nephropathy, *Acta Med. Jug.* **31**:189.

Apostolov, K., Spasic, P., and Alexander, D. J., 1977*b*, Comparative ultrastructural studies on endemic (Balkan) nephropathy and chicken embryo nephritis caused by infectious bronchitis virus. II. Chick embryo nephritis, *Acta Med. Jug.* **31**:205.

Atkins, G. J., Samuels, J., and Kennedy, S. I. T., 1974, Isolation and preliminary characterization of temperature-sensitive mutants of Sindbis virus strain AR 339, *J. Gen. Virol.* **25**:371.

Bailey, O. T., Pappenheimer, A. M., Sargent, F., Cheever, M. D., and Daniels, J. B., 1949, A murine virus (JHM) causing disseminated encephalomyelitis with extensive destruction of myelin. II. Pathology, *J. Exp. Med.* **90**:195.

Berry, D. M., and Almeida, J. D., 1968, The morphological and biological effects of various antisera on avian infectious bronchitis virus, *J. Gen. Virol.* **3**:97.

Bhatt, P. N., and Jacoby, R. O., 1977, Experimental infection of adult axenic rats with Parker's rat coronavirus, *Arch. Virol.* **54**:345.

Bingham, R. W., 1975, The polypeptide composition of avian infectious bronchitis virus, *Arch. Virol.* **49**:207.

Bingham, R. W., and Almeida, J. D., 1977, Studies on the structure of a coronavirus-avian infectious bronchitis virus, *J. Gen. Virol.* **36**:495.

Binn, L. N., Lazar, E. C., Keenan, K. P., Huxsoll, D. L., Marchwicki, R. H., and Strano, A. J., 1974, Recovery and characterization of a coronavirus from military dogs with diarrhea, *Proc. Annu. Meet. U.S. Anim. Health Assoc.* **78**:359.

Bond, C. W., and Robb, J. A., 1979, Pathogenic murine coronaviruses. II. Characterization of virus-specific intracellular proteins: JHMV and A59V, *Virology* **94**:371.

Broderson, J. R., Murphy, F. A., and Hierholzer, J. C., 1976, Lethal enteritis in infant mice caused by mouse hepatitis virus, *Lab. Anim. Sci.* **26**:824.

Brown, T. T., DeLahunta, A., Bistner, S. I., Scott, F. W., and McEntee, K., 1974, Pathogenetic studies of infection of the bovine fetus with bovine viral diarrhea virus. I. Cerebellular atrophy, *Vet. Pathol.* **11**:486.

Caul, E. O., and Clarke, S. K. R., 1975, Coronavirus propagated from patient with non-bacterial gasteroenteritis, *Lancet* **2**:7942.

Caul, E. O., and Egglestone, S. I., 1977, Further studies on human enteric coronaviruses, *Arch. Virol.* **54**:107.

Chasey, D., and Alexander, D. J., 1976, Morphogenesis of avian infectious bronchitis virus in primary chick kidney cells, *Arch. Virol.* **52**:101.

Chasey, D., and Lucas, M., 1977, A bovine coronavirus identified by thin-section electron microscopy, *Vet. Rev.* **100**:530.

Cheever, F. S., Daniels, J. B., Pappenheimer, A. M., and Bailey, O. T., 1949, A murine virus (JHM) causing disseminated encephalomyelitis with extensive destruction of myelin. I. Isolation and biological properties of the virus, *J. Exp. Med.* **90**:181.

Collins, M. S., Alexander, D. J., and Harkness, J. W., 1976, Heterogeneity of infectious bronchitis virus grown in eggs, *Arch. Virol.* **50**:55.

Cook, J. K. A., Darbyshire, J. H., and Peters, R. W., 1976, Growth kinetic studies of avian infectious bronchitis virus in tracheal organ cultures, *Res. Vet. Sci.* **20**:348.

Cowen, B. S., and Hitchner, S. B., 1975, Serotyping of avian infectious bronchitis viruses by the virus-neutralization test, *Avian Dis.* **19**:583.

Cowen, B. S., Hitchner, S. B., and Lucio, B., 1971, Characterization of a new infectious bronchitis virus isolate. I. Serological and pathogenicity studies of Clark 333, *Avian Dis.* **15**:517.

Darbyshire, J. H., Cook, J. K. A., and Peters, R. W., 1975, Comparative growth kinetic studies on avian infectious bronchitis virus in different systems, *J. Comp. Pathol.* **85**:623.

Darbyshire, J. H., Cook, J. K. A., and Peters, R. W., 1976, Organ culture studies on the efficiency of infection of chicken tissues with avian infectious bronchitis virus, *Br. J. Exp. Pathol.* **57**:443.

Deshmukh, D. R., Sautter, J. H., Patel, B. L., and Pomeroy, B. S., 1976, Histopathology of fasting and bluecomb disease in turkey poults and embryos experimentally infected with bluecomb disease coronavirus, *Avian Dis.* **20**:631.

Doughri, A. M., and Storz, J., 1977, Light and ultrastructural pathologic changes in intestinal coronavirus infection of newborn calves, *Zentralbl. Veterinaermed.* **24**:367.

Doughri, A. M., Storz, J., Hajer, I., and Fernando, H. S., 1976, Morphology and morphogenesis of a coronavirus infecting intestinal epithelial cells of newborn calves, *Exp. Mol. Pathol.* **25**:355.

Dupuy, J. M., Levey-Leblond, E., and Le Prevost, C., 1975, Immunopathology of mouse hepatitis virus type 3 infection. II. Effect of immunosuppression in resistant mice, *J. Immunol.* **114**:226.

Dutta, S. K., 1974, Morphological changes in chicken tracheas and tracheal organ cultures infected with avian infectious bronchitis virus studied in scanning electron microscope, *Avian Dis.* **19**:429.

Egan, J. A., and Tannock, G. A., 1978, A comparative evaluation of chicken embryo tracheal organ cultures for the assay of avian infectious bronchitis virus, *J. Biol. Stand.* **6**:205.

England, J. J., Frye, C. S., and Enright, E. A., 1975, Negative contrast electron microscopic diagnosis of viruses of neonatal calf diarrhea, *Cornell Vet.* **66**:172.

Fabricant, J., and Levine, P. P., 1951, The persistence of infectious bronchitis virus in eggs and tracheal exudates of infected chickens, *Cornell Vet.* **41**:240.

Fleissner, E., 1971, Chromatographic separation and antigenic analysis of proteins of the oncornaviruses, *J. Virol.* **8**:778.

Flewett, T. H., and Boxall, E., 1976, The hunt for viruses in infections of the alimentary system: An immunoelectron-microscopical approach. *Clin. Gastroenterol.* **5**:359.

Fox, J. G., Murphy, J. C., and Igras, V. E., 1977, Adverse effects of mouse hepatitis virus on ascites myeloma passage in the BALB/cJ mouse, *Lab. Anim. Sci.* **27**:173.

Frederick, G. T., and Bohl, E. H., 1976, Local and systemic cell-mediated immunity against transmissible gastroenteritis, an intestinal viral infection of swine, *J. Immunol.* **116**:1000.

Fujiwara, K., Tamura, T., Hirano, N., and Takenaka, S., 1975, Implication pancréatique chez la souris infectée avec le virus de l'hépatite murine, *C. R. S. Soc. Biol.* **169**:477.

Fujiwara, K., Tamura, T., Taguchi, F., Machii, K., and Suzuki, K., 1976, Immunisation de la Souris "nude" contre le virus de l'hépatite murine par transfert de lymphocytes sensibilisés, *C. R. Soc. Biol.* **170**:509.

Gard, G. P., Acland, H. M., and Plant, J. W., 1976, A mucosal disease virus as a cause of abortion, hairy birth coat and unthriftiness in sheep. 2. Observation on lambs surviving for longer than seven days, *Aust. Vet. J.* **52**:64.

Garwes, D. J., and Pocock, D. H., 1975, The polypeptide structure of transmissible gastroenteritis virus, *J. Gen. Virol.* **29**:25.

Garwes, D. J., Pocock, D. H., and Wijaszka, T. M., 1975, Identification of heat-dissociable RNA complexes in two porcine coronaviruses, *Nature (London)* **257**:508.

Garwes, D. J., Pocock, D. H., and Pike, B. V., 1976, Isolation of subviral components from transmissable gastroenteritis virus, *J. Gen. Virol.* **32**:283.

Giambrone, J. J., Eidson, C. S., and Kleven, S. H., 1977, Effect of infectious bursal disease on the response of chickens to *Mycoplasma synoviae*, Newcastle disease virus, and infectious bronchitis virus, *Am. J. Vet. Res.* **38**:251.

Gonder, E., Patel, B. L., and Pomeroy, B. S., 1976, Scanning electron, light, and immunofluorescent microscopy of coronaviral enteritis of turkeys (bluecomb), *Am. J. Vet. Res.* **37**:1435.

Goto, N., Hirano, N., Aiuchi, M., Hayashi, T., and Fujiwara, K., 1977, Nasoencephalopathy of mice infected intranasally with a mouse hepatitis virus, JHM strain, *Jpn. J. Exp. Med.* **47**:59.

Greig, A. S., and Bouillant, A. M. P., 1977, Binding effects of cancanavalin A on a coronavirus, *Can. J. Comp. Med.* **41**:122.

Greig, A. S., Johnson, C. M., and Bouillant, A. M. P., 1971, Encephalomyelitis of swine caused by a haemagglutinating virus, *Res. Vet. Sci.* **12**:305.

Gump, D. W., Phillips, C. A., Forsythe, B. R., McIntosh, K., Lamborn, K. R., and Stouch, W. H., 1976, *Am. Rev. Res. Dis.* **113**:465.

Hafez, S. M., Liess, B., and Frey, H.-R., 1976, Studies on the natural occurrence of neutralizing antibodies against six strains of bovine viral diarrhea virus in field sera of cattle, *Zentralbl. Veterinaermed.* **23**:669.

Herndon, R. M., Griffin, D. E., McCormick, U., and Weiner, L. P., 1975, Mouse hepatitis virus-induced recurrent demyelination. A preliminary report, *Arch. Neurol.* **32**:32.

Hidalgo, H., and Raggi, L. G., 1976, Identification of seven isolants of infectious bronchitis virus by interference with the B-1 isolant of Newcastle disease virus, *Avian Dis.* **20**:167.

Hierholzer, J. C., 1976, Purification and biophysical properties of human coronavirus 229E, *Virology* **75**:155.

Hierholzer, J. C., and Tannock, G. A., 1977, Quantitation of antibody to nonhemagglutinating viruses by single radial hemolysis: Serological test for human coronaviruses, *J. Clin. Microbiol.* **5**:613.

Hierholzer, J. C., Palmer, E. L., Whitfield, S. G., Kaye, H. S., and Dowdle, W. R., 1972, Protein composition of coronavirus OC43, *Virology* **48**:516.

Hirano, N., Fujiwara, K., Hino, S., and Matumoto, M., 1974, Replication and plaque formation of mouse hepatitis virus (MHV-2) in mouse cell line DBT culture, *Archiv. Gesamti. Virusforsch.* **44**:298.

Hirano, N., Takenaka, S., and Fujiwara, K., 1975a, Pathogenicity of mouse hepatitis virus for mice depending upon host age and route of infection, *Jpn. J. Exp. Med.* **45**:285.

Hirano, N., Tamura, T., Taguchi, F., Ueda, K., and Fujiwara, K., 1975b, Isolation of low-virulent mouse hepatitis virus from nude mice with wasting syndrome and hepatitis, *Jpn. J. Exp. Med.* **45**:429.

Hirano, N., Fujiwara, K., and Matumoto, M., 1976, Mouse hepatitis virus (MHV-2) Plaque assay and propagation in Mouse cell line DBT cells, *Jpn. J. Microbiol.* **20**:219.

Holmes, K. V., and Allen, R., 1977, Chronic infection *in vitro* with the corona virus MHV, *Abstr. Annu. Meet. Am. Soc. Microbiol.* ISSN 0067-2777:345.

Horzinek, M. C., Osterhaus, A. D. M. E., and Ellens, D. J., 1977, Feline infectious peritonitis virus, *Zentralbl. Veterinaermed. Reihe B* **24**:398.

Huang, A. S., and Baltimore, D., 1977, Defective interfering animal viruses, in: *Comprehensive Virology*, Vol. 10 (H. Fraenkel-Conrat and R. R. Wagner, eds.), pp. 73–116, Plenum, New York.

Hunter, T., and Garrells, J. I., 1977, Characterization of the mRNAs for α, β and γ actin, *Cell* **12**:767.

Inaba, Y., Sato, K., Kurogi, H., Takahashi, E., Ito, Y., Omori, T., Goto, Y., and Matumoto, M., 1976, Replication of bovine coronavirus in cell line BEK-1 culture, *Arch. Virol.* **50**:339.

Ishii, A., Yago, A., Nariuchi, H., Shirasaka, A., Wada, Y., and Matushasi, T., 1974, Some aspects on the transmission of hepatitis B antigen; model experiments by mosquitoes with murine hepatitis virus, *Jpn. J. Exp. Med.* **44**:495.

Jackson, G. G., and Muldoon, R. L., 1975, *Viruses Causing Common Respiratory Infections in Man*, pp. 132–141, University of Chicago Press, Chicago.

Jacoby, R. O., Bhatt, P. N., and Jonas, A. M., 1975, Pathogenesis of sialodacryo-adenitis in gnotobiotic rats, *Vet. Pathol.* **12**:196.

Kapikian, A. Z., 1975, The coronaviruses, *Dev. Biol. Stand.* **28**:42.

Kaye, H. S., Yarbrough, W. B., Reed, C. J., Harrison, A. K., 1977, Antigenic relationship between human coronavirus strain OC43 and hemagglutinating encephalomyelitis virus strain 67N of swine: Antibody responses in human and animal sera, *J. Infect. Dis.* **135**:201.

Keenan, K. P., Jervis, H. R., Marchwicki, R. H., and Binn, L. N., 1976, Intestinal infection of neonatal dogs with canine coronavirus 1-71: Studies by virologic, histologic, histochemical and immunofluorescent techniques, *Am. J. Vet. Res.* **37**:247.

Kemeny, L. J., 1976, Antibody response in pigs inoculated with transmissible gastroenteritis virus and cross reactions among ten isolates, *Can J. Comp. Med.* **40**:209.

Kemeny, L. J., and Woods, R. D., 1977, Quantitative transmissible gastroenteritis virus shedding patterns in lactating sows, *Am. J. Vet. Res.* **38**:307.

Kemeny, L. J., Wiltsey, V. L, and Riley, J. L., 1974, Upper respiratory infection of lactating sows with transmissible gastroenteritis virus following contact exposure to infected piglets, *Cornell Vet.* **65**:352.

Kennedy, D. A., and Johnson-Lussenberg, 1975/1976, Isolation and morphology of the internal component of human coronavirus, strain 229E, *Intervirology* **6**:197.

Kerzner, B., Kelley, M. H., Gall, D. G., Butler, D. G., and Hamilton, J. R., 1977,

Transmissible gastroenteritis: Sodium transport and the intestinal epithelium during the course of viral enteritis, *Gastroenterology* **72**:457.

King, A. A., and Harkness, J. W., 1975, Viral contamination of foetal bovine serum, *Vet. Rec.* **97**:16.

Kiuchi, Y., Yamanaka, H., Miyamoto, S., and Fujiwara, K., 1974, Susceptibility to mouse hepatitis virus of mice from infected and non-infected breeding colonies, *Exp. Anim.* **24**:25.

Krum, S., Johnson, K., and Wilson, J., 1975, Hydrocephalus associated with the noneffusive form of feline infectious peritonitis, *J. Am. Vet. Med. Assoc.* **167**:746.

Lai, M. M. C., and Stohlman, S. A., 1978, The RNA of mouse hepatitis virus, *J. Virol.* **26**:236.

Lai, Y.-L., Jacoby, R. O., Bhatt, P. N., and Jonas, A. M., 1976, Keratoconjunctivitis associated with sialodacryoadenitis in rats, *Invest. Ophthalmol.* **15**:538.

Lampert, P. W., 1978, Autoimmune and virus-induced demyelinating diseases, *Am. J. Pathol.* **91**:176.

Lampert, P. W., Sims, J. K., and Kniazeff, A. J., 1973, Mechanism of demyelination in JHMV virus encephalomyelitis. Electron microscopic studies, *Acta Neuropathol.* **24**:76.

LePrévost, C., Levy-Leblond, E., Virelizier, J. L., and Dupuy, J. M., 1975a, Immunopathology of mouse hepatitis virus type 3 infection. 1. Role of humoral and cell-mediated immunity in resistance mechanisms, *J. Immunol.* **114**:221.

LePrévost, C., Virelizier, J. L., and Dupuy, J. M., 1975b, Immunopathology of mouse hepatitis virus type 3 infection, III. Clinical and virologic observation of a persistent viral infection, *J. Immunol.* **115**:640.

Lomniczi, B., 1977, Biological properties of avian coronavirus RNA, *J. Gen. Virol.* **36**:531.

Lomniczi, B., and Kennedy, I., 1977, Genome of infectious bronchitis virus, *J. Virol.* **24**:99.

Lucas, A., Flintoff, W., Anderson, R., Percy, D., Coulter, M., and Dales, S., 1977, *In vivo* and *in vitro* models of demyelinating diseases: Tropism of the JHM strain of murine hepatitis virus for cells of glial origin, *Cell* **12**:553.

Lucio, B., and Hitchner, S. T., 1970, Differentiation and detection of infectious bronchitis virus subtypes by immunofluorescence, *Avian Dis.* **14**:9.

MacNaughton, M. R., and Madge, M. H., 1977a, The polypeptide composition of avian infectious bronchitis virus, *Arch. Virol.* **55**:47.

MacNaughton, M. R., and Madge, M. H., 1977b, The characterization of the virion RNA of avian infectious bronchitis virus, *FEBS Lett.* **77**:311.

MacNaughton, M. R., Madge, M. H., Davies, H. A., and Dourmashkin, R. R., 1977, Polypeptides of the surface projections and the ribonucleoprotein of avian infectious bronchitis virus, *J. Virol.* **24**:821.

Matsuno, S., Inouye, S., and Kono, R., 1977, Plaque assay of neonatal calf diarrhea virus and the neutralizing antibody in human sera, *J. Clin. Microbiol.* **5**:1.

McClung, H. J., Butler, D. G., Kerzner, B., Gall, D. G., and Hamilton, J. R., 1976, Transmissible gastroenteritis. Mucosal ion transport in acute viral enteritis, *Gastroenterology* **70**:1091.

McIntosh, K., 1974, Coronaviruses: A comparative review, *Curr. Top. Microbiol. Immunol.* **63**:86.

McIntosh, K., Chao, R. K., Krause, H. E., Wasil, R., Mocega, H., and Mufson, M.,

1974, Coronavirus infection in acute lower respiratory tract disease of infants, *J. Infect. Dis.* **130**:502.

Mengeling, W. L., and Cutlip, R. C., 1976, Pathogenicity of field isolants of hemagglutinating encephalomyelitis virus for neonatal pigs, *J. Am. Vet. Med. Assoc.* **168**:236.

Mishra, N. K., and Ryan, W. L., 1973, Ribonucleic acid synthesis in porcine cell cultures infected with transmissable gastroenteritis virus, *Am. J. Vet. Res.* **34**:185.

Monto, A. S., 1974, Coronaviruses, *Yale J. Biol. Med.* **47**:234.

Monto, A. S., 1976, Coronaviruses, in: *Viral Infections of Humans* (A. S. Evans, ed.), pp. 127–141, Plenum, New York.

Monto, A. S., and Rhodes, L. M., 1977, Detection of coronavirus infection of man by immunofluorescence, *Proc. Soc. Exp. Biol. Med.* **155**:143.

Moore, B., Lee, P., Hewish, M., Dixon, B., and Mukherjee, T., 1977, Coronaviruses in training centre for intellectually retarded, *Lancet* **1**:261.

Morin, M., Morehouse, L. G., Solorzano, R. F., and Olson, L. D., 1973, Transmissible gastroenteritis in feeder swine: Clinical immunofluorescence and histopathological observations, *Can. J. Comp. Med.* **37**:239.

Morin, M., Laiviere S., and Lallier, R., 1976, Pathological and microbiological observations made on spontaneous cases of acute neonatal calf diarrhea, *Can. J. Comp. Med.* **40**:228.

Namiki, M., Takayama, H., and Fujiwara, K., 1977, Viral growth in splenic megakaryocytes of mice experimentally infected with mouse hepatitis virus, MHV-2, *Jpn. J. Exp. Med.* **47**:41.

Naqi, S. A., Panigrahy, B., and Hall, C. F., 1975, Purification and concentration of viruses associated with transmissible (coronaviral) enteritis of turkeys (bluecomb), *Am. J. Vet. Res.* **36**:548.

Nelson, J. B., 1952, Acute hepatitis associated with mouse leukemia. I. Pathological features and transmission of the disease, *J. Exp. Med.* **96**:293.

Norman, J. O., McClurkin, A. W., and Bachrach, H. L., 1968, Infectious nucleic acid from a transmissable agent causing gastroenteritis in pigs, *J. Comp. Pathol.* **78**:227.

Oth, D., Achille, E., Levy-LeBlond, E., and Dupuy, J. M., 1976, H-2 Influence on the chronic disease due to mouse hepatitis virus type 3, *Folia Biol.* **22**:409.

Patel, B. L., Pomeroy, B. S., Gonder, E., and Cronkite, C. E., 1976, Indirect fluorescent antibody tests for the diagnosis of coronaviral enteritis of turkeys (bluecomb), *Am. J. Vet. Res.* **37**:1111.

Patel, B. L., Gonder, E., and Pomeroy, B. S., 1977, Detection of turkey coronaviral enteritis (bluecomb) in field epiornithics, using the direct and indirect fluorescent antibody tests, *Am. J. Vet. Res.* **38**:1407.

Patterson, S., and Bingham, R. W., 1976, Electron microscope observations on the entry of avian infectious bronchitis virus into susceptible cells, *Arch. Virol.* **52**:191.

Pedersen, N. C., 1976, Morphologic and physical characteristics of feline infectious peritonitis virus and its growth in autochthonous peritoneal cell cultures, *Am. J. Vet. Res.* **37**:567.

Pfefferkorn, E. R., and Shapiro, D., 1974, Reproduction of togaviruses, in: *Comprehensive Virology* (H. Fraenkel-Conrat and R. R. Wagner, eds.), pp. 171–230, Plenum, New York.

Piazza, M., 1969, *Experimental Viral Hepatitis*, Thomas, Springfield, Ill.

Pike, B. V., and Garwes, D. J., 1977, Lipids of transmissible gastroenteritis virus and their relation to those of two different host cells, *J. Gen. Virol.* **34**:531.

Plant, J. W., Acland, H. M., and Gard, G. P., 1976, A mucosal disease virus as a cause of abortion hairy birth coat and unthriftiness in sheep. I. Infection of pregnant ewes and observations on aborted foetuses and lambs dying before one week of age, *Aust. Vet. J.* **52**:57.

Pocock, D. H., and Garwes, D. H., 1977, The polypeptides of hemagglutinating encephalomyelitis virus and isolated subviral particles, *J. Gen. Virol.* **37**:487.

Powell, H. C., and Lampert, P. W., 1975, Oligodendrocytes and their myelinplasma membrane connections in JHM mouse hepatitis virus encephalomyelitis, *Lab. Invest.* **33**:440.

Purcell, D. A., Tham, V. L., and Surman, P. G., 1976, The histopathology of infectious bronchitis in fowls infected with a nephrotropic "T" strain of virus, *Aust. Vet. J.* **52**:85.

Reed, J. M., Schiff, L. J., Shefner, A. M., and Poiley, S. M., 1975, Murine virus susceptibility of cell cultures of mouse, rat, hamster, monkey and human origin, *Lab. Anim. Sci.* **25**:420.

Reynolds, D. J., Garwes, D. J., and Gaskell, C. J., 1977, Detection of transmissible gastroenteritis virus neutralising antibody in cats, *Arch. Virol.* **55**:77.

Rinaldo, C. R., Isackson, D. W., Overall, J. C., Glasgow, L. A., Brown, T. T., Bistner, S. I., Gillespie, J. H., and Scott, F. W., 1976, Fetal and adult bovine interferon production during bovine viral diarrhea virus infection, *Infect. Immun.* **14**:660.

Riski, H., Hovi, T., Väänänen, P., and Penttinen, K., 1977, Antibodies to human coronavirus OC43 measured by radial haemolysis in gel. *Scand. J. Infect. Dis.* **9**:75.

Robb, J. A., 1977, Virus cell interactions: A classification for virus-caused human disease, *Prog. Med. Virol.* **23**:51.

Robb, J. A., and Bond, C. W., 1979*a*, Pathogenic murine coronaviruses. I. Characterization of biological behavior *in vitro* and virus-specific intracellular RNA of strongly neurotropic JHMV and weakly neurotropic A59V viruses, *Virology* **94**:352.

Robb, J. A., Bond, C. W., and Leibowitz, J., 1979*b*, Pathogenic murine coronaviruses. III. Biological and biochemical characterization of temperature-sensitive mutants of JHMV, *Virology* **94**:385.

Sabesin, S. M., 1972, Isolation of a latent murine hepatitis virus from cultured mouse liver cells, *Am. J. Gastroenterol.* **58**:259.

Saif, L. J., Bohl, E. H., Kohler, E. M., and Hughes, J. H., 1977, Immune electron microscopy of transmissible gastroenteritis virus and rotavirus (reovirus-like agent) of swine, *Am. J. Vet. Res.* **38**:13.

Schochetman, G., Stevens, R. H., and Simpson, R. W., 1977, Presence of infectious polyadenylated RNA in the coronavirus avian bronchitis virus, *Virology* **77**:772.

Sebesteny, A., and Hill, A. C., 1974, Hepatitis and brain lesions due to mouse hepatitis virus accompanied by wasting in nude mice, *Lab. Anim.* **8**:317.

Sharpee, R. L., Mebus, C. A., and Bass, E. P., 1976, Characterization of a calf diarrheal coronavirus, *Am. J. Vet. Res.* **37**:1031.

Shope, R. E., Muscoplat, C. C., Chen, A. W., and Johnson, D. W., 1976, Mechanism of protection from primary bovine viral diarrhea virus infection. I. The effects of dexamethasone, *Can. J. Comp. Med.* **40**:355.

Smith, G. C., Kalter, S. S., Heberling, R. L., and Helmke, R. J., 1975/1976, Particles morphologically resembling mouse hepatitis virus in nude mouse uterus, *Intervirology* **6**:90.

Snowdon, W. A., Parsonson, I. M., and Broun, M. L., 1975, The reaction of pregnant ewes to inoculation with mucosal disease virus of bovine origin, *J. Comp. Pathol.* **85**:241.

Sprino, P. H., Morilla, A., and Ristic, M., 1976, Intestinal immune response of feeder pigs to infection with transmissible gastroenteritis, *Am. J. Vet. Res.* **37**:171.

Stark, S. L., Fernelius, A. L., Booth, G. D., and Lambert, G., 1974, Transmissible gastroenteritis (TGE) of swine: Effect of age of swine testes cell culture monolayers on plaque assays of TGE virus, *Can. J. Comp. Med.* **39**:466.

Stohlman, S. A., and Frelinger, J. A., 1978, Resistance to fatal central nervous system disease by mouse hepatitis virus, strain JHM. I. Genetic analysis, *Immunogenetics* **6**:277.

Stohlman, S. A., and Weiner, L. P., 1978, Stability of neurotropic mouse hepatitis virus (JHM strain) during chronic infection of neuroblastoma cells, *Arch. Virol.* **57**:53.

Stone, S. S., Jensen, M. T., Kemeny, L. J., and Wiltsey, L., 1976, Chromatographic separation of gram quantities of immunoglobulins from porcine colostrum against transmissible gastroenteritis virus, *J. Immunol. Methods* **11**:333.

Stone, S. S., Kemeny, L. J., Woods, R. D., and Jensen, M. T., 1977, Efficacy of isolated colostral IgA, IgG, and IgM(A) to protect neonatal pigs against the coronavirus of transmissible gastroenteritis, *Am. J. Vet. Res.* **38**:1285.

Sturman, L. S., 1977, Characterization of a coronavirus. I. Structural proteins: Effects of preparative conditions on the migration of protein in polyacrylamide gels, *Virology* **77**:637.

Sturman, L. S., and Holmes, K. V., 1977, Characterization of a coronavirus. II. Glycoproteins of the viral envelope: Tryptic peptide analysis, *Virology* **77**:650.

Sturman, L. S., and Takemoto, K. K., 1972, Enhanced growth of a murine coronavirus in transformed mouse cells, *Infect. Immun.* **6**:501.

Taguchi, F., Hirano, N., Kiuchi, Y., and Fujiwara, K., 1976, Difference in response to mouse hepatitis virus among susceptible mouse strains, *Jpn. J. Microbiol.* **20**:293.

Taguchi, F., Aiuchi, M., and Fujiwara, K., 1977, Age-dependent response of mice to a mouse hepatitis virus, MHV-S, *Jpn. J. Exp. Med.* **47**:109.

Takayama, J., and Kirn, A., 1976, An improved method for titration of mouse hepatitis virus type 3 in a mouse cell culture, *Arch. Virol.* **52**:347.

Takeuchi, A., Binn, L. N., Jervis, H. R., Keenan, K., Hildebrandt, P. K., Valas, R. B., and Bland, F. F., 1976, Electron microscope study of experimental enteric infection in neonatal dogs with a canine coronavirus, *Lab. Invest.* **34**:539.

Tamura, T., Ueda, K., Hirano, N., and Fujiwara, K., 1976, Response of nude mice to a mouse hepatitis virus isolated from a wasting nude mouse, *Jpn. J. Exp. Med.* **46**:19.

Tamura, T., Taguchi, I., Ueda, K., and Fujiwara, K., 1977, Persistent infection with mouse hepatitis virus of low virulence in nude mice, *Microbiol. Immunol.* **21**:683.

Tanaka, R., Iwasaki, Y., and Koprowski, H., J., 1976, Intracisternal virus-like particles in brain of a multiple sclerosis patient, *J. Neurol. Sci.* **28**:121.

Tannock, G. A., 1973, The nucleic acid of infectious bronchitis virus, *Arch. Gesamte Virusforsch.* **43**:259.

Tannock, G. A., and Hierholzer, J. C., 1977, The RNA of human coronavirus OC43, *Virology* **78**:500.

Tannock, G. A., and Hierholzer, J. C., 1978, Presence of genomic polyadenylate and absence of detectable virion transcriptase in human coronavirus OC43, *J. Gen. Virol.* **39**:29.

Thomas, F. C., and Dulac, G. C., 1976, Transmissible gastroenteritis virus: Plaques and a plaque neutralization test, *Can. J. Comp. Med.* **40**:171.

Thornton, D. H., and Muskett, J. C., 1975, Effect of infectious bronchitis vaccination on the performance of live Newcastle disease vaccine, *Vet. Rec.* **96**:467.

Timoney, J. F., 1976, Feline infectious peritonitis, *Vet. Clin. N. Am.* **6**:391.

Traavik, T., Mehl, R., and Kjeldsberg, E., 1977, "Runde" Virus, a coronavirus-like agent associated with seabirds and ticks, *Arch. Virol.* **55**:25.

Tyrrell, D. A. J., Almeida, J. D., Cunningham, C. H., Dowdle, W. R., Hofstad, M. S., McIntosh, K., Tajima, M., Zakstelskaya, L. Y., Esterday, B. C., Kapikian, A., and Bingham, R. W., 1975, Coronaviridae, *Intervirology* **5**:76.

Underdahl, N. R., Mebus, C. A., Stair, E. L., Rhodes, M. B., McGill, L. D., and Twiehaus, M. J., 1974, Isolation of transmissible gastroenteritis virus from lungs of market-weight swine, *Am. J. Vet. Res.* **35**:1209.

Underdahl, N. R., Melbus, C. A., and Torres-Medina, A., 1975, Recovery of transmissible gastroenteritis virus from chronically infected experimental pigs, *Am. J. Vet. Res.* **36**:1473.

Virelizier, J. L., and Gresser, I., 1978, Role of interferon in the pathogenesis of viral diseases of mice as demonstrated by the use of anti-interferon serum. IV. Protective role in mouse hepatitis virus type 3 infection of susceptible and resistant strains of mice, *J. Immunol.* **120**:1616.

Virelizier, J. L., Dayan, A. D., and Allison, A. C., 1975, Neuropathological effects of persistent infection of mice by mouse hepatitis virus, *Infect. Immun.* **12**:1127.

Virelizier, J. L., Virelizier, A. M., and Allison, A. C., 1976. The role of circulating interferon in the modifications of immune responsiveness by mouse hepatitis virus (MHV-3), *J. Immunol.* **117**:748.

Ward, J. M., Collins, M. J., and Parker, J. C., 1977, Naturally occurring mouse hepatitis virus infection in the nude mouse, *Lab. Anim. Sci.* **27**:372.

Watkins, H., Reeve, P., and Alexander, D. J., 1975, The ribonucleic acid of infectious bronchitis virus, *Arch. Virol.* **47**:279.

Weiner, L. P., 1973, Pathogenesis of demyelination induced by a mouse hepatitis virus (JHM virus), *Arch. Neurol.* **28**:298.

Weisbroth, S. H., and Peress, N., 1977, Ophthalmic lesions and dacryoadenitis: A naturally occurring aspect of sialodacryoadenitis virus infection of the laboratory rat, *Lab. Anim. Sci.* **27**:466.

Weiser, W., and Bang, F. B., 1976, Macrophages genetically resistant to mouse hepatitis virus converted in vitro to susceptible macrophages. *J. Exp. Med.* **143**:690.

Weiser, W. Y., and Bang, F. B., 1977, Blocking of *in vitro* and *in vivo* susceptibility to mouse hepatitis virus, *J. Exp. Med.* **146**:24.

Weiser, W., Vellisto, I., and Bang, F. B., 1976, Congenic strains of mice susceptible and resistant to mouse hepatitis virus, *Proc. Soc. Exp. Biol. Med.* **152**:499.

Werdin, R. E., Sorensen, D. K., and Stewart, W. C., 1976, Porcine encephalomyelitis caused by hemagglutinating encephalomyelitis virus, *J. Am. Vet. Med. Assoc.* **168**:240.

Whitmore, H. L., and Archbald, L. F., 1977, Demonstration and quantitation of immunoglobulins in bovine serum, follicular fluid, and uterine and vaginal secretions with reference to bovine viral diarrhea and infectious bovine rhinotrachietis, *Am. J. Vet. Res.* **38**:455.

Woods, R. D., 1977, Leukocyte migration-inhibition procedure for transmissible gastroenteritis viral antigens, *Am. J. Vet. Res.* **38**:1267.

Wooley, R. E., and Brown, J., 1977, Correlation of cytopathic effect, fluorescent-antibody microneutralization, and plaque reduction test results for determining avian infectious bronchitis virus antibodies, *J. Clin. Microbiol.* **5**:361.

Yogo, Y., Hirano, N., Hino, S., Shibuta, H., and Matumoto, M., 1977, Polyadenylate in the virion RNA of mouse hepatitis virus, *J. Biochem.* **82**:1103.

Zuckerman, A. J., 1978, A new human hepatitis virus, *Nature (London)* **271**:113.

CHAPTER 4

Caliciviruses

Frederick L. Schaffer

Naval Bioscience Laboratory, School of Public Health
University of California
Berkeley, California 94720

1. INTRODUCTION AND CLASSIFICATION

The name "calicivirus" is derived from the cup-shaped (chalice or kalyx) indentations observed on the surface of virions negatively stained with phosphotungstate. The caliciviruses, whose recognized members include vesicular exanthema of swine virus, feline calicivirus (formerly feline picornavirus), and San Miguel sea lion virus, were provisionally classified as a genus of the family Picornaviridae (Melnick *et al.*, 1974; Fenner, 1976). Based on the difference in morphology and the observation that caliciviruses contain only one major polypeptide, Burroughs and Brown (1974) suggested that they constitute a separate family, Caliciviridae. Although this suggestion met with some opposition (Cooper, 1974), newer information indicates that the genome strategy of caliciviruses differs significantly from that of typical picornaviruses. Consequently, the Picornavirus Study Group of the ICTV has recently recommended that the caliciviruses be excluded from the Picornaviridae and that a new study group be formed to consider them as a separate family (Cooper *et al.*, 1978).

Caliciviruses are considered briefly in comparison with picornaviruses in Volume 6 of *Comprehensive Virology* (Rueckert, 1976). A recent review on caliciviruses by Studdert (1978) and this chapter cover much of the same material. Studdert's coverage of pathology and epizootiology is more extensive, whereas molecular biological aspects, to the extent of limited current knowledge, are emphasized here. To date, the diseases caused by caliciviruses have been almost exclusively of veterinary interest. However, recent findings in humans broadens interest in them as disease agents.

2. NATURAL HISTORY AND DISEASE ASPECTS

2.1. Vesicular Exanthema of Swine Virus (VESV)

Vesicular exanthema of swine (VES) was first observed in 1932, when it was thought to be foot and mouth disease. Based on a host range virtually restricted to swine, as opposed to a wider host range for foot and mouth disease virus (FMDV), it was recognized that VES was caused by a different virus, VESV. VESV is not to be confused with swine vesicular disease virus, which is an enterovirus antigenically related to Coxsackie B5 (Nardelli *et al.*, 1968; Moore, 1977). VES as observed in the 1930s–1950s was a highly infectious disease in swine, affecting primarily the snout, mouth parts, and feet. Although overall mortality was not high, severe economic losses were suffered by hog raisers in California, where the disease originated, and subsequently in other states in the United States as the disease spread. Spread of VESV was attributed to the feeding of garbage containing infected pork scraps to swine; institution and strict enforcement of regulations requiring cooking of garbage fed to swine were credited for eradication of the disease. The last outbreak of VES occurred in 1956. Numerous antigenically distinct serotypes of VESV,* with varying virulence, were isolated, but many of the early stocks of infectious material were destroyed when they were believed to be FMDV. History, epizootiology, and pathogenesis of VESV have been well reviewed (Madin and Traum, 1955; Bankowski, 1965; Madin, 1975). The U.S. Department of Agriculture declared VESV an exotic virus, and subsequent work with VESV has been confined to laboratories in the United States with special permits and to the Pirbright Animal Disease Research Laboratories in England.

2.2. San Miguel Sea Lion Virus (SMSV)

In 1972, several isolates of a calicivirus were made by A. W. Smith and co-workers from California sea lions on San Miguel Island. The

---

* See Bankowski (1965) or Studdert (1978) for a listing of VESV serotypes and an explanation of their designations, e.g., A_{48}, E_{54}.

virus, called San Miguel sea lion virus (SMSV), was indistinguishable from VESV by several criteria including morphology, biophysical properties, and host range (Smith *et al.*, 1973). The SMSV isolates were not all of one serotype, and were serotypically distinct from VESV (Section 3.1). Further studies of marine mammal populations yielded additional isolates from California sea lions and from two other pinnipeds, Alaskan fur seals and elephant seals, whose ranges in the Pacific Ocean overlap that of the sea lions (Smith *et al.*, 1978*a*). Additionally, SMSV has been isolated from a lower vertebrate food source of the sea lion, opal eye perch, and from a sea lion's invertebrate parasite, a liver fluke (Smith *et al.*, 1978*a*). Serological evidence has indicated that SMSV has been prevalent in additional pinniped species and several species of whales in the same geographic area since at least 1961 (Akers *et al.*, 1974; Smith *et al.*, 1976; Smith and Latham, 1978). Neutralizing antibodies to SMSV have also been found in terrestrial mammals, including wild foxes, and feral swine, donkeys, and sheep, leading to suggestions of transmission of SMSV between marine and terrestrial species (Prato *et al.*, 1974, 1977; Smith *et al.*, 1976; Smith and Latham, 1978). There were eight serotypes of SMSV at the time of writing this chapter (A. W. Smith, personal communication).

Lesions on flippers are the only clear manifestation of SMSV as a etiological agent of disease in marine mammals, but reproductive failure may be a more serious manifestation. The original isolations of SMSV, along with *Leptospira*, were made during a study of abortions in California sea lions; it was suggested that an interrelation of one or both of these agents with environmental pollutants could have caused the abortions (Smith *et al.*, 1974; Gilmartin *et al.*, 1976). SMSV did not infect small laboratory animals (Smith *et al.*, 1977*a*), but evidence of infection of a monkey has been obtained (Smith *et al.*, 1978*b*). No confirmed disease in man has been observed, but some persons involved in field plus laboratory studies with the virus showed antibodies to SMSV (Smith *et al.*, 1978*b*; Soergel *et al.*, 1978).

2.3. Relationship between VESV and SMSV

The possibilities that VESV came from a marine source and that nonmammalian marine species may have played a role in the natural history of both viruses have been discussed (Madin, 1973, 1975; Madin *et al.*, 1976; Smith and Akers, 1976; Sawyer, 1976; Studdert, 1978; Smith and Latham, 1978). Experimental infection of swine with SMSV produces a disease clinically indistinguishable from VES (Breese and

Dardiri, 1977). In addition, SMSV and VESV show a close antigenic relationship by methods other than neutralization (Section 3.1). Because of the virtual identity of SMSV and VESV, except for the species from which they were isolated, the U.S. Department of Agriculture has applied restrictions on work with SMSV as with VESV. Recent isolations of virus of a SMSV serotype from asymptomatic domestic swine, together with the presence of SMSV and VESV antibodies in marine mammals and current feral and domestic swine populations, suggest that VES as a virus disease may not have been eradicated even though clinical disease has not been seen in over 20 years (Smith and Latham, 1978; Sawyer, 1976, and personal communication).

2.4. Feline Calicivirus (FCV)

The first reported isolation of FCV was made during an attempt to cultivate feline panleukopenia virus; the FCV was cytopathic in cell culture but was of low virulence in cats (Fastier, 1957). Subsequently, numerous strains, with varying virulence, have been isolated from domestic cats throughout the world. FCV has also been isolated from captive cheetahs (Sabine and Hyne, 1970). Gillespie and Scott (1973), who have reviewed the history and pathology of FCV and FCV infections, consider FCV to be a major health hazard to feline populations. FCV is primarily an upper respiratory infection in cats, but some strains cause pneumonia; FCV has also been implicated in urolithiasis. In experimental infections, typical symptoms include a febrile response, conjunctivitis, rhinitis, and oral ulcerations; mortality may be as high as 30% in kittens. Cats may carry FCV asymptomatically for prolonged periods, probably in tonsils, and may serve as foci of infection of susceptible animals (Wardley, 1976; Wardley and Povey, 1977a,b). To avoid complications due to other agents, specific pathogen-free cats have been used in various experimental studies; these have included investigations of pathogenesis (Hoover and Kahn, 1973; Povey and Hale, 1974) and immunity (Olsen et al., 1974; Povey and Ingersoll, 1975; Bittle and Rubic, 1976; Kahn and Hoover, 1976; Scott, 1977).

2.5. Human Calicivirus

Evidence for calicivirus in humans is based on electron microscopic observations of stool specimens. Madeley and Cosgrove (1976) first mentioned "calicivirus" from nonbacterial infantile gastroenteritis patients. Subsequently, other observations of "calicivirus" in infant stools have been reported (Flewett and Davies, 1976; Middleton *et al.*, 1977). Considering the nature of the specimens and the difficulties in obtaining good electron micrographs of known caliciviruses, it is possible that other observations of virus-like particles, perhaps including "astroviruses," may have represented caliciviruses (see Section 8). These purported viruses have not been cultivated, nor has a role as a causative agent in infantile gastroenteritis been proven. Other viruses, such as Norwalk virus and similar agents which are known to cause gastroenteritis but have not been cultured (Kapikian *et al.*, 1975; Thornhill *et al.*, 1977), appear to have some properties similar to caliciviruses. Classification of these various human agents remains uncertain pending serological evidence of antigenic relatedness to known viruses or laboratory propagation and determination of molecular biological properties. Human calicivirus will not be considered outside this section (except in Fig. 3, Section 5.2, and Section 8).

3. ANTIGENIC ASPECTS

3.1. VESV and SMSV

In early studies with VESV (reviewed by Madin and Traum, 1955; Bankowski, 1965; Madin, 1975), serotypes were readily distinguished by lack of cross-reactivity in neutralization tests and in immunity of naturally or experimentally infected animals. Attempts to apply hemagglutination to VESV were unsuccessful, but complement fixation did reveal common antigens among the serotypes. The complement fixation test has not been widely applied, in part because of difficulties with the reaction with swine serum. Lack of cross-reactivity in neutralization tests has also distinguished SMSV serotypes from each other and from VESV (Smith *et al.*, 1977*b*; Burroughs *et al.*, 1978*a*). Strictly, there is not a total lack of cross-reactivity, but high levels of antiserum (relative to homotypic neutralization) must be used to detect any cross-neutralization. Since other immunological criteria (below), nucleic acid homology (Section 5.6.6), and similarities in diseases produced indicate close relatedness among serotypes of VESV and SMSV, the observed specificity of neutralization and *in vivo* immunity suggest that highly specific antigenic sites are critical in immunity to these viruses.

Antigenic relatedness among VESV and SMSV serotypes has been demonstrated by immunodiffusion (Burroughs *et al.*, 1978*a*), immuno-electron microscopy (Smith *et al.*, 1978*a*), and radioimmune precipitation with protein-A-bearing staphylococci as immunoadsorbent (St-

RIP test) (Soergel *et al.*, 1978). There would appear to be differences in relative cross-reactivities among the serotypes, but more work is needed to quantitate the differences. The polypeptide from SMSV (Section 5.7.1) obtained by heating in sodium dodecylsulfate (SDS) and mercaptoethanol was immunogenic, eliciting antibodies reacting in homotypic and to a somewhat lesser extent in heterotypic St-RIP tests with intact virion antigens (Soergel *et al.*, 1978). A virion subunit from VESV consisting of a polypeptide trimer (Section 5.2) reacts with homologous antiserum in the complement fixation test (Burroughs *et al.*, 1978*b*).

3.2.   FCV

In contrast to clear serotypic differentiation with VESV/SMSV, neutralization tests with FCV isolates revealed considerable cross-reactivity, making designation of serotypes difficult. Early studies have been reviewed by Gillespie and Scott (1973). The more recent careful studies have led to a conclusion that all FCV isolates are variants of a single serotype, although some strains show only one-way crosses with others (Povey, 1974; Kalunda *et al.*, 1975; Burki *et al.*, 1976). Those studies showed that the strains or variants could usually be distinguished from each other; in a similar study of cross-neutralization, Chappuis and Stellmann (1974) developed a biomathematical system to ascertain relationships. Hemagglutination has not been found with FCV.

Homotypic and heterotypic antibody responses in experimental cats infected with virulent strain 255 and avirulent strain F-9 were followed by neutralization, complement fixation, and complement-fixation inhibition tests (Olsen *et al.*, 1974). Antibodies reacting in the various tests differed in sedimentation characteristics (7 S and 19 S) and in times of appearance. By immunodiffusion, one to three lines were observed with homologous cat sera; a single line of identity between the two FCV strains was found with hyperimmune goat serum. Kalunda *et al.* (1975) reported that a number of FCV strains were indistinguishable by immunodiffusion.

In early studies, doubt was expressed that a practical FCV vaccine could be developed. However the F-9 strain, which showed broad cross-neutralization, was effective in cross-protection against virulent FCV, leading to development of a commercial vaccine (Kahn *et al.*, 1975; Povey and Ingersoll, 1975; Bittle and Rubic, 1976; Scott, 1977).

3.3.   Relation between FCV and VESV/SMSV

There is limited information on antigenic relationships between FCV and VESV/SMSV. Burroughs *et al.* (1978*a*) found no cross-reaction between FCV strain K-1 and three serotypes of VESV and SMSV by immunodiffusion. In contrast, immunoelectron microscopy showed cross-reaction between FCV F-9 and two serotypes of VESV (Smith *et al.*, 1978*a*). Staphylococcal radioimmune precipitation (St-RIP) tests showed reaction of two SMSV serotypes and antiFCV cat sera; however, hyperimmune goat sera to two FCV strains showed no reaction (Table 1). The highest reactivity was with strain F-9, which, perhaps coincidently, also shows broad cross-neutralization with other FCV strains (Section 3.2).

4.   CALICIVIRUSES IN CULTURED CELLS

Available evidence indicates that calicivirus replication and maturation occur entirely within the cytoplasm of infected cells.

TABLE 1

St-RIP (Staphylococcal Radioimmune Precipitin) Reactions of SMSV with Anti-FCV Sera[a]

Antiserum[b]		Radiolabeled virions precipitated (%)[c]	
FCV strain	Species	SMSV-4	SMSV-5
Pooled[d]	Cat	60	48
F-9	Cat	69 (4)	62 (6)
F-17	Cat	28 (4)	20 (3)
F-19	Cat	17 (5)	14 (5)
KCD	Goat	5	4
FRI	Goat	5	4

[a] Previously unpublished results of M. E. Soergel and F. L. Schaffer; details of the St-RIP test and reactions of the SMSV antigens with homologous and heterologous (SMSV and VESV) antisera are presented elsewhere (Soergel *et al.*, 1978).
[b] Antisera were kindly provided by D. F. Holmes (*cf.* Kalunda *et al.*, 1975).
[c] One microliter of undiluted serum was used in each test; numbers in parentheses are for preimmune serum from the same animal.
[d] Pooled sera from individual cats immunized with FCV strains KCD, 255, F-9, F-17, and F-19.

4.1. Growth and Host Range

The host range of FCV in cell culture is quite narrow. The virus is readily propagated in primary cultures and cell lines from domestic cats and in a lion kidney cell line; some strains have been grown in nonfeline cells, including Vero monkey kidney cells and dolphin kidney cells (reviewed by Studdert, 1978). Good replication of FCV in organ cultures of kitten tongue and trachea was reported by Love and Donaldson-Wood (1975), whereas Milek et al. (1976) reported poor replication in tracheal ring organ cultures when compared to cell culture.

VESV was originally thought to have a very restricted host range in cell culture as in vivo, but subsequently some cell lines from primates and a few other species were found to be susceptible (Madin, 1975; Smith et al., 1977a). SMSV has an in vitro host range similar to that of VESV, replicating well in pig kidney and Vero monkey cell lines; some SMSV strains also replicate in cell lines from ruminants (Smith et al., 1977a). An overlap with FCV in host range (in addition to aforementioned Vero cells) is the replication of several serotypes of SMSV and at least one VESV serotype in feline cells (Smith et al., 1977a).

The caliciviruses are characterized by rapid cytolytic effects in cultured cells. Although there may be differences in details depending on the virus–cell system and input multiplicity, typically intracellular virus titer begins to increase 1.5–3 hr after infection, reaching a maximum by 6–8 hr; the extracellular virus curve follows the intracellular curve by about 1–2 hr (Wawrzkiewicz et al., 1968; Zee et al., 1968a,b; Studdert et al., 1970; Smith et al., 1977b).

In experiments relating to viral growth cycles, VESV photosensitized with acridine orange lost photosensitivity on establishment of eclipse; newly synthesized virus acquired photosensitivity in the presence of the dye early during the growth phase, but not after maturation had occurred (Hackett, 1962).

Replication of caliciviruses is not appreciably inhibited by actinomycin D (Oglesby et al., 1971), halogenated uridine deoxyribosides (Bürki, 1965; Studdert et al., 1970; Smith et al., 1977b), guanidine, or hydroxybenzyl benzimidizole (Bürki and Pichler, 1971). Little is known of effects of concurrent infection with other viruses or mycoplasma. In one study, Wooley et al. (1976) found that FCV replication was enhanced in cells infected an hour later with feline herpesvirus. A reciprocal effect on herpesvirus yield was found also, and these authors suggested concurrent infections in vivo may be important in feline viral diseases.

4.2. Cytopathology

As one might expect, there are variations in reports on cytopathology of calicivirus-infected cells. These may be attributable to differences in techniques, multiplicities of infection, and times of observations, as well as to differences in virus strains and cells.

4.2.1. Light Microscopy

Typical gross cytopathic changes in calicivirus-infected cells, occur more or less in synchrony with intracellular virus production; the cells become refractile, rounded, and shrunken. Finer details revealed by light microscopy include cytoplasmic basophilia, with granules showing typical RNA staining with acridine orange (Hackett, 1961; Zee et al., 1967; Adldinger et al., 1969). Viral antigen in the cytoplasm is detectable with fluorescent antibody (Zee et al., 1967, 1968b). Nuclear changes include condensation of chromatin, nucleolar alterations, and abnormal mitotic figures (Hackett, 1961; Studdert et al., 1970; Studdert and O'Shea, 1975).

4.2.2. Electron Microscopy

Electron microscopy of thin sections reveals nuclear changes starting as early as 2 hr after infection; later effects may include condensation of chromatin or "nuclear masses," dispersion of nucleolar material, and nuclear membrane alteration (Zee et al., 1968a; Love and Sabine, 1975; Studdert and O'Shea, 1975). Golgi apparatus alteration is an early cytoplasmic manifestation, and numerous vesicles appear later; virions may be observed in the cytoplasm as early as 4 hr after infection. Virions accumulate in irregular clusters and in crystalline arrays; they may also be associated with cisternae or with cytoplasmic microfibrils (Zee et al., 1968a,b; Peterson and Studdert, 1970; Love and Sabine, 1975; Studdert and O'Shea, 1975; Breese and Dardiri, 1977; Smith et al., 1977b). Cytoplasmic granular accumulations or "viroplasmic foci," closely associated with smooth membrane-bound vesicles, have been suggested as sites of synthesis and accumulation of viral material (Zee et al., 1968a; Studdert and O'Shea, 1975). Figure 1 shows intracellular calicivirions in selected thin-section electron micrographs.

Scanning electron microscopy revealed surface changes in infected cells; numerous microvilli and delicate transluscent pseudopodia,

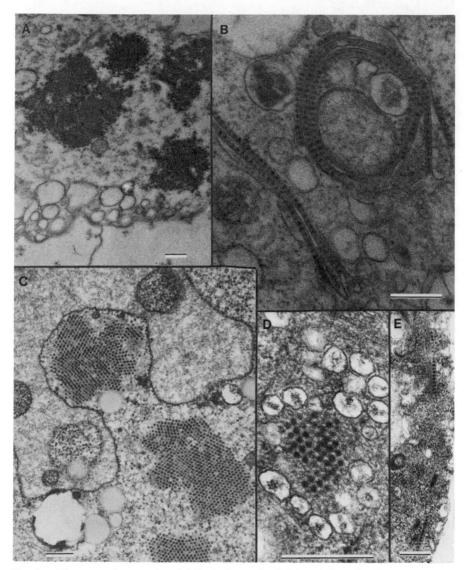

Fig. 1.   Electron micrographs of thin sections of calicivirus-infected cells. A: Intracyto-plasmic crystalline arrays of VESV-A$_{48}$, and a "viroplasmic focus" in a pig kidney cell (Zee *et al.*, 1968*a*). B: VESV-H$_{54}$ virions aligned along cytoplasmic cisternae in a pig kidney cell (Zee *et al.*, 1968*b*). C: Intracytoplasmic crystalline arrays of SMSV-4 in a Vero cell (Smith *et al.*, 1977*b*; reproduced by permission of S. Karger AG, Basel). D,E: Small crystalline array and microfibril-associated linear array, respectively, of FCV-10/66 (Studdert and O'Shea, 1975). Note cytoplasmic vesicles in the various sections. Each bar represents 300 nm.

present in uninfected cells, were lost, and cells became shrunken (Smith and Skilling, 1977).

4.3. Genetics

VESV shows a correlation between plaque size and pathogenicity in swine, large plaque-forming virus being more virulent than small plaque formers (McClain *et al.*, 1958; Walen *et al.*, 1966). Mutation from one plaque type to another occurred in cell culture and in the pig (Walen, 1963; Walen *et al.*, 1966). Although it has often been suggested that mutations from one serotype to another were responsible for the sequential appearance of multiple serotypes of VESV in the swine population, no firm evidence for this exists. Modern techniques of animal virus genetics (chemical mutagens, temperature-sensitive mutant selection, etc.) have not been applied to caliciviruses.

4.4. Viral RNA

The following account is taken primarily from the work of Ehresmann in the author's laboratory (Ehresmann and Schaffer, 1977; Ehresmann, 1978); some of the intracellular components have also been observed by others (Love, 1976; Black and Brown, 1978). There are two major single-stranded (ss) RNAs. The larger appears to be identical to virion RNA, with a sedimentation rate of 36 S, a molecular weight of 2.6×10^6 (by gel electrophoresis), and a polyadenylated 3' end. The smaller ssRNA, present in lesser quantity, sediments at 22 S, has a molecular weight of 1.1×10^6, and is also polyadenylated. Synthesis of both was detected by 3 hr after infection, and continued until at least 7 hr. In addition to the two ssRNAs, two or more components suggestive of double-stranded (ds) RNA and partially double-stranded replicative intermediate (RI) RNA were observed by polyacrylamide gel electrophoresis. These components, which sediment in the same region as the 22 S ssRNA, were fractionated from pooled 18–22 S RNA by 2 M LiCl precipitation and chromatography on CF-11 cellulose. Most of the dsRNA sedimented at 18 S, and yielded 36 S ssRNA on denaturation with dimethyl sulfoxide. A minor dsRNA component separated by electrophoresis on a polyacrylamide gel slab contained 22 S single-strand components. RI from 18–22 S RNA sedimented at 20 S and was

56% resistant to RNase. After RNase treatment, the resistant portion cosedimented with 18 S dsRNA, indicating that it contained a 36 S strand backbone. The findings on the intracellular viral RNAs are summarized in Table 2.

The presence of poly(A) on both 36 S and 22 S ssRNA suggests that both serve as mRNA. However, association with polysomes has not yet been demonstrated. (Much of the 36 S RNA is probably in mature but unreleased virions late in infection.) Information on the 5′ ends of the two ssRNAs was collected by heavy labeling with ^{32}P, digestion with RNase T2, and chromatography on DEAE-cellulose (final steps of analysis were done in Aaron Shatkin's laboratory). No oligonucleotides typical of methylated 5′ caps were found, suggesting that calicivirus mRNA, along with picornavirus mRNA, lacks the 5′ cap typical of eukaryotic cell and viral mRNAs (Shatkin, 1976). No information is available on the possible presence of covalently linked proteins on the two calicivirus mRNAs, but, by analogy to picornaviruses (Nomoto *et al.*, 1977), protein might be expected on virion RNA (Section 5.6.7), dsRNA, and RI, but not mRNA (see Section 8).

The function of 22 S RNA as mRNA has not been established, but it has been suggested that it codes for synthesis of the virion polypeptide (Ehresmann and Schaffer, 1977; Ehresmann, 1978; Black and Brown, 1978; see also Section 4.5). Black and Brown (1978) cited unpublished experiments indicating that it was translated *in vitro*, the major product being similar to the virion polypeptide (see Section 8). Black and Brown also mentioned a 0.7×10^6 dalton polyadenylated

TABLE 2
Viral RNA Components in Calicivirus-Infected Cells[a]

Property	Major ssRNA	Minor ssRNA	Major dsRNA	Minor dsRNA	RI[b]
Sedimentation rate, S	36	22	18	nd	20
Molecular weight, $\times 10^{-6}$	2.6	1.1	5.2[c]	2.2[c]	nd[d]
RNase resistant	No	No	Yes	nd	Partial
Poly(A)	Yes	Yes	Yes	nd	Yes
5′-Methylated cap	No	No	nd	nd	nd

[a] From studies with SMSV (Ehresmann and Schaffer, 1977; Ehresmann 1978); incomplete information indicates that similar components are present in cells infected with VESV and FCV. nd, not determined.
[b] Only RI from 18–22 S RNA was examined.
[c] Calculated from denatured product.
[d] RNase-resistant core cosediments with dsRNA of 5.2×10^6 molecular weight.

ssRNA that was nonfunctional in the *in vitro* translation system. We have observed a minor component of similar size in various preparations, but think it may be a breakage product from virion-sized RNA (*cf.* Section 5.6.2).

Infectivity was associated with 36 S and 18–22 S RNA fractions from SMSV-infected cells; the 36 S infectious RNA was RNase sensitive, whereas infectivity presumably associated with the dsRNA in the slower-sedimenting fraction was resistant to RNase (Ehresmann and Schaffer, unpublished).

In addition to the usual components, RNA sedimenting at approximately 42 S was present in some but not all preparations of RNA from infected cells (Ehresmann and Schaffer, unpublished). The 42 S RNA was converted to 36 S on denaturation, and returned to 42 S on high-salt (0.5 M NaCl) treatment. The 42 S form was the predominant component present in high-salt extracts of infected cells. It would appear that the 42 S RNA, which has not been investigated further, is a configurational variant of the 2.6×10^6 dalton ssRNA.

The scheme of calicivirus RNA replication has not been elucidated, but Ehresmann (1978) has suggested it resembles that of alphaviruses (Strauss and Strauss, 1977).

4.5. Viral Protein

The virion polypeptide is the predominant product of protein synthesis in calicivirus-infected cells (Black and Brown, 1975/76, 1978; Fretz, 1978; Fretz and Schaffer, 1978). In their earlier experiments, Black and Brown (1975/1976) found that VESV noncapsid proteins were not readily detectable, in contrast to easily demonstrable multiple polypeptides and precursor–product relationships in picornavirus-infected cells. More recently, Black and Brown (1978) demonstrated polypeptides with molecular weights of approximately 100,000 and 80,000 in addition to the capsid polypeptide (molecular weight 65,000) in VESV- and FCV-infected cells. The virion polypeptide was seen as early as 2 hr after infection; the others were first observed 30 min to 1 hr later, and appeared to be shut off at about 4 hr after infection. Pulse-chase and inhibitor experiments showed neither evidence of precursor–product relationship among the three polypeptides nor evidence for sequential synthesis. However, protease inhibitors (iodoacetamide and Trasylol) did reveal an additional polypeptide, molecular weight *ca.* 120,000, that was a probable precursor of the 100,000 molecular weight polypeptide.

Findings in the author's laboratory (Fretz, 1978; Fretz and Schaffer, 1978) differ in detail from those of Black and Brown. In polyacrylamide slab gels, we have observed at least five bands from SMSV-infected cells that appear to be nonstructural viral polypeptides (Fig. 2). Similar patterns have been obtained from cells infected with VESV and FCV. Pulse-chase and chemical protease inhibitor experiments were not very revealing. After incubation of infected cells at 43°C, a band at 86,000 apparent molecular weight (P86) and three bands with molecular weights greater than 140,000 were observed. A prolonged "chase" at 37°C indicated that P86 was the precursor of the capsid polypeptide (apparent molecular weight 60,000 in this slab gel system). Substantiating evidence for the P86 → capsid relationship was provided by tryptic peptide mapping; the patterns were essentially identical except for an additional spot on the P86 map. It would appear that P86 (or a slightly larger short-lived precursor of P86) is the prime candidate as the translation product of the 1.1×10^6 molecular weight mRNA (*cf.* Section 4.4). P115 would then be the candidate for the translation product of the remaining 1.5×10^6 portion of the genome. The elevated-temperature experiments and peptide mapping also indicated that P115 is the precursor of P80. Why P115, if it is the precursor of P80 (and some of the smaller polypeptides), appears to be partially stable under our experimental conditions remains to be answered. Also remaining to be answered is the nature of the larger polypeptides (molecular weight > 140,000) observed at elevated temperatures and occasionally under other conditions. Their size appears to exceed the coding capacity of the 1.5×10^6 dalton genome segment. Peptide mapping showed no relationship to P86 or capsid protein, arguing against readthrough of an overlapping portion of the entire viral genome. On the other hand, the three large polypeptides appeared to be related to each other and to P115. The sources of the polypeptides smaller than capsid polypeptide (Fig. 2) have not been clearly revealed by mapping, but most of them appear to be related to P115 and/or the larger units rather than to P86.

The discrepancies in number and molecular weights of polypeptides observed in the two laboratories may reflect technical rather than fundamental differences. The findings of both laboratories show that the capsid polypeptide is predominant; also, other polypeptides are synthesized, among which precursor–product relationships exist. Functions of nonstructural proteins have not been elucidated, but among them an RNA replicase(s) would be expected.

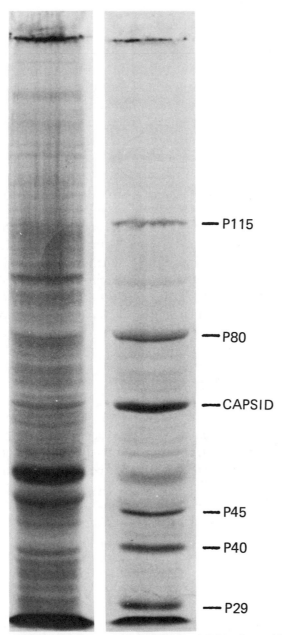

Fig. 2. Polyacrylamide gel electrophoretic patterns of [^{35}S]polypeptides from SMSV-infected (right) and control uninfected (left) Vero cells. Numbers are apparent molecular weights $\times 10^{-3}$; the capsid polypeptide is 60,000 molecular weight in this slab gel system.

5. THE VIRION

5.1. Purification

Calicivirus virions can be purified from cell culture fluids with relative ease to a purity sufficient for studies of physiocochemical properties. Purification procedures have included various combinations of treatment with deoxycholate, freon, or chloroform; precipitation with polyethylene glycol, alcohol, or $(NH_4)_2SO_4$; differential ultracentrifugation; velocity sedimentation in sucrose or glycerol density gradients; and isodensity ultracentrifugation in CsCl (Adldinger *et al.*, 1969; Bachrach and Hess, 1973; Love, 1976; Oglesby *et al.*, 1971; Schaffer and Soergel, 1976; Soergel *et al.*, 1976; Wawrzkiewicz *et al.*, 1968). Virions may readily be labeled extrinsically with ^{125}I (Schaffer and Soergel, 1976) or intrinsically with [^3H] or [^{14}C]amino acids, [^{35}S]methionine, [^3H]uridine, or [^{32}P]orthophosphate in cell culture medium (Wawrzkiewicz *et al.*, 1968; Bachrach and Hess, 1973; Schaffer and Soergel, 1973; Love, 1976; Burroughs *et al.*, 1978b). Crystallization of purified virions of SMSV has been reported (Schaffer and Soergel, 1973).

5.2. Morphology and Structure

Calicivirions negatively stained with phosphotungstate present an appearance of cup-shaped depressions (hence the name "calicivirus") arranged in characteristic patterns on the surface. Representative electron micrographs of virions of the three recognized caliciviruses and of a probable human calicivirus are shown in Fig. 3. Measurement of the diameter of negatively stained virions is subject to technical variations, but is usually stated to be 35–40 nm. In preparation of caliciviruses for electron microscopy, technique is often critical for clear demonstration of morphology. Uniformly good results have been obtained with SMSV by using the Ritchie-Fernelius (1969) spray droplet technique (A. W. Smith, personal communication).

Zwillenberg and Bürki (1966) were the first to examine calicivirus morphology, pointing out that FCV differed from the usual picornaviruses. They suggested a double-shell structure with 32 morphological units in an outer capsid. Almeida *et al.* (1968) rejected the double-shell idea, and proposed a single-shell structure with 32 morphological units in pentamer/hexamer icosahedral arrangement. To

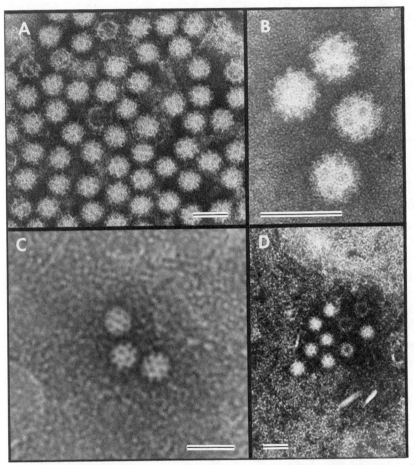

Fig. 3. Electron micrographs of caliciviruses negatively stained with phosphotungstate. A: FCV (Almeida *et al.*, 1968. B: VESV (Wawrzkiewicz *et al.*, 1968). C: SMSV (Smith *et al.*, 1977*b*; reproduced by permission of S. Karger AG, Basel). D: Human calicivirus (Madeley and Cosgrove, 1976). Each bar represents 50 nm.

account for the dark-staining features, they suggested a variation from the usual arrangement of structural units in the morphological units; these were called "negameres." Peterson and Studdert (1970) pointed out certain features indicative of 5,3,2 symmetry (*cf.* Fig. 3): four dark areas in a rhomboid pattern, a central dark area surrounded by six others, and a central dark area surrounded by five others (the latter is more difficult to discern; *cf.* Burroughs *et al.*, 1978*b*). Peterson and Studdert also suggested that the frequently observed ten "projections" are artifacts of the arrangements of the dark areas. They proposed a model with 20 identical morphological units consisting of 60 identical structural units.* Based on a suggestion by Mattern that 60 structural units and 32 "holes" could be arranged with icosahedral symmetry, we (Schaffer and Soergel, 1976) also proposed a 60-subunit model, each with polypeptide dimers or trimers. Mattern (1977) has formally developed the concept of "holes" in icosahedral viral structures, in which the usual triangulation number, T, is augmented by a triangulation number, t, for symmetry of the "holes." In this scheme, $T = 9$, $t = 3$ would represent our proposed 60-unit calicivirus structure. Either 180 or 120 polypeptide units would fit symmetry requirements, but we preferred the latter (60 dimers) based on polypeptide molecular weight and original estimates of RNA content (*cf.* Section 5.8). A different 180-structural-unit calicivirus model is presented on p. 7 of the book by Fenner *et al.* (1974). This model, in which 60 of the structural units are positioned as dimers on the 2-fold axes (= icosahedron edges), can be considered to fit either a $T = 3$ or a $T = 12$, $t = 3$ lattice (Mattern, personal communication).

Convincing evidence that the calicivirion is made up of 180 polypeptides, probably arranged in trimers, has recently been presented by Burroughs *et al.* (1978*b*). Virions were treated at pH 3.5, yielding subunits which sedimented at 6–7 S. These subunits were fixed with formaldehyde and analyzed by polyacrylamide gel electrophoresis. A significant portion migrated with a molecular weight of about 200,000, corresponding to three linked polypeptides (monomers were seen, but there was no peak corresponding to dimers). Based on model construction and electron micrographs, with and without rotational superposition, Burroughs *et al.* suggested a virion with trimeric clustering in a $T = 3$ lattice. The 180-polypeptide model also fits well with new data on virion mass based on RNA content (Section 5.8).

5.3. Sedimentation

Early reports of the sedimentation rate of VESV varied from 160 S (Wawrzkiewicz *et al.*, 1968) to 207 S (Oglesby *et al.*, 1971). The discrepancy probably reflects differences in marker viruses, gradient medium, and method of calculation. Better consistency has been

---

* Peterson and Studdert suggested that each structural unit could consist of one or more than one polypeptide. Symmetry in the 60 structural units in a 20 × 3 arrangement on the 3-fold axes (or an essentially equivalent 12 × 5 arrangement on the 5-fold axes) would require the number of polypeptides, if identical, to be 1, 2, 4, etc., resulting in 60, 120, 240, etc., polypeptides per virion; 180 would be prohibited (Mattern, personal communication). Mattern (1977) has recently reviewed viral icosahedral symmetry requirements.

obtained in more recent estimates. Is the authors' laboratory, SMSV-1 sedimented at 183 S relative to a poliovirus marker (Schaffer and Soergel, 1973), and three additional serotypes of SMSV had identical S values on cosedimentation (Soergel *et al.*, 1975). Bachrach and Hess (1973) observed identical rates, consistent with the 183 S estimate, for VESV, SMSV, and FCV on cosedimentation. Burroughs and Brown (1974), however, reported a difference between VESV (180 S) and FCV (170 S). Whether the discreprancy with FCV is attributable to technical factors or to differences in strain of virus is not known.

5.4. Buoyant Density

Most reported values of bouyant density of caliciviruses in CsCl fall in the 1.36–1.39 g/ml range. Small differences were found among serotypes of VESV (Oglesby *et al.*, 1971) and SMSV (Soergel *et al.*, 1975), and similarly among strains of FCV (Pichler, 1972). Some calicivirus preparations have yielded very sharp homogeneous peaks in CsCl, while others have shown broad or heterogeneous peaks (Pichler, 1972; Soergel *et al.*, 1975; Wawrzkiewicz *et al.*, 1968). Oglesby *et al.* (1971) found two major bands of VESV with a density difference of 0.02 g/ml in crude and in purified preparations. Specific infectivities (PFU/A_{260}) of both bands were of similar magnitude, but infectivity of the more dense band appeared to be less stable. Single peaks of intermediate or high density were obtained by alternative purification procedures using chloroform or ethanol and chloroform. An effect of pH was noted by Rowlands *et al.* (1971); VESV had a higher density at pH 9 than at pH 7. When centrifuged for 6 hr in preformed CsCl gradients, densities of VESV (Burroughs and Brown, 1974) and SMSV (Soergel *et al.*, 1975) were lower than when centrifugation was prolonged in self-formed gradients. A similar shift was observed with FCV by Love and Jones (1974), who also found an increase in buoyant density to 1.42 g/ml with increasing storage (4–8 weeks) at 20°C. With a different strain of FCV, Burroughs and Brown (1974) observed no increase in buoyant density on prolonged centrifugation nor on fixation with gluteraldehyde, whereas VESV showed increased density. The anion also has an effect on buoyant density; VESV bands at 1.32 g/ml in Cs_2SO_4 (Rowlands *et al.*, 1971). These facets of behavior of caliciviruses in Cs salts probably reflect variations in binding of Cs^+ ion among the caliciviruses and among differing conditions. Binding of Cs^+ in relation to similar observations with picornaviruses has been discussed by Rueckert in

Volume 6 of *Comprehensive Virology* (1976). As with enteroviruses (Jamison and Mayor, 1966), the buoyant density of caliciviruses is less in potassium tartrate than in Cs salts; we (Soergel and Schaffer, unpublished) recently determined it to be about 1.27 g/ml for two serotypes of SMSV.

5.5. Inactivation and Stability

Most observations of inactivation and stability of caliciviruses have been made with crude preparations from cell culture. Absence of a lipid envelope is indicated by resistance to ether, chloroform, and phospholipase C (Bürki, 1965; Wawrzkiewicz *et al.*, 1968; Studdert *et al.*, 1970; Bürki and Pichler, 1971; Oglesby *et al.*, 1971). Wawrzkiewicz *et al.* (1968) reported resistance to deoxycholate and Tween 80, but variable inactivation among VESV serotypes by the anionic detergent SDS (see also Section 5.6.2). Caliciviruses differ from enteroviruses in being labile at low pH; they are stable at pH 5, but considerable variation among strains or serotypes is observed between pH 3 and pH 5 (Wawrzkiewicz *et al.*, 1968; Bürki and Pichler, 1971; Lee and Gillespie, 1973). VESV was reported to be inactivated at pH 12.6 in early studies (quoted by Bankowski, 1965), but to my knowledge subsequent studies at high pH have not been made. Thermal inactivation of caliciviruses at 37°C has not been extensively reported, but the observation of 1 $\log_{10}$ loss of infectivity in 8 hr (Wawrzkiewicz *et al.*, 1968) is representative of its magnitude. In contrast to some of the picornaviruses, caliciviruses are rapidly inactivated at 50°C in high concentrations of Mg salts; high concentrations of Na and K salts may exert a slight stabilizing effect (Bürki, 1965; Zee and Hackett, 1967; Studdert *et al.*, 1970; Oglesby *et al.*, 1971; Lee and Gillespie, 1973). With regard to resistance to enzymes, ribonuclease and trypsin have been used in purification of VESV (Oglesby *et al.*, 1971). However, some other caliciviruses are inactivated by trypsin (Bürki and Pichler, 1971; Burroughs *et al.*, 1978a).

Purified caliciviruses appear to be much less stable under a variety of storage conditions than are unpurified preparations (Oglesby *et al.*, 1971). Doubly labeled preparations of one SMSV serotype, on long-term storage at 4°C, lost RNA, probably in a degraded form, leaving a protein-containing unit sedimenting at about 118 S (Schaffer and Soergel, 1976). Cross-linking of the protein with dimethylsuberimidate retarded the RNA loss. This is probably another example of differences among caliciviruses, since another SMSV serotype (not cross-linked) was reasonably stable under similar conditions (unpublished).

Photodynamic inactivation of VESV propagated in the presence of acridine orange (Hackett, 1962) or other dyes such as proflavine and neutral red (Schaffer, unpublished) has been observed.

"Reactivation" of apparently inactive VESV in vesicle fluids by prolonged incubation with cysteine was observed by Madin and Traum (1953, 1955). The biochemical basis for this phenomenon has not been investigated.

5.6. Virion RNA

5.6.1. RNA Content

Oglesby *et al.* (1971), using orcinol reagent, estimated the RNA content of VESV to be 20–22%, and assumed the remainder to be protein. Recently, more precise analyses, including ultraviolet absorbance of hydrolysis products from dried and weighed virus, were carried out by Burroughs *et al.* (1978*b*). They obtained a value of 18% RNA. The UV absorbance ratio, $A_{260}/A_{280} = 1.48$–1.54, of purified calicivirions (Oglesby *et al.*, 1971; Newman *et al.*, 1973; Love, 1976) is in accord with the chemical determinations of RNA content.

5.6.2. RNA Extraction

Difficulties in obtaining homogenous preparations of high-molecular-weight RNA from purified virions in the author's laboratory (Oglesby *et al.*, 1971; Schaffer and Soergel, 1973; Ehresmann, 1978) and elsewhere (Love, 1976) have been mentioned. Others (Wawrzkiewicz *et al.*, 1968; Newman *et al.*, 1973; Burroughs *et al.*, 1978*b*) have reported high molecular weight RNA without mentioning such difficulties. Love found that brief treatment of FCV virions with SDS yielded 32–35 S RNA, but, with more prolonged SDS treatment, the RNA was degraded to predominantly 16–20 S. We (Ehresmann and Schaffer, 1977) found that virion RNA extracted by SDS in the presence of proteinase K was not degraded, suggesting that action of traces of ribonuclease contributed to the earlier difficulties. Additionally, preferential sites of breakage are suggested by the observation of predominant size classes in degradation products (Schaffer and Soergel, 1973; Love, 1976; Ehresmann and Schaffer, unpublished). Although these RNA fragments from virions overlap the size of intracellular 1.1 million dalton ssRNA (Section 4.4), there is probably no functional relationship to that subgenomic mRNA. A 0.7 million dalton ssRNA from cell extracts may be a degradation product of virion-sized RNA, as previously mentioned. If so, it probably represents the 3' end, since it is polyadenylated (Black and Brown, 1978).

5.6.3. Sedimentation

The sedimentation rate of RNA from VESV and from SMSV has been found to be 36–38 S (Wawrzkiewicz *et al.*, 1968; Oglesby *et al.*, 1971; Schaffer and Soergel, 1973; Ehresmann and Schaffer, 1977). Newman *et al.* (1973) reported that FCV RNA sedimented at 30–32 S, significantly less than that of VESV RNA (and somewhat less than Love's value mentioned above). However, Ehresmann (1978) found that RNA from FCV-infected cells cosedimented at 36 S with virion-sized RNA from SMSV-infected cells, suggesting that the reported difference in sedimentation rates of the virion RNAs may not be real. Newman *et al.* (1973) also reported sedimentation rates for RNA in formaldehyde, where configurational effects (at least for RNAs of similar base composition) are supposedly abolished. Under these conditions, FCV RNA again had a slightly lower S rate, 16 S, than VESV and several picornaviruses, 17 S.

5.6.4. Gel Electrophoresis

The molecular weight of SMSV RNA was estimated to be 2.6×10^6 by coelectrophoresis with cell rRNA and EMC virus RNA markers in polyacrylamide gel electrophoresis (Schaffer and Soergel, 1973; Ehresmann and Schaffer, 1977). A slightly higher molecular weight, 2.8×10^6, was reported for VESV RNA by Burroughs *et al.* (1978*b*), who used swine vesicular disease virus RNA as a marker.

5.6.5. Infectivity

Infectious RNA, sensitive to ribonuclease, has been obtained from various caliciviruses (Adldinger *et al.*, 1969; Bachrach and Hess, 1973; Love, 1973; Wawrzkiewicz *et al.*, 1968). The efficiency of infection with calicivirus RNA is quite low when compared to RNA from picornaviruses; for example, Bachrach and Hess obtained (usually) less than 0.05% infectivity of calicivirus RNA relative to that of intact virus, whereas about 3% was obtained with FMDV. The low efficiency may be a reflection of the previously mentioned sensitivity to RNase or breakage. Use of DEAE-dextran in assay of FCV RNA has produced conflicting reports; Love was unable to detect infectivity without DEAE-dextran, while Adldinger *et al.* found no enhancement.

5.6.6. Base Composition and Homology

Base ratio analyses of calicivirus RNAs have been conducted at the Pirbright laboratories. Earlier work indicated a difference in base composition between VESV and FCV (Newman *et al.*, 1973; Burroughs and Brown, 1974), but with improved methodology, recent results revealed no significant differences among the caliciviruses (Burroughs *et al.*, 1978a). These latter results are shown in Table 3. The Pirbright group did find FCV differed from VESV and SMSV by RNA hybridization. Excess unlabeled virion RNA was hybridized with labeled double-stranded RNA (*cf.* Section 4.4) from cells infected with VESV-E or SMSV-1. Results showed 70–80% homology among four VESV serotypes, 80–90% between two SMSVs, and 60–70% between SMSV and VESV; FCV-K1 RNA hybridized to only 10–15% with VESV, and not at all with SMSV (Burroughs *et al.*, 1978a).

5.6.7. End Groups

Since calicivirus RNA is infectious, indicating it must serve as mRNA on entering a cell, it should possess other attributes of mRNA.

TABLE 3
Calicivirus RNA Base Composition[a]

Virus	Mole %			
	A	C	G	U
SMSV-1	27.7	24.2	22.2	25.8
VESV-D	27.6	23.9	21.8	26.3
VESV-E	28.9	22.8	22.0	26.1
FCV-K1	28.5	22.3	22.4	27.5

[a] From data of Burroughs *et al.* (1978a).

SMSV virion RNA bound to oligo(dT)-cellulose, showing that it had polyadenylic acid sequences, presumably at the 3' end (Ehresmann and Schaffer, 1977). The 5' end probably does not have a typcial methylated cap (discussed in Section 4.4), but may have a small protein similar to the picornaviruses (Lee *et al.*, 1977; Flanegan *et al.*, 1977; Sanger *et al.*, 1977). Preliminary evidence for such a protein has been obtained in the author's laboratory (Schaffer, Ehresmann, and Fretz, unpublished; see Section 8).

5.7. Virion Protein

5.7.1. Major Polypeptide

A unique feature of the caliciviruses among viruses of vertebrates is the presence of only one major virion polypeptide (Bachrach and Hess, 1973; Burroughs and Brown, 1974). Experimental evidence indicates the polypeptide is not phosphorylated (Schaffer and Soergel, 1976), and the *N*-terminal end is blocked (Burroughs *et al.*, 1978*b*). Estimates of the molecular weight of the polypeptide have ranged from 60,000 to 71,000 by gel electrophoresis. Some differences may be attributed to the virus used (discussed below), but major differences in the estimates are due to variations in polyacrylamide gel electrophoresis techniques. Bachrach and Hess (1973), using a "disc" buffer system with and without 8 M urea, found molecular weights of 60,000–62,000. Burroughs and co-workers obtained a similar molecular weight, *ca.* 61,000, in disc buffer, and molecular weights from 60,000 to 68,000 in phosphate buffer gel systems (Burroughs and Brown, 1974; Burroughs *et al.*, 1978*b*). In the author's laboratory, the molecular weight of SMSV-4 polypeptide appeared to be 64,000 in tube gels with disc buffer and 71,000 with phosphate buffer (Schaffer and Soergel, 1976). The difference between the two buffer systems was less apparent in slab gel electrophoresis with SMSV-2 polypeptide (Fretz, 1978). Small differences in migration on coelectrophoresis of polypeptides of different caliciviruses have been reported (Bachrach and Hess, 1973; Burroughs and Brown, 1974). Fretz (1978) observed a clearly separated doublet on gel electrophoresis of polypeptide from a SMSV-5 stock derived from a single plaque. This may have been the result of mutation during passage (*cf.* Section 4.3), although contamination has not been ruled out. Repeated plaque purifications resolved this stock into two populations with differing apparent molecular weights. Whether the differences among the caliciviruses reflect true differences in molecular weight or in polypeptide configuration remains to be resolved. If there are actual differences in molecular weight among the caliciviruses, they may relate to the site of precursor cleavage (Section 4.5).

To obtain an estimate of molecular weight independent of gel electrophoresis, Burroughs *et al.* (1978*b*) used 6 M guanidine-Sepharose chromatography. The molecular weight for VESV-E$_{54}$ polypeptide was 76,000–80,000 by this method. They considered that a mean value from the two methods, *ca.* 70,000, to be the most realistic estimate. It would appear that a precise determination of the molecular weight must await further work.

5.7.2. Minor Polypeptide

A small polypeptide, molecular weight *ca.* 15,000, accounting for less than 2% of the total protein, has been observed in preparations of purified virus labeled with ^{14}C-amino acids (Bachrach and Hess, 1973; Burroughs and Brown, 1974; Burroughs *et al.*, 1978*b*). It does not label with [^{35}S]methionine, indicating it lacks that amino acid (Burroughs *et al.*, 1978*b*). The minor polypeptide was not detected in ^{125}I-labeled virions, nor was there any evidence for cross-linking of a small polypeptide to ^{125}I-major polypeptide in virions treated with dimethyl suberimidate (Schaffer and Soergel, 1976). Whether the minor polypeptide is an essential virion component or a tenacious host cell contaminant has not been resolved. If it is a virion component, a possible capsid site might be at the base of "holes," as in some plant viruses (discussed by Mattern, 1977). The quantity present, about 12 copies per virion, would allow for one molecule for each 5-fold axis "hole." Alternatively, the minor polypeptide might be associated (noncovalently) with the RNA (see Section 8). It is highly unlikely that a single small polypeptide covalently linked to the RNA (Section 5.6.7) would be detected by the techniques used to examine the major polypeptide.

5.7.3. Amino Acids and Peptides

The amino acid compositions of three serotypes of SMSV and one VESV have been analyzed (Soergel *et al.*, 1976). The compositions were quite similar, but statistical tests indicated differences among the SMSVs with respect to six of the amino acids (Table 4). (VESV was not included in the statistical tests since only a single sample was analyzed). The Pirbright group has taken different approaches to

TABLE 4

Amino Acid Composition of Caliciviruses[a]

Amino acid[b]	Mole %	
	SMSV[c]	VESV[d]
Lys	5.1–6.0	5.8
His	2.2–2.6	2.4
Arg	3.4–3.6	3.1
Asp	10.5–10.9	12.1
Thr*	8.4–10.9	9.2
Ser	8.4–8.8	8.8
Glu	8.9–9.8	8.8
Pro	6.4–7.4	7.3
Gly	8.0–8.1	7.9
Ala*	5.8–6.7	6.2
Val*	6.7–7.4	6.2
Met	1.1–1.5	1.0
Ile*	4.9–5.8	5.8
Leu*	7.2–7.8	7.7
Tyr	3.3–3.7	3.5
Phe*	4.4–4.9	4.4

[a] Summarized from data of Soergel et al. (1976).
[b] Only 16 amino acids were analyzed; asterisks indicate amino acids for which statistical tests show significant difference (at least at the 5% level) among SMSV serotypes.
[c] Range for SMSV serotypes 1, 4, and 5.
[d] VESV serotype A_{48}.

demonstrate similarities and differences among caliciviruses. When chromatographed on hydroxyapatite, FCV polypeptide eluted at a higher buffer concentration than VESV polypeptide (Burroughs and Brown, 1974). Tryptic peptide mapping on Chromobead P ion exchange resin revealed at least one, and as many as four, peptides in common for various pairs of four caliciviruses (Burroughs et al., 1978a). The relatedness was in accord with their RNA hybridization data (Section 5.6.6). The number of peptides labeled with ^{35}S or ^{125}I appeared to correspond to the number of methionines and tyrosines, respectively, in a 70,000 molecular weight polypeptide (Burroughs et al., 1978b).

5.8. Virion Mass

Estimates of virion mass based on the newer, more precise value of an 18% RNA content (Section 5.6.1) are higher than earlier approximations. Thus the virion mass is 14.4–15.6 million daltons based on RNA molecular weight estimates of $2.6–2.8 \times 10^6$ (Section 5.6.4). A figure of about 15 million is also obtained by adding the mass of RNA and 180 polypeptides of molecular weight 70,000 (Section 5.7.1), assuming no contribution of minor polypeptides (Section 5.7.2). Calculation of mass from the sedimentation rate is subject to considerable uncertainty unless precise data for other hydrodynamic properties are known (*cf.* Rueckert, 1976). Nevertheless, a calicivirion mass of 15 million daltons can be estimated via the Svedberg equation by assuming data relative to those for poliovirus—183 S and 160 S (from cosedimentation, Section 5.3), 37-nm and 27-nm diameters (from electron microscopy), 0.713 ml/g and 0.687 ml/g partial specific volumes (theoretical from composition, adjusting for a discrepancy between experimental and theoretical, Rueckert, 1976), respectively, and a poliovirion mass of 8.96×10^6 (from 29% RNA of 2.6×10^6 molecular weight, Rueckert, 1976)—and canceling contributions of solvent viscocity and density. An estimate of about 15 million was also calculated by Burroughs *et al.* (1978*b*) by direct application of the Svedberg equation and certain assumptions of hydrodynamic parameters.

6. DEFECTIVE INTERFERING VIRUS

There has been little investigation of caliciviruses with regard to the defective interfering (DI) phenomenon. Jensen and Coates (1976, and personal communication) serially passaged FCV at high multiplicity and obtained DI particles with a buoyant desnity of 1.30 g/ml (standard virions = 1.37) and RNA sedimenting at 14–19 S. The DI particles interfered with replication of standard virus. In an effort to elicit the DI phenomenon in our laboratory, SMSV was serially passed ten times at high multiplicity without effect of RNA patterns in cells (Ehresmann and Schaffer, unpublished).

7. CONCLUDING REMARKS

Much of the information in this chapter, particularly regarding RNA and protein in infected cells, is of a preliminary nature and needs confirmation and further elucidation. Nevertheless, sufficient is known of the unique charcteristics of caliciviruses to justify taxonomic classification as a distinct family. With picornaviruses, they share attributes of virion RNA, namely, molecular weights, function as mRNA, and lack of a 5'-methylated cap. However, calicivirions are slightly larger in size than picornavirions, and their structures, in both morphology and number and size of polypeptides, differ markedly. With respect to protein–protein and protein–RNA interactions in virion structure (Tikchonenko, 1975), differences between caliciviruses and picornaviruses probably exist also. The genome strategy of caliciviruses, with respect to subgenomic mRNA and protein cleavage, resembles that of alphaviruses (Togaviridae) more closely than picornaviruses.* However, caliciviruses differ from alphaviruses in that the latter have an envelope with glycoproteins, of which the protein portions are cleaved from the translation product of the subgenomic RNA, along with the nucleocapsid protein. Tobacco mosaic virus (TMV) has a genome strategy that uses a subgenomic mRNA for synthesis of a single virion polypeptide (Hunter *et al.*, 1976; Siegel *et al.*, 1976). TMV and caliciviruses appear to differ in that cleavage of a precursor to yield virion protein occurs with calicivirus but not with TMV. Also, TMV RNA has a 5'-methylated cap (Keith and Fraenkel-Conrat, 1975). Other differences between these two viruses, in addition to obvious virion structure and host differences, are the subgenomic mRNA molecular weight and polypeptide molecular weight.

Of the recognized caliciviruses, SMSV and VESV are very closely related, if not identical, and strong evidence points to a common marine source. Immune precipitation, RNA homology, and peptide maps indicate that FCV is more distantly related. A marine source for FCV has also been postulated by Studdert (1978). Relatedness of these recognized caliciviruses to caliciviruses from humans and possibly other species remains to be determined.

8.   ADDENDUM

New information pertinent to the subject has become available since this chapter was written. Insect viruses that superficially resemble caliciviruses were not mentioned since their properties appeared to differ significantly from those of the accepted caliciviruses. Data on this group of insect viruses have now been summarized by Reinganum *et al.*

---

* Replication of togaviruses and picornaviruses has been reviewed by Pfefferkorn and Shapiro and by Levintow, respectively, in Volume 2 of Comprehensive Virology (1974), and more recently by Strauss and Strauss (1977) and Rekosh (1977), respectively.

(1978). In a careful morphological study of particles in human feces, Madeley (1979) has pointed out criteria for distinguishing caliciviruses from astroviruses. It is unfortunate that inability to culture such agents from humans remains as an obstacle to their further characterization.

Black *et al.* (1978) have provided further information on intracellular RNAs. Three species of ssRNA, 37 S, 22 S, and 18 S, exhibited binding to oligo(dt)cellulose and hybridization to dsRNA. On the basis of these findings and observations of several viral polypeptides in infected cells, Black *et al.* suggested that each of the three was a distinct mRNA. However, under *in vitro* translation conditions only the 22 S RNA yielded detectable products, the predominant component being the size of virion polypeptide. The 37 S RNA from cells was inactive, whereas 37 S virion RNA was translated to yield heterogeneous polypeptides; this surprising difference remains to be explained.

The presence of a small protein, VPg, covalently linked to calicivirus RNA has been established. The Pirbright group (Black *et al.*, 1978; Burroughs and Brown, 1978) reported the absence of a 5' cap and presence of a protein of molecular weight about 10,000 on VESV virion RNA. The VPg ([³H]lysine label) sedimented sharply with the 37 S peak of a somewhat heterogeneous RNA ([¹⁴C]uridine label) preparation. VPg did not dissociate from RNA under denaturing conditions but was eliminated by proteinase K treatment. VESV RNA was not infectious after treatment with proteinase K, which differs from the picornavirus situation where VPg is not necessary for infectivity. VPg with an apparent molecular weight of 15,000 linked to SMSV RNA has been found in the author's laboratory (Schaffer *et al.*, 1979). RNA labeled with ³²P was exhaustively digested with RNases, revealing a ³²P-labeled residue that was susceptible to proteinase K. The quantity of ³²P approached that expected for a protein–nucleoside diphosphate residue. We also found VPg by iodination of a preparation of 36 S RNA from SMSV-infected cells (extracted at a time when much of the RNA was from unreleased virions). The VPg, which was proteinase K sensitive, banded with the RNA under denaturing conditions in a cesium trichloroacetate (CsTCA) gradient. Another iodinated protein associated with the RNA was separable by electrophoresis and by CsTCA centrifugation. It appeared to have a slightly higher molecular weight than VPg; its identity has not been established, but it may be the minor virion polypeptide. The possibility that this RNA-associated (noncovalent) protein could be an endonuclease such as that in FMDV virions (Denoya *et al.*, 1978) should be considered in view of similarities in instability of calicivirus RNA and FMDV RNA.

ACKNOWLEDGMENTS

The author's research was supported by the Office of Naval Research. Drs. June Almeida, Fred Brown, Adeline Hackett, C. R. Madeley, Alvin W. Smith, Michael Studdert, and Y. C. Zee kindly provided electron micrographs. Drs. Brown, Smith, and Studdert also graciously provided manuscripts prior to publication.

9. REFERENCES

Adldinger, H. K., Lee, K. M., and Gillespie, J. H., 1969, Extraction of infectious ribonucleic acid from a feline picornavirus, *Arch. Gesamte Virusforsch.* **28**:245.

Akers, T. G., Smith, A. W., Latham, A. B., and Watkins, H. M. S., 1974, Calicivirus antibodies in California gray whale (*Eschrichtius robustus*) and Steller sea lions (*Eumetopias jupatus*), *Arch. Gesamte Virusforsch.* **46**:175.

Almeida, J. D., Waterson, A. P., Prydie, J., and Fletcher, E. W. L., 1968, The structure of a feline picornavirus and its relevance to cubic viruses in general, *Arch. Gesamte Virusforsch.* **25**:105.

Bachrach, H. L., and Hess, W. R., 1973, Animal picornaviruses with a single major species of capsid protein, *Biochem. Biophys. Res. Commun.* **55**:141.

Bankowski, R. A., 1965, Vesicular exanthema, *Adv. Vet. Sci. Comp. Med.* **10**:23.

Bittle, J. L., and Rubic, W. J., 1976, Immunization against feline calicivirus infection, *Am. J. Vet. Res.* **37**:275.

Black, D., and Brown, F., 1975/1976, A major difference in the strategy of the calici- and picornaviruses and its significance in classification, *Intervirology* **6**:57.

Black, D. N., and Brown, F., 1978, Proteins induced by infection with caliciviruses, *J. Gen. Virol.* **38**:75.

Black, D. N., Burroughs, J. N., Harris, T. J. R., and Brown, F., 1978, The structure and replication of calicivirus RNA, *Nature (London)*, **274**:614.

Breese, S. S., Jr., and Dardiri, A. H., 1977, Electron microscope observations on a virus transmissible from pinnipeds to swine, *J. Gen. Virol.* **36**:221.

Bürki, F., 1965, Picornaviruses of cats, *Arch. Gesamte Virusforsch.* **15**:690.

Bürki, F., and Pichler, L., 1971, Further biochemical testing of feline picornaviruses, *Arch. Gesamte Virusforsch.* **33**:126.

Burki, F., Starustka, B., and Ruttner, O., 1976, Attempts to serologically classify feline caliciviruses on a national and an international basis, *Infect. Immun.* **14**:876.

Burroughs, J. N., and Brown, F., 1974, Physico-chemical evidence for re-classification of the caliciviruses, *J. Gen. Virol.* **22**:281.

Burroughs, J. N., and Brown, F., 1978, Presence of a covalently linked protein on calicivirus RNA, *J. Gen. Virol.* **41**:443.

Burroughs, N., Doel, T., and Brown, F., 1978a, Relationship of San Miguel sea lion virus to other members of the calicivirus group, *Intervirology* **10**:51.

Burroughs, J. N., Doel, T. R., Smale, C. J., and Brown, F., 1978b, A model for vesicular exanthema virus, the prototype of the calicivirus group, *J. Gen. Virol.* **40**:161.

Chappuis, G., and Stellmann, C., 1974, Biomathematical system of relationship and dominance for classification of feline picornavirus, *J. Biol. Stand.* **2**:319.

Cooper, P. D., 1974, Towards a more profound basis for the classification of viruses, *Intervirology* **4**:317.

Cooper, P. D., Agol, V. I., Bachrach, H. L., Brown, F., Ghendon, Y., Gibbs, A. J., Gillespie, J. H., Lonberg-Holm, K., Mandel, B., Melnick, J. L., Mohanty, S. B., Povey, R. C., Rueckert, R. R., Schaffer, F. L., and Tyrrell, D. A. J., 1978, *Picornaviridae:* Second report, *Intervirology* **10**:165.

Denoya, C. D., Scodeller, E. A., Vasquez, C., and La Torre, J. L., 1978, Foot and mouth disease virus. II. Endoribonuclease activity within purified virions, *Virology* **89**:67.

Ehresmann, D. W., 1978, Studies on calicivirus genomic replication and transcription: Characterization of RNA from virions and infected cells, thesis, University of California, Berkeley.

Ehresmann, D. W., and Schaffer, F. L., 1977, RNA synthesized in calicivirus-infected cells is atypical of picornaviruses, *J. Virol.* **22**:572.

Fastier, L. B., 1957, A new feline virus isolated in tissue culture, *Am. J. Vet. Res.* **18**:382.

Fenner, F., 1976, Classification and nomenclature of viruses. Second report of the international committee on taxomy of viruses, *Intervirology* **7**:1.

Fenner, F., McAuslan, B. R., Mims, C. A., Sambrook, J., and White, D. O., 1974, *The Biology of Animal Viruses*, 2nd ed., Academic Press, New York.

Flanegan, J. B., Pettersson, R. F., Ambros, V., Hewlett, M. J., and Baltimore, D., 1977, Covalent linkage of a protein to a defined nucleotide sequence at the 5'-terminus of virion and replicative intermediate RNAs of poliovirus, *Proc. Natl. Acad. Sci. USA* **74**:961.

Flewett, T. H., and Davies, H., 1976, Caliciviruses in man, *Lancet* **1**:31.

Fretz, M. K., 1978, Characterization of the virus-specific proteins synthesized in cells infected with caliciviruses, thesis, University of California, Berkeley.

Fretz, M., and Schaffer, F. L., 1978, Calicivirus proteins in infected cells: Evidence for a capsid polypeptide precursor, *Virology* **89**:318.

Gillespie, J. H., and Scott, F. W., 1973, Feline viral infections, *Adv. Vet. Sci. Comp. Med.* **17**:163.

Gilmartin, W. G., Delong, R. L., Smith, A. W., Sweeney, J. C., De Lappe, B. W., Risebrough, R. W., Griner, L. A., Dailey, M. D., and Peakall, D. B., 1976, Premature parturition in the California sea lion, *J. Wildl. Dis.* **12**:104.

Hackett, A. J., 1961, The cellular changes produced by two variants within type E54 of vesicular exanthema of swine virus in tissue culture, *Virology* **15**:102.

Hackett, A. J., 1962, The photodynamic effects of acridine orange on an RNA virus (vesicular exanthema), *Photochem. Photobiol.* **1**:147.

Hoover, E. A., and Kahn, D. E., 1973, Lesions produced by feline picornaviruses of different virulence in pathogen-free cats, *Vet. Pathol.* **10**:307.

Hunter, T. R., Hunt, T., Knowland, J., and Zimmern, D., 1976, Messenger RNA for the coat protein of tobacco mosaic virus, *Nature (London)* **260**:759.

Jamison, R. M., and Mayor, H. D., 1966, Comparative study of seven picornaviruses of man, *J. Bacteriol.* **91**:1971.

Jensen, M., and Coates, S. R., 1976, Defective interfering particles of feline calicivirus, *Abstr. Annu. Meet. Am. Soc. Microbiol.* **S41**:211.

Kahn, D. E., and Hoover, E. A., 1976, Feline caliciviral disease: Experimental immunoprophylaxis, *Am. J. Vet. Res.* **37**:279.

Kahn, D. E., Hoover, E. A., and Bittle, J. L., 1975, Induction of immunity to feline caliciviral disease, *Infect. Immun.* **11**:1003.

Kalunda, M., Lee, K. M., Holmes, D. F., and Gillespie, J. H., 1975, Serologic classification of feline caliciviruses by plaque-reduction neutralization and immunodiffusion, *Am. J. Vet. Res.* **36**:353.

Kapikian, A. Z., Feinstone, S. M., Purcell, R. H., Wyatt, R. G., Thornhill, T. S., Kalica, A. R., and Chanock, R. M., 1975, Detection and identification by immune electron microscopy of fastidious agents associated with respiratory illness, acute nonbacterial gastroenteritis, and hepatitis A, in: *Perspectives in Virology*, Vol. 9 (M. Pollard, ed.), pp. 9–47, Academic Press, New York.

Keith, J., and Fraenkel-Conrat, H., 1975, Tobacco mosaic virus RNA carries 5′-terminal triphosphorylated guanosine blocked by 5′-linked 7-methyl-guanosine, *FEBS Lett.* **57**:31.

Lee, K. M., and Gillespie, J. H., 1973, Thermal and pH stability of feline calicivirus, *Infect. Immun.* **7**:678.

Lee, Y. F., Nomoto, A., Detjen, B. M., and Wimmer, E., 1977, A protein covalently linked to poliovirus genome RNA, *Proc. Natl. Acad. Sci. USA* **74**:59.

Levintow, L. 1974, The reproduction of picornaviruses, in: *Comprehensive Virology*, Vol. 2 (H. Fraenkel-Conrat and R. R. Wagner, eds.), pp. 109–171, Plenum, New York.

Love, D. N., 1973, The effect of DEAE-dextran on the infectivity of a feline calicivirus and its RNA, *Arch. Gesamte Virusforsch.* **41**:52.

Love, D. N., 1976, Feline calicivirus: Purification of virus and extraction and characterization of its ribonucleic acid, *Cornell Vet.* **66**:498.

Love, D. N., and Donaldson-Wood, C., 1975, Replication of a strain of feline calicivirus in organ culture, *Arch. Virol.* **47**:167.

Love, D. N., and Jones, R. F., 1974, Studies on the buoyant density of a feline calicivirus, *Arch. Gesamte Virusforsch.* **44**:142.

Love, D. N., and Sabine, M., 1975, Electron microscopic observation of feline kidney cells infected with a feline calicivirus, *Arch. Virol.* **48**:213.

Madeley, C. R., 1979, A comparison of the features of astroviruses and caliciviruses seen in samples of feces by electron microscopy, *J. Infect. Dis.* **139**:519.

Madeley, C. R., and Cosgrove, B. P., 1976, Caliciviruses in man, *Lancet* **1**:199.

Madin, S. H., 1973, Pigs, sea lions, and vesicular exanthema, in: *Second International Conference on Foot and Mouth Disease* (M. Pollard, ed.), pp. 78–81, Academic Press, New York.

Madin, S. H., 1975, Vesicular exanthema, in *Diseases of Swine*, 4th ed., (H. W. Dunne and A. D. Leman, eds.), pp. 286–307, Iowa State University Press, Ames, Ia.

Madin, S. H., and Traum, J., 1953, Experimental studies with vesicular exanthema of swine, *Vet. Med.* **48**:443.

Madin, S. H., and Traum, J., 1955, Vesicular exanthema of swine, *Bacteriol. Rev.* **19**:6.

Madin, S. H., Smith, A. W., and Akers, T. G., 1976, Current status caliciviruses isolated from marine mammals and their relationship to caliciviruses of terrestrial animals, in: *Wildlife Diseases* (L. A. Page, ed.), pp. 197–204, Plenum, New York.

Mattern, C. F. T., 1977, Symmetry in virus architecture, in: *The Molecular Biology of Animal Viruses*, Vol. 1 (D. P. Nayak, ed.), pp. 1–39, Dekker, New York.

McClain, M. E., Hackett, A. J., and Madin, S. H., 1958, Plaque morphology and pathogenicity of vesicular exanthema virus, *Science* **127**:1391.

Melnick, J. L., Agol, V. I., Bachrach, H. L., Brown, F., Cooper, P. D., Fiers, W., Gard, S., Gear, J. H. S., Ghendon, Y., Kasza, L., LaPlaca, M., Mandel, B., McGregor, S., Mohanty, S. B., Plummer, G., Rueckert, R. R., Schaffer, F. L., Tagaya, I., Tyrrell, D. A. J., Voroshilova, M., and Wenner, H. A., 1974, Picornaviridae, *Intervirology* **4**:303.

Middleton, P. J., Szymanski, M. T., and Petric, M., 1977, Viruses associated with acute gastroenteritis in young children, *Am. J. Dis. Child.* **131**:733.

Milek, M., Wooley, R. E., and Blue, J. L., 1976, Replication of feline herpesvirus and feline calicivirus in cell and organ cultures, *Am. J. Vet. Res.* **37**:723.

Moore, D. M., 1977, Characterization of three antigenic particles of swine vesicular disease virus, *J. Gen. Virol.* **34**:431.

Nardelli, L., Lodetti, E., Gualandi, G. L., Burrows, R., Goodridge, D., Brown, F., and Cartwright, B., 1968, A foot and mouth disease syndrome in pigs caused by an enterovirus, *Nature (London)* **219**:1275.

Newman, J. F. E., Rowlands, D. J., and Brown, F., 1973, A physico-chemical subgrouping of the mammalian picornaviruses, *J. Gen. Virol.* **18**:171.

Nomoto, A., Detjen, B., Pozzatti, R., and Wimmer, E., 1977, The location of the polio genome protein in viral RNAs and its implication for RNA synthesis, *Nature (London)* **268**:208.

Oglesby, A. S., Schaffer, F. L., and Madin, S. H., 1971, Biochemical and biophysical properties of vesicular exanthema of swine virus, *Virology* **44**:329.

Olsen, R. G., Kahn, D. E., Hoover, E. A., Saxe, N. J., and Yohn, D. S., 1974, Differences in acute and convalescent-phase antibodies of cats infected with feline picornaviruses, *Infect. Immun.* **10**:375.

Peterson, J. E., and Studdert, M. J., 1970, Feline picornavirus. Structure of the virus and electron microscopic observations on infected cell cultures, *Arch. Gesamte Virusforsch.* **32**:249.

Pfefferkorn, E. R., and Shapiro, D., 1974, Reproduction of togaviruses, in: *Comprehensive Virology* Vol. 2 (H. Fraenkel-Conrat and R. R. Wagner eds.), pp. 171–230, Plenum, New York.

Pichler, L., 1972, Bestimmung der Dichte feliner Picornaviren im CsCl-Gradienten, *Zentralbl. Bakteriol. Parasitenkd. Infectionskr. Hyg. Abt. Orig. Reihe A* **222**:162.

Povey, R. C., 1974, Serological relationships among feline caliciviruses, *Infect. Immun.* **10**:1307.

Povey, R. C., and Hale, C. J., 1974, Experimental infections with feline caliciviruses (picornaviruses) in specific-pathogen-free kittens, *J. Comp. Pathol.* **84**:245.

Povey, R. C., and Ingersoll, J., 1975, Cross-protection among feline caliciviruses, *Infect. Immun.* **11**:877.

Prato, C. M., Akers, T. G., and Smith, A. W., 1974, Serological evidence of calicivirus transmission between marine and terrestrial mammals, *Nature (London)* **249**:255.

Prato, C. M., Akers, T. G., and Smith, A. W., 1977, Calicivirus antibodies in wild fox populations, *J. Wildl. Dis.* **13**:448.

Reinganum, C., Robertson, J. S., and Tinsley, T. W., 1978, A new group of RNA viruses from insects, *J. Gen. Virol.* **40**:195.

Rekosh, D. M. K., 1977, The molecular biology of picornaviruses, in: *The Molecular Biology of Animal Viruses*, Vol. 1, pp. 63–110, Dekker, New York.

Ritchie, A. E., and Fernelius, A. L., 1969, Characterization of bovine viral diarrhea viruses. V. Morphology of characteristic particles studied by electron microscopy, *Arch. Gesamte Virusforsch.* **28**:369.

Rowlands, D. J., Sangar, D. V., and Brown, F., 1971, Buoyant density of picornaviruses in caesium salts, *J. Gen. Virol.* **13**:141.

Rueckert, R. R., 1976, On the structure and morphogenesis of picornaviruses, in: *Comprehensive Virology*, Vol. 6 (H. Fraenkel-Conrat and R. R. Wagner, eds.), pp. 131–213, Plenum, New York.

Sabine, M., and Hyne, R. H. J., 1970, Isolation of a feline picornavirus from cheetahs with conjunctivitis and glossitis, *Vet. Rec.* **87**:794.

Sangar, D. V., Rowlands, D. J., Harris, T. J. R., and Brown, F., 1977, Protein covalently linked to foot-and-mouth disease virus RNA, *Nature (London)* **268**:648.

Sawyer, J. C., 1976, Vesicular exanthema of swine and San Miguel sea lion virus, *J. Am. Vet. Med. Assoc.* **169**:707.

Schaffer, F. L., and Soergel, M. E., 1973, Biochemical and biophysical characterization of calicivirus isolates from pinnipeds, *Intervirology* **1**:210.

Schaffer, F. L., and Soergel, M. E., 1976, Single major polypeptide of a calicivirus: Characterization by polyacrylamide gel electrophoresis and stabilization of virions by cross-linking with dimethyl suberimidate, *J. Virol.* **19**:925.

Schaffer, F. L., Ehresmann, D. W., Fretz, M. K., and Soergel, M. E., 1979, A protein, VPg, covalently linked to 36 S calicivirus RNA, submitted for publication.

Scott, F. W., 1977, Evaluation of a feline viral rhinotracheitis-feline calicivirus disease vaccine, *Am. J. Vet. Res.* **38**:229.

Shatkin, A. J., 1976, Capping of eucaryotic mRNAs, *Cell* **9**:645.

Siegel, A., Hari, V., Montgomery, I., and Kolacz, K., 1976, A messenger RNA for capsid protein isolated from tobacco mosaic virus infected tissue, *Virology* **73**:363.

Smith, A. W., and Akers, T. G., 1976, Vesicular exanthema of swine, *J. Am. Vet. Med. Assoc.* **169**:700.

Smith, A. W., and Latham, A. B., 1978, Prevalence of vesicular exanthema of swine antibodies among feral mammals associated with the Southern California coastal zones, *Am. J. Vet. Res.* **39**:291.

Smith, A. W., and Skilling, D. E., 1977, Scanning electron microscopy of calicivirus infected monkey kidney (Vero) cells, *Microbios Lett.* **4**:17.

Smith, A. W., Akers, T. G., Madin, S. H., and Vedros, N. A., 1973, San Miguel sea lion virus isolation, preliminary characterization and relationship to vesicular exanthema of swine virus, *Nature (London)* **244**:108.

Smith, A. W., Prato, C. M., Gilmartin, W. G., Brown, R. J., and Keyes, M. C., 1974, A preliminary report on potentially pathogenic microbiological agents recently isolated from pinnipeds, *J. Wildl. Dis.* **10**:54.

Smith, A. W., Akers, T. G., Prato, C. M., and Bray, H., 1976, Prevalence and distribution of four serotypes of SMSV serum neutralizing antibodies in wild animal populations, *J. Wildl. Dis.* **12**:326.

Smith, A. W., Madin, S. H., Vedros, N. A., and Bankowski, R. A., 1977a, Host range comparisons of five serotypes of caliciviruses, *Am. J. Vet. Res.* **38**:101.

Smith, A. W., Prato, C. M., and Skilling, D. E., 1977b, Characterization of two new serotypes of San Miguel sea lion virus, *Intervirology* **8**:30.

Smith, A. W., Skilling, D. E., and Ritchie, A. E., 1978a, Immuno-electron microscopic comparisons of caliciviruses, *Am. J. Vet. Res.* **39**:1531.

Smith, A. W., Prato, C., and Skilling, D. E., 1978b, Caliciviruses infecting monkeys and possibly man, *Am. J. Vet. Res.* **39**:287.

Soergel, M. E., Smith, A. W., and Schaffer, F. L., 1975, Biophysical comparisons of calicivirus serotypes isolated from pinnipeds, *Intervirology* **5**:239.

Soergel, M. E., Akers, T. G., Schaffer, F. L., and Noma, A. T., 1976, Amino acid composition of three immunological types of a calicivirus, San Miguel sea lion virus, *Virology* **72**:527.

Soergel, M. E., Schaffer, F. L., Sawyer, J. C., and Prato, C. M., 1978, Assay of antibodies to caliciviruses by radioimmune precipitation using staphylococcal protein A as IgG adsorbent, *Arch. Virol.* **57**:271.

Strauss, J. H., and Strauss, E. G., 1977, Togaviruses, in: *The Molecular Biology of Animal Viruses*, Vol. 1 (D. P. Nayak, ed.), pp. 111–166, Dekker, New York.

Studdert, M. J., 1978, Caliciviruses. *Arch. Virol.* **58**:157.

Studdert, M. J., and O'Shea, J. D., 1975, Ultrastructural studies of the development of feline calicivirus in a feline embryo cell line, *Arch. Virol.* **48**:317.

Studdert, M. J., Martin, M. C., and Peterson, J. E., 1970, Viral diseases of the respiratory tract of cats: Isolation and properties of viruses tentatively classified as picornaviruses, *Am. J. Vet. Res.* **31**:1723.

Thornhill, T. S., Wyatt, R. G., Kalica, A. R., Dolin, R., Chanock, R. M., and Kapikian, A. Z., 1977, Detection by immune electron microscopy of 26- to 27-nm viruslike particles associated with two family outbreaks of gastroenteritis, *J. Infect. Dis.* **135**:20.

Tikchonenko, T. I., 1975, Structure of viral nucleic acis *in situ*, in: *Comprehensive Virology*, Vol. 5 (H. Fraenkel-Conrat and R. R. Wagner, eds.), pp. 1–117, Plenum, New York.

Walen, K. H., 1963, Demonstration of inapparent heterogeneity in a population of an animal virus by single-burst analyses, *Virology* **20**:230.

Walen, K. H., Madin, S. H., and Hackett, A. J., 1966, *In vivo* and *in vitro* studies of plaque type mutants of an RNA virus, *Arch. Gesamte Virusforsch.* **18**:316.

Wardley, R. C., 1976, Feline calicivirus carrier state: A study of the host/virus relationship, *Arch. Virol.* **52**:243.

Wardley, R. C., and Povey, R. C., 1977a, The clinical disease and patterns of excretion associated with three different strains of feline caliciviruses, *Res. Vet. Sci.* **23**:7.

Wardley, R. C., and Povey, R. C., 1977b, The pathology and sites of persistence associated with three different strains of feline calicivirus, *Res. Vet. Sci.* **23**:15.

Wawrzkiewicz, J., Smale, C. J., and Brown, F., 1968, Biochemical and biophysical characteristics of vesicular exanthema virus and the viral ribonucleic acid, *Arch. Gesamte Virusforsch.* **25**:337.

Wooley, R. E., Blue, J. L., and Milek, M. 1976, Enhancement effect of feline herpesvirus and feline calicivirus infections in Crandell feline kidney cells, *Bull. Ga. Acad. Sci.* **34**:171.

Zee, Y. C., and Hackett, A. J., 1967, The influence of cations on the thermal inactivation of vesicular exanthema of swine virus, *Arch. Gesamte Virusforsch.* **20**:473.

Zee, Y. C., Hackett, A. J., and Madin, S. H., 1967, A study of the cellular pathogenesis of vesicular exanthema of swine virus in pig kidney cells, *J. Infect. Dis.* **117**:229.

Zee, Y. C., Hackett, A. J., and Madin, S. H., 1968a, Electron microscopic studies on vesicular exanthema of swine virus: Intracytoplasmic viral crystal formation in cultured pig kidney cells, *Am. J. Vet. Res.* **29**:1025.

Zee, Y. C., Hackett, A. J., and Talens, L. T., 1968*b*, Electron microscopic studies on the vesicular exanthema of swine virus. II. Morphogenesis of VESV Type H_{54} in pig kidney cells, *Virology* **34**:596.

Zwillenberg, L. O., and Bürki, F., 1966, On the capsid structure of some small feline and bovine RNA viruses, *Arch. Gesamte Virusforsch.* **19**:373.

CHAPTER 5

Orbiviruses

D. W. Verwoerd, H. Huismans, and B. J. Erasmus

Veterinary Research Institute
Onderstepoort
0110 Republic of South Africa

1. INTRODUCTION

The genus orbivirus has been formed only recently, although the type species, bluetongue virus of sheep (BTV), as well as African horsesickness virus (AHSV) have been known since the turn of the century. Both of these viruses are important animal pathogens that were originally limited to Africa but have later spread to the Middle East and other continents. Because they were known to be transmitted by insects, both BTV and AHSV were historically classified as arboviruses (Casals, 1959). It later became clear that they, and some other isolates from insects, did not show the extreme sensitivity to lipid solvents characteristic of the enveloped, lipid-containing arboviruses now classified as togaviruses. This group was therefore often referred to as ungrouped or unclassified arboviruses.

Early electron microscopic studies (Polson and Deeks, 1963; Studdert *et al.*, 1966) first suggested a reoviruslike structure, and the discovery that BTV possesses a segmented double-stranded RNA genome (Verwoerd, 1969) seemed to confirm their provisional classification as reoviruses (Andrewes and Pereira, 1967).

It soon became apparent, however, that these viruses, although obviously related to reovirus, could be distinguished as a separate group on the basis of some characteristic differences. The most important of these differences include a smaller size, the absence of a clearly structured second capsid layer, greater sensitivity toward pH, temperature, and lipid solvents, as well as the involvement of an intermediate insect host in their transmission to mammalian hosts. They were therefore grouped together into a genus (Verwoerd, 1970; Murphy *et al.*, 1971), for which the name "orbiviruses" was proposed (Borden *et al.*, 1971).

During recent years a large number of orbiviruses have been isolated from insects, mainly in Australia. This interest in insect-borne orbiviruses stems mainly from the potential hazard that bluetongue disease constitutes for the Australian sheep industry. Fortunately, most isolates have so far proved to be nonpathogenic viruses serologically distinct from both BTV and AHSV. The important fact emerged, however, that there exist a large number of insect orbiviruses. The majority of these are in all probability primarily insect viruses, and those pathogenic to mammals are the exception rather than the rule. It is also becoming clear that the existence of so many closely related viruses is at least partly due to the facility with which these viruses can exchange genetic information. Although any attempt to group them is complicated by this characteristic, they can be classified into serological subgroups, based on complement fixation. A catalogue of these subgroups is given in Table 1. Certain orbiviruses are not listed separately but are regarded as serotypes of a subgroup, e.g., Ibaraki virus, which is considered to be an EHDV serotype. Some subgroups such as EHDV and BTV are listed separately, although they show some degree of relatedness.

The purpose of the present chapter is to collate all the information presently available on the various orbiviruses and to attempt a generalized description of the genus. Reviews have previously been published on African horsesickness virus (Mornet and Gilbert, 1968), on diplornaviruses (Verwoerd, 1970), and on bluetongue virus (Howell and Verwoerd, 1971). In addition, orbiviruses have been included in more general reviews dealing with double-stranded RNA containing viruses (Wood, 1973) and with the reproduction of the Reoviridae (Joklik, 1974).

2. PROPAGATION AND ASSAY SYSTEMS

2.1. Primary Isolation

With few exceptions, the primary isolation of orbiviruses has been achieved by the intracerebral inoculation of suckling mice. Newborn

TABLE 1

Orbivirus Classification

Virus or subgroup	Number of serotypes	Abbreviation	Mammalian host	Insect host
Bluetongue virus	20	BTV	Ungulates	*Culicoides*
Epizootic hemorrhagic disease subgroup	8	EHDV	Ungulates	—
African horsesickness virus	9	AHSV	Equines	*Culicoides*
Equine encephalosis virus	4	—	Equines	—
Wallal subgroup	2	—	Marsupials	—
Warrego subgroup	2	—	Marsupials	*Culicoides*
Palyam subgroup	6	—	Ungulates	Mosquitoes
Eubenangee subgroup	3	—	Marsupials	Mosquitoes
Corriparta subgroup	2	—	Ungulates	Mosquitoes
Colorado tick fever subgroup	2	CTFV	Humans, rodents	Ticks
Changuinola subgroup	8	—	—	*Phlebotomines*
Kemerovo subgroup	18	—	Humans	Ticks
Ungrouped: Japanaut	—	—	—	Mosquitoes
Lebombo	—	—	—	Mosquitoes
Orungo	—	—	—	Mosquitoes
Umatilla	—	—	—	Mosquitoes
Ug MP 359	—	—	—	Mosquitoes

(1–4 days old) mice are routinely used since an inverse relationship exists between age and susceptibility to most orbiviruses. Incubation periods usually range from 3 to 7 days but can be as long as 17 days. The symptoms exhibited by infected mice are by no means pathognomonic but merely signify encephalitis. Initially the mice cease suckling, leave the nest, and become scattered. This stage may be followed by one of hyperactivity or by alternating periods of lethargy and hyperactivity. As the disease progresses, their movements become more uncoordinated and spastic, finally followed by a comatose state of variable duration with eventual death.

Although adult mice have in certain instances been used for the primary isolation of an orbivirus, e.g., AHSV (Alexander, 1933), this host is seldom used in view of its insusceptibility to most viruses of the group.

Embryonating chicken eggs proved particularly useful for the primary isolation of bluetongue virus. The yolk sac route of inoculation was employed by Mason *et al.* (1940) and by Alexander (1947), who also demonstrated the importance of a low temperature of incubation. A most significant contribution was made by Goldsmit and Barzilai (1965, 1968, 1969) and by Foster and Luedke (1968), who demonstrated that intravascular inoculation of embryonating eggs enhanced the susceptibility to bluetongue virus about a hundredfold as compared to the yolk sac route and gave more reproducible results.

It is of particular interest that EHDV, although similar to BTV in many respects, does not multiply in chicken embryos irrespective of the route of inoculation. However, certain EHD-like viruses were isolated from wild-caught *Culicoides* spp. in South Africa by intravenous inoculation of embryonated eggs (Erasmus, unpublished observation).

African horsesickness virus can also be isolated in embryonating eggs following yolk sac (Goldsmit, 1967) as well as intravascular (Boorman *et al.*, 1975) inoculation. However, since more sensitive host systems are available for the primary isolation of AHSV, embryonated eggs are seldom used.

Cell cultures are nowadays increasingly used for the primary isolation of orbiviruses. Cells most commonly used for this purpose include primary cultures such as chicken embryo and lamb kidney cells as well as established cell lines such as BHK-21, Vero, LLC-MK$_2$, and HeLa, and lines of insect cells. BHK-21 cells are used routinely for the isolation of AHSV (Erasmus, 1972) and equine encephalosis viruses (Erasmus *et al.*, 1976a). A particular subline of Vero cells has proved very useful for the primary isolation of BTV and EHDV (Bando, 1975; Luedke *et al.*, 1975). KB cells have been used for the direct isolation of CTFV from ticks and from blood.

2.2. Cultivation

For primary isolation, newborn mice are still commonly used in the routine cultivation of many orbiviruses. After adaptation most viruses will kill mice within 2–4 days following intracerebral inoculation. Infected mouse brain generally serves as a very useful source of complement-fixing antigens.

Whenever large volumes of virus with relatively low concentrations of extraneous protein are required, e.g., for biophysical and biochemical studies or for vaccine production, cell cultures and line cells in particular are the host systems of choice. In view of their extremely wide spectrum of susceptibility, BHK-21 and Vero cells are most commonly used for this purpose. Other cell lines used include

L929, LLC-MK$_2$, KB, HEp-2, HeLa, MS (monkey stable), and PS (pig stable).

Certain orbiviruses have been shown to replicate in Singh's mosquito cell lines, particularly in the *Aedes albopictus* cell line (Buckley, 1969, 1972), without the production of cytopathic effects. Viruses of the Kemerovo group, however, produce plaques in these cells (Yunker and Cory, 1975).

Of particular interest is the development of persistently infected cultures of *Aedes albopictus* cells carrying African horsesickness virus (Mirchamsy *et al.*, 1970) and Irituia, Palyam, and Lebombo viruses (Buckley, 1972).

2.3. Cytopathology

Most orbiviruses produce fairly characteristic cytopathic effects in cell cultures. These effects consist mainly of focal or disperse rounding off of cells accompanied by increased refractivity and eventual detachment from the glass. In the case of BTV and most of the others, cytopathic changes extend rapidly to involve the entire cell sheet, whereas in a few (e.g., the equine encephalosis serogroup) changes tend to remain localized with the formation of macroscopically visible foci or plaques (Erasmus, unpublished). Stained cell cultures generally show condensation of the cytoplasm, sometimes with the formation of intracytoplasmic inclusion bodies, pyknosis of the nucleus, karyorrhexis, and, finally, disintegration of the cell structure.

The cytopathic changes produced by BTV in lamb kidney cells were first described by Haig *et al.* (1956). Fernandes (1959) observed similar effects in a number of cell lines he surveyed. Livingston and Moore (1962) described the presence of inclusion bodies in the cytoplasm of infected McCoy synovial cells. Bowne and Jochim (1967) described two types of intracytoplasmic inclusion bodies in BTV-infected lamb kidney and McCoy synovial cells. Type I inclusions originated from the perinuclear space within the nuclear envelope. Material accumulated within this space and eventually was pinched off from the outer nuclear membrane, resulting in an intracytoplasmic body surrounded by a single membrane. The significance of these inclusions is unknown. Type II inclusions were granular, not membrane bound, were RNA positive, fluoresced in response to specific conjugated BTV antiserum, and were associated with BT virions electron microscopically.

Cytopathic changes largely similar to those produced by BTV have been described for AHSV (Mirchamsy and Taslimi, 1963; Erasmus, 1964; Ozawa and Hazrati, 1964), EHDV (Tsai and Karstad, 1970; Fosberg *et al.*, 1977), Orungo virus (Tomori *et al.*, 1976), equine encephalosis virus (Erasmus *et al.*, 1970), and various other orbiviruses.

2.4. Assay Systems

Orbiviruses can be titrated in various ways such as by intracerebral inoculation of baby mice, by inoculation of embryonating eggs by the intravascular or yolk sac routes, or in cell cultures. Although the dilution end-point method based on the appearance of cytopathic effects in roller tube cell cultures is still used, it has been replaced by the more accurate plaque assay in many instances.

Plaque techniques have been described for BTV in L929 cells (Howell *et al.*, 1967; Thomas and Trainer, 1970), in BHK-21 cells (Jochim and Jones, 1976), and in Vero cells (Barber and Jochim, 1973). Similar techniques have also been described for EHDV (Willis *et al.*, 1970; Barber and Jochim, 1975; Jochim and Jones, 1976), Ibaraki virus (Suzuki *et al.*, 1977), AHSV (Ozawa and Hazrati, 1964; Oellermann, 1970; Erasmus, 1972), CTFV (Deig and Watkins, 1964), the Kemerovo group of viruses (Libíková and Buckley, 1971), and various other orbiviruses. A few orbiviruses were among the large number of viruses shown to produce plaques in Vero and LLC-MK$_2$ cells by Stim (1969).

3. THE VIRION

3.1. Morphology

Some of the viruses included in Table 1, especially those isolated from insect hosts, are difficult to cultivate and purify in sufficient quantities for biochemical studies. Morphological features have therefore remained one of the most important criteria, and sometimes the only one, for their classification as orbiviruses. In fact, the name of the genus is derived from a morphological feature, namely the characteristic ringlike capsomere structure (*orbis* is Latin for "ring") seen on the surface of the viral capsid. This feature clearly distinguishes members of the genus orbivirus from the other Reoviridae.

3.1.1. Size

Most orbiviruses have been studied electron microscopically in thin sections of infected cells using positive staining techniques with electron-dense metal salts such as uranyl acetate and lead citrate after fixation in glutaraldehyde and/or osmium tetroxide. A diameter of 65–70 nm was found in most cases, but slight differences may exist between the various subgroups. For AHSV the diameter was estimated to be about 70 nm (Polson and Deeks, 1963; Lecatsas and Erasmus, 1967). Murphy *et al.* (1971) recorded diameters of 65–75 nm for Lebombo virus, 60–65 nm for the Changuinola subgroup, 60–65 nm for BTV and EHDV, and 65–70 nm for Palyam virus. Average diameters of 63–71 nm were found for all five groups of Australian isolates (Corriparta, Eubenangee, Palyam, Warrego, and Wallal) by Carley and Standfast (1969), Schnagl and Holmes (1971), and Lecatsas and Gorman (1972).

Size determinations of negatively stained virions yielded more variable results, and a range of particle sizes from 40 to 80 nm has been reported. Negative staining with phosphotungstate does not involve fixation and virions generally appear somewhat larger than positively stained particles. Because they are seen as translucent particles with an indistinct outline against an electron-dense background (see Fig. 1), these particles are difficult to measure accurately, contributing to the discrepancy introduced by the preparative technique.

Two other phenomena have caused considerable confusion about the size of orbivirus particles, especially in the early literature. The first is the occurrence of "enveloped" particles resulting from the release of virus from the infected cell by a budding process. This method of release seems to predominate in the case of certain viruses such as Eubenangee (Schnagl and Holmes, 1971), but in most others only a few membrane-associated virions are found. As these membranes can be removed by treatment with Tween 80 and ether without loss of infectivity, they are not considered part of the virion and were termed "pseudoenvelopes" (Els and Verwoerd, 1969).

The second cause of confusion was associated with the method used for purification of orbiviruses. For example, in the case of BTV, particles with a diameter of 68–70 nm were found in nonpurified preparations or in virus purified on sucrose gradients whereas most particles purified by isopyknic centrifugation on neutral CsCl gradients had a diameter of 54 nm (Els and Verwoerd, 1969; Verwoerd *et al.*, 1972). This discrepancy was resolved when it was demonstrated that

BTV possesses a double-layered capsid. Complete virions consist of core particles, with a clearly defined capsomere structure, surrounded by a diffuse outer layer. This outer layer, which causes its "fuzzy" appearance and was first thought to be of cellular origin, was shown to be essential for infectivity and coded for by the viral genome (Verwoerd *et al.*, 1972; Martin and Zweerink, 1972).

Core particles with diameters close to that of BTV have also been demonstrated in the case of AHSV (Breese *et al.*, 1969; Oellermann *et al.*, 1970), various Australian isolates (Lecatsas and Gorman, 1972), Ibaraki virus (EHDV group) (Ito *et al.*, 1973), and EHDV (Kontor and Welch, 1976).

3.1.2.   Structure

The presence of a diffuse, structureless outer capsid layer has been demonstrated in all the viruses mentioned so far and seems to be characteristic of the orbiviruses, distinguishing them morphologically from the reoviruses and rotaviruses. One possible exception is Colorado tick fever virus, which, although closer to reovirus both in size (80 nm) and in morphology (Murphy *et al.*, 1968), is nevertheless included in the orbivirus group on the strength of its biological and physicochemical properties (Borden *et al.*, 1971).

The differences between the orbiviruses, reoviruses, and rotaviruses are illustrated in Fig. 1, where the indistinct diffuse outer layer of BTV is compared with the structured but featureless outer capsid of reovirus and the sharply defined outer layer characteristic of the rotaviruses (Palmer *et al.*, 1977).

Regarding the structure of the core particle, there now seems to be general agreement that the inner capsid layer consists of 32 capsomeres arranged in icosahedral symmetry with the triangulation number T-3 (Els and Verwoerd, 1969; Bowne and Ritchie, 1970; Oellermann *et al.*, 1970; Murphy *et al.*, 1971), although earlier papers (Polson and Deeks, 1963; Owen and Munz, 1966; Studdert *et al.*, 1966; Breese *et al.*, 1969) often proposed an icosahedron consisting of 92 capsomeres, analogous to the suggested structure for reovirus (Luftig *et al.*, 1972). The capsomeres are tubelike hollow structures 10–12 nm wide with an axial hole about 4 nm in diameter. They are about 8 nm in length and consist of smaller structural units arranged in regular hexagonal and pentagonal patterns. These measurements have been carried out for BTV (Els and Verwoerd, 1969), AHSV (Oellermann *et al.*, 1970), and EHDV (Tsai and Karstad, 1970). In a study of XBM/67 virus (EHDV

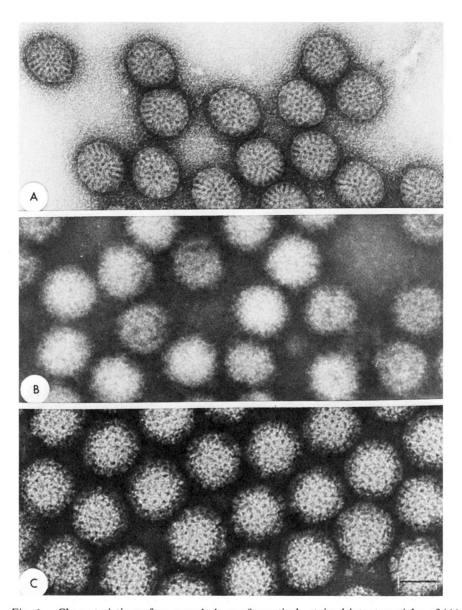

Fig. 1. Characteristic surface morphology of negatively stained intact particles of (A) rotaviruses, (B) orbiviruses (BTV), and (C) reoviruses (type 3). For the typical capsomere structure of orbivirus core particles, revealed by the removal of the diffuse outer layer, see Fig. 2. ×200,000. Bar equals 75 nm.

group) in thin sections, Lecatsas and Erasmus (1973) proposed a substructure of 12 spherical subunits for the core particles.

Electron micrographs of a number of other orbiviruses suggest a structure very similar, if not identical, to that of the prototype BTV. For comparison, the morphology of some representatives of the orbivirus genus is presented in Fig. 2, showing both core particles and complete virions.

In conclusion, it should be noted that, although morphology will probably remain the primary criterion for the preliminary classification of newly discovered orbiviruses, it can sometimes be misleading and should always be used in conjunction with other characteristics of this genus. A case in point is the etiological agent of Gumboro or infectious bursal disease of chickens. Morphologically these viruses are very similar to the orbiviruses, but a lower density, reflecting a lower RNA content, and possibly a differently structured RNA genome preclude inclusion of this agent in the genus orbivirus at present.

3.2. Physicochemical Properties

3.2.1. Physical Properties

The determination of the physical properties of the orbiviruses is complicated by the fact that the complete particle can readily lose both polypeptide and nucleic acid components and be converted to core particles, empty particles, and intermediate forms. This is particularly true when the virus is highly purified and studied under artificial experimental conditions. For example, the BT virion can be converted on neutral CsCl gradients to core particles or to an intermediate form by the loss of one or two polypeptides. Somewhat conflicting values have been reported for the densities of the virion and core particle of BTV (Martin and Zweerink, 1972; Verwoerd et al., 1972). In a recent reinvestigation of these densities in which labeled reovirus cores and virions were used as internal control markers, values of 1.36 for the virion and 1.40 for the core were found (van Dijk and Huismans, unpublished results). This result agrees with the values found for EHDV cores and virions (Huismans et al.. 1979) and is also in close agreement with values reported for AHSV (Bremer, 1976).

Sedimentation constants have been determined only for BTV. Verwoerd (1969) used partially purified material and reported a biphasic sedimentation pattern with an approximate sedimentation constant of 650 S for the fastest-moving component. Martin and Zweerink (1972)

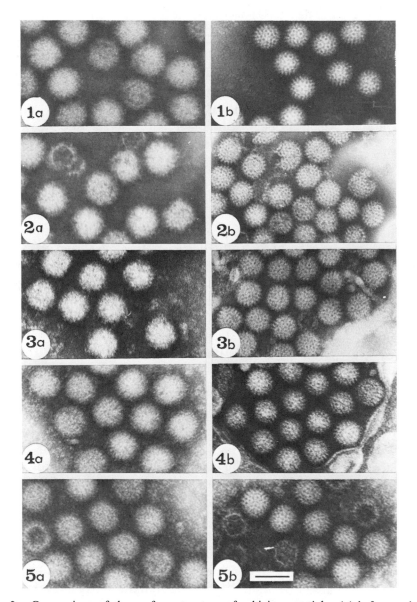

Fig. 2. Comparison of the surface structure of orbivirus particles (a) before and (b) after removal of the outer protein layer. Note the difference in size between the particles in (a) and (b), both negatively stained with phosphotungstate. Viruses illustrated are 1, BTV; 2, AHSV; 3, Wallal virus; 4, equine encephalosis virus; 5, EHDV. ×120,000. Bar equals 75 nm.

found sedimentation constants of 550 S and 470 S, respectively, for their light (L) and dense (D) particles.

3.2.2. Chemical Composition

The only data available are those reported for BTV purified on sucrose gradients (Verwoerd, 1969). Chemical analysis of these preparations, which probably contained a low percentage of cores and empty particles, indicated that the virion is composed of approximately 20.0% RNA and 80.0% protein. A small amount of phospholipid (1–2%), consisting mainly of cholesterol, was also found but was considered to be due to contamination with cellular material.

From these figures and the independently determined molecular weights of the individual nucleic acid components (see Section 3.3), a total complement of 11.8×10^6 daltons of dsRNA and 47.2×10^6 daltons of protein can be calculated, from which an approximate particle mass of 60×10^6 daltons can be estimated for BTV (Verwoerd et al., 1972). The base composition of the viral RNA yielded a G+C value of 42.4 and a (A+G)/(U+C) ratio of 1.00, indicating complete base paring (Verwoerd, 1969). Further proof of its double-strandedness is discussed in Section 3.3 dealing with the viral genome.

3.2.3. Stability

Much attention has been focused on the relative stability of the orbiviruses to lipid solvents and sodium deoxycholate and on their lability at a low pH, since these characteristics served to distinguish them from the other arthropod-borne viruses on the one hand and from reovirus on the other. In a study of a group of so-called uncategorized arboviruses, including BT, CTF, AHS, Irituia (Changuinola group), EHD, Chenuda, Tribec, Wad Medani, Lebombo, Palyam, Eubenangee, and Corriparta viruses, Borden et al. (1971) found that, in contrast to the absolute sensitivity of togaviruses, the reduction in infectivity of these viruses caused by lipid solvents or sodium deoxycholate was less than $10^{1.5}$ suckling mouse intracerebral LD_{50}. This degree of sensitivity was also significantly different from the absolute resistance of reovirus. Resistance to treatment with ether at 1°C for 22 hr was also recently demonstrated for representatives of four of the five Australian orbivirus groups, Wallal being the exception. On the other hand, in the case of chloroform only Corriparta virus resisted treatment at 1°C for 22 hr

(Gorman, 1978). It is not known what the mechanism of inactivation by lipid solvents is in the case of orbiviruses, since they do not possess a lipid-containing envelope. It is known, however, that most of the viruses in this group are closely associated with cellular membranes in the infected cell and that their infectivity is stabilized by external material. One can therefore conjecture that treatment with lipid solvents acts through removal of these external stabilizers or through denaturation of viral proteins.

Much the same applies to the temperature stability of the orbiviruses. Although some subgroups, e.g., Palyam, are less stable than others, orbiviruses on the whole are regarded as reasonably thermostable viruses. The demonstration of viable bluetongue virus in blood stored for 25 years at room temperature indicated a marked thermostability (Neitz, 1948). Svehag (1963a), also using nonpurified virus, confirmed this in a study of the thermal inactivation of BTV at pH 7.0. On the other hand, Howell et al. (1967) found that purified virus was extremely unstable at higher temperatures when all extraneous protein was removed. Stabilization could be achieved by the addition of 1% albumin, serum, or other protein.

It is important to note that stability in these studies was solely determined by measuring infectivity. The significance of this was realized when Verwoerd et al. (1972) demonstrated that removal of the outer capsid layer of BTV reduces its infectivity by at least 5 orders of magnitude. Instability in the context of loss of infectivity therefore reflects the loss of the outer polypeptides rather than instability of the core particle. The role of extraneous protein in stabilizing infectivity can probably be explained in terms of prevention of the dissociation of the outer polypeptides.

In their study of the group of viruses quoted above, Borden et al. (1971) found that exposure to pH 3.0 for 3 hr completely abolished all infectivity. In a study of the stability of BTV, Owen (1964) found a marked loss of infectivity below pH 6.5, and Svehag et al. (1966) found a narrow zone of stability for BTV between pH 6.0 and 8.0. Similar results were obtained for CTV (Murphy et al., 1968) and for six Australian orbiviruses (Gorman, 1978). Removal of the diffuse outer layer is probably not the main mechanism for the inactivation of orbiviruses at low pH values. When investigating the loss of the outer layer polypeptides from BT virions on CsCl gradients, Verwoerd et al. (1972) observed that the core particle remained essentially intact above pH 5.0, but a further increase in acidity led to a complete disruption of the virions. The acid sensitivity of orbiviruses is in stark contrast to the pronounced resistance to inactivation shown by reovirus at low pH values (Stanley, 1967).

3.3. The Viral Genome

3.3.1. Double-Strandedness

BTV was the first orbivirus found to possess a double-stranded RNA genome (Verwoerd, 1969). Since then many more viruses have been isolated and provisionally classified as orbiviruses. Only a limited number of these have, however, been shown to contain dsRNA. There are several criteria that have been used to establish the double-strandedness of Reoviridae (Joklik, 1974). Of these the most commonly used in the studies on orbiviruses are:

1. The heterochromatic staining of the inclusion bodies in infected cells by acridine orange.
2. The characteristic sharp melting profile of the isolated RNA.
3. Its relative resistance to degradation by pancreatic ribonuclease.
4. A base composition reflecting base pairing of A and U as well as G and C.

Apart from BTV, the following orbiviruses were shown to contain dsRNA on the basis of one or more of these criteria: CTFV (Green, 1970), AHSV (Oellermann, 1970), EHDV (Tsai and Karstad, 1973), Kemerovo virus (Rosenbergová and Slávik, 1975; Kontor and Welch, 1976), Warrego and Mitchell River viruses (Gorman *et al.*, 1977*a*), and Ibaraki virus (Suzuki *et al.*, 1977). In the case of other members of the Eubenangee, Palyam, Wallal, and Corriparta groups, the characteristic electrophoretic profiles of their RNA suggest double-strandedness (Schnagl and Holmes, 1975; Gorman *et al.*, 1976; Gorman and Taylor, 1978).

Purified orbiviruses, e.g., BTV (Verwoerd *et al.*, 1970) and AHSV (Bremer, 1976), contain dsRNA as the only nucleic acid component. This is in contrast to reovirus, in which as much as 20–25% of the total RNA is present as low molecular weight, single-stranded oligonucleotides (Bellamy and Joklik, 1967; Shatkin and Sipe, 1968*a*), for which no biological function is known (Nichols *et al.*, 1972).

The molecular weights reported for the RNA genomes of orbiviruses vary between 11.0×10^6 and 12.0×10^6 (Verwoerd *et al.*,

1972; Schnagl and Holmes, 1975; Bremer, 1976; Gorman *et al.*, 1977*a*). This is significantly lower than the molecular weights of the other members of the Reoviridae family such as cytoplasmic polyhedrosis virus (CPV) (Payne and Rivers, 1976), rice dwarf virus (RDV) (Fujii-Kawata *et al.*, 1970), wound tumor virus (WTV) (Reddy and Black, 1973), and reovirus (Shatkin *et al.*, 1968), all of which possess a dsRNA genome with a molecular weight of the order of 15×10^6.

3.3.2. Segmentation

The most characteristic feature of the dsRNA genome of the Reoviridae is the fact that it is composed of a number of differently sized segments. Sucrose gradient sedimentation analyses of the RNA extracted from orbiviruses show a heterogeneous size distribution ranging from 8.5 to 15.5 S. This was first shown for BTV (Verwoerd *et al.*, 1970) and later for AHSV (Oellermann, 1970). The dsRNA of CTFV virus (Green, 1970) and Kemerovo virus (Rosenbergová and Slaŭik, 1975) sediments with a peak region at 14 S.

The separation of the RNA into size classes is greatly improved by electrophoretic fractionation on polyacrylamide gels. A typical fractionation pattern of the dsRNA of two of the Australian orbiviruses, Warrego and Tilligerry viruses, is shown in Fig. 3. Ten different genome segments can be distinguished, separated into a distinctive pattern. Genome segments are numbered in each case in order of decreasing size.

Figure 4 shows the size distribution of dsRNA segments of most of the orbiviruses that have been studied so far. Also shown is the electrophoretic fractionation pattern of the reovirus genome.

The ten segments found in all orbiviruses investigated are typically distributed into three groups of three segments each, with the tenth and smallest segment in a size class of its own. The differences in size between the members of the three groups are generally larger than those within the reovirus size groups. However, in some cases, e.g., EHDV and AHSV, the third size group can be resolved into three segments only with difficulty.

The orbivirus RNA pattern is quite distinct from that of reovirus, which can, in turn, be easily distinguished from other members of the Reoviridae such as CPV (Payne and Rivers, 1976), RDV (Fujii-Kawata *et al.*, 1970), and rotaviruses (Rodger *et al.*, 1975; Obijeski *et al.*, 1977). The size distribution of the RNA segments of an unknown dsRNA virus can therefore be used as a preliminary criterion for its classification.

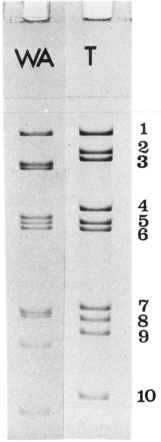

Fig. 3.   Gel electrophoretic separation of the dsRNA segments of Warrego (WA) and Tilligerry (T) viruses.

3.3.3.   Linkage of the Genome Segments

The observed segmentation of the dsRNA genome raises the question of whether or not the segments are linked inside the virion. Evidence of linkage in the case of reovirus was found in the electron microscope when mildly disrupted virions occasionally showed long RNA filaments, corresponding in size to the total molecular weight of the genome, after spreading by the Kleinschmidt technique (Dunnebacke and Kleinschmidt, 1967; Granboulan and Niveleau, 1967). This was also shown for CPV (Nishimura and Hosaka, 1969). In the orbivirus group electron microscopic evidence of linkage has been reported for EHDV (Tsai and Karstad, 1973) and BTV (Els, 1973; Foster *et al.*, 1978). Linkage by means of normal covalent phosphodiester bonds is unlikely because of the reproducible fragmentation pattern obtained after extraction of the RNA. Furthermore, the fact that the BTV segments are transcribed individually (Huismans and Verwoerd, 1973) would suggest that the segments are functionally distinct inside the intact virion. Evidence that the RNA of reovirus is present as segments inside the virion is summarized by Silverstein *et al.* (1976).

The 5'- or 3'-terminal sequences of the RNA segments of orbiviruses have not yet been determined. The only information available is for other double-stranded RNA viruses such as reovirus (Banerjee *et al.*, 1971; Chow and Shatkin, 1975; Furuichi *et al.*, 1975), CPV (Furuichi and Miura, 1973), and WTV (Lewandowski and Leppla, 1972).

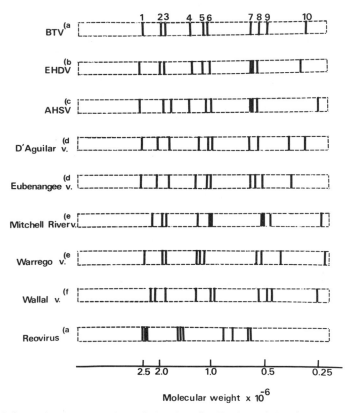

Fig. 4. Schematic representation of the size distribution of the dsRNA genome segments of a number of orbiviruses on polyacrylamide gels. The original separations were carried out by (a) Verwoerd *et al.* (1972), (b) Huismans *et al.* (1979), (c) Bremer (1976), (d) Schnagl and Holmes (1975), (e) Gorman *et al.* (1977a), and (f) Gorman *et al.* (1977b).

3.3.4. Homology between Viral Genomes

Serological techniques have been widely used to study and classify the large number of orbiviruses isolated (see Table 1 and Section 5.2). Many of these isolations were made from the same insects that transmit BTV and AHSV, the two members causing economically important stock diseases. For those countries free of these diseases it is important to be able to determine the relationship of new isolates to the known pathogens as accurately as possible. This has stimulated the exploration of other means of studying the relationship between these viruses, such as determining possible sequence homologies in their genomes. It is also of considerable academic interest to study the degree of homology existing (1) between the various genera of the Reoviridae, (2) between the various serological subgroups of the genus orbivirus, and (3) between the individual members or serotypes. Such studies could yield interesting data concerning the origin and evolution of these viruses. Furthermore, by providing answers to such questions as whether serologically related viruses possess common genome segments, or whether certain genome segments are more likely to be heterologous than others, it may be possible to elucidate the functions coded for by some of the genome segments.

The orbiviruses with their segmented, double-stranded RNA genomes are uniquely suited for homology studies. Not only can the individual corresponding segments of different viruses be compared in size and homology, but also the fact that most of the polypeptides coded for by these segments can be identified gives such homology studies even greater relevance.

Comparing the size of corresponding genome segments constitutes a first step in studying sequence homology. Gorman *et al.* (1977*b*) compared dsRNA derived from a number of isolates belonging to the Wallal group. They found major size differences only between corresponding segments 2 and 5, suggesting that these segments code for polypeptides that constitute the serological determinants of these viruses. In the case of BTV serotypes similar size differences were found between segments 2 and 6 (Huismans, unpublished results).

Homology of the base sequences of different genome segments can be determined by means of molecular hybridization. When single-stranded mRNA, derived from BTV-infected cells, is hybridized with denatured BTV dsRNA, the resulting hybrid is indistinguishable from normal dsRNA (Verwoerd and Huismans, 1972; Huismans and Verwoerd, 1973). This indicates that the mRNA is an exact copy of one of the strands of the dsRNA from which it was transcribed. Homology between genera has been investigated by cross-hybridization of the mRNA and dsRNA of BTV and reovirus. No homology was observed (Verwoerd and Huismans, 1969). The degree of homology between different subgroups is also low and was found to be less than 5% in cross-hybridization of BTV with EHDV and with AHSV (Verwoerd and Huismans, 1969; Huismans *et al.*, 1979).

A much higher degree of cross-hybridization was found between members of subgroups such as the different BTV serotype strains (Huismans and Howell, 1973). Electrophoretic characterization of the hybrids yielded the following results:

1. Complete homology between corresponding genome segments of different serotypes was generally found in only one of the ten genome segments of BTV. In the majority of cases segment 5 was involved which appears to be identical in as many as 80% of all BTV serotypes investigated. This would indicate a remarkable resistance to mutation in this genome segment.

2. Incomplete cross-hybridization of corresponding genome segments, which results in a reduction of the mobility of the hybrid dsRNA segment relative to normal dsRNA (Ito and Joklik, 1972; Schuerch and Joklik, 1973), was generally observed in six of the ten BTV genome segments.

3. Three of the ten genome segments generally showed no cross-hybridization at all with the corresponding segment from another serotype. In almost all of these cases both segments 2 and 6 were involved. Segment 2 never showed cross-hybridization and segment 6 only in a few cases. This result suggests that segment 2 codes for the major serotype-specific polypeptide of the virus and segment 6 for a minor determinant. It is supported by the fact that genome segments 2 and 6 code for the polypeptides forming the outer layer of the virus particle (Verwoerd *et al.*, 1972).

3.4. The Viral Capsid

The original classification of many members of the orbivirus group was not based on their double-strandedness but on morphological and serological evidence, both of which are exclusively determined by the protein coat or capsid of the virus. The morphology of the orbiviruses has been described in Section 3.1. Two differently sized particles are found (Martin and Zweerink, 1972; Verwoerd *et al.*, 1972). The larger of these two particles (L particle) can be converted to the smaller one (core or D particle) by the removal of its outer protein layer.

Only a few of the orbiviruses have been studied with regard to their protein composition, and little work has been done beyond the electrophoretic characterization of the polypeptides. Most of the available data have been obtained in studies involving BTV. Nevertheless, an attempt will be made to point out those features of their protein composition that seem to be characteristic for all orbiviruses and to discuss how differences between certain members of the orbivirus group as well as between members of subgroups are reflected in the protein coat of the virus.

3.4.1. Polypeptide Composition

Polyacrylamide gel electrophoresis of the protein components of purified BTV indicates the presence of seven polypeptides, numbered P1–P7 in the sequence of increasing electrophoretic mobilities (Martin and Zweerink, 1972; Verwoerd *et al.*, 1972). Four of these are major polypeptides that together contribute as much as 94% of the total protein content. The other three are minor components each of which represents about 2% of the total.

The molecular weights of the polypeptides, estimated by comparing their mobilities with those of markers of known molecular weight, range from 30,000 to 140,000 (Verwoerd *et al.*, 1972). The slightly higher values reported by Martin and Zweerink (1972) can probably be ascribed to differences in the molecular weights assigned to the markers used for calibration. The whole question of molecular weights determined in this way must, however, be approached with caution. Cross and Fields (1976) pointed out that a change in the gel and buffer system reverses the electrophoretic mobilities of certain reovirus polypeptides. They suggested that protein modifications such as phosporylation (Krystal *et al.*, 1975) and glycosylation (Krystal *et al.*, 1976) are responsible for these effects. Similar effects would probably have to be taken into account in the case of orbiviruses if a similar gel and buffer system is used.

The proteins of only a few other orbiviruses, including AHSV (Bremer, 1976) and EHDV (Huismans *et al.*, 1979), have been studied. A schematic representation of their electrophoretic mobilities compared with that of BTV is shown in Fig. 5. The electrophoretic fractionation

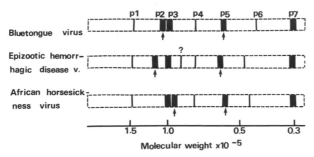

Fig. 5. Schematic representation of the size distribution of the capsid polypeptides of three different orbiviruses on polyacrylamide gels. Major capsid polypeptides are indicated by the broad bands. The arrows indicate polypeptides in the outer capsid layers of the viruses. The question mark indicates a minor polypeptide component found in the outer capsid layer of EHDV which appears to be virus specified. Results shown are those obtained by Huismans *et al.* (1979) and Bremer (1976).

patterns of the proteins of the three orbiviruses are very similar, although EHDV seems to contain an additional minor component. This orbivirus pattern can be distinguished quite easily from that of reovirus, however, even more so than in the case of the dsRNA fractionation patterns. Equally distinctive are the polypeptide patterns of other Reoviridae such as the rotaviruses (Rodger *et al.*, 1975) and CPV (Payne and Rivers, 1976).

3.4.2. Polypeptides in the Outer Capsid

The large L particles of BTV can be converted to cores by centrifugation on CsCl gradients at pH 7.0 (Verwoerd *et al.*, 1972). The conversion is accompanied by the removal of two polypeptides, P2 and P5, which form a protein layer surrounding the smaller core particle. In this layer P2 is probably on the outside because an intermediate form in which P2 is lost but P5 remains attached to the core particle can also be found.

Other orbiviruses display a similar pattern. It was shown that in the case of AHSV the outer protein layer is composed of P3 and P5 (Bremer, 1976) whereas in EHDV polypeptides P2 and P5, as well as an additional polypeptide called P3A, are involved (Huismans *et al.*, 1979). Figure 5 also illustrates that the polypeptide on the outside of the surrounding protein layer (P2 in the case of EHDV and BTV and P3 in AHSV) is the most variable of all the major orbivirus capsid polypeptides with regard to size. In EHDV this polypeptide is much larger than the corresponding one in BTV, whereas it is much smaller in AHSV. The accommodation of polypeptides of various sizes in the loosely structured layer on the outside of these virions may be responsible for the divergence found among different members of the orbivirus group.

These results are substantiated by an experiment in which a comparison was made of the capsid polypeptides present in 12 of the different BTV serotypes (de Villiers, 1974). The largest variation in size was found in polypeptide P2, with smaller variations in a few of the others including the second polypeptide of the outer protein layer, P5. The size variations observed in P2 derived from different serotypes were not so great as those between P2 from different orbiviruses. Polypeptides P2 and P5 are coded for by genome segments 2 and 6 (Verwoerd *et al.*, 1972), and these segments show a similar variability in cross-hybridization experiments (Section 3.3).

3.4.3.   Polypeptides of the Core Particle

The core or D particle of BTV contains two major and three minor polypeptides. The major polypeptides, P3 and P7 in the case of BTV and EHDV and P2 and P7 in the case of AHSV, show very little variation in size. These polypeptides are likely to be the main structural components of the characteristic core capsomers. The symmetry of these structures might require that only polypeptides of a very specific size can be used in their construction. The core particles of orbiviruses differ morphologically from those of other Reoviridae. This difference is also reflected in the size of equivalent major and minor core polypeptides (Verwoerd *et al.*, 1972). Different orbiviruses are therefore mainly distinguished by differences in the outer protein layer, whereas the various genera of the Reoviridae can probably be distinguished also by differences in the polypeptide composition and structure of their core particles.

The location of the polypeptides within the BTV core particle was studied by Martin *et al.* (1973) using an iodination technique. They found that major polypeptide P3 and minor polypeptides P1, P4, and P6 are easily iodinated and therefore located close to the surface of the particle, whereas P7 is less reactive and therefore probably located internally. It is not known which and how many core polypeptides are involved in the transcriptase activity associated with intact BTV core particles (Verwoerd and Huismans, 1972).

3.4.4. Possible Coding Relationship between the Genome Segments and Polypeptides

It was first shown by Zweerink and Joklik (1970) that a remarkable relationship exists between the size of the reovirus genome segments and its polypeptides. If the molecular weight of the theoretical polypeptide which would be coded for by each genome segment is calculated, each of the seven capsid polypeptides coincides almost exactly in size with one of these. This suggested that each genome segment codes for the synthesis of a specific polypeptide and that each of the segments is transcribed and translated in its entirety.

Similar coding relationships were demonstrated for BTV (Martin and Zweerink, 1972; Verwoerd *et al.*, 1972) and AHSV (Bremer, 1976). Since the assumption of complete translation of genome segments has not been proven yet and because of uncertainties about the exact molecular weights of both RNA segments and virus polypeptides, one can regard these assignments only as an approximation. Nevertheless, the relationships lead to the important concept that each genome segment be regarded as a separate gene (or cistron) coding for the synthesis of a specific viral polypeptide.

3.5. Viral Enzymes

3.5.1. RNA Polymerase

A dsRNA-dependent RNA polymerase or RNA transcriptase was first discovered in reovirus (Shatkin and Sipe, 1968b; Borsa and Graham, 1968; Skehel and Joklik, 1969). The possession of such an enzyme is probably a characteristic of all viruses containing a dsRNA genome, however, since known cellular enzymes do not transcribe dsRNA.

Of all the known orbiviruses, an RNA polymerase has been demonstrated only in BTV (Verwoerd *et al.*, 1972; Martin and Zweerink, 1972). In reovirus the enzyme is activated by the removal of the outer capsid proteins by means of heat shock, low concentrations of SDS, or treatment with chymotrypsin (Silverstein *et al.*, 1976). Similarly, the enzyme can be demonstrated in the case of BTV after removal of the outer layer polypeptides. This has been achieved by centrifugation in CsCl gradients at pH 7.0 (Verwoerd *et al.*, 1972) or by isolation of naturally occurring core particles (Martin and Zweerink, 1972). It has recently been found, however, that BTV virions can also be activated by chymotrypsin in the presence of Mg ions. It was demonstrated that the removal of outer capsid polypeptide P5 is Mg^{2+} dependent (Van Dijk and Huismans, unpublished results).

The enzyme activity is associated with the intact core particle. Further dissociation of the particle completely eliminates all activity (Verwoerd and Huismans, 1972), and it is therefore not known which of the five core polypeptides are associated with the enzyme.

The activity of the enzyme can be assayed *in vitro* by measuring the incorporation of nucleotide triphosphates into acid-precipitable RNA (Martin and Zweerink, 1972; Verwoerd and Huismans, 1972). This assay showed that the reaction is dependent on Mg ions, is stimulated by the presence of Mn ions, and has an optimum pH range of 8.1–8.5.

An interesting characteristic of the enzyme is its maximum *in vitro* activity at 28°C. This is in sharp distinction to both reoviruses and rotaviruses, for which an optimum temperature of 45–50°C has been demonstrated (Cohen, 1977).

This low optimum temperature is possibly related to the fact that BTV is transmitted by and can replicate in an insect host. It might even by regarded as an indication that BTV is basically an insect and not a mammalian virus. If this is true, it could be a common characteristic of all orbiviruses, distinguishing them from other members of the Reoviridae. Some support for this hypothesis is the observation that a number of orbiviruses can replicate in *Aedes albopictus* cell cultures, whereas reovirus cannot (Buckley, 1969).

The product of the *in vitro* transcription was shown to consist of ten segments of RNA which can be hybridized with the RNA genome isolated from purified BTV. The absence of any self-hybridization indicated that it is single-stranded (Verwoerd and Huismans, 1972).

3.5.2. Other Enzymes

In the case of reovirus, a number of other enzyme activities associated with the virion have been demonstrated, including capping and methylating enzymes and nucleotide phosphohydrolases (Silverstein *et al.*, 1976). None of these activities has so far been demonstrated in any orbivirus.

4. REPLICATION

4.1. Adsorption and Penetration

BTV can replicate in a wide variety of cell types (Haig *et al.*, 1956; Fernandes, 1959). Adsorption kinetics, however, have only been studied in the case of L strain mouse fibroblasts infected with BTV (Howell *et al.*, 1967). Under the conditions used (pH 7.4 and a temperature of 37°C) the adsorption rate was rapid. During the first 15 min it was approximately exponential, and adsorption was essentially complete after 30 min.

Penetration of BTV and AHSV into the cell interior was shown to proceed by a process of pinocytosis (Lecatsas and Erasmus, 1967; Lecatsas, 1968). Virus is transported into the cell interior in pinocytotic vesicles. The appearance of lysozymelike bodies with dense inclusions shortly after infection suggests that the particles are partly degraded in these structures.

4.2. Site of Replication

Orbiviruses generally seem to replicate in the perinuclear area of the cytoplasm in association with granular to reticular inclusions or matrices. These intracytoplasmic viral "factories" are common to all Reoviridae, but the morphogenesis of the orbiviruses is not so closely associated with the spindle tubules of the mitotic apparatus as that of reovirus. Association of maturing virions with fine filaments and with tubules of approximately the same diameter as the virus or smaller is commonly found. After maturation, virions are often seen associated with membranous structures and are eventually liberated from the cell either by a process of dissolution of the cell membrane or rarely by extrusion in which case the virion may be surrounded by a membranous "pseudoenvelope." These features have been described, with minor variations, for AHSV (Lecatsas and Erasmus, 1967), BTV (Bowne and Jochim, 1967; Lecatsas, 1968), CTFV (Murphy *et al.*, 1968), Corriparta virus (Lecatsas *et al.*, 1969), EHDV (Tsai and Karstad, 1970), and for the Kemerovo group (Murphy *et al.*, 1971; Karmysheva *et al.*, 1973), five Australian isolates (Schnagl and Holmes, 1971), Wallal virus (Gorman and Lecatsas, 1972), equine encephalosis virus (Lecatsas *et al.*, 1973), and Ibaraki virus (Ito *et al.*, 1973).

4.3. Synthesis of Viral Nucleic Acids

4.3.1. *In Vivo* Synthesis of mRNA

The first important step in the replication of orbiviruses after the virus has penetrated into the cell is the transcription of the dsRNA genome segments into ten species of single-stranded mRNA containing all the information encoded in the corresponding dsRNA segments. Little is known about the initial steps leading to *in vivo* transcription in orbivirus-infected cells. By analogy to reovirus, one can assume that the virus particles are never fully uncoated but are modified by full or partial removal of one or more of the proteins in the outer capsid layer of the virus. This conversion to subviral particles (SVP) has been studied extensively in reovirus-infected cells, and recent reviews by Silverstein *et al.* (1976) and Joklik (1974) summarize the results. An analogy between orbiviruses and reovirus in this respect is suggested by the fact that transcriptase activity in BTV particles is also unmasked *in vitro* after partial removal of the outer protein layer of the virus (Verwoerd *et al.*, 1972).

Information on the transcription process in orbivirus-infected cells has been derived mainly from experiments with BTV (Huismans, 1970*a*). The rate of mRNA synthesis is low during the first 6 hr after infection but gradually increases until a maximum is reached 8–13 hr after infection. Subviral particles derived from parental virus are probably involved in synthesis of ssRNA during the early period of infection whereas progeny SVP are responsible for late ssRNA synthesis. The ssRNA synthesized is heterogeneous with regard to size, with S values on sucrose gradients ranging from 12 S to 23 S (Huismans, 1970*a*). Proof that all ten genome segments are transcribed *in vivo* is derived from hybridization experiments (Verwoerd and Huismans, 1972).

4.3.2. Regulation of Transcription

Specific regulation of protein synthesis at the level of transcription has been studied by determining the ratio of mRNA species formed in BTV-infected cells (Huismans and Verwoerd, 1973).

In Table 2 the molar ratio of *in vivo* synthesized mRNA is compared to the molar ratio of *in vitro* synthesized mRNA. Also shown is the ratio that would be expected if the ten different genome segments

TABLE 2

Molar Ratio in Which the BTV mRNA Species Are Synthesized *in Vivo* and *in Vitro* Compared to the Predicted Molar Ratio If the Ten Genome Segments Are Transcribed at a Molar Proportion Inversely Proportional to Their Molecular Weight

RNA species	Molecular weight $\times 10^{-6}$	Molar ratio (%)		
		Predicted[a]	*In vivo*[b]	*In vitro*[b]
1	2.50	3.1	3.8	4.0
2	1.99	3.9	5.3	4.2
3	1.82	4.2	4.2	3.8
4	1.31	5.9	8.0	6.6
5	1.16	6.7	18.2	18.2
6	1.08	7.2	8.1	7.0
7	0.60	13.0	12.8	12.0
8	0.54	14.4	16.5	20.1
9	0.50	15.4	12.0	12.1
10	0.30	26.0	11.1	11.9

[a] Calculated by normalizing the reciprocal of the molecular weight of the different dsRNA species to a percentage.
[b] Huismans and Verwoerd (1973).

are individually transcribed at a constant rate of chain growth. Under these conditions the molar proportion of mRNA species would be inversely proportional to the molecular weights of the ten genome segments. Only in the case of two segments is a significant deviation from the anticipated result apparent. Genome segment 5 is transcribed more than twice as frequently and segment 10 with half the expected frequency.

Since the molar ratio obtained during *in vitro* transcription is very similar, the factors controlling the process are probably an inherent property of the transcriptase particle itself. This is supported by the observation that the *in vivo* regulation of transcription is unaffected by inhibition of protein synthesis (Huismans and Verwoerd, 1973). In the case of EHDV, genome segment 5 is also transcribed much more frequently than expected (Huismans *et al.*, 1979).

These results are at variance with those obtained for reovirus, where the ratio of mRNA species found *in vivo* differs significantly from the *in vitro* result (Skehel and Joklik, 1969; Banerjee and Shatkin, 1970; Zweerink and Joklik, 1970).

4.3.3.   Synthesis of dsRNA

Apart from its involvement in translation, orbivirus mRNA probably also plays an important role as a template for the synthesis of dsRNA. No work has been done on this aspect of orbivirus replication. It has been intensively studied in the case of reovirus, however, and there is no reason to doubt the validity of these results for other members of the Reoviridae. The most important point about the replication of the dsRNA genome is that it is fully conservative. Replication takes place by using single-stranded mRNA (plus strands) as the template for the synthesis of complementary minus strands (Schonberg *et al.*, 1971).

A particle possessing ssRNA-dependent dsRNA polymerase activity and representing the active site of dsRNA synthesis has been partially purified and characterized by Zweerink *et al.* (1972), Zweerink (1974), and Morgan and Zweerink (1975). According to Acs *et al.* (1971), most of the precursor plus strands are formed early in the replicative cycle, but Morgan and Zweerink (1977) claim that any ssRNA synthesized during the infection cycle can function as the template for dsRNA synthesis. It remains an intriguing question how one copy of each of the ten mRNA species is correctly assembled inside this replicase particle which is a precursor of the progeny virion.

4.4.   Synthesis of Viral Proteins

Two important questions should be considered regarding the synthesis of viral proteins. The first is whether or not all ten mRNA species are translated into corresponding polypeptides. The other concerns the frequency of translation and the possible involvement of a regulatory system for the process of translation.

4.4.1.   Synthesis of Capsid and Noncapsid Polypeptides

It has been demonstrated by Verwoerd *et al.* (1972) that the BTV capsid contains seven polypeptides. Three of the mRNA species are therefore either not translated or code for nonstructural polypeptides. In order to distinguish between these two possibilities, a study was made of the synthesis of BTV-specific polypeptides in infected cells.

Synthesis of BTV proteins can first be demonstrated in infected cells during the period 2–4 hr after infection at 31°C (Huismans, 1979).

The rate of synthesis increases rapidly until 11 hr after infection; thereafter it remains at about the same level until 26 hr after infection. During this period synthesis of all seven capsid polypeptides is demonstrable. In addition, two polypeptides called P5A and P6A, with respective molecular weights of 54,000 and 40,000, are synthesized. These polypeptides are not found in uninfected cells.

Polypeptide P5A is synthesized in very large quantities, especially late in the infection cycle. Most of it is associated with a complex that sediments on sucrose gradients as a heterogeneous peak with a sedimentation constant in the region of 400 S. Electron microscopy (Huismans and Els, 1979) indicates that the complex consists of hollow tubular structures that contain P5A as the only protein component. The tubules found in AHSV- and EHDV-infected cells have also been characterized. The size of the respective tubule polypeptides is very close to that of P5A in BTV-infected cells, but the diameter of the tubules is characteristic for each virus and is on average 18 nm for AHSV and 54 nm for EHDV as compared to 68 nm for BTV (Huismans and Els, 1979). The difference is illustrated in the electron micrographs shown in Fig. 6. In the EHDV- and BTV-associated tubules there is a striking linear periodicity, giving the tubules a ladder-like appearance with steps 9 nm apart.

Nothing is known about the role of these tubular structures in replication. They were first observed in BTV-infected cells (Lecatsas, 1968) and later also in cells infected with other orbiviruses such as EHDV (Tsai and Karstad, 1970; Thomas and Miller, 1971), CTFV (Murphy et al., 1968), the Kemerovo and Changuinola groups (Murphy et al., 1971), and AHSV (Oellermann et al., 1970; Lecatsas and Erasmus, 1967).

Most of the available evidence (Huismans and Els, 1979) suggests that the tubules in orbivirus-infected cells are virus specified and quite different from microtubules seen in uninfected cells and from the spindle tubules associated with reovirus replication (Spendlove et al., 1963; Dales et al., 1965). Tubules have also been described in association with rotaviruses (Holmes et al., 1975; Kimura and Murakami, 1977). These workers proposed that they are formed by aberrant assembly of viral capsid material, which is not the case with the orbivirus-associated tubules since they are composed of a noncapsid polypeptide.

Little is known about P6A, the other noncapsid polypeptide found in BTV-infected cells. Evidence for virus specificity is based mainly on the fact that it is precipitated from the soluble protein fraction of BTV-

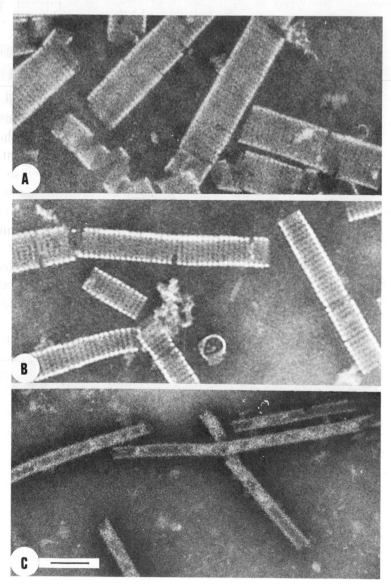

Fig. 6. Electron micrographs of negatively stained tubular structures associated with (A) BTV, (B) EHDV, and (C) AHSV. Note the differences in diameter. ×150,000. Bar equals 75 nm.

infected cells by BTV antiserum (Huismans, 1979). However, the possibility that P6A is a modified form of one of the capsid polypeptides cannot be ruled out at this stage. Recent results (Bremer and Huismans, unpublished observations) indicate the P6A is a phosphorylated polypeptide.

If both polypeptides p6A and P5A are primary gene products it would leave the translation product of the smallest mRNA segment (10) unaccounted for. This mRNA is capable of coding for a polypeptide of about 16,000 daltons (Verwoerd et al., 1972), but no such polypeptide has as yet been found in infected cells.

4.4.2. Control of Translation

In BTV-infected cells the mRNA species are associated with polyribosomes in a ratio corresponding to that in which they are synthesized (Huismans and Verwoerd, 1973). The same observation was made in the case of reovirus (Ward et al., 1972). This could be interpreted to indicate the absence of translation control. However, all mRNA species isolated from the polyribosome fractions are not necessarily involved in translation (Joklik, 1974).

Regulation of the translation process would be reflected by the synthesis of viral polypeptides in a ratio other than that in which the corresponding mRNA's are transcribed, or by selective translation during the early and late stages of the infection cycle.

There is no evidence in BTV-infected cells of "early" and "late" protein synthesis. The ratio in which polypeptides are synthesized very early after infection is much the same as late in the infection cycle (Huismans, 1979). Neither is there any convincing evidence that the rate of translation of the different mRNA species is controlled. Only the noncapsid polypeptide P5A is synthesized at a rate markedly increased above those of the other polypeptides (Huismans, 1979). However, this result is not necessarily an indication of translation control. It could also be explained by a relative excess of the mRNA coding for polypeptide P5A. If the coding assignment between genome segments and polypeptides as proposed by Martin and Zweerink (1972) and Verwoerd et al. (1972) is correct, polypeptide P5A could only be coded for by genome segment 5. As shown in Table 2, segment 5 is transcribed with a frequency at least twice as high as any of the others. No evidence therefore exists for the selective control of translation.

This result differs from what has been reported in the case of reovirus (Joklik, 1974; Both et al., 1975). Neither the in vivo nor the in *vitro* translation of the reovirus polypeptides was directly related to the relative abundance of corresponding mRNA species.

The *in vitro* translation of BTV mRNA species into corresponding polypeptides has not been carried out as yet. Such an experiment should prove interesting, both to clarify the question of possible translation control and to provide additional evidence that the noncapsid polypeptides P5A and P6A are virus specified.

4.5. Mutants and Defective Particles

Both temperature-sensitive (*ts*) mutants and defective particles (deletion mutants) have been widely used in the study of the replication of reovirus (Joklik, 1974; Silverstein *et al.*, 1976). The use of mutants in the study of orbivirus replication is, by comparison, still in its infancy, since mutants have been isolated only in the case of BTV and some of the Australian orbiviruses. Their use in the study of viral replication has also been very limited so far.

4.5.1. Temperature-Sensitive Mutants

Shipham and De la Rey (1976) isolated 19 stable *ts* mutants of BTV which they were able to classify genetically into six recombination classes. *N*-Methyl-*N*-nitroso-*N*-nitroguanidine, 5-fluorouracil, and nitrous acid were found to be the most effective mutagens. As in the case of reovirus, exchange of genetic material between BTV *ts* mutants is believed to take place by independent assortment of genome segments, probably at the level of assembly of the ten ssRNA segments into a viral precursor particle. Complementation studies have also been carried out, but the results are not conclusive.

Gorman *et al.* (1976) isolated 13 stable *ts* mutants of Wallal virus, falling into three recombination classes, and four of Mudjinbarry virus, which belongs to the same serological group. They found recombination between some of the Mudjinbarry viruses and members of groups II and III of the Wallal *ts* mutants. Considerable variation in recombination frequencies occurred, similar to that described for BTV. An interesting result was obtained in a study of the RNA patterns of recombinant Mudjinbarry and Wallal *ts* mutants (Gorman *et al.*, 1978). The RNA isolated from such a recombinant contained nine segments indistinguishable from those of Wallal virus and one segment (segment 5) identical in size to its equivalent in Mudjinbarry virus. This observation supports the proposed mechanism of recombination by exchange of genome segments in orbiviruses.

In the case of BTV *ts* mutants some further characterization has been carried out. In temperature-shift experiments, Shipham and De la Rey (1979) found that two groups could be classified as early and four groups as late mutants. One late mutant was found to lack the ability to synthesize ssRNA during the late period of infection at the nonpermissive temperature. A shift from 28°C (permissive temperature) to 38°C resulted in an immediate inhibition of ssRNA synthesis in cells infected by the *ts* mutant. This result suggested that the synthesis of ssRNA by progeny virus particles was involved. A second mutant was found to accumulate corelike particles at a late stage of infection at the nonpermissive temperatures. Outer capsid polypeptides P2 and P5 were synthesized, but no fully infectious virions were assembled.

4.5.2. Defective Particles

Preliminary studies (Hellig and Jennings, personal communication) indicate that defective particles are formed in BTV-infected cells. Plaque-purified BTV passaged at a high multiplicity of infection undergoes a 2 log reduction in yield between the 16th and 20th passages. The high-passage tissue culture material is highly inhibitory for the replication of normal low-passage virus. Purification and preliminary characterization of the inhibitory factor indicated that it consists of defective particles.

Similar effects will probably also be found in the case of other orbiviruses, and many of the reported low yields may be related to interference by defective particles.

4.6. Effect of Viral Infection on Cellular Functions

The synthesis of virus-specific components in orbivirus-infected cells has been dealt with in the sections on RNA and protein synthesis. One remaining question is how host-specific cellular synthesis is affected by viral replication.

4.6.1. Host-Cell Macromolecular Synthesis

Infection of a suspension culture of L cells results in a rapid shutoff of host cell protein and DNA synthesis shortly after infection

(Huismans, 1970*b*). There is no inhibition of RNA synthesis before 7 hr after infection. The length of the lag phase before the inhibition of protein synthesis is initiated depends on the multiplicity of infection. Suspension cultures of L cells infected with reovirus under exactly the same conditions show no such effect (Huismans, 1971).

No viral replication or protein synthesis is required for inhibition (Huismans, 1970*b*). One possible mechanism for the rapid inhibition of protein synthesis in L cells is related to the fact that dsRNA is an extremely potent inhibitor of protein synthesis both *in vivo* and *in vitro*. (Ehrenfeld and Hunt, 1971; Robertson and Mathews, 1973; Hunter *et al.*, 1975). It is conceivable that infection with an abnormally large number of BTV particles results in abnormal uncoating of the virions. Some of the RNA may leak out of partially uncoated particles and subsequently cause the inhibition of protein synthesis. Reovirus is much more stable than orbiviruses and may not be affected in the same way.

The inhibition of host cell macromolecular synthesis is much less marked in infected monolayers of L cells than in suspension cultures. This could be due to the fact that monolayer cultures probably adsorb smaller numbers of virus particles compared to suspension cultures.

4.6.2. Interferon Synthesis

A further response of cells to infection with orbiviruses is the synthesis of interferon. BTV can induce interferon synthesis in both primary mouse embryo cells and mice (Huismans, 1969; Eksteen and Huismans, 1972). The most interesting aspect is, however, a report by Jameson *et al.* (1978) that described BTV as one of the most potent interferon inducers ever found. They found that injection of mice with a high dose of purified virus ($10^{8.3}$ plaque-forming units) resulted in an interferon yield of as much as 680,000 units/ml, which is more than a tenfold increase above the yield obtained with reovirus type 3.

5. ANTIGENIC PROPERTIES

5.1. Serological Reactions

5.1.1. Neutralization

The serum–virus neutralization test is generally accepted as the most sensitive serological technique to demonstrate minor antigenic differences between orbiviruses and to assay type-specific neutralizing antibodies. Standard procedures are generally used, sometimes with minor modifications.

The neutralization test with BTV has been performed in a number of host systems with varying success (Howell and Verwoerd, 1971). Roller tube cell cultures have been used by Haig *et al.* (1956) and by Howell (1960), who was able to recognize 12 distinct serotypes of BTV. Embryonated eggs and suckling mice have also been used (Goldsmit and Barzilai, 1968; Klontz *et al.*, 1962; Svehag, 1963b, 1966). All these tests had the disadvantages, however, of being very laborious and unsuitable for the detection of low levels of antibody. The plaque-inhibition technique described by Howell *et al.* (1970) greatly facilitated and simplified the serotyping of BT viruses. The test has since been further improved by the substitution of fish-spine beads with filter paper disks (Erasmus, 1977). Whatman antibiotic assay disks (6 mm) are saturated with serotype-specific guinea pig serum and lyophilized in screw cap bottles. Whenever required, these dry disks are placed in appropriate positions on the agarose overlay of BTV-infected petri dish cell cultures. The handling of dry disks greatly facilitates the procedure and results in a more economical use of typing reagents.

Although the plaque-inhibition technique can be used for the demonstration of neutralizing antibodies in test sera, it has the disadvantages of not being strictly quantitative and of not being very sensitive in that low levels of antibody cannot be detected. These disadvantages were overcome by the development of highly sensitive plaque-reduction techniques (Barber and Jochim, 1973, 1975; Erasmus, 1977; Jochim and Jones, 1976; Thomas *et al.*, 1976; Thomas and Trainer, 1970, 1971). The test can be performed in multiwell disposable plastic panels and thus lends itself to some degree of automation. Yet, despite the obvious advantages of the plaque-reduction neutralization test, the results obtained by various workers show certain discrepancies. In the hands of the American and South African workers the test is highly serotype specific, whereas a considerable degree of cross-neutralization between heterologous serotypes is obtained by the Canadian workers (Thomas *et al.*, 1976).

Plaque-reduction neutralization tests have also been described for the identification and serotyping of EHD virus (Barber and Jochim, 1975; Jochim and Jones, 1976; Thomas and Trainer, 1971).

The neutralization test for the identification of AHSV or antibody can be conducted in mice (Alexander, 1935; McIntosh, 1958), in roller tube cell cultures (Hazrati and Ozawa, 1965), by plaque inhibition (Erasmus, 1977), and by plaque-reduction neutralization (Hopkins *et al.*, 1966). Neutralization tests in roller tube cell cultures or plaque-inhibition tests were used for the identification of the equine encephalosis viruses and for the demonstration of antibodies specific for this virus (Erasmus *et al.*, 1970, 1976*a*).

Few details are available regarding neutralization tests for the lesser-known orbiviruses, but it is conceivable that the standard techniques would be applicable to most members of the genus.

5.1.2. Complement Fixation (CF)

Complement fixation is probably the most commonly used serological technique for the identification of orbiviruses and their classification into serogroups. Standard procedures are generally employed, and with few exceptions CF antigens are prepared from infective mouse brains by sucrose–acetone extraction as described by Clarke and Casals (1958). Sera and ascitic fluids are usually prepared by hyperimmunization of laboratory animals.

The CF test generally detects group-specific rather than type-specific antigens and antibodies and is therefore very useful to demonstrate wider relationships between viruses. CF antibodies are usually relatively short lasting, and high CF titers are therefore indicative of recent infections and may thus often be of great diagnostic and epidemiological significance.

A CF test for BTV using mouse brain extracts was first described by Van den Ende *et al.* (1954), and an improved method, particularly suitable for the testing of bovine sera, has been developed by Robertson *et al.* (1965) and by Boulanger *et al.* (1967). Shone *et al.* (1956) have shown that a satisfactory BTV CF antigen could be prepared from infected cell cultures. CF antigens prepared by these procedures still contain high titers of infective virus, and the use of such antigens may pose a risk to countries free of the disease. It was, however, possible to prepare a safe but effective inactivated antigen by exposure to low pH and ultraviolet irradiation (Erasmus and French, unpublished observations).

CF tests have also been described for AHS virus (McIntosh, 1956), equine encephalosis virus (Erasmus *et al.*, 1970, 1976*a*), Kemerovo viruses (Libíková and Casals, 1971), and various other orbiviruses (Borden *et al.*, 1971).

5.1.3. Immunodiffusion

Immunodiffusion tests generally involve soluble antigens and their antibodies and are therefore group specific rather than type specific. In contrast to the CF test, immunodiffusion is technically very simple, and very small volumes of reagents are required for the microimmunodiffusion technique. This test is therefore ideally suited for large-scale serological surveys.

An agar gel precipitin (AGP) technique for BTV was first described by Klontz *et al.* (1962) and later also by Jochim and Chow (1969), Metcalf and Jochim (1970), Boulanger *et al.* (1970), and Boulanger and Frank (1975). Wang *et al.* (1972) have described a method for the purification and concentration of a BTV soluble antigen from infected lamb kidney cells.

Despite its obvious advantages, the immunodiffusion technique has not been widely applied to the remaining members of the orbivirus genus.

5.1.4. Immunofluorescence

The fluorescent antibody technique is particularly useful for the rapid identification of viruses in cells and for studies on viral pathogenesis.

Immunofluorescence was used extensively in the study of BTV (Bowne and Jochim, 1967; Ruckerbauer *et al.*, 1967). It was applied very elegantly by Stair (1968) in a study of the pathogenesis of BT.

Fluorescent antibody procedures were also used for EHDV (Jochim *et al.*, 1974*a*) and AHSV (Davies and Lund, 1974; Ozawa, 1966; Tessler, 1972) as well as for other orbiviruses.

5.1.5. Hemagglutination

Unlike the togaviruses, orbiviruses do not readily hemagglutinate erythrocytes. However, hemagglutinins have been demonstrated in brain extracts of mice infected with AHSV (Pavri, 1961; Pavri and Anderson, 1963). The same authors also proved that hemagglutination could be inhibited by homologous type-specific antisera.

It has recently been demonstrated that purified BTV does agglutinate erythrocytes of various species and that the hemagglutination can be inhibited by homologous antibodies (Van der Walt, 1979). This test may therefore provide a simple method for the serotyping of BTV or for the detection of type-specific antibodies. It may well be that other orbiviruses may similarly cause specific hemagglutination after virus purification and concentration.

A passive hemagglutination test for the detection of BTV antibodies has been described by Blue *et al.* (1974), but little is known at present with regard to the practical value of the procedure.

5.2. Serological Classification

Orbiviruses are presently grouped on the basis of serological relationships and viruses that are related by CF are grouped together. However, as with other arboviruses, orbiviruses do not always fit neatly into their respective serogroups, and the problem of intergroup relationships or intragroup variation is becoming more pertinent. Clear directives concerning the magnitude of the differences required to create a new serogroup should be formulated. It may well be, however, that the attempt to group orbiviruses into well-defined serogroups is too artificial and that an absolutely satisfactory classification on this basis may be unattainable as the relationships between these viruses may be more spatial than linear.

The BTV serogroup presently consists of 20 serotypes which show complete cross-reactions in CF tests but can be distinguished by means of neutralization tests. The 20 serotypes are composed of the 16 types previously described by Howell *et al.* (1970), type 17, which represents one of the four American serotypes (Barber and Jochim, 1975), types 18 and 19, which were isolated in South Africa (Erasmus, 1977), and type 20, which was recently isolated in Australia (Erasmus, unpublished observations; St. George *et al.*, 1978).

The members of the EHDV serogroup show considerable crossing in CF but are distinct in neutralization tests. In addition to the New Jersey and Alberta serotypes, the group includes viruses isolated from *Culicoides* in Nigeria (Lee *et al.*, 1974) and South Africa (Erasmus, unpublished observations). Ibaraki virus has also been shown to be related to EHDV (Campbell *et al.*, 1977), and XBM/67 (Lecatsas and Erasmus, 1973) similarly falls in this group.

The AHSV serogroup is composed of nine serotypes (Howell, 1962), and the equine encephalosis subgroup consists of four serologically distinct viruses (Erasmus *et al.*, 1976*a*).

Other recognized subgroups are:

Palyam (Palyam, Kasba, Vellore, Abadina, D'Aguilar, and Nyabira)
Warrego (Warrego and Mitchell River)
Wallal (Wallal and Mudjinbarry)
Corriparta (Corriparta and Acado)
Eubenangee (Eubenangee, Pata, and Tilligerry)

Changuinola (Changuinola, Irituia, and others)
Colorado tick fever (CTF, Eyach)

The Kemerovo subgroup is a very heterogeneous serogroup, and certain viruses such as Chenuda and Wad Medani show very little relationship to the rest of the group (Libíková and Casals, 1971).

Certain other orbiviruses which show no relationship to any of the established serogroups or which have not been adequately characterized are presently regarded as ungrouped orbiviruses (see Table 1).

5.3. Antigens Involved in Antigenic Variation

Antigenic variation in viruses reflects differences in the protein coat. It should therefore be possible to relate the observed antigenic variation in orbiviruses to specific polypeptides in the virus capsid.

One approach in attempting such a study has been described in the section on capsid polypeptides. It is based on a comparison of the polypeptide compositions of different antigenic variants by gel electrophoresis. The results indicate that the polypeptide on the outside of the protein layer which surrounds the core particle (P2) is mainly implicated in antigenic variation (De Villiers, 1974). However, these experiments provide only indirect evidence because the results reflect differences in the size of the polypeptides and not differences between the antigenic determinants actually responsible for the variation. A more direct approach would be to compare the specificity of antibodies for homologous and heterologous serotype protein. Such experiments require a source of soluble virus proteins, which, in the case of orbiviruses, is readily available in the soluble protein fraction of infected cells.

Antigenic variation among the different serotypes of BTV was studied by precipitating ^{14}C-labeled BTV proteins with homologous and heterologous antisera and comparing the immune precipitates by means of electrophoresis and autoradiography. In such experiments the main difference between homologous and heterologous immune precipitates was the fact that polypeptide P2 is precipitated only with homologous antiserum (Huismans and Erasmus, unpublished results). This indicates that P2 is the main serotype-specific antigen in BTV. This result confirms previous conclusions drawn from hybridization experiments (Huismans and Howell, 1973).

P2 was also identified as serotype specific when a similar experiment was carried out using the EHDV strains Alberta and New Jersey

(Huismans, unpublished observation), and the same result will probably be obtained for the other orbiviruses.

In order to identify the antigen(s) in the group-specific CF reaction in the case of BTV, attempts were made to correlate CF titers in sera with the ability to precipitate soluble virus proteins (Huismans and Erasmus, unpublished results).

In all cases investigated the CF titers seemed to correlate with ability to precipitate P7. From this result it was concluded that P7 is the main determinant of group specificity. Other polypeptides may, however, also be involved.

5.4. Immunity

Infection with orbiviruses is generally followed by the appearance of a variety of antibodies and by an immune state. Immunity associated with specific neutralizing antibodies is usually long lasting and in many instances of lifelong duration. CF antibodies, on the other hand, are usually of relative short duration and may reach low or undetectable levels within a few months.

Immunity can also be artificially induced by the administration of live or inactivated viral vaccines. The first orbivirus vaccine, consisting of virus attenuated by serial intracerebral passage in mice, was prepared against AHSV (Alexander, 1936). Its use also represented one of the first applications of the concept of multivalent immunization. However, despite its obvious value, the neurotropic mouse brain vaccine had a number of disadvantages (Erasmus, 1966), most of which could be eliminated by the attenuation of AHSV in various mammalian cell culture systems (Erasmus, 1965, 1976; Mirchamsy and Taslimi, 1964). Mirchamsy *et al.* (1972) also achieved attenuation of AHSV in mosquito cell cultures. Inactivated vaccines have been described by Bourdin *et al.* (1969), Mirchamsy *et al.* (1969), Ozawa and Bahrami (1966), and Parker (1975).

BTV was attenuated by serial passage in embryonating eggs by Alexander (1947), and a polyvalent attenuated vaccine has been used extensively (for references, see Howell and Verwoerd, 1971). Its application and some of the problems associated with the use of attenuated BTV vaccine have been discussed, and the need for an inactivated vaccine as well as for a vaccine for cattle has been indicated (Erasmus, 1975c).

Immunization of bighorn sheep against BTV was attempted both by inoculation and by the use of experimentally-infected *Culicoides* gnats (Robinson *et al.*, 1974).

Ibaraki virus was attenuated by serial passage in chick embryo cell cultures, and administration of the attenuated virus to cattle induced neutralizing antibodies that persisted for at least 3 years (Omori, 1970). Koprowski *et al.* (1950) used a live chick embryo-adapted CTFV as a vaccine, but it proved to be insufficiently attenuated and a formalized vaccine has since been developed (Thomas *et al.*, 1963).

Bovine fetuses were shown to respond immunologically to BTV, even when inoculated at 5 months' gestation, but such calves were not fully resistant to challenge exposure after birth (Jochim *et al.*, 1974*b*).

The finding that the development of specific antibodies does not necessarily lead to the termination of viremia is of great practical concern. Erythrocyte-associated BTV in the presence of demonstrable antibodies has been observed in cattle and sheep (Luedke, 1969, 1970; Luedke *et al.*, 1969, 1977*d*). Similar associations have been described for AHSV in horses (Ozawa *et al.*, 1972) and in zebra (Erasmus *et al.*, 1976*b*) and for CTFV in man (Hughes *et al.*, 1974). It is very likely that association with erythrocytes is a basic phenomenon common to most orbiviruses, and it evidently plays a very significant epidemiological role by prolonging viremia.

Administration of orbiviruses to animals does not invariably lead to a state of immunity. Luedke and Jochim (1968) demonstrated that oral administration of BTV to sheep followed by parenteral inoculation of the homologous virulent virus resulted in an intensified clinical reaction. A similar state of "sensitization" has been observed in horses immunized with poorly immunogenic AHSV and subsequently challenged with homologous virulent virus. This phenomenon could be very important in nature, where transmission of very low levels of virus by insect vectors may sensitize animals to subsequent exposure (Erasmus, 1976).

6. EPIZOOTIOLOGY

6.1. Host Range

Since most if not all orbiviruses replicate in and are biologically transmitted by insect vectors, these viruses could perhaps be considered as insect viruses with the potential to infect mammalian hosts as well. However, information regarding the natural mammalian host range for the various orbiviruses is as yet very incomplete. Available data are largely limited to (1) hosts which develop overt clinical disease and which can therefore not be regarded as true natural hosts but merely as accidental or indicator hosts, and (2) hosts which develop inapparent infections and which are incriminated on serological evidence or on account of fortuitous virus isolations.

It is not intended to present a complete checklist of hosts for the various orbiviruses but merely to draw attention to some of the more pertinent virus–host relationships. More detailed information is to be found in the *International Catalogue of Arboviruses* (Berge, 1975).

Bluetongue had traditionally been regarded as a disease of sheep and to a lesser degree of cattle and goats (for references, see Erasmus, 1975a,b; Hourrigan and Klingsporn, 1975a,b; Howell and Verwoerd, 1971). In more recent years it became evident that the natural host range of BTV is extremely wide and includes species such as deer, big-horn sheep, and most species of African antelope (for details, see Davies and Walker, 1974; Hoff *et al.*, 1973; Hoff and Hoff, 1976; Hourrigan and Klingsporn, 1975b). The outcome of infection may range from fatal to inapparent, with the latter situation prevailing in African game species which have been exposed to this virus for centuries. The duration and level of viremia vary among different species as well as among individuals of the same species. In sheep the viremia reaches a relatively high peak and usually coincides with a febrile reaction, although on occasion it has been possible to isolate virus from the first day after infection to as late as 31 days after infection (Luedke, 1969). Essentially the same applies to cattle and goats since virus could readily be isolated from blood samples collected up to 28 days after infection (Luedke, 1970). However, the Denver workers have made very interesting observations on latent or chronic BTV infection in cattle which is characterized by a viremia, albeit sometimes sporadic, for an indeterminate time (Bowne *et al.*, 1968; Luedke *et al.*, 1970). Of particular interest and practical significance were the findings that biological recovery of BTV from latently infected animals could often be effected only by feeding of the insect vector following prior stimulation of virus ("showering") by insect bites (Luedke *et al.*, 1977d). These observations corroborated the earlier views of Du Toit (1962) and Nevill (1971) regarding the role of cattle as overwintering hosts for BTV.

EHDV infects various species of deer (white-tailed, black-tailed, mule, and elk) and pronghorn antelope (Hoff and Hoff, 1976; Stauber *et al.*, 1977). Serological evidence of infection with EHD-related viruses isolated in South Africa was found in cattle and sheep, and experimental infection of sheep with these viruses resulted in inapparent infection (Erasmus, unpublished observations). Ibaraki virus is pathogenic for cattle but merely produces a low-grade viremia and antibody formation in experimentally infected sheep (Inaba, 1975).

The host range of AHSV includes horses, mules, donkeys, and zebra. Infection of zebra is essentially subclinical but in contrast to other Equidae virus could still be isolated from the blood 27 days after artificial infection and from organs after 40 days (Erasmus *et al.*, 1976*b*). A very high percentage of elephant sera react positively in complement-fixation tests (Davies and Otieno, 1977; Erasmus *et al.*, 1976b), but the significance of these findings is still not clear. No unequivocal evidence of AHSV replication could be obtained by the artificial infection of young elephants (Erasmus *et al.*, 1976*b*). Dogs can also become infected by the ingestion of infective carcass material but apparently play no epizootiological role (Dardiri and Ozawa, 1969).

The viruses of the equine encephalosis subgroup were all isolated from horses, and serological surveys have indicated a high incidence of antibody in horses but not in other domestic animals (Erasmus, unpublished observations).

Antibodies to Warrego and Eubenangee viruses were found in cattle, kangaroos, and wallabies, to Wallal virus in kangaroos and wallabies, and to Corriparta virus in man, cattle, horses, wallabies, kangaroos, domestic fowls, and wild birds (Doherty, 1972).

The viruses of the Palyam subgroup seem to be associated with cattle. Nyabira virus was isolated on several occasions from aborted bovine fetuses (Swanepoel and Blackburn, 1976), and D'Aguilar virus has been isolated from the blood of a cow (St. George and Dimmock, 1976). Serological evidence of infection was obtained for D'Aguilar virus in cattle and sheep (Doherty, 1972) and for Abadina virus in cattle and goats (Moore and Kemp, 1974).

CTFV is a very important pathogen of man, but its host range also includes rodents such as ground squirrels, chipmunks, and deer mice (Burgdorfer and Eklund, 1959, 1960). Very little is known about the host range of the Kemerovo serogroup, but evidence of infection has been found in man (Kemerovo, Lipovnik, Tribec), cattle (Kemerovo, Seletar, Tribec), and small mammals and birds (Berge, 1975).

6.2. Transmission

The role of bloodsucking insects as vectors of certain orbiviruses (e.g., AHSV, BTV) was surmised long ago. The biological transmission of certain orbiviruses by insects has been proved only in more recent years, however, and the arbovirus status of many orbiviruses is based on incomplete evidence such as isolation of the particular virus from wild-caught insects or replication of virus in insects following artificial infection. For a large number of orbiviruses the vectorial role of insects is merely surmised on the grounds of circumstantial epizootiological data or by extrapolation of evidence obtained for closely related viruses. Nevertheless, insect transmission as the mode of spread can be postulated with confidence for most if not all orbiviruses. Orbiviruses comply with the prerequisites for insect transmission (high viremia for relatively long periods and replication over a wide temperature range). Transmission by other means (e.g., contact) has not been demonstrated and is unlikely in view of the low concentration of virus in body secretions or excretions.

Du Toit (1944) first focused attention on biting midges (*Culicoides*) as biological vectors of bluetongue, and his findings have since been conclusively confirmed with colonized *C. variipennis* (Foster *et al.*, 1963, 1968; Luedke *et al.*, 1976). *Culicoides* has also been shown to transmit AHSV (Mellor *et al.*, 1975) and EHDV (Foster *et al.*, 1977; Jones *et al.*, 1977). In addition, EHD-related viruses have been isolated from wild-caught *Culicoides* in Nigeria (Lee *et al.*, 1974) and in South Africa (Erasmus, unpublished observations). Based on virus isolations, *Culicoides* has been incriminated as a vector for viruses of the Warrego and Wallal serogroups (Doherty, 1972).

Mosquitoes have been incriminated as nonvertebrate hosts for the Corriparta, Eubenangee, and Palyam serogroups and for certain unclassified orbiviruses (Berge, 1975; Doherty, 1972). It is of interest, however, that two members of the Palyam serogroup (Abadina and D'Aguilar) have been isolated from *Culicoides* only (Doherty, 1972) or from *Culicoides* as well as from mosquitoes (Lee *et al.*, 1974).

Most of the members of the Changuinola serogroup have been isolated from *Phlebotomines*, and these insects conceivably act as biological vectors for these viruses.

CTFV probably constitutes the best-known example of an orbivirus transmitted biologically by ticks. All the members of the Kemerovo group are transmitted by or have at least been isolated from ticks of the following genera: *Argas, Boophilus, Ixodes, Ornithodoros,* and *Rhipicephalus* (Berge, 1975).

Mechanical transmission of orbiviruses by hematophagous insects such as *Tabanidae, Stomoxys, Simulium, Melophagus, Haematopinus,* and others should also be considered in the epizootiology of orbiviruses, although it is probably of lesser significance than biological transmission.

6.3. Ecological Factors

On account of the involvement of insect vectors, the incidence and distribution of orbiviruses will be governed to a very large extent by ecological factors which favor optimal insect breeding and activity. The most important ecological factors are rainfall, temperature, relative altitude, and wind. Consequently, the seasonal occurrence of many orbivirus diseases is not unexpected.

The incidence of viruses transmitted by midges (*Culicoides*) and mosquitoes is influenced more directly and to a much greater extent by optimal climatic conditions than that of viruses transmitted by ticks. This is probably related to the shorter life-span of midges and mosquitoes, and hence diseases transmitted by these vectors will tend to have more of an epidemic (epizootic) nature than tick-borne diseases.

High rainfall alternating with very hot, humid conditions is optimal for most insects. Insect numbers and activity and hence the incidence of orbiviruses will therefore generally start increasing during late spring, reach a climax toward late summer or autumn, and diminish abruptly within days of the first frost or onset of winter weather.

The role of prevailing winds has seldom been considered in epizootiological studies of orbiviruses. Sellers (1977) and Sellers *et al.* (1977), however, presented interesting data to incriminate strong prevailing winds as a very important factor in the spread of diseases such as BT and AHS. Infected midges can be blown over vast distances in a matter of a few hours. In this way outbreaks in previously uninfected areas or countries can be initiated. This fact poses a grave problem for international disease control.

6.4. Pathogenesis

Knowledge about the pathogenesis of orbivirus infections is limited to a few members of the group. This paucity of knowledge can, at least partially, be ascribed to the fact that relatively few orbiviruses produce serious disease in man or domestic animals.

The first symptom of BTV infection in sheep is a febrile reaction accompanied or even preceded by a viremia. In the blood, virus is primarily associated with the erythrocyte component and to a much lesser degree with the buffy coat fraction (Hoff and Trainer, 1974; Luedke, 1970). Vascular lesions are considered to be the primary injury (Thomas and Neitz, 1947), and the results of some well-executed experiments allowed Stair (1968) to postulate that BTV multiplies in vascular endothelial cells with eventual vascular occlusion, stasis, and exudation. This in turn leads to hypoxia of overlying epithelium with secondary development of lesions in the epithelium. The severity of secondary lesions is greatly influenced by mechanical stress, abrasion, and bacterial infection. A correlation between the distribution of the lesions and the temperature gradients within the host is also suggested. The most severe lesions are invariably observed in tissues exposed to the environment (e.g., oral mucosa, hooves) and hence with a temperature lower than that of the internal structures (Stair, 1968). Lymphoid tissues have also been implicated as an important site of BTV replication (Pini, 1976). The mortality rate in BT varies markedly and is influenced by factors such as pathogenicity of the infecting virus, exposure to sunlight or to adverse weather conditions, and the breed of sheep. African breeds of sheep generally develop a milder form of the disease than others.

Congenital malformation in lambs has been associated with naturally occurring BTV infection as well as with modified live BTV vaccine (Cordy and Shultz, 1961; Griner et al., 1964; Osburn et al., 1971a,b; Richards and Cordy, 1967; Schmidt and Panciera, 1973; Shultz and DeLay, 1955). Lambs infected at 50–58 days of gestation developed a severe necrotizing encephalopathy which presented as hydranencephaly at birth. Lambs infected at 75–78 days developed multifocal encephalitis and vacuolation of the white matter while infection at 100 days of gestation resulted in a mild focal encephalitis with minimal pathological sequelae (Osburn et al., 1971a).

Hydranencephaly and other congenital deformities as a result of natural or experimental BTV infection have also been observed in calves (Barnard and Pienaar, 1976; Luedke et al., 1970, 1977a; Richards et al., 1971). Depending on fetal age at the time of infection, newborn calves may either remain immunologically competent or become tolerant to BTV and may become latently infected after exposure to bites of BTV-infected Culicoides midges (Luedke et al., 1977b,c).

The mortality rate in deer infected with BTV is extremely high, but the gross pathology and pathogenesis are essentially similar to those in sheep (Karstad and Trainer, 1967; Stair et al., 1968). EHDV infection in white-tailed deer is clinically indistinguishable from BT, and its pathogenesis is considered to be a combination of damage to vascular walls and abnormalities of platelets resulting in extensive hemorrhages, tissue degeneration, and necrosis (Debbie and Abelseth, 1971; Fletch and Karstad, 1971). Viremia is also associated with the erythrocyte fraction of the blood (Hoff and Trainer, 1974). Ibaraki disease of cattle resembles BT clinically, and their pathogenesis could conceivably also be similar (Inaba, 1975; Omori, 1970).

The pathogenesis of AHS bears some similarity to that of BT. Virus replication occurs mainly in the lungs, spleen, and lymph nodes (Erasmus, 1972). The most significant effect of virus replication is the development of a state of increased permeability of capillaries in specific organs or regions of the body, which explains not only the symptomatology but also the outcome of the disease. Evidence has been obtained that field strains of AHSV are composed of a mixed population with regard to tissue tropism. Some virus particles apparently multiply selectively in endothelial cells lining pulmonary capillaries, while others replicate in lymphoid tissue such as lymph nodes, spleen, thymus, and pharyngeal mucosa (Erasmus, 1972).

Equine encephalosis virus produces a very low incidence of clinical disease in horses and is characterized by marked nervous symptoms and peracute death. Histopathological examination reveals extensive brain edema but no classical evidence of encephalitis (Erasmus et al., 1970). It is conceivable that the virus causes an increased permeability of cerebral capillaries and that death as a result of the cerebral edema follows peracutely before perivascular white cell infiltrations, characteristic of viral encephalitis, can develop. The closely related Bryanston virus has also been associated with brain edema and with cardiac muscle degeneration leading to eventual cardiac fibrosis and sudden death from cardiac arrest (Erasmus et al., 1976a).

Certain orbiviruses have been associated with fetal death and abortion. These include BTV (Luedke et al., 1977a) and Nyabira virus (Swanepoel and Blackburn, 1976) in cattle and Bryanston virus in horses (Erasmus et al., 1976a). It is very likely that infection of pregnant animals with other orbiviruses likewise results in abortion or fetal malformations, and orbiviruses may eventually prove to be very important pathogens in this respect.

7. CONCLUDING REMARKS

Biological and biochemical studies on orbiviruses have revealed some characteristics unique for this group. Although orbiviruses were initially regarded as mammalian viruses, it is becoming clear that only a few are pathogenic to mammals and that the vast majority are probably nonpathogenic viruses of invertebrates. Serological studies have revealed a complicated pattern of relationships based on antigenic determinants common to certain serogroups on the one hand and type-specific antigens within the groups on the other.

The various orbiviruses are morphologically very similar, and all have the same basic structure consisting of ten segments of dsRNA and a double-layered capsid composed of seven polypeptides, each probably coded for by one of the genome segments or "genes." The structure of the viral genome and the mechanism by which it is replicated facilitate genetic reassortment, and this enhanced exchange of genetic information is probably partly responsible for the very existence of so many closely related orbiviruses.

The fact that both the polypeptides and the genome segments involved in this antigenic variation could be identified makes the orbivirus genus eminently suitable for studies of the evolution of viral serogroups and serotypes. Similarly, the availability of such a large genetic pool in a group of viruses with widely different host specificities and pathogenicities should facilitate the study of these important biological phenomena on a molecular level.

Further comparative studies of the various orbiviruses can therefore be expected to contribute significantly to our understanding of some basic problems in virology.

Acknowledgments

The authors wish to acknowledge the collaboration of Mr. H. J. Els in all electron microscopic studies and in contributing the electron micrographs in Figs. 1, 2, and 6, with the exception of Fig. 1A, which was kindly supplied by Dr. E. L. Palmer, Centre for Disease Control, Atlanta, Georgia, and Fig. 2 (4), which was obtained from Dr. G. Lecatsas, University of Pretoria, South Africa. We also wish to thank Dr. B. Gorman, Queensland Institute of Medical Research, Australia, for providing Fig. 3 as well as unpublished material.

8. REFERENCES

Acs, G., Klett, H., Schonberg, M., Christman, J., Levin, D. H., and Silverstein, S. C., 1971, Mechanism of reovirus double-stranded ribonucleic acid synthesis *in vivo* and *in vitro*, *J. Virol.* **8:**684.

Alexander, R. A., 1933, Preliminary note on the infection of white mice and guinea-pigs with the virus of horsesickness, *J. S. Afr. Vet. Med. Assoc.* **4**:1.

Alexander, R. A., 1935, Studies on the neurotropic virus of horsesickness. III. The intracerebral protection test and its application to the study of immunity, *Onderstepoort J. Vet. Sci.* **4**:349.

Alexander, R. A., 1936, Studies on the neurotropic virus of horsesickness. V. The antigenic response of horses to simultaneous trivalent immunization, *Onderstepoort J. Vet. Sci.* **7**:11.

Alexander, R. A., 1947, The propagation of bluetongue virus in the developing chick embryo with particular reference to the temperature of incubation, *Onderstepoort J. Vet. Sci.* **22**:7.

Andrewes, C. H., and Pereira, H. G., 1967, *Viruses of Vertebrates*, Bailliére, Tindall and Cassell, Ltd. London.

Bando, B. M., 1975, Isolation of bluetongue and epizootic hemorrhagic disease viruses in cell culture, *Proc. 18th Annu. Meet. Am. Assoc. Vet. Lab. Diagn.*, Portland, Ore.

Banerjee, A. K., and Shatkin, A. J., 1970, Transcription *in vitro* by reovirus-associated ribonucleic acid-dependent polymerase, *J. Virol.* **6**:1.

Banerjee, A. K., Ward, R. L., and Shatkin, A. J., 1971, Cytosine at the 3′-termini of reovirus genome and *in vitro* RNA, *Nature (London) New Biol.* **232**:114.

Barber, T. L., and Jochim, M. M., 1973, Serological characterization of selected bluetongue virus strains from the United States, *Proc. 77th Annu. Meet. U.S. Anim. Hlth. Assoc.*, pp. 352–359.

Barber, T. L., and Jochim, M. M., 1975, Serotyping bluetongue and epizootic hemorrhagic disease virus strains, *Proc. 18th Annu. Meet. Am. Assoc. Vet. Lab. Diagn.*, Portland, Ore., pp. 149–162.

Barnard, B. J. H., and Pienaar, J. G., 1976, Bluetongue virus as a cause of hydranencephaly in cattle, *Onderstepoort J. Vet. Res.* **43**:155.

Bellamy, A. R., and Joklik, W. K., 1967, Studies on the A-rich RNA of reovirus, *Proc. Natl. Acad. Sci. USA* **58**:1389.

Berge, T. O., ed., 1975, *International Catalogue of Arboviruses*, 2nd ed., DHEW Publication No. (CDC) 75-8301, Washington, D.C.

Blue, J. L., Dawe, D. L., and Gratzek, J. B., 1974, The use of passive hemagglutination for the detection of bluetongue viral antibodies, *Am. J. Vet. Res.* **35**:139.

Boorman, J., Mellor, P. S., Penn, M., and Jennings, M., 1975, The growth of African horsesickness virus in embryonated hen eggs and the transmission of virus by *Culicoides variipennis* Coquillett (Diptera, Ceratopogonidae), *Arch. Virol.* **47**:343.

Borden, E. C., Shope, R. E., and Murphy, F. A., 1971, Physicochemical and morphological relationships of some arthropod-borne viruses to bluetongue virus—a new taxonomic group. Physicochemical and serological studies, *J. Gen. Virol.* **13**:261.

Borsa, J., and Graham, A. F., 1968, Reovirus: RNA polymerase activity in purified virions, *Biochem. Biophys. Res. Commun.* **33**:896.

Both, G. W., Lavi, S., and Shatkin, A. J., 1975, Synthesis of all the gene products of the reovirus genome *in vivo* and *in vitro*, *Cell* **4**:173.

Boulanger, P., and Frank, J. F., 1975, Serological methods in the diagnosis of bluetongue, *Austr. Vet. J.* **51**:185.

Boulanger, P., Ruckerbauer, G. M., Bannister, G. L., Gray, D. P., and Girard, A., 1967, Studies on bluetongue III Comparison of two complement-fixation methods, *Can. J. Comp. Med.* **31**:166.

Boulanger, P., Girard, A., Bannister, G. L., and Ruckerbauer, G. M., 1970, Serological studies in bluetongue, *Proc. 74th Annu. Meet U.S. Anim. Hlth. Assoc.*, pp. 537–548.

Bourdin, P., Monnier-Cambon, J., Rioche, M., and Laurent, A., 1969, Vaccination against African horsesickness in Tropical Africa: Evaluation of an inactivated vaccine, *Proc. 2nd Int. Conf. Equine Infect. Dis.* , Paris, pp. 202–206, Karger, Basel.

Bowne, J. G., and Jochim, M. M., 1967, Cytopathologic changes and development of inclusion bodies in cultured cells infected with bluetongue virus, *Am. J. Vet. Res.* **28**:1091.

Bowne, J. G., and Ritchie, A. E., 1970, Some morphological features of bluetongue virus, *Virology* **40**:903.

Bowne, J. G., Luedke, A. J., Jochim, M. M., and Metcalf, H. E., 1968, Bluetongue disease in cattle, *J. Am. Vet. Med. Assoc.* **153**:662.

Breese, S. S., Jr., Ozawa, Y., and Dardiri, A. H., 1969, Electron microscopic characterization of African Horse-sickness viruses, *J. Am. Vet. Med. Assoc.* **155**:391.

Bremer, C. W., 1976, A gel electrophoretic study of the protein and nucleic acid components of African horsesickness virus, *Onderstepoort J. Vet. Res.* **43**:193.

Buckley, S. M., 1969, Susceptibility of *Aedes albopictus* and *A. aegypti* cell lines to infection with arboviruses, *Proc. Soc. Exp. Biol. Med.* **131**:625.

Buckley, S. M., 1972, Propagation of 3 relatively solvent-resistant arboviruses in Singh's *Aedes albopictus* and *A. aegypti* cell lines, *J. Med. Entomol.* **9**:168.

Burgdorfer, W., and Eklund, C. M., 1959, Studies on the ecology of Colorado tick fever virus in Western Montana, *Am. J. Hyg.* **69**:127.

Burgdorfer, W., and Eklund, C. M., 1960, Colorado tick fever I. Further ecological studies in western Montana, *J. Infect. Dis.* **107**:379.

Campbell, C. H., Barber, T. L., and Jochim, M. M., 1977, The antigenic relationship of Ibaraki, bluetongue and epizootic hemorrhagic disease viruses, *Int. Symp. Reoviridae*, Guelph, May 1977.

Carley, J. G., and Standfast, H. A., 1969, Corriparta virus: Properties and multiplication in experimentally inoculated mosquitoes, *Am. J. Epidemiol.* **89**:583.

Casals, J., 1959, Antigenic classification of arthropod-borne viruses, *Proc. 6th Int. Congr. Trop. Med. Malaria* **5**:34.

Chow, N.-L., and Shatkin, A. J., 1975, Blocked and unblocked 5′ termini in reovirus genome RNA, *J. Virol.* **15**:1057.

Clarke, D. H., and Casals, J., 1958, Techniques for haemagglutination and haemagglutination inhibition with arthropod-borne viruses, *Am. J. Trop. Med. Hyg.* **7**:561.

Cohen, J., 1977, Ribonucleic acid polymerase activity, associated with purified calf rotavirus, *J. Gen. Virol.* **36**:395.

Cordy, D. R., and Shultz, G., 1961, Congenital subcortical encephalopathies in lambs, *J. Neuropathol. Exp. Neurol.* **20**:554.

Cross, R. K., and Fields, B. N., 1976, Reovirus-specific polypeptides: Analysis using discontinuous gel electrophoresis, *J. Virol.* **19**:162.

Dales, S., Gomatos, P. J., and Hsu, K. C., 1965, The uptake and development of reovirus in strain L cells followed with labeled viral ribonucleic and ferritin-antibody conjugates, *Virology* **25**:193.

Dardiri, A. H., and Ozawa, Y., 1969, Immune and serologic response of dogs to neurotropic and viscerotropic African horsesickness viruses, *J. Am. Vet. Med. Assoc.* **155**:400.

Davies, F. G., and Lund, L. J., 1974, The application of fluorescent antibody techniques to the virus of African horsesickness, *Res. Vet. Sci.* **17**:128.

Davies, F. G., and Otieno, S., 1977, Elephants and zebras as possible reservoir hosts for African horsesickness virus, *Vet. Rec.* **100**:291.

Davies, F. G., and Walker, A. R., 1974, The distribution in Kenya of bluetongue virus and antibody, and the *Culicoides* vector, *J. Hyg.* **72**:265.

Debbie, J. G., and Abelseth, M. K., 1971, Pathogenesis of epizootic hemorrhagic disease I. Blood coagulation during viral infection, *J. Infect. Dis.* **124**:217.

Deig, E. F., and Watkins, H. M. S., 1964, Plaque assay procedure for Colorado tick fever virus, *J. Bacteriol.* **88**:42.

De Villiers, E.-M., 1974, Comparison of the capsid polypeptides of various bluetongue virus serotypes, *Intervirology* **3**:47.

Doherty, R. L., 1972, Arboviruses of Australia, *Aust. Vet. J.* **48**:172.

Dunnebacke, T. H., and Kleinschmidt, A. K., 1967, Ribonucleic acid from reovirus as seen in protein monolayers by electron-microscopy, *Z. Naturforsch.* **22b**:159.

Du Toit, R. M., 1944, The transmission of bluetongue and horsesickness by *Culicoides*, *Onderstepoort J. Vet. Sci.* **19**:7.

Du Toit, R. M., 1962, The role played by bovines in the transmission of bluetongue in sheep, *J. S. Afr. Vet. Med. Assoc.* **33**:483.

Ehrenfeld, E., and Hunt, T., 1971, Double-stranded poliovirus RNA inhibits initiation of protein synthesis by reticulocyte lysates, *Proc. Natl. Acad. Sci. USA.* **68**:1075.

Eksteen, P. A. L., and Huismans, H., 1972, Interferon induction by bluetongue virus and bluetongue virus ribonucleic acid, *Onderstepoort J. Vet. Res.* **39**:125.

Els, H. J., 1973, Electron microscopy of bluetongue virus RNA, *Onderstepoort J. Vet. Res.* **40**:73.

Els, H. J., and Verwoerd, D. W., 1969, Morphology of bluetongue virus, *Virology* **38**:213.

Erasmus, B. J., 1964, Some observations on the propagation of horsesickness virus in tissue culture, *Bull. Off. Int. Epiz.* **64**:697.

Erasmus, B. J., 1965, The attenuation of viscerotropic horsesickness virus in tissue culture, *Bull. Off. Int. Epiz.* **64**:697.

Erasmus, B. J., 1966, The attenuation of horsesickness virus: Problems and advantages associated with the use of different host systems, *Proc. 1st Int. Conf. Equine Infect. Dis.*, pp. 208–213, Stresa.

Erasmus, B. J., 1972, The pathogenesis of African horsesickness, *Proc. 3rd Int. Conf. Equine Infect. Dis.* Paris, pp. 1–11, Karger, Basel.

Erasmus, B. J., 1975a, Bluetongue in sheep and goats, *Aust. Vet. J.* **51**:165.

Erasmus, B. J., 1975b, The epizootiology of bluetongue: The African situation, *Aust. Vet. J.* **51**:196.

Erasmus, B. J., 1975c, The control of bluetongue in an enzootic situation, *Aust. Vet. J.* **51**:209.

Erasmus, B. J., 1976, A new approach to polyvalent immunization against African horsesickness, *Proc. 4th Int. Conf. Equine Infect. Dis.* Lyon, pp. 401–403, Veterinary Publications, Inc., Princeton, N.J.

Erasmus, B. J., 1977, Bluetongue and African Horsesickness viruses, *Int. Symp. Reoviridae*, Guelph, May 1977.

Erasmus, B. J., Adelaar, T. F., Smit, J. D., Lecatsas, G., and Toms, T., 1970, The isolation and characterization of equine encephalosis virus, *Bull. Off. Int. Epiz.* **74**:781.

Erasmus, B. J., Boshoff, S. T., and Pieterse, L. M., 1976a, The isolation and characterization of equine encephalosis and serologically related orbiviruses from horses, *Proc. 4th Int. Conf. Equine Infect. Dis.* Lyon, pp. 447–450, Veterinary Publications, Inc., Princeton, N.J.

Erasmus, B. J., Young, E., Pieterse, L. M., and Boshoff, S. T., 1976b, The susceptibility of zebra and elephants to African horsesickness virus, *Proc. 4th Int. Conf. Equine Infect. Dis.* Lyon, pp. 409–413, Veterinary Publications, Inc., Princeton, N.J.

Fernandes, M., 1959, Isolation and propagation of bluetongue virus in tissue culture, *Am. J. Vet. Res.* **20**:398.

Fletch, A. L., and Karstad, L. H., 1971, Studies on the pathogenesis of experimental epizootic hemorrhagic disease of white-tailed deer, *Can. J. Comp. Med.* **35**:224.

Fosberg, S. A., Stauber, E. H., and Renshaw, H. W., 1977, Isolation and characterization of epizootic hemorrhagic disease virus from white-tailed deer (*Odocoileus virginianus*) in Eastern Washington, *Am. J. Vet. Res.* **38**:361.

Foster, N. M., and Luedke, A. J., 1968, Direct assay for bluetongue virus by intravascular inoculation of embryonating chicken eggs, *Am. J. Vet. Res.* **29**:749.

Foster, N. M., Jones, R. H., and McCrory, B. R., 1963, Preliminary investigations on insect transmission of bluetongue virus in sheep, *Am. J. Vet. Res.* **24**:1195.

Foster, N. M., Jones, R. H., and Luedke, A. J., 1968, Transmission of attenuated and virulent bluetongue virus with *Culicoides variipennis* infected orally via sheep, *Am. J. Vet. Res.* **29**:275.

Foster, N. M., Breckon, R. D., Luedke, A. J., Jones, R. H., and Metcalf, H. E., 1977, Transmission of two strains of epizootic hemorrhagic disease virus in deer by *Culicoides variipennis*, *J. Wildl. Dis.* **13**:9.

Foster, N. M., Alders, M. A., and Walton, T. E., 1978, Continuity of the dsRNA genome of bluetongue virus, *Current Microbiol.* **1**:171.

Fujii-Kawata, I., Miura, K.-I., and Fuke, M., 1970, Segments of genome of viruses containing double-stranded ribonucleic acid, *J. Mol. Biol.* **51**:247.

Furiuchi, Y., and Miura, K.-I., 1973, Identity of the 3′-terminal sequence in ten genome segments of silkworm cytoplasmic polyhedrosis virus, *Virology* **55**:418.

Furuichi, Y., Morgan, M., Muthukrishnan, S., and Shatkin, A. J., 1975, Reovirus messenger RNA contains a methylated blocked 5′ terminal structure: 7 m $G^{5′}$ ppp $^{5′}G^m$ pCp . . ., *Proc. Natl. Acad. Sci. USA* **72**:362.

Goldsmit, L., 1967, Growth characteristics of six neurotropic and one viscerotropic African horsesickness virus strains in fertilized eggs, *Am. J. Vet. Res.* **28**:19.

Goldsmit, L., and Barzilai, E., 1965, Isolation and propagation of a bluetongue virus strain in embryonating chicken eggs by the intravenous route of inoculation—preliminary report, *Refu. Vet.* **22**:285.

Goldsmit, L., and Barzilai, E., 1968, An improved method for the isolation and identification of bluetongue virus by intravenous inoculation of embryonating chicken eggs, *J. Comp. Pathol.* **78**:477.

Goldsmit, L., and Barzilai, E., 1969, Multiplication of bluetongue virus in experimentally inoculated sheep assayed by intravenous inoculation of embryonating chicken eggs, *Refu. Vet.* **26**:44.

Gorman, B. M., 1978, Susceptibility of orbiviruses to low pH and to organic solvents, *Aust. J. Exp. Biol. Med. Sci.* **56**:359.

Gorman, B. M., and Lecatsas, G., 1972, Formation of Wallal virus in cell culture, *Onderstepoort J. Vet. Res.* **39**:229.

Gorman, B. M., and Taylor, J., 1978, The RNA genome of Tilligerry virus, *Aust. J. Exp. Biol. Med. Sci.* **56**:369.

Gorman, B. M., Walker, P. J., Sorensen, J., Melzer, A. J., and Smith, D., 1976, Laboratory studies of arboviruses. Structure and genetics of orbiviruses, *Annu. Rep. Qld. Inst. Med. Res.* **31**:19.

Gorman, B. M., Walker, P. J., and Taylor, J., 1977*a*, Electrophoretic separation of double-stranded RNA genome segments from Warrego and Mitchell River viruses, *Arch. Virol.* **54**:153.

Gorman, B. M., Taylor, J., Brown, K., and Melzer, A. J., 1977*b*, Laboratory studies of arboviruses. Structure and genetics of orbiviruses, *Annu. Rep. Qld. Inst. Med. Res.* **32**:15.

Gorman, B. M., Taylor, J., Walker, P. J., and Young, P. R., 1978, The isolation of recombinants between related orbiviruses, *J. Gen. Virol.* **41**:333.

Granboulan, N., and Niveleau, A., 1967, Étude au microscope electronique du RNA de reovirus, *J. Microsc. (Oxford)* **6**:23.

Green, I. J., 1970, Evidence for the double-stranded nature of the RNA of Colorado tick fever virus, an ungrouped arbovirus, *Virology* **49**:878.

Griner, L. A., McCrory, B. R., Foster, N. M., and Meyer, H., 1964, Bluetongue associated with abnormalities in newborn lambs, *J. Am. Vet. Med. Assoc.* **145**:1013.

Haig, D. A., McKercher, D. G., and Alexander, R. A., 1956, the cytopathogenic action of bluetongue virus on tissue cultures and its application to the detection of antibodies in the serum of sheep, *Onderstepoort J. Vet. Res.* **27**:171.

Hazrati, A., and Ozawa, Y., 1965, Serologic studies of African horsesickness virus with emphasis on neutralization test in tissue culture, *Can. J. Comp. Med. Vet. Sci.* **29**:173.

Hoff, G. L., and Hoff, D. M., 1976, Bluetongue and epizootic hemorrhagic disease: A review of these diseases in nondomestic artiodactyles, *J. Zoo. Anim. Med.* **7**:26.

Hoff, G. L., and Trainer, D. O., 1974, Observations on bluetongue and epizootic hemorrhagic disease viruses in white-tailed deer: (1) Distribution of virus in the blood (2) Crosschallenge, *J. Wildl. Dis.* **10**:25.

Hoff, G. L., Griner, L. A., and Trainer, D. O., 1973, Bluetongue virus in exotic ruminants, *J. Am. Vet. Med. Assoc.* **163**:565.

Holmes, I. H., Ruck, B. J., Bishop, R. F., and Davidson, G. P., 1975, Infantile enteritis viruses: Morphogenesis and morphology, *J. Virol.* **16**:937.

Hopkins, I. G., Hazrati, A., and Ozawa, Y., 1966, Development of plaque techniques for titration and neutralization tests with African horsesickness virus, *Am. J. Vet. Res.* **27**:96.

Hourrigan, J. L., and Klingsporn, A. L., 1975*a*, Bluetongue: The disease in cattle, *Aust. Vet. J.* **51**:170.

Hourrigan, J. L., and Klingsporn, A. L., 1975*b*, Epizootiology of bluetongue: The situation in the United States of America, *Aust. Vet. J.* **51**:203.

Howell, P. G., 1960, A preliminary antigenic classification of strains of bluetongue virus, *Onderstepoort J. Vet. Res.* **28**:357.

Howell, P. G., 1962, The isolation and identification of further antigenic types of African horsesickness virus, *Onderstepoort J. Vet. Res.* **29**:139.

Howell, P. G., and Verwoerd, D. W., 1971, Bluetongue virus, in: *Virology Monographs* (S. Gard, C. Hallauer, and K. F. Meyer, eds.), pp. 35–74, Springer-Verlag, New York.

Howell, P. G., Verwoerd, D. W., and Oellermann, R. A., 1967, Plaque formation by bluetongue virus, *Onderstepoort J. Vet. Res.* **34**:317.

Howell, P. G., Kümm, N. A., and Botha, M. J., 1970, The application of improved techniques to the identification of strains of bluetongue virus, *Onderstepoort J. Vet. Res.* **37**:59.

Hughes, L. E., Casper, E. A., and Clifford, C. M., 1974, Persistence of Colorado tick fever virus in red blood cells, *Am. J. Trop. Med. Hyg.* **23**:530.

Huismans, H., 1969, Bluetongue virus induced interferon synthesis, *Onderstepoort J. Vet. Res.* **36**:181.

Huismans, H., 1970*a*, Macromolecular synthesis in bluetongue virus-infected cells, I. Virus-specific ribonucleic acid synthesis, *Onderstepoort J. Vet. Res.* **37**:191.

Huismans, H., 1970*b*, Macromolecular synthesis in bluetongue virus-infected-cells. II. Host cell metabolism, *Onderstepoort J. Vet. Res.* **37**:199.

Huismans, H., 1971, Host cell protein synthesis after infection with bluetongue virus and reovirus, *Virology* **46**:500.

Huismans, H., 1979, Protein synthesis in bluetongue virus-infected cells, *Virology* **92**:385.

Huismans, H., and Els, H. J., 1979, Characterization of the microtubules associated with the replication of three different orbiviruses, *Virology* **92**:397.

Huismans, H., and Howell, P. G., 1973, Molecular hybridization studies on the relationships between different serotypes of bluetongue virus and on the difference between virulent and attenuated strains of the same serotype, *Onderstepoort J. Vet. Res.* **40**:93.

Huismans, H., and Verwoerd, D. W., 1973, Control of transcription during the expression of the bluetongue virus genome, *Virology* **52**:81.

Huismans, H., Bremer, C. W., and Barber, T. L., 1979, The nucleic acid and proteins of epizootic hemorrhagic disease virus, *Onderstepoort J. Vet. Res.* **46**:95.

Hunter, T., Hunt, T., and Jackson, R. J., 1975, Characteristics of inhibition of protein synthesis by double-stranded RNA in reticulocyte lysates, *J. Biol. Chem.* **250**:409.

Inaba, Y., 1975, Ibaraki disease and its relationship to bluetongue, *Aust. Vet. J.* **51**:178.

Ito, Y., and Joklik, W. K., 1972, Temperature-sensitive mutants of reovirus. II. Anomalous electrophoretic migration behaviour of certain hybrid RNA molecules composed of mutant plus strands and wild-type minus strands, *Virology* **50**:202.

Ito, Y., Tanaka, Y., Inaba, Y., and Omori, T., 1973, Electron microscopy of Ibaraki virus, *Arch. Gesamte Virusforsch.* **40**:29.

Jameson, P., Schoenherr, C. K., and Grossberg, S. E., 1978, Bluetongue virus, an exceptionally potent interferon inducer in mice, *Infect. Immun.* **20**:321.

Jochim, M. M., and Chow, T. L., 1969, Immunodiffusion of bluetongue virus, *Am. J. Vet. Res.* **30**:33.

Jochim, M. M., and Jones, S. C., 1976, Plaque neutralization of bluetongue virus and epizootic hemorrhagic disease virus in BHK21 cells, *Am. J. Vet. Res.* **37**:1345.

Jochim, M. M., Barber, T. L., and Bando, B. M., 1974*a*, Identification of bluetongue and epizootic hemorrhagic disease viruses by the indirect fluorescent antibody procedure, *Proc. 17th Annu. Meet. Am. Assoc. Vet. Lab. Diagn. 1974*, pp. 91–103.

Jochim, M. M., Luedke, A. J., and Chow, T. L., 1974*b*, Bluetongue in cattle: Immunogenic and clinical responses in calves inoculated *in utero* and after birth, *Am. J. Vet. Res.* **35**:517.

Joklik, W. K., 1974, Reproduction of Reoviridae, in: *Comprehensive Virology*, Vol. 2 (H. Fraenkel-Conrat and R. R. Wagner, eds.) pp. 231–334, Plenum, New York.

Jones, R. H., Roughton, R. D., Foster, N. M., and Bando, B. M., 1977, *Culicoides*, the vector of epizootic hemorrhagic disease in white-tailed deer in Kentucky in 1971, *J. Wildl. Dis.* **13**:2.

Karmysheva, V. YA., Semashko, I. V., Borisov, V. M., and Chumakov, M. P., 1973, Comparative study of cytopathology produced by some Kemerovo group viruses, *Acta Virol.* **17**:479.

Karstad, L., and Trainer, D. O., 1967, Histopathology of experimental bluetongue disease of white-tailed deer, *Can. Vet. J.* **8**:247.

Kimura, T., and Murakami, T., 1977, Tubular structures associated with acute nonbacterial gastroenteritis in young children, *Infect. Immun.* **17**:157.

Kontz, G. W., Svehag, S.-E., and Gorham, J. R., 1962, A study by the agar diffusion technique of precipitating antibody directed against bluetongue virus and its relation to homotypic neutralizing antibody, *Arch. Gesamte Virusforsch.* **12**:259.

Kontor, E. J., and Welch, A. B., 1976, Characterization of an epizootic haemorrhagic disease virus, *Res. Vet. Sci.* **21**:190.

Koprowski, H., Cox, H. R., Miller, M. S., and Florio, L., 1950, Response of man to egg-adapted Colorado tick fever virus, *Proc. Soc. Exp. Biol. Med.* **74**:126.

Krystal, G., Winn, P., Millward, S., and Sakuma, S., 1975, Evidence for phospho-proteins in reovirus, *Virology* **64**:505.

Krystal, G., Perrault, J., and Graham, A. F., 1976, Evidence for a glycoprotein in reovirus, *Virology* **72**:308.

Lecatsas, G., 1968, Electron microscopic study of the formation of bluetongue virus, *Onderstepoort J. Vet. Res.* **35**:139.

Lecatsas, G., and Erasmus, B. J., 1967, Electron microscopic study of the formation of African horsesickness virus, *Arch. Gesamte Virusforsch.* **22**:442.

Lecatsas, G., and Erasmus, B. J., 1973, Core structure in a new virus, XBM/67, *Arch. Gesamte Virusforsch.* **42**:264.

Lecatsas, G., and Gorman, B. M., 1972, Visualization of the extra capsid coat in certain bluetongue-type viruses, *Onderstepoort J. Vet. Res.* **39**:193.

Lecatsas, G., Erasmus, B. J., and Els, H. J., 1969, Electron microscopic studies on Corriparta virus, *Onderstepoort J. Vet. Res.* **36**:321.

Lecatsas, G., Erasmus, B. J., and Els, H. J., 1973, Electron microscopic studies on equine encephalosis virus, *Onderstepoort J. Vet. Res.* **40**:53.

Lee, V. H., Causey, O. R., and Moore, D. L., 1974, Bluetongue and related viruses in Ibadan, Nigeria: Isolation and preliminary identification of viruses, *Am. J. Vet. Res.* **35**:1105.

Lewandowski, L. J., and Leppla, S. H., 1972, Comparison of the 3'-termini of discrete segments of the double-stranded ribonucleic acid genomes of cytoplasmic polyhedrosis virus, wound tumor virus, and reovirus, *J. Virol.* **10**:965.

Libíková, H., and Buckley, S. M., 1971, Serological characterization of Eurasian Kemerovo group viruses. II. Cross plaque neutralization tests, *Acat Virol.* **15**:79.

Libíková, H., and Casals, J., 1971, Serological characterization of Eurasian Kemerovo group viruses. I. Cross complement fixation tests, *Acta Virol.* **15**:65.

Livingston, C. W., and Moore, R. W., 1962, Cytochemical changes of bluetongue virus in tissue culture, *Am. J. Vet. Res.* **23**:701.

Luedke, A. J., 1969, Bluetongue in sheep: Viral assay and viremia, *Am. J. Vet. Res.* **30**:499.

Luedke, A. J., 1970, Distribution of virus in blood components during viremia of bluetongue, *Proc. 74th Annu. Meet. U.S. Anim. Hlth. Assoc.* pp. 9–21.

Luedke, A. J., and Jochim, M. M., 1968, Bluetongue virus in sheep. Intensification of the clinical response by previous oral administration, *Cornell Vet.* **58**:48.

Luedke, A. J., Jochim, M. M., and Jones, R. H., 1969, Bluetongue in cattle: Viremia, *Am. J. Vet. Res.* **30**:511.

Luedke, A. J., Jochim, M. M., Bowne, J. G., and Jones, R. H., 1970, Observations on latent bluetongue virus infection in cattle, *J. Am. Vet. Med. Assoc.* **156**:1871.

Luedke, A. J., Walton, T. E., and Jones, R. H., 1975, Detection of bluetongue virus in bovine semen, *Proc. 20th W. Vet. Congr.*, Thessaloniki **3**:2039.

Luedke, A. J., Jones, R. H., and Jochim, M. M., 1976, Serial cyclic transmission of bluetongue virus in sheep and *Culicoides variipennis*, *Cornell Vet.* **66**:536.

Luedke, A. J., Jochim, M. M., and Jones, R. H., 1977a, Bluetongue in cattle: Effects of *Culicoides variipennis*-transmitted bluetongue virus on pregnant heifers and their calves, *Am. J. Vet. Res.* **38**:1687.

Luedke, A. J., Jochim, M. M., and Jones, R. H., 1977b, Bluetongue in cattle: Effects of calves previously infected *in utero*, *Am. J. Vet. Res.* **38**:1697.

Luedke, A. J., Jochim, M. M., and Jones, R. H., 1977c, Bluetongue in cattle: Repeated exposure of two immunologically tolerant calves to bluetongue virus by vector bites, *Am. J. Vet. Res.* **38**:1701.

Luedke, A. J., Jones, R. H., and Walton, T. E., 1977d, Overwintering mechanism for bluetongue virus: Biological recovery of latent virus from a bovine by bites of *Culicoides variipennis*, *Am. J. Trop. Med. Hyg.* **26**:313.

Luftig, R. B., Kilham, S., Hay, A. J., Zweerink, H. J., and Joklik, W. K., 1972, An ultrastructural study of virions and cores of reovirus type 3, *Virology* **48**:170.

Martin, S. A., and Zweerink, H. J., 1972, Isolation and characterization of two types of bluetongue virus particles, *Virology* **50**:495.

Martin, S. A., Pett, D. M., and Zweerink, H. J., 1973, Studies on the topography of reovirus and bluetongue virus capsid polypeptides, *J. Virol.* **12**:194.

Mason, J. H., Coles, J. D. W. A., and Alexander, R. A., 1940, Cultivation of bluetongue virus in fertile eggs produced on a vitamin deficient diet, *Nature (London)* **145**:1022.

McIntosh, B. M., 1956, Complement fixation with horsesickness virus, *Onderstepoort J. Vet. Res.* **27**:165.

McIntosh, B. M., 1958, Immunological types of horsesickness virus and their significance in immunization, *Onderstepoort J. Vet. Res.* **27**:465.

Mellor, P. S., Boorman, J., and Jennings, M., 1975, The multiplication of African horsesickness virus in two species of *Culicoides* (Diptera, Ceratopogonidae), *Arch. Virol.* **47**:351.

Metcalf, H. E., and Jochim, M. M., 1970, Bluetongue in cattle: Efficacy of the agar gel precipitin tests, *Am. J. Vet. Res.* **31**:1743.

Mirchamsy, H., and Taslimi, H., 1963, Adaptation of horsesickness virus to tissue culture, *Nature (London)* **198**:704.

Mirchamsy, H., and Taslimi, H., 1964, Attempts to vaccinate foals with living tissue culture adapted horsesickness virus, *Bull. Off. Int. Epiz.* **62**:911.

Mirchamsy, H., Taslimi, H., and Bahrami, S., 1969, Recent advances in immunization of horses against African horsesickness, *Proc. 2nd Int. Conf. Equine Infect. Dis.*, Paris, pp. 212–221, Karger, Basel.

Mirchamsy, H., Hazrati, A., Bahrami, S., and Shafyi, 1970, Growth and persistent infection of African horsesickness virus in a mosquito cell line, *Am. J. Vet. Res.* **31**:1755.

Mirchamsy, H., Hazrati, A., Bahrami, S., Shafyi, A., and Mahinpoor, M., 1972, Comparative attenuation of African horsesickness virus in mosquitoe (*Aedes albopictus*) and in hamster kidney (BHK21) cell lines, *Proc. 3rd Int. Conf. Equine Infect. Dis.*, Paris, pp. 45–57, Karger, Basel.

Moore, D. L., and Kemp, G. E., 1974, Bluetongue and related viruses in Abadan, Nigeria: Serologic studies of domesticated and wild animals, *Am. J. Vet. Res.* **35**:1115.

Morgan, E. M., and Zweerink, H. J., 1975, Characterization of transcriptase and replicase particles isolated from reovirus-infected cells, *Virology* **68**:455.

Morgan, E. M., and Zweerink, H. J., 1977, Characterization of the double-stranded RNA in replicase particles in reovirus-infected cells, *Virology* **77**:421.

Mornet, P., and Gilbert, Y., 1968, *La Peste Equine*, L'Expansion Scientifique Française, Paris.

Murphy, F. A., Coleman, P. H., Hansen, A. K., and Gray, G. W., 1968, Colorado tick fever virus, an electron microscope study, *Virology* **35**:28.

Murphy, F. A., Borden, E. C., Shope, R. E., and Harrison, A., 1971, Physicochemical and morphological relationships of some arthropod-borne viruses to bluetongue virus—A new taxonomic group. Electron microscopic studies, *J. Gen. Virol.* **13**:273.

Neitz, W. O., 1948, Immunological studies on bluetongue in sheep, *Onderstepoort J. Vet. Sci. Anim. Ind.* **23**:93.

Nevill, E. M., 1971, Cattle and *Culicoides* biting midges as possible overwintering hosts of bluetongue virus, *Onderstepoort J. Vet. Res.* **38**:65.

Nichols, J. L., Bellamy, A. R., and Joklik, W. K., 1972, Identification of the nucleotide sequences of the oligonucleotides present in reovirus, *Virology* **49**:562.

Nishimura, A., and Hosaka, Y., 1969, Electron microscopic study of RNA of cytoplasmic polyhedrosis virus of the silkworm, *Virology* **38**:550.

Obijeski, J. F., Palmer, E. L., and Martin, M. L., 1977, Biochemical characterization of infantile gastroenteritis virus (IGV), *J. Gen. Virol.* **34**:485.

Oellermann, R. A., 1970, Plaque formation by African horsesickness virus and characterization of its RNA, *Onderstepoort J. Vet. Res.* **37**:137.

Oellermann, R. A., Els, H. J., and Erasmus, B. J., 1970, Characterization of African horsesickness virus, *Arch. Gesamte Virusforsch.* **29**:163.

Omori, T., 1970, Ibaraki disease: A bovine epizootic disease resembling bluetongue, *Natl. Inst. Anim. Health Q.* **10**(Supp.):45.

Osburn, B. I., Silverstein, A. M., Prendergast, R. A., Johnson, R. T., and Parshall, C. J., 1971*a*, Experimental viral-induced congenital encephalopathies I. Pathology of hydranencephaly and porencephaly caused by bluetongue vaccine virus, *Lab. Invest.* **25**:197.

Osburn, B. I., Johnson, R. T., Silverstein, A. M., Prendergast, R. A., Jochim, M. M., and Levy, S. E., 1971*b*, Experimental viral-induced congenital encephalopathies. II. The pathogenesis of bluetongue vaccine virus infection in fetal lambs, *Lab. Invest.* **25**:206.

Owen, N. C., 1964, Investigation into the pH stability of bluetongue virus and its survival in mutton and beef, *Onderstepoort J. Vet. Res.* **31**:109.

Owen, N. C., and Munz, E. K., 1966, Observations on a strain of bluetongue virus by electron microscopy, *Onderstepoort J. Vet. Res.* **33**:9.

Ozawa, Y., 1966, Growth of African horsesickness virus in African green monkey cells, *Proc. 1st Int. Conf. Equine Infect. Dis.* pp. 214–223, Stresa.

Ozawa, Y., and Bahrami, S., 1966, African horsesickness killed virus tissue culture vaccine, *Can. J. Comp. Med.* **30**:311.

Ozawa, Y., and Hazrati, A., 1964, Growth of African horsesickness virus in monkey kidney cell cultures, *Am. J. Vet. Res.* **25**:505.

Ozawa, Y., Salama, S. A., and Dardiri, A. H., 1972, Methods for recovering African horsesickness virus from horse blood, *Proc. 3rd Int. Conf. Equine Infect. Dis.* Paris pp. 58–68, Karger, Basel.

Palmer, E. L., Martin, M. L., and Murphy, F. A., 1977, Morphology and stability of infantile gastroenteritis virus: Comparison with reovirus and bluetongue virus, *J. Gen. Virol.* **35**:403.

Parker, J., 1975, Inactivation of African horsesickness virus by betapropiolactone and by pH, *Arch. Virol.* **47**:357.

Pavri, K. M., 1961, Haemagglutination and haemagglutination-inhibition with African horsesickness virus, *Nature* (London) **189**:249.

Pavri, K. M., and Anderson, C. R., 1963, Haemagglutination-inhibition tests with different types of African horsesickness virus, *Indian J. Vet. Sci.* **33**:113.

Payne, C. C., and Rivers, C. F., 1976, A provisional classification of cytoplasmic polyhedrosis viruses based on the sizes of the RNA genome segments, *J. Gen. Virol.* **33**:71.

Pini, A., 1976, A study on the pathogenesis of bluetongue: Replication of the virus in the organs of infected sheep, *Onderstepoort J. Vet. Res.* **43**:159.

Polson, A., and Deeks, D., 1963, Electron microscopy of neurotropic African horsesickness virus, *J. Hyg.* **61**:149.

Reddy, D. V. R., and Black, L. M., 1973, Electrophoretic separation of all components of the double-stranded RNA of wound tumor virus, *Virology* **54**:557.

Richards, W. P. C., and Cordy, D. R., 1967, Bluetongue virus infection: Pathologic responses of nervous systems in sheep and mice, *Science* **156**:530.

Richards, W. P. C., Crenshaw, G. L., and Bushnell, R. B., 1971, Hydranencephaly of calves associated with natural bluetongue virus infection, *Cornell Vet.* **61**:336.

Robertson, A., Appel, M., Bannister, G. L., Ruckerbauer, G. M., and Boulanger, P., 1965, Studies on bluetongue II. Complement-fixing activity of ovine and bovine sera, *Can. J. Comp. Med. Vet. Sci.* **29**:113.

Robertson, H. D., and Mathews, M. B., 1973, Double-stranded RNA as an inhibitor of protein synthesis and as a substrate for a nuclease in extracts of Krebs II ascites cells, *Proc. Natl. Acad. Sci. USA.* **70**:225.

Robinson, R. M., Hailey, T. L., Marburger, R. G., and Weishuhn, L., 1974, Vaccination trials in desert bighorn sheep against bluetongue virus, *J. Wildl. Dis.* **10**:228.

Rodger, S. M., Schnagl, R. D., and Holmes, I. H., 1975, Biochemical and biophysical characteristics of diarrhea viruses of human and calf origin, *J. Virol.* **16**:1229.

Rosenbergová, M., and Slávik, I., 1975, Ribonuclease-resistant RNA of Kemerovo virus, *Acta Virol.* **19**:67.

Ruckerbauer, G. M., Gray, D. P., Girard, A., Bannister, G. L., and Boulanger, P., 1967, Studies on bluetongue V. Detection of the virus in infected materials by immunofluorescence, *Can. J. Comp. Med. Vet. Sci.* **31**:175.

Schmidt, R. E., and Panciera, R. J., 1973, Cerebral malformation in fetal lambs from a bluetongue-enzootic flock, *J. Am. Vet. Med. Assoc.* **162**:567.

Schnagl., R. D., and Holmes, I. H., 1971, A study of Australian arboviruses resembling bluetongue virus, *Aust. J. Biol. Sci.* **24**:1151.

Schnagl, R. D., and Holmes, I. H., 1975, Polyacrylamide gel electrophoresis of the genomes of two orbiviruses: D'Aguilar and Eubenangee, *Intervirology* 5:300.

Schnagl, R. D., Holmes, I. H., and Doherty, R. L., 1969, An electron microscope study of Eubenangee, an Australian arbovirus, *Virology* 38:347.

Schonberg, M., Silverstein, S. C., Levin, D. H., and Acs, G., 1971, Asynchronous synthesis of the complementary strands of the reovirus genome, *Proc. Natl. Acad. Sci. USA* 68:505.

Schuerch, A. R., and Joklik, W. K., 1973, Temperature-sensitive mutants of reovirus. IV. Evidence that anomalous electrophoretic migration behaviour of certain double-stranded RNA hybrid species is mutant group-specific, *Virology* 56:218.

Sellers, R. F., 1977, Spread of African horsesickness and bluetongue in North African and Middle Eastern countries, *International Symposium on Reoviridae*, May 1977, Guelph.

Sellers, R. F., Pedgley, D. E., and Tucker, M. R., 1977, Possible spread of African horse sickness on the wind, *J. Hyg.* 79:279.

Shatkin, A. J., and Sipe, J. D., 1968a, Single-stranded adenine-rich RNA from purified reoviruses, *Proc. Natl. Acad. Sci. USA* 59:246.

Shatkin, A. J., and Sipe, J. D., 1968b, RNA polymerase activity in purified reoviruses, *Proc. Natl. Acad. Sci. USA* 61:1462.

Shatkin, A. J., Sipe, J. D., and Loh, P. C., 1968, Separation of ten reovirus genome segments by polyacrylamide gel electrophoresis, *J. Virol.* 2:986.

Shipham, S. O., and De la Rey, M., 1976, The isolation and preliminary genetic classification of temperature-sensitive mutants of bluetongue virus, *Onderstepoort J. Vet. Res.* 43:189.

Shipham, S. O., and De la Rey, M., 1979, Temperature-sensitive mutants of bluetongue virus: Genetic and physiological characterization, *Onderstepoort J. Vet. Res.* 46:87.

Shone, D. K., Haig, D. A., and McKercher, D. G., 1956, The use of tissue culture propagated bluetongue virus for complement fixation studies on sheep sera, *Onderstepoort J. Vet. Res.* 27:179.

Shultz, G., and DeLay, P. D., 1955, Losses in new-born lambs associated with bluetongue vaccination of pregnant ewes, *J. Am. Vet. Med. Assoc.* 127:224.

Silverstein, S. C., Christman, J. K., and Acs, G., 1976, The reovirus replicative cycle, *Annu. Rev. Biochem.* 45:921.

Skehel, J. J., and Joklik, W. K., 1969, Studies on the *in vitro* transcription of reovirus RNA catalyzed by reovirus cores, *Virology* 39:822.

Spendlove, R. S., Lennette, E. H., and John, A. C., 1963, The role of mitotic apparatus in the intracellular location of reovirus antigen, *J. Immunol.* 90:554.

Stair, E. L., 1968, The pathogenesis of bluetongue in sheep: A study by immunofluorescence and histopathology, Dissertation, Texas A & M University.

Stair, E. L., Robinson, R. M., and Jones, L. P., 1968, Spontaneous bluetongue in Texas white-tailed deer, *Pathol. Vet.* 5:164.

Stanley, N. F., 1967, Reoviruses, *Br. Med. Bull.* 23:50.

Stauber, E. H., Farrell, R. K., and Spencer, G. R., 1977, Nonlethal experimental inoculation of Columbia black-tailed deer (*Odocoileus hemionus columbianus*) with virus of epizootic hemorrhagic deer disease, *Am. J. Vet. Res.* 38:411.

St. George, T. D., and Dimmock, C. K., 1976, The isolation of D'Aguilar virus from a cow, *Aust. Vet. J.* 52:598.

St. George, T. D., Standfast, H. A., and Cybinski, D. H., 1978, The isolation of a blue-tongue virus from *Culicoides* collected in the Northern Territory of Australia, *Aust. Vet. J.* **54:**153.

Stim, T. B., 1969, Arbovirus plaquing in two simian kidney cell lines, *J. Gen. Virol.* **5:**329.

Studdert, M. J., Pangborn, J., and Addison, R. B., 1966, Bluetongue virus structure, *Virology* **29:**509.

Suzuki, Y., Saito, Y., and Nakagawa, S., 1977, Double-stranded RNA of Ibaraki virus, *Virology* **76:**670.

Svehag, S. E., 1963a, Thermal inactivation of bluetongue virus, *Arch. Gesamte Virus-forsch.* **13:**499.

Svehag, S. E., 1963b, Effect of different "contact conditions" on the bluetongue virus-antibody reaction and on the validity of the "Percentage Law," *Arch. Gesamte Virusforsch.* **12:**678.

Svehag, S. E., 1966, Quantal and graded dose-responses of bluetongue virus: A comparison of their sensitivity as assay methods for neutralizing antibody, *J. Hyg.* **64:**231.

Svehag, S. E., Leendertsen, L., and Gorham, J. R., 1966, Sensitivity of bluetongue virus to lipid solvents, trypsin and pH changes and its serological relationship to arboviruses, *J. Hyg.* **64:**339.

Swanepoel, R., and Blackburn, N. K., 1976, A new member of the Palyam serogroup of orbiviruses, *Vet. Rec.* **99:**360.

Tessler, J., 1972, Detection of African horsesickness viral antigens in tissues by immunofluorescence, *Can. J. Comp. Med.* **36:**167.

Thomas, A. D., and Neitz, W. O., 1947, Further observations on the pathology of blue-tongue in sheep, *Onderstepoort J. Vet. Sci. Anim. Ind.* **22:**27.

Thomas, F. C., and Miller, J., 1971, A comparison of bluetongue virus and EHD virus: Electronmicroscopy and serology, *Can. J. Comp. Med.* **35:**22.

Thomas, F. C., and Trainer, D. O., 1970, Bluetongue virus: (1) In pregnant white-tailed deer (2) A plaque reduction neutralization test, *J. Wildl. Dis.* **6:**384.

Thomas, F. C., and Trainer, D. O., 1971, Bluetongue virus: Some relationships among North American isolates and further comparisons with EHD virus, *Can. J. Comp. Med.* **35:**187.

Thomas, F. C., Girard, A., Boulanger, P., and Ruckerbauer, G., 1976, A comparison of some serological tests for bluetongue virus infection, *Can. J. Comp. Med.* **40:**291.

Thomas, L. A., Eklund, C. M., Philip, R. N., and Casey, M., 1963, Development of a vaccine against Colorado tick fever for use in man, *Am. J. Trop. Med. Hyg.* **12:**678.

Tomori, O., Fabiyi, A., and Murphy, F., 1976, Characterization of Orungo virus, an orbivirus from Uganda and Nigeria, *Arch. Virol.* **51:**285.

Tsai, K.-S., and Karstad, L., 1970, Epizootic hemorrhagic disease virus of deer: An electron microscopic study, *Can. J. Microbiol.* **16:**427.

Tsai, K.-S., and Karstad, L., 1973, Ultrastructural characterization of the genome of epizootic hemorrhagic disease virus, *Infect. Immun.* **8:**463.

Van den Ende, M., Linder, A., and Kaschula, V. R., 1954, Experiments with the Cyprus strain of bluetongue virus: Multiplication in the central nervous system of mice and complement fixation, *J. Hyg.* **52:**155.

Van der Walt, N. T., 1979, A hemagglutination and hemagglutination inhibition test for bluetongue virus, *Onderstepoort J. Vet. Res.* (in press).

Verwoerd, D. W., 1969, Purification and characterization of bluetongue virus, *Virology* **38**:203.

Verwoerd, D. W., 1970, Diplornaviruses: A newly recognized group of double-stranded RNA viruses, *Prog. Med. Virol.* **12**:192.

Verwoerd, D. W., and Huismans, H., 1969, On the relationship between bluetongue, African horsesickness, and reoviruses: Hybridization studies, *Onderstepoort J. Vet. Res.* **36**:175.

Verwoerd, D. W., and Huismans, H., 1972, Studies on the *in vitro* and *in vivo* transcription of the bluetongue virus genome, *Onderstepoort J. Vet. Res.* **39**:185.

Verwoerd, D. W., Louw, H., and Oellermann, R. A., 1970, Characterization of bluetongue virus ribonucleic acid, *J. Virol.* **5**:1.

Verwoerd, D. W., Els, H. J., de Villiers, E.-M., and Huismans, H., 1972, Structure of the bluetongue virus capsid, *J. Virol.* **10**:783.

Wang, C. S., Lueker, D. C., and Chow, T. L., 1972, Soluble antigen of bluetongue virus, *Infect. Immun.* **5**:467.

Ward, R., Banerjee, A. K., La Fiandra, A., and Shatkin, A. J., 1972, Reovirus-specific ribonucleic acid from polysomes of infected L cells, *J. Virol.* **9**:61.

Willis, N. G., Corey, P. N., Campbell, J. B., and Macpherson, L. W., 1970, Development and statistic evaluation of a plaque assay for the virus of epizootic hemorrhagic disease of deer, *Can. J. Microbiol.* **16**:1293.

Wood, H. A., 1973, Viruses with double-stranded RNA genomes, *J. Gen. Virol.* **20**:61.

Yunker, C. E., and Cory, J., 1975, Plaque production by arboviruses in Singh's *Aedes albopictus* cells, *Appl. Microbiol.* **29**:81.

Zweerink, H. J., 1974, Multiple forms of SS → DS RNA polymerase activity in reovirus-infected cells, *Nature (London)* **247**:313.

Zweerink, H. J., and Joklik, W. K., 1970, Studies on the intracellular synthesis of reovirus-specified proteins, *Virology* **41**:501.

Zweerink, H. J., Ito, Y., and Matsuhisa, T., 1972, Synthesis of reovirus double-stranded RNA within virionlike particles, *Virology* **50**:349.

Icosahedral Cytoplasmic Deoxyriboviruses

Rakesh Goorha and Allan Granoff

St. Jude Children's Research Hospital
Division of Virology
Memphis, Tennessee 38101

1. INTRODUCTION

Deoxyriboviruses having an apparent icosahedral symmetry and replicating in the cytoplasm have been titled "icosahedral cytoplasmic deoxyriboviruses" (ICDVs) (Kelly and Robertson, 1973; McAuslan and Armentrout, 1974). Members of this group are widely distributed in nature in a variety of hosts and include iridescent viruses from insects, lymphocystis virus from fish, amphibian viruses, African swine fever virus, and cauliflower mosaic and related viruses from plants (Granoff, 1969; Stoltz, 1971; Plowright, 1972; Kelly and Robertson, 1973). In this chapter we have chosen to retain the term "icosahedral cytoplasmic deoxyribovirus," but because of the diversity of properties of these viruses this term is inadequate for classification and nomenclature purposes. We might compare this term to grouping papovaviruses, adenoviruses, and herpesviruses under the heading of "icosahedral nuclear deoxyriboviruses." Our usage of this term merely defines those viruses that have or may have icosahedral symmetry, appear to replicate in the cytoplasm, and contain DNA. It does not imply any taxonomic relationships and includes viruses from plants, invertebrates, and vertebrates. The designation "ICDV" is useful in distinguishing these viruses from the morphologically distinct and structurally complex poxviruses, which also replicate in the cytoplasm (Moss, 1974). A number of the viruses to be discussed in this chapter have been the main subjects of previous reviews and include iridescent viruses (Bellett, 1968), African swine fever virus (Hess, 1971), amphibian icosahedral cytoplasmic deoxyriboviruses (Granoff, 1969), and general reviews on these viruses (Kelly and Robertson, 1973; McAuslan and Armentrout, 1974). In this chapter we will review available information on ICDVs and the biochemistry of their replication, concentrating mainly on frog virus 3, which has provided most of the biochemical information.

2. CLASSIFICATION AND GENERAL BIOLOGICAL PROPERTIES OF ICOSAHEDRAL CYTOPLASMIC DEOXYRIBOVIRUSES

Table 1, modified and updated from Kelly and Robertson (1973) provides the names of ICDVs, the host from which the original isolate was made, and an appropriate reference. Clearly, a wide variety of plants and animals are hosts for these viruses. Insect ICDVs have mainly been grown in the intact host. However, several will grow in insect cells cultured *in vitro* (Kelly, 1972b). In general, ICDVs from invertebrates do not replicate in vertebrate cells. An interesting exception is *Chilo* iridescent virus (CIV), which replicates in vertebrate (viper spleen) cells and, unlike other insect ICDVs, buds through the plasma membrane in these cells (McIntosh and Kimura, 1974). African swine fever virus is the only member of ICDVs known to agglutinate erythrocytes (Malmquist and Hay, 1960), and it has a much more restricted host range in cell culture than frog virus 3 (FV3) (Enjuanes *et al.*, 1977). FV3 replicates in cells of amphibian, avian, piscine, and mammalian origin (Granoff, 1969). Lymphocystis virus replicates in cultures of marine fish cells (Sigel *et al.*, 1971). Structural protein(s) of FV3 (Aubertin *et al.*, 1973) as well as *Chilo* iridescent virus (M. Cerutti, personal communication) causes rapid inhibition of cellular DNA, RNA, and protein synthesis. Inhibition of cellular macromolecular synthesis by the structural protein(s) of FV3 occurs at a temperature (37°C) that is restrictive for the replication of virus (Granoff, 1969). CIV inhibits host macromolecular synthesis in both permissive (*Aedes aegypti*) and nonpermissive (*Aedes albopictus* and HeLa) cells, presumably also via its structural protein(s) (C. Monnier, personal communication).

ICDVs that have been studied generally cause a systemic infection in susceptible hosts, with the apparent exception of lymphocystis disease of fish (Weissenberg, 1965) and *Octopus vulgaris* disease virus (Rungger *et al.*, 1971). Insect ICDVs, because of the lethal effect on their hosts, have been considered as potentially useful in the biological control of insects. Among the animal ICDVs, FV3 is highly lethal for developing frog embryos (Tweedell and Granoff, 1968; Granoff *et al.*, 1969) but not for adult animals. The virus multiplies in various tissues of Fowler toads inoculated with FV3, produces a histopathology of the kidney compatible with acute glomerular nephritis, and is lethal. FV3 virions, or a soluble viral protein extract from them, produce a rapid inhibition of DNA, RNA, and protein synthesis in liver cells of mice and an accompanying acute degenerative hepatitis (Kirn *et al.*, 1972; Elharrar, 1973; Aubertin *et al.*, 1977). These results show that neither FV3 replication nor the presence of its genome is requisite for disease production in mice. ASFV produces a highly lethal disease of domestic swine (Hess, 1971). In contrast to the ICDVs just mentioned, which are cytocidal, lymphocystis disease virus of fish cause a marked hypertrophy (10 times normal) of target cells (Weissenberg, 1965). This phenomenon can also be demonstrated by infection of cultured fish cells, which reach diameters of up to 300 μm (Wolf *et al.*, 1966). Although lymphocystis disease virus is a benign infection of fish, *Octopus vulgaris* disease virus, which regularly causes tumors, kills the host (Rungger *et al.*, 1971).

3. SIZE, MORPHOLOGY, AND STRUCTURE

3.1. Size

ICDVs range widely in size, from 50 nm to 300 nm in their longest axis (Fig. 1), and comprise two distinct classes based on size distribution (Fig. 1). Plant ICDVs—dahlia mosaic virus, cauliflower mosaic virus, and carnation etched ring virus—are all approximately 50 nm (Shepherd *et al.*, 1970; Brunt, 1971; Rubio-Huertos *et al.*, 1972). Other ICDVs range from 130 nm to 300 nm; the largest and the one with the greatest reported size differences is lymphocystis virus. The sizes include 130–150 nm (Walker and Weissenberg, 1965), 200 nm (Midlige and Malsberger, 1968), 240–260 nm (Howse and Christmas, 1971), and 300 nm (Zwillenberg and Wolf, 1968). This wide variation in size has several explanations: (1) the viruses measured were isolated from lymphocystis tumors of different species of fish and hence may represent different ICDVs associated with lymphocystis tumors; (2) dif-

TABLE 1

Catalogue of Icosahedral Cytoplasmic Deoxyriboviruses[a]

Host	Virus name	Authority
Vertebrates		
Mammals		
Phacochoerus aethiopicus (warthog)		
Potamochoerus porcus (bushpig)	African swine fever	Hess (1971)
Hylochoerus meinertzhageni (giant forest hog)		
Sus scrofa (swine)		
Amphibians		
Rana pipiens (leopard frog)	None	Bernard *et al.* (1969)
R. pipiens	Frog virus 1 + 2	Granoff *et al.* (1969)
R. pipiens	Frog virus 3	Granoff *et al.* (1969)
R. pipiens	Frog virus 5–24	Granoff *et al.* (1969)
R. pipiens	L4 + L5	Clark *et al.* (1968)
R. catesbiana (bull frog)	Tadpole edema virus (TEV)	Wolf *et al.* (1968)
R. pipiens/*Diemictylus viridescens* (newt)	LT1–4	Clark *et al.* (1969)
Diemictylus viridescens	T6–20	Clark *et al.* (1969)
Xenopus laevis (toad)/*Diemictylus viridescens*	T21	Balls and Ruben (1968)
Reptiles		
Gehyra variegata (gecko)	None	Stebhens and Johnston (1966)
Fish		
Over 50 species, including		
Micropogon undulatus (Atlantic croaker)	Lymphocystis	Christmas and Howse (1970)
Lepomis macrochirus (bluegill)		
Cynoscion arenarius (sand seatrout)		
Invertebrates		
Insects		
Tipula paludosa (leatherjacket)	Iridescent, type 1	Glitz *et al.* (1968)
Sericesthis pruinosa (scarabaeid beetle)	Iridescent, type 2	Kelly (1972b)
Aedes taeniorhyncus (mosquito)	Iridescent, type 3	Matta and Lowe (1970)
Aedes cantans	Iridescent, type 4	Weiser (1965)
Aedes annulipes	Iridescent, type 5	Weiser (1965)

Chilo suppressalis (rice stem borer)	Iridescent, type 6	Kelly (1972*b*)
Simulium ornatum (blackfly)	Iridescent, type 7	Weiser (1968)
Culicoides sp. (midge)	Iridescent, type 8	Chapman *et al.* (1971)
Wiseana cervinata	Iridescent, type 9	D. C. Kelly and J. S. Robertson (unpublished results)
Witlesia sabulosella	Iridescent, type 10	Fowler and Robertson (1971)
Aedes stimulans	Iridescent, type 11	Anderson (1970)
Aedes cantans	Iridescent, type 12	Tinsley *et al* (1971)
Corethrella brakeleyi	Iridescent, type 13	Chapman *et al.* (1971)
Aedes detritus	Iridescent, type 14	Hasan *et al.* (1970)
Aedes detritus	Iridescent, type 15	Vago *et al.* (1969)
Costelytra zealandica	Iridescent, type 16	Kalmakoff *et al.* (1972)
Pterostrictus madidus	Iridescent, type 17	J. S. Robertson (unpublished results)
Opogonia sp.	Iridescent, type 18	J. S. Robertson (unpublished results)
Odontria striata	Iridescent, type 19	J. Kalmakoff (unpublished results)
Simocephalus expinosus	Iridescent, type 20	Federici and Hazard (1975)
Chironomus plumosus	None	Stoltz *et al.* (1968)
Molluscs		
Octopus vulgaris (common octopus)	None	Rungger *et al.*(1971)
Protozoa		
Entamoeba histolytica	None	Mattern *et al.* (1972)
Higher plants		
Brassica oleracea	Cauliflower mosaic virus	Shepherd (1970)
Dahlia sp.	Dahlia mosaic virus	Brunt (1971)
Dianthus caryophyllus	Carnation etched virus	(Hollings and Stone (1969)
Fragaria vesca	Strawberry vein-banding virus	Kitajima *et al.* (1973)
Lower plants		
Phycomycetes		
Aphelidium sp.	None	Schnepf *et al.* (1970)
Algae		
Oedogonium sp.	None	Pickett-Heaps (1972)
Chorda tomentosa	None	Toth and Wilce (1972)

[a] The list of insect ICDVs is a partial one. An additional ten types have been isolated from various insect hosts.

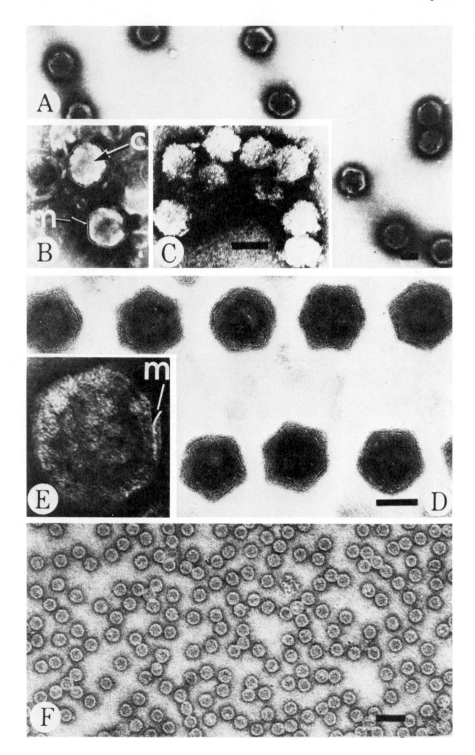

ferent methods of negative staining or of measuring thin sections were used, complicating the interpretation of results; and (3) lymphocystis virus may be inherently variable in size. Amphibian ICDVs (Granoff, 1969), octopus ICDV (Rungger *et al.*, 1971), and iridescent viruses (types 1–19) (Chapman *et al.*, 1968) are approximately 130 nm in size. The reported sizes of other iridescent viruses range from 130 to 170 nm (Bellet, 1968) and from 175 to 215 nm for African swine fever virus (Breese and DeBoer, 1966).

3.2. Morphology and Structure

Apparent icosahedral symmetry is a major feature of ICDVs. *Tipula* iridescent virus (TIV) was the first virus to be shown conclusively to possess icosahedral symmetry, having 812 surface subunits (Smith and Hill, 1962). Subsequently, Wrigley (1970) provided evidence that TIV probably had 1472 subunits, although 1292 and 1562 could not be excluded. Stoltz (1971, 1973) found similar structural arrangements in *Scironomus plumosus* virus and TIV and in the "T" strain of a mosquito iridescent virus. The faces of TIV particles are approximately equilateral, and triangular and trisymmetrons (regular triangular arrays) of hexagonally packed subunits in their shells can be observed (Wrigley, 1970; Stoltz, 1971, 1973) (Fig. 2). Similarly detailed substructure of *Sericesthis* iridescent virus (SIV) (type 2) was shown to have around 1562 morphological subunits (Wrigley, 1969, 1970). Almeida *et al.* (1967) using negative staining techniques compared the structures of iridescent type 1 and ASFV. The structures of both of these viruses were quite complex, but similar, and were composed of about 812 subunits. ICDV particles appear isometric and hexagonal in thin sections.

The structural details of plant ICDVs have not been satisfactorily resolved, although the capsid structure is easily demonstrated (Shepherd, 1970; Brunt, 1971), and icosahedral structures have not been rigorously demonstrated for many ICDVs. The presence of numerous

←——————————————————————————————————————

Fig. 1.   Morphology of icosahedral cytoplasmic DNA viruses. A: Purified frog virus 3 (FV3) particles negatively stained. B: Higher-magnification electron micrograph showing FV3 membrane (m) and core (c) structure. C: FV3 cores prepared by NP-40 treatment of the purified virus particles. D: Electron micrograph of a thin section of *Tipula* iridescent virus (TIV) infected cells. E: Higher magnification of negatively stained TIV showing membrane. F: Electron micrograph of a negatively stained preparation of cauliflower mosaic virus. Bar in all photos equals 0.1 μm.

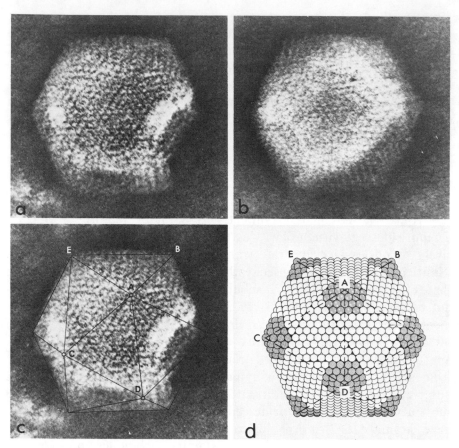

Fig. 2. (a,b) Two samples of TIV particles after 24-hr treatment with "Afrin." Rows of subunits can be clearly seen in parts. (c) Same particles as in (a) but with a possible interpretation of the icosahedron edges superimposed. (d) 1562-subunit model proposed for *Sericethis* iridescent virus (SIV), for comparison with (c). The size scale for these pictures is given by the icosahedron edge length 824 Å (lengths *A* to *B*, *B* to *E*, etc.) determined for TIV. From Wrigley (1970).

fibers trailing from the icosahedron has been described for the *Chironomus* virus and other iridescent viruses (Stoltz, 1971, 1973). Similar fibers about 200 nm long and 4 nm wide have been found in lymphocystis virus preparations (Zwillenberg and Wolf, 1968) and FV3 (Lunger and Came, 1966). The viral specificity and significance of these fibers remain to be established.

The mammalian ICDVs possess envelopes derived by budding into cytoplasmic vacuoles or through the plasma membrane (Fig. 3) (Walker, 1962; Granoff *et al.*, 1965; Granoff, 1969; Breese and DeBoer,

1966; Kelly, 1975). At least with FV3 the outer viral envelope is not needed for infectivity as nonenveloped particles are infectious (Willis and Granoff, 1974). In addition to the outer cell-derived envelope, mammalian ICDVs have a "limiting membrane" as a structural component of the icosahedral particle (Fig. 1B) (Willis and Granoff, 1974). This membrane is essential for infectivity since lipid solvents render virions noninfectious.

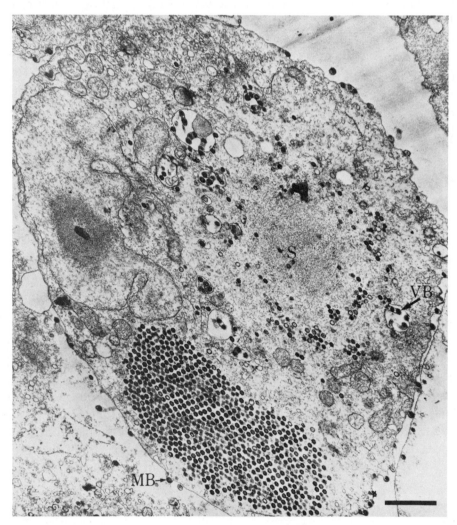

Fig. 3.   Electron micrograph of a thin section of an FHM cell infected with FV3. Virus synthesis site (S) in center has displaced nucleus to the left. A loosely packed virus crystal is in the lower center. Virus particles may be seen budding either from the cytoplasmic membrane (MB) or in the cytoplasmic vacuoles (VB). Bar represents 1 μm. From Granoff (1969).

In contrast to the mammalian ICDVs, insect ones do not have a cell-derived envelope but do have a lipid-containing structure, the location of which appears to be internal (Fig. 1E) (Day and Mercer, 1964; Stoltz, 1971). Iridescent viruses are not ether sensitive (Day and Mercer, 1964), suggesting that the lipid membrane is not essential for infectivity or that because of its internal nature it is inaccessible to the lipid solvent.

Thin sections of virus particles of several ICDVs show an electron-dense irregularly shaped core that presumably contains DNA (Fig. 1B). In iridescent virions the cores, as noted above, are apparently surrounded by one or more "membranes" (Fig. 1E). Detergent treatment of FV3 results in a subunit structure referred to as a "core" (Fig. 1C) (Aubertin et al., 1971; Willis and Granoff, 1974). However, the structural and compositional relationship between cores produced by detergent treatment and those seen by electron microscopy is not known.

4. PHYSICAL PROPERTIES

Most of the information on the physical properties of ICDVs is derived from studies with the iridescent viruses, frog virus 3, and the plant viruses. The $s_{20,w}$ values for several of the iridescent viruses (types 1, 2, 6, and 9) are around 2200 (reviewed by Kelly and Robertson, 1973), in contrast to the value obtained for iridescent virus type 3, which is 4450 (Matta, 1970). The differences in values obtained between these viruses probably reflect differences in their sizes. In cesium chloride the density of these virus particles ranges from 1.354 g/cm³ for iridescent virus type 3 (Matta, 1970) to 1.32 g/cm³ for iridescent virus types 1 and 2 and 1.30 g/cm³ for iridescent virus type 9 (Robertson and Longworth, 1973). Enveloped virus particles of frog virus 3 have a buoyant density of 1.28 g/cm³ and unenveloped particles 1.32 g/cm³ (Morris et al., 1966). Information on plant ICDVs is limited to a sedimentation coefficient of 220 S for cauliflower mosaic virus (Pirone et al., 1961) and 254 S for dahlia mosaic virus (Brunt, 1971).

5. CHEMICAL COMPOSITION

5.1. DNA

The DNA of large ICDVs is double-stranded and linear, and in the iridescent viruses types 2, 6, 9, and 18 its molecular weight ranges from

114 to 160 × 10⁶ (Bellett, 1968; Kelly and Avery, 1974a). Wagner and Paschke (1977), however, reported a much higher molecular weight of DNA of mosquito iridescent virus (MIV). Two strains of MIV—R and T—have DNA with molecular weights of 243.3 × 10⁶ and 287.7 × 10⁶, respectively, the largest reported for any viruses. The R strain of MIV may contain two identical duplex DNA molecules per virion. The molecular weight of African swine fever virus DNA has been estimated to be 100 × 10⁶ (Enjuanes et al., 1976). The molecular weight of FV3 DNA was first estimated as 130 × 10⁶ on the basis of velocity sedimentation and electron microscopy (Smith and McAuslan, 1969; Houts et al., 1970), but Kelly and Avery (1974b) have reported a lower estimate, 100 × 10⁶, based on reannealing kinetics of DNA and velocity sedimentation analysis of viral DNA after careful removal of all structural proteins. This is probably the most reliable value. FV3 DNA has alkali-labile, single-strand interruptions in both strands (Kelly and Avery, 1974b; R. Goorha and A. Granoff, unpublished observations). It appears, however, that these interruptions are produced during the purification of virus particles and the extraction of DNA. DNA extracted from unfrozen and unsonicated freshly prepared virions has considerably fewer interruptions under conditions when nucleases are least active (R. Goorha and A. Granoff, unpublished results). Moreover, genome-size uninterrupted DNA is readily obtained from the infected cells by alkaline sucrose gradient centrifugation (Goorha et al., 1978). Sonication followed by freezing and thawing of freshly prepared virus preparations introduces nicks in the FV3 genome, although infectivity titers after these treatments are not reduced (R. Goorha and A. Granoff, unpublished results). Therefore, it appears that single-strand interruptions in FV3 genomes are repaired in the cells before DNA replication occurs. A similar interpretation has been given to other DNA viruses with single-strand interruptions, such as herpesviruses (Ben-Porat et al., 1976).

In small iridescent viruses the base composition ranges from 30% G+C in types 2 and 6 to 40% in type 9 (Kelly and Avery, 1974a); in MIV it is 53.9% (Wagner and Paschke, 1977). The base composition of FV3 DNA is 53% G+C (Houts et al., 1970). Repetitious DNA has been demonstrated in several ICDVs. The amount of repetitious DNA in R and T strains of MIV (17–30%) is higher than reported for iridescent virus types 2 and 6 (5–15%) (Kelly and Avery, 1974a; Wagner and Paschke, 1977). Reiterated sequences in FV3 comprise 7% of the genome (Kelly and Avery, 1974b). The function of repetitive sequences in ICDVs, as in other DNA viruses, remains speculative. Quantitative analysis of DNA-DNA homology showed no sequence homology between FV3 and iridescent virus type 2, 6, or 9 (Kelly and Avery, 1974a).

As expected from their small diameter, plant ICDVs have a much smaller genome (4.3×10^6) than their mammalian counterparts. The DNA of these viruses is double-stranded and, in contrast to that of large ICDVs, is circular (Shepherd et al., 1968, 1970; Russel et al., 1971). The nicked, circular form of cauliflower mosaic virus DNA is infectious (Hull and Shepherd, 1977). A physical map of the genome of cauliflower mosaic virus has been constructed on the basis of the cleavage of the DNA by restriction endonucleases (Meagher et al., 1977). Evidence for nucleotide sequence heterogeneity in the native viral DNA population is the presence of uncommon restriction endonuclease sites found only in a small portion of the DNA molecules.

5.2. Proteins and Enzyme Activities

5.2.1. Proteins

Proteins of the ICDV group have been analyzed by polyacrylamide gel electrophoresis or serological techniques. Available information from polyacrylamide gel electrophoresis suggests that the number of polypeptides present in virus particles of ICDVs is quite different and not correspondingly related to virus size. African swine fever virus apparently contains only five structural proteins (Black and Brown, 1976). Frog virus 3 contains about 20 structural polypeptides (Tan and McAuslan, 1971; Goorha and Granoff, 1974a; Willis et al., 1977), the most prevalent having a molecular weight of 55,000 and accounting for nearly 26% of the total proteins. None of the proteins appears to be glycosylated (R. Goorha and A. Granoff, unpublished observation). Iridescent virus types 2 and 6 contain about 20 proteins each; the major structural protein of both viruses has a molecular weight of 65,000, with the molecular weights of other proteins ranging from 10,000 to 200,000 (Kelly and Tinsley, 1972). Polyacrylamide gel analysis of mosquito iridescent virus disclosed nine proteins, none of which reacted with Schiff's reagent, consistent with a lack of glycoproteins in these virions (Wagner et al., 1974). *Tipula* iridescent virus was found to contain 28 polypeptides ranging in molecular weight from 17.5 to 300×10^3; none was a glycoprotein (Krell and Lee, 1974). In keeping with their small size, plant ICDVs have a simple electrophoretic profile of protein; cauliflower mosaic virus contains only two structural proteins, having molecular weights of 68,000 and 33,000 (Tezuka and Taniguchi, 1972).

Serological techniques have provided information on the presence of common antigens among certain ICDVs. On the basis of complement-fixation, gel diffusion, and neutralization tests, amphibian ICDVs can be divided into two groups. FV1, FV2, FV3, LT1, LT3, LT4, L4, L5, TEV, T6, T8, and T15 are very similar and perhaps represent one serotype, whereas isolate L2 differs from the other isolates and can be considered a separate serotype (Lehane *et al.*, 1968; Clark *et al.*, 1969; Kaminski *et al.*, 1969). Although several serotypes of ASFV exist (Coggins, 1968; Hess, 1971), there has not been a concerted effort to establish the relationship between the various isolates. African swine fever virus does not cross-react serologically with FV3 (Came and Dardiri, 1969), iridescent virus type 1, or lymphocystis virus (Clark *et al.*, 1969; Kaminski *et al.*, 1969). Iridescent virus types 1, 2, 9, 10, 16, 17, 18, and 19 show cross-reactivity but are not identical when examined by immunoprecipitation tests (Cunningham and Tinsley, 1968; Kalmakoff and Robertson, 1970; Glitz *et al.*, 1968; Kalmakoff *et al.*, 1972). Iridescent virus types 3 and 12 are related to each other but do not possess antigens in common with types 1, 2, 6, 9, and 10 (Tinsley *et al.*, 1971; Cunningham and Tinsley, 1968). Type 6 is not serologically related to type 1, 2, 3, 9, 10, 12, or 16 (Kelly and Robertson, 1973). There does appear to be a serological relationship among the plant ICDVs (Brunt, 1966; Hollings and Stone, 1969).

5.2.2. Enzyme Activities Associated with Virions

Some ICDVs contain an assortment of enzyme activities associated with purified virions. Purified particles of FV3, for example, have been shown to contain at least five enzyme activities, including nucleotide phosphohydrolase, which exhibits a high specificity for ATP (Vilagines and McAuslan, 1971); ribonucleasae, which cleaves both single- and double-stranded RNA (Kang and McAuslan, 1972); deoxyribonuclease activities having pH optimum of 5 and 7.5 (Kang and McAuslan, 1972); protein kinase, which is not dependent on cyclic nucleotide and which is the only enzyme established as virus coded (Silberstein and August, 1973, 1976); and protein phosphatase (Silberstein and August, 1973). *Chilo* iridescent virus particles contain a nucleotide phosphohydrolase activity (Monnier and DeVauchelle, 1976) as well as protein kinase activity which has been purified to apparent homogeneity from the virus particles (C. Monnier, personal communication).

Whether or not DNA-dependent RNA polymerase activity is present in FV3 and iridescent viruses is controversial. Gaby and Kucera

(1974) reported a transcriptase activity in FV3 particles, but they used an exogenous template ("activated" calf thymus DNA) to stimulate transcription. The enzyme activity was very low, and the viral specificity of the RNA synthesized was not established. Other workers (D. Willis, personal communication; A. Aubertin, personal communication) have failed to detect RNA polymerase activity under the conditions described by Gaby and Kucera (1974). Kelly and Tinsley (1973) reported an RNA polymerase activity in iridescent virus, SIV and CIV types 2 and 6 particles, but C. Monnier (personal communication) has not been able to confirm these results.

Although a number of ICDVs contain an impressive array of enzyme activities, especially FV3, their role in virus replication is not clear. The observation that DNA extracted from African swine fever virus is infectious (Adldinger *et al.*, 1966) further obscures the role of viral enzymes in the replication process of this virus.

5.3.   Lipids

As mentioned in the preceding section, ICDVs that have been studied contain lipid. Smith and McAuslan (1969) reported that the composition of FV3 is 14% extractable lipid, but this estimate was probably too high because of inadequate purification of virions. Willis and Granoff (1974) reported that about 9% of the unenveloped FV3 virions is lipid, mainly phospholipid. The ratios of the various phospholipid classes of the virion and of those of host cells, as well as the low amount of cholesterol present in the virions, led to the conclusion that the viral membrane was not derived from preexisting host membranes. Early reports (Thomas, 1961; Glitz *et al.*, 1968) of the presence of lipid (5%) in iridescent viruses were considered to represent casual cellular contaminant (Bellett, 1968). However, recently, lipid extracted from purified iridescent virus type 2 and type 6 and analyzed by thin-layer chromatography was found to be different from that of the host cell (Kelly and Vance, 1973). A minor lipid component of the virus was found to be sphingomyelin, a lipid abundant in the plasma membrane. The virus particles contained 9% lipid by weight, which could account for the amount required to form a continuous bilayer at an internal site within the virus particle. Wagner *et al.* (1973) reported between 3% and 4% lipid for two strains of mosquito iridescent virus. To our knowledge, there is no information on the plant ICDVs regarding the presence or absence of lipid.

6. REPLICATION

Studies on the replication of many ICDVs have been limited to electron microscopic observations. The biological and biochemical aspects of ICDV replication have been studied mainly in FV3-infected cells and to a lesser extent in iridescent virus types 2 and 6 and in cells infected with African swine fever virus. After some general considerations of ICDV replication, we will discuss in detail information on the replication of FV3, and, wherever possible, we will compare it with results for other ICDVs.

Since only morphological changes can be identified with electron microscopy, such studies have been limited to very early and late events in the replicative cycle of ICDVs. The results of electron microscopic studies have frequently provided the basis for identifying the cytoplasm as the site of ICDV replication (Figs. 3 and 4). In FV3-infected cells, virions are adsorbed on the cell membrane and enter the cell through pinocytosis (Fig. 5A–E) (Houts *et al.*, 1974; Kelly, 1975). Once inside the cells, virus particles are rapidly uncoated in phagocytic vacuoles and lose their morphological identity. The first morphological event apparently related to virus replication is the appearance of discrete areas in the cytoplasm which have been termed "inclusion bodies." These are round, finely granulated, with an electron-translucent matrix (Fig. 3), and usually devoid of ribosomes—in sharp contrast to the surrounding cytoplasm (Darlington *et al.*, 1966; Bingen-Brendel *et al.*, 1971; Kelly, 1975). Cytoplasmic inclusion bodies have been shown to contain newly synthesized DNA, presumably viral, in cells infected with FV3 (Maes and Granoff, 1967; McAuslan and Smith, 1968; Guir *et al.*, 1970), iridescent virus type 1 (Morris, 1970), or carnation etched-ring virus (Rubio-Huertos *et al.*, 1972). The presence of inclusion bodies in the cytoplasm of infected cells precedes the appearance and accumulation of virus particles.

Although accumulation of virus particles in a paracrystalline array in the cytoplasm is readily seen (Fig. 3), the morphogenetic and maturational events during the replication of ICDVs are poorly understood. In cells infected with iridescent type 1 virus, the presence of "empty" (incompletely stained) particles has led to opposing views on the assembly of these virions: (1) viral DNA first condenses and then is encapsidated by proteins (Bird, 1961, 1962; Kelly, 1972a) or (2) empty virus particles are formed first, followed by the entry of viral DNA (Xeros, 1964; Smith, 1958, 1967). Available data are not adequate to permit a choice between these alternatives. In FV3-infected cells, virus-

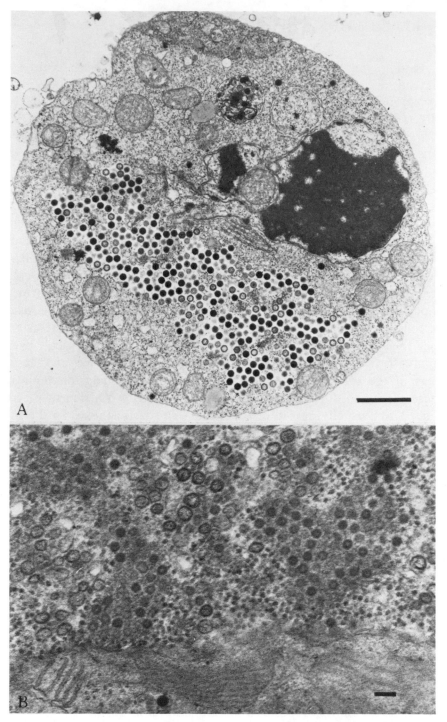

Fig. 4.   Electron micrograph of a thin section of *Tipula* iridescent virus (A) or cauliflower mosaic virus (B) infected cells showing the site of replication for these viruses.

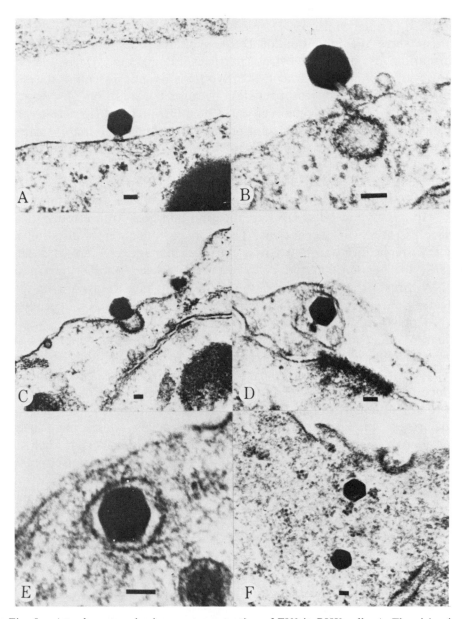

Fig. 5.   Attachment and subsequent penetration of FV3 in BHK cells. A: The virion is attached at a vortex, and there appears to be a stalklike structure between the point of attachment and the vortex. B: A vesicle immediately beneath the point of virus attachment. C: A virion partly engulfed by a vesicle. D: Almost complete engulfment of a virion by an undulating cell fold. The virus appears to be bound to the vacuole wall by a structure resembling that seen at the attachment site. E: A completely engulfed virion. F: Two particles of FV3 lying free in the cytoplasm of an FHM cell that may have entered by direct penetration. From Houts *et al.* (1974).

specific structures are not observed unless viral DNA synthesis has been initiated (Tripier *et al.*, 1977), in contrast to cells infected with vaccinia virus, where the inhibition of DNA synthesis does not prevent the formation of immature virus particles (Pogo and Dales, 1971). However, continuous viral DNA synthesis is not essential for the formation of empty virus particles, because the addition of cytosine arabinoside to FV3-infected cells at 3 hr after infection (to arrest subsequent DNA synthesis) does not prevent formation of immature particles in paracrystalline arrays (Tripier *et al.*, 1977). Encapsidation of viral DNA occurs soon after its synthesis in FV3-infected cells (McAuslan and Smith, 1968; Kucera, 1970; Purifoy *et al.*, 1973), although the process by which virus particles mature is still unknown.

In eukaryotic cells, DNA replication and gene transcription take place essentially in the nucleus. Therefore, a fundamental question in ICDV replication is how these viruses manage to replicate and transcribe genomes in the cytoplasm. Poxviruses, another group of DNA viruses that replicate in the cytoplasm, have evolved a unique strategy of replication. Incoming virus particles have a DNA-dependent RNA polymerase that transcribes a portion of the viral genome. A segment of the transcribed genome codes for a DNA polymerase—an enzyme required for DNA replication. Apparently, this strategy bypasses a requirement for host machinery in nucleic acid synthesis, which presumably is confined to the nucleus. The strategy of replication of FV3, although much less clear, is quite different from that of poxviruses. In FV3, evidence for several steps which have been considered essential for cytoplasmic replication of vaccinia, such as uncoating of virions in two stages and virion-associated transcriptase, either has not been found or is equivocal as discussed above. We will discuss the results obtained with FV3 and, as mentioned earlier, compare them wherever possible with results from other ICDVs.

6.1. Replication of Frog Virus 3

6.1.1. General Characteristics

Although FV3 replicates in a wide variety of cells of piscine, amphibian, avian, or mammalian origin (Granoff, 1969), most of the biochemical aspects of its replication have been studied in fathead minnow (FHM) or baby hamster kidney (BHK-21/13) cells (McAuslan and Armentrout, 1974). The temperature range for growth of the virus is between 12°C and 32°C (Gravell and Granoff, 1970). Above

32°C, infectious virus is not produced, although some virus-specific macromolecular synthesis does occur (Kucera and Granoff, 1969; Kucera, 1970; Goorha and Granoff, 1974b). The time course of infectious virus production is quite variable, depending on the type of cells, temperature of incubation, multiplicity of infection, conditions of growth, and strain of the virus (Gravell and Granoff, 1970; Goorha and Granoff, 1974a; Kelly, 1975; Tripier et al., 1977). In FHM cells, the life cycle of FV3 is over in 12–16 hr (Fig. 6). The duration of eclipse in these cells is about 4 hr, which represents a minimum eclipse period, one that cannot be decreased by increasing the multiplicity of infection. The yield of virus from infected cells increases exponentially between 4 and 12 hr, and almost all of the infectious progeny are produced by 16 hr after infection. Under optimal conditions, the yield of FV3 is 100–200 PFU/cell. Since routine preparations of FV3 contain 50–100 particles PFU (G. Murti, personal communication), each cell produces between 5000 and 20,000 virus particles. Around 80% of the infectious virus remains cell associated and only 20% of the progeny are released into the medium (Gravell and Granoff, 1970).

In most viral infections, virus-specific macromolecules are difficult to detect because host macromolecular synthesis continues, albeit at a reduced rate, especially during the early stages of virus replication. Unequivocal evidence for the viral origin of these macromolecules can be obtained in two ways: (1) by demonstrating that infected cells are incapable of expressing their own genetic information or (2) by showing

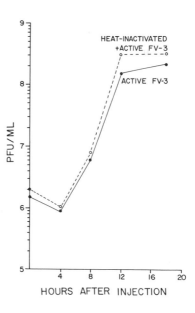

Fig. 6. Growth of FV3 at 30°C in FHM monolayers exposed or not exposed to heat-inactivated (△) FV3. At various intervals the total virus yield (cell-associated plus released virus) was determined by suspending the cells in culture medium and releasing the cell-associated virus into it by sonic oscillation. Virus titers were determined by plaque assay. ●——●, Active virus alone; ○---○, active virus in cells preexposed to △FV3 for 4 hr. From Goorha and Granoff (1974a).

that macromolecules are genetically determined by the virus. In practice, the viral specificity of macromolecules is established indirectly, i.e., by nucleic acid hybridization or by immunoprecipitation of proteins; thus the quantitation of viral macromolecules becomes especially difficult and inaccurate. In this regard, FV3 offers a unique advantage as, eventually, may other ICDVs. As mentioned earlier, a structural protein(s) of FV3 severely inhibits host macromolecular synthesis. Furthermore, FV3 inactivated at 56°C for 20–30 min loses its infectivity and its ability to initiate viral macromolecular synthesis, but still inhibits host macromolecular synthesis by 90% or more (Goorha and Granoff, 1974a; Goorha et al., 1978). However, the inhibition of host macromolecular synthesis is selective; i.e., preexposure of cells to heat-inactivated (Δ) FV3 does not affect either the kinetics of replication or the final yield of virus on subsequent infection with active FV3 (Fig. 6). Therefore, in these cells, newly synthesized DNA, RNA, and proteins are almost exclusively of viral origin (Goorha and Granoff, 1974a; Willis and Granoff, 1978; Goorha et al., 1978) and can be readily analyzed.

A number of FV3 temperature-sensitive (ts) mutants have been obtained and placed into seven complementation groups (Naegele and Granoff, 1971; R. F. Naegele, unpublished data). Several of these mutants have been further characterized (Purifoy et al., 1973) and have provided insight into the virus specificity of regulatory mechanisms of protein (Goorha et al., 1975; Silberstein and August, 1976) and RNA synthesis (D. Willis, R. Goorha, and A. Granoff, unpublished observations). They have also been useful in identifying the FV3 protein kinase as a virus-specific enzyme (Silberstein and August, 1976). High recombination frequencies have been found in all crosses between ts mutants (Naegele and Granoff, 1971). Like poxviruses (for review, see McAuslan, 1969), FV3 is capable of "nongenetic" reactivation (Gravell and Naegele, 1970; Gravell and Cromeans, 1971). If heat-inactivated and UV-inactivated virus particles are aggregated before adsorption to the host cell, there is a seventyfold or more reactivation in their infectivity. Structural complementation has been proposed as the basis for nongenetic reactivation. Virus particles inactivated with UV light have a nonfunctional genome but can supply structural protein(s) required for infection, while heat-inactivated virus particles have denatured structural proteins but possess a normal genome. A normal infection is initiated when both types of particles are in close proximity within a cell. This mechanism was first proposed to explain the nongenetic reactivation of poxviruses (for review, see McAuslan, 1969). The phenomenon of nongenetic reactivation has been interpreted as indirect evidence for the presence of an RNA polymerase in FV3 virions. However, alternative explanations for nongenetic reactivation, such as the requirement of an established virion-associated enzyme or a requirement for a functional structural protein for uncoating of heat-inactivated virions, are equally plausible.

6.1.2. Adsorption, Penetration, and Uncoating

Early events in FV3 infection have been studied by two different techniques: electron microscopy and analysis of the fate of radioactively labeled virus after inoculation. Since the ratio of particles to plaque-forming units in FV3 is between 50 and 100, available methods for examining early events in infection do not reveal the fate of all particles, making it difficult to identify the true infectious pathway. Nevertheless, studies on early virus–cell interaction can provide clues to the strategy of virus replication. For example, in vaccinia infection, virus uncoating has a controlling influence on the phases of viral transcription. Preexisting cellular enzymes remove the outer coat of the virion, and the resulting "core" transcribes the early genes. A second stage of uncoating, requiring protein and viral DNA synthesis, precedes the transcription of "late" genes (Kates and McAuslan, 1967a,b; McAuslan, 1969).

Electron microscopic studies have shown that attachment of FV3 virions to the host cell membrane at the vertex of the icosahedron and pinocytosis appeared to be a predominant mode of entry (Fig. 5A–E) (Houts et al., 1974; Kelly 1975). Soon after penetration, virions were uncoated in cytoplasmic vacuoles and lost their morphological identity. For subsequent steps in the infectious cycle to occur, the vacuolar contents have to be released into the cytoplasm. However, evidence that virions may enter the cell by direct penetration was also obtained (Fig. 5F), and it is not known with certainty which mode of entry leads to a productive infection.

Uncoating of radioactively labeled FV3 has been measured by the conversion of DNase-resistant DNA (coated virion) to a DNase-sensitive form (uncoated virion) (Smith and McAuslan, 1969). Virions were rapidly uncoated, and within an hour approximately 50% of the viral DNA became DNase sensitive. Whether half of the virus particles are completely uncoated or whether all particles are only partially uncoated cannot be ascertained from these experiments. The extent and rate of uncoating of FV3 virions were similar in the presence or absence of a protein synthesis inhibitor, suggesting that the uncoating process does not require protein synthesis. Therefore, unlike the transcriptional control exerted by uncoating of vaccinia virus, uncoating of FV3 does not appear to exert a controlling influence on its trancription.

6.1.3.   Transcription (RNA Synthesis)

After entry and uncoating, transcription of viral DNA is the first major event in the growth cycle of FV3. The question of how FV3 initiates transcription has not been settled, although there are only three possible alternatives: (1) presence of RNA polymerase in the virion, (2) use of cellular RNA polymerase, and (3) presence of mRNA in the virion, which is then translated into RNA polymerase. The third possibility has been excluded by the observation that, in infected cells, viral RNA is synthesized in the presence of cycloheximide (Armentrout and McAuslan, 1974; Willis and Granoff, 1978). A great deal of effort has been spent attempting to find an RNA polymerase in the virions, but, as mentioned earlier, the results have been equivocal. A low level of transcriptase activity associated with the virion was reported (Gaby and Kucera, 1974), although activity was detected only when exogenous template ("activated" calf thymus DNA) was added. Low levels of DNA polymerase activity have also been observed by Tan and Mc-Auslan (1972), who believed that the low activity was caused by the small amounts of cellular polymerase adsorbed to the virus particles. Other workers have also failed to find any polymerase activity in FV3 virions (A. Aubertin, personal communication; D. Willis, personal communication). To establish firmly the presence of polymerase in the virion, it must be shown that RNA synthesized *in vitro* hybridizes to FV3 DNA, has the same size class as viral RNA isolated from the polysomes of the infected cells, and is translated into viral proteins *in vitro*. To date, none of these conditions has been fulfilled.

There are three lines of indirect evidence favoring the presence of virion-associated polymerase. The first two, nongenetic reactivation of FV3 (discussed earlier) and synthesis of viral RNA in the absence of protein synthesis (Armentrout and McAuslan, 1974; Willis and Granoff, 1978), suggest that a preexisting enzyme is utilized for transcription, but neither observation distinguishes between the utilization of host and viral polymerase. The reduction of FV3 transcription in BHK cells at 37°C (Gravell and Cromeans, 1971; D. Willis and A. Granoff, unpublished results), a temperature compatible with the normal function of cellular enzymes but not for FV3, has been interpreted as evidence for a virion-associated polymerase. However, the reduction of transcription could reflect the unavailability of viral template rather than inactivation of the polymerase. Thus the source of enzyme (viral or cellular) for early transcription in FV3-infected cells remains to be established.

Studies on the transcription of the FV3 genome have been concerned mainly with qualitative, quantitative, and temporal control. Posttranscriptional modification of viral RNA has also been examined. A unique advantage of the FV3 system, as noted earlier, is that it allows direct detection and quantitation of infected-cell RNA (ICR) species because pretreatment of cells with heat-inactivated FV3 (ΔFV3) almost completely abolishes host RNA synthesis (Guir *et al.*, 1970; Willis and Granoff, 1976a) without affecting the subsequent replication of infectious FV3 (Goorha and Granoff, 1974a). Additionally, the absence of poly(A) on FV3 RNAs (Willis and Granoff, 1976b) has facilitated their resolution and quantitation in polyacrylamide gels (Willis *et al.*, 1977).

Viral RNA species from wild-type and *ts* mutant-infected cells have been examined at various times after infection to determine to what extent qualitative, quantitative, and temporal controls of RNA synthesis are operative during FV3 replication (Willis and Granoff, 1976a, 1978; Willis *et al.*, 1977; D. Willis and A. Granoff, unpublished observations). Results obtained thus far, accounted for in the preceding references, are now summarized.

6.1.3a. Qualitative Control

Forty-seven species of viral RNA have been resolved in polyacrylamide gels under denaturing conditions (Figs. 7 and 8). Only ten of the 47 RNA bands were plainly visible after electrophoresis of extracts from cells labeled from 1.0 to 1.5 hr after infection; these ten RNAs were designated as "early" RNA (Fig. 8b). By 3–4 hr after infection, all of the remaining RNA species that could be detected were synthesized and were termed "late" RNA (Fig. 8d). As will be discussed in the following section, these RNAs can be further subdivided based on their temporal relationships. The above results establish the presence of qualitative controls during FV3 transcription. An important aspect of the FV3 transcription pattern is that the classical definition of "early" and "late" RNA, i.e., RNA synthesis tightly coupled to viral DNA replication (Ginsberg, 1969), was not entirely applicable. When

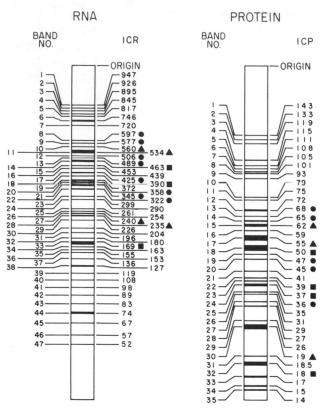

Fig. 7. Schematic representation of FV3 intracellular RNAs (ICR) and proteins (ICP). This drawing is a composite of all bands seen on both short- and long-term exposure of polyacrylamide gels and at every interval examined. The symbols represent the time during the virus growth cycle at which various ICPs are maximally synthesized. ●, Early; ■, intermediate; ▲, late. The ICRs postulated to code for ICPs were assigned identical symbols (see Table 5). From Willis *et al.* (1977).

DNA synthesis was prevented for 6 hr, either by cytosine arabinoside or by growth of a DNA-negative mutant (*ts6642*) at nonpermissive temperature, RNA synthesized under these conditions contained 80–85% of the sequences present late in normal infection. In contrast, RNA extracted at 2.0 hr after infection (viral DNA synthesis is initiated within 2 hr of infection) contained only 40–45% of sequences present late in normal infection.

6.1.3b. Quantitative Control

The relative molar rates of RNA species synthesized at various times after infection have been determined, and the results suggest the

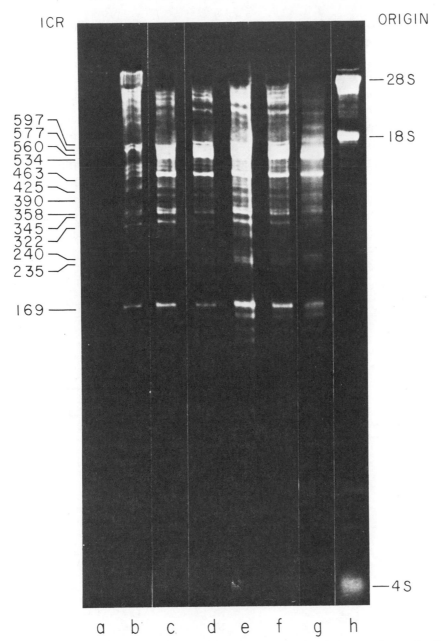

Fig. 8. Fluorograph of polyacrylamide gel containing RNAs from FV3-infected cells. RNA, labeled for 30 min with [³H]uridine at various times after the infection, was extracted from the cytoplasm of the infected cells. Heat-inactivated (Δ) FV3 was used to inhibit host cell RNA synthesis except for the 6- or 8-hr samples. By these times active virus alone sufficiently reduced host synthesis. (a) 4-hr ΔFV3; (b) 3-hr ΔFV3, 1-hr active FV3; (c) 3-hr ΔFV3, 2-hr active FV3; (d) 3-hr ΔFV3, 4-hr active FV3; (e) 6-hr active FV3; (f) 8-hr active FV3; (g) 6-hr FV3 RNA hybridized to and eluted from FV3 DNA; (h) uninfected FHM RNA. From Willis *et al.* (1977).

presence also of complex quantitative controls (Table 2). Thus most of the RNA species synthesized 1.0–1.5 hr after infection were produced in approximately equimolar amounts; at most there was only a three- to four-fold difference in molar rates of synthesis. By 4 hr after infection, not only were additional species synthesized but also there was as much as a fiftyfold difference between the relative molar rates of synthesis of the most scarce and the most abundant RNAs.

Similarly, the rate of synthesis of certain RNA species varied markedly during the replication cycle. For example, the molar rate of synthesis of ICR 534 increased at least tenfold form 2 to 4 hr after infection (Table 2). Analysis of *ts* mutants has shown that the rates of synthesis of ICR 534 increased at least tenfold from 2 to 4 hr after regulatory protein. Synthesis of most species of RNA, once initiated, continued at the same or higher rates. Thus the synthesis of all early RNA species continued unabated throughout the infection.

The extent of transcription of viral DNA during the replication cycle of FV3 represents about one-half of the available nucleotide

TABLE 2
Molar Ratios of Viral RNAs Synthesized at Various Times after Infection[a]

Band No.	ICR molecular weight ($\times 10^{-3}$)	Molar ratio (hr)				
		1	2	4	6	8
2	926	1.22	0.49	0.62	0.79	1.14
7	720	1.50	0.48	0.63	0.97	1.16
8	597	1.28	1.34	3.50	2.49	2.15
9	577	2.44	3.00	4.64	5.14	4.80
11	534	ND	2.17	23.65	14.54	9.76
12	506	1.42	0.96	1.46	1.84	1.69
13	489	1.55	1.30	1.54	2.26	1.54
14	463	1.30	4.65	7.05	6.81	5.43
17	425	1.36	0.92	0.91	1.05	0.75
18	390	ND	0.92	1.46	2.35	1.33
21	345	0.75	0.97	1.33	3.63	1.74
22	322	1.00	0.96	1.57	2.57	1.46
23	299	ND	0.62	1.18	1.28	1.09
24	290	ND	0.65	2.96	0.81	0.73
27	240 ⎫	0.57	0.72	2.03	3.22	2.09
28	235 ⎭					
32	180	ND	0.43	0.69	1.10	0.49
33	169	3.16	4.19	5.01	10.10	8.25
34	163	ND	0.64	0.70	1.16	0.85
35	155 ⎫	ND	0.87	2.51	3.68	2.55
36	153 ⎭					

[a] These data have been selected from Willis *et al.* (1977). ND, nondetectable.

sequences. This conclusion is based on the fact that the RNA present in infected cells late in infection is complementary, by molecular hybridization, to 50% of the viral DNA. The datum suggests that only half of the genome, or the equivalent of one strand, is transcribed. It does not distinguish between the possibilities that one strand is transcribed exclusively or that both strands are partially transcribed.

6.1.3c. Temporal Control

In an earlier section on qualitative analysis, we divided viral RNA synthesis into early and late classes. However, detailed analysis of viral RNA synthesis in the presence of protein synthesis inhibitors or amino acid analogues, and the use of several temperature-sensitive mutants, has allowed further dissection of early and late RNAs into three subclasses each (Table 3) for operational purposes.

Early

1. *"Early early" RNA.*   Immediately after infection, part of the incoming genome is transcribed by a host- or virion-associated enzyme. "Early early" RNA is transcribed from about 32% of a single-strand equivalent of the FV3 genome, and its synthesis is not affected by the presence of protein synthesis inhibitors, such as cycloheximide.

2. *"Intermediate early" RNA.*   A virus-induced polypeptide, presumably not requiring phenylalanine for its function, allows the synthesis of a few additional "intermediate early" RNAs during the first 2 hr of infection. "Early early" and "intermediate early" RNA species represent approximately 70% of the single-strand equivalent of FV3 DNA. They are synthesized in the presence of the amino acid analogue fluorophenylalanine (FPA).

3. *"Late early" RNA.*   The presence of this class of RNA was established with a temperature-sensitive mutant, *ts 9467*. Late in infection, at the nonpermissive temperature, the mutant produces all of the RNAs found in wild-type infected cells treated with FPA. However, the rate of synthesis of some of the RNAs made by *ts 9467* differs from those of wild type. For example, infected-cell RNA (ICR) 169 is strikingly overproduced.

Late

1. *"Early late" RNA.*   Another mutant, *ts 2436*, was used to identify the "early late" class of RNA. This mutant appears to be

TABLE 3

Proposed Sequence of Events in Transcription of Frog Virus 3 mRNA

RNA class	Subdivision of each class	Experimental conditions	Viral DNA synthesis
Early			
	Early early	Cycloheximide addition	–
	Intermediate early	Fluorophenylalanie addition	–
	Late early	*ts9467* at nonpermissive temperature	+
Late			
	Early late	*ts2436* at nonpermissive temperature	+
	Intermediate late	*ts6642* at nonpermissive temperature	–
	Late late	Wild type	+

blocked at a later stage than *ts 9467* and primarily synthesizes early classes of RNA species. At the nonpermissive temperature, it makes a very small amount of "late" RNA species. Both *ts9467* and *ts2436* synthesize functional viral DNA at the nonpermissive temperature (Purifoy *et al.*, 1973).

2. *"Intermediate late" RNA.* A DNA-negative mutant (*ts6642*) establishes the presence of this class of RNAs. At nonpermissive temperature, the transcriptional pattern of *ts6642*, as analyzed by gel electrophoresis, does not show any qualitative or temporal differences from that of wild-type FV3. Nevertheless, qualitative differences do exist, since RNA synthesized by *ts6642* at nonpermissive temperature, when analyzed by DNA–RNA hybridization, contained only 80–85% of the sequences present late in the normal infection. Furthermore, the rate of synthesis of late RNAs is lower in *ts6642* at the nonpermissive temperature.

3. *"Late late" RNA.* This class of RNA represents the sequences which are present late in normal infection but are missing in *ts6642*-infected cells at nonpermissive temperature.

6.1.3d.   Posttranscriptional Modification of Viral RNA

The majority of mRNAs from eukaryotic cells and their viruses are modified at both ends. At the 3′ end, there is usually a poly(A) tract of variable length—up to 200 nucleotides. Although the function of poly(A) on mRNA is not known, its presence might increase the stability of mRNA. FV3 is the only known animal DNA virus that lacks poly(A) on its messages (Willis and Granoff, 1976b), and its absence appears to allow a sharper resolution of viral RNA on polyacrylamide gel electrophoresis.

The 5′ ends of the majority of eukaryotic cell and viral RNAs are "capped" and methylated (Rottman *et al.*, 1974). The term "cap" refers to an unusual 5′-5′ phosphodiester linkage between the last and penultimate nucleotide of mRNA. Methylation of mRNA occurs internally as well as at the 5′ end, and both bases as well as the sugar moiety of the nucleotides are modified. The internal methylation is usually in the form of 6-methyladenosine. Methylation of the 5′ end can generate as many as three oligonucleotide structures: m7G (5′)-ppp(5′)Xp_1, m7G (5′)-ppp(5′) X^mp Np, and m7G (5′)-ppp(5′)X^mp Y^mp NP, where X^m and Y^m represent 2′-O^--methylated derivatives of all four nucleotides (Rottman *et al.*, 1974). Preliminary results from our laboratory suggest that FV3 mRNAs are capped and methylated at the 5′ end and that the cap structure of these messages is heterogeneous, i.e., all three oligonucleotide structures are present. There is also internal methylation (R. Raghow, R. Goorha, D. Willis, and A. Granoff, unpublished data). No evidence for the posttranscriptional cleavage of FV3 messages has been obtained (D. Willis, personal communication).

6.1.4. Translation (Viral Protein Synthesis)

Selective inhibition of host protein synthesis by ΔFV3 prior to infection with active FV3 has greatly facilitated the examination of virus-specific protein synthesis as well as RNA (Goorha and Granoff, 1974*a,b*; Willis *et al.*, 1977). Electrophoresis in gradient polyacrylamide slab gels of cytoplasmic extracts of infected cells pulse-labeled with [^{35}S]methionine has led to the resolution of 35 infected cell protein (ICP) bands, ranging in molecular weight from 14,000 to 143,000 (Figs. 7 and 9). Inhibition of host protein synthesis by ΔFV3 was more than 90%. Quantitative data were obtained by determining the relative molar rates of synthesis of each polypeptide at various times during the infectious cycle (Table 4). The following conclusions are supported by our work, both published (Goorha and Granoff, 1974*a,b*; Goorha *et al.*, 1975; Willis *et al.*, 1977) and unpublished.

6.1.4a. Qualitative Control

FV3 protein synthesis is controlled at the qualitative level. However, since all detectable proteins are synthesized within 2 hr of

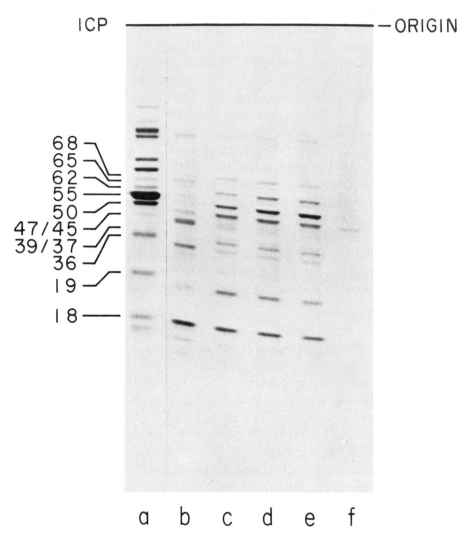

Fig. 9. Autoradiograph of polyacrylamide gel containing virus-specific polypeptides from FV3-infected cells. Proteins were labeled for 30 min with [³⁵S]methionine, and the cytoplasmic extracts were prepared and subjected to electrophoresis. (a) Purified FV3 structural proteins; (b) 3-hr ΔFV3, 2-hr active FV3; (c) 3-hr ΔFV3, 4-hr active FV3; (d) 6-hr active FV3; (e) 8-hr active FV3; (f) 5-hr ΔFV3. Heat-inactivated FV3 was used to inhibit host cell protein synthesis except for the 6- or 8-hr samples, at which time active virus alone was inhibitory to host synthesis. From Willis *et al.* (1977).

infection, analysis of qualitative control is difficult. This difficulty can be overcome by use of the amino acid analogue fluorophenylalanine (FPA). When FPA is added at the beginning of the infection, only a subset of viral proteins is synthesized. This subset can be broadly classified as "early" proteins. Proteins that are not made in the presence of FPA but are synthesized in its absence have been termed "late" proteins. As will be discussed later in this section, this subset of early proteins can be further divided into two groups based on the time of their maximal rates of synthesis. Data obtained with FPA imply that a viral protein(s) is responsible for the synthesis of late proteins. Apparently, substitutions of FPA in place of phyenylalanine renders the protein(s) required for late transcription nonfunctional; therefore, no late messages or proteins are made.

Unlike most other DNA viruses such as SV40, adenovirus, and vaccinia virus, the appearance of late proteins is not dependent on the

TABLE 4

Molar Ratios of Viral Polypeptides Synthesized at Various Times after Infection[a]

Band No.	ICR molecular weight ($\times 10^{-3}$)	Molar ratio (hr)				
		1	2	4	6	8
5	111	0.115	0.20	ND	ND	ND
6	108	0.088	0.24	0.24	0.11	0.19
11	75	0.19	0.48	1.10	0.96	0.71
13	68	0.47	1.18	0.47	0.34	ND
15	62	ND	0.40	2.36	2.89	2.4
16	59	0.29	1.0	0.68	0.79	0.75
17	55	0.39	1.08	4.8	5.71	5.7
18	50	1.01	2.46	7.3	5.69	4.47
19 20	47 45 }	2.10	7.2	3.78	1.73	0.76
22 23	39 37 }	0.61	1.82	6.75	5.53	4.38
24	36	1.64	6.12	4.38	3.57	2.83
25 26	35 31 }	0.76	2.72	1.20	1.32	ND
29	26	ND	1.20	2.86	1.79	ND
30	19	0.63	5.88	12.99	16.96	8.4
32	18	4.32	20.65	26.48	16.3	12.0
33	17	0.65	5.2	5.41	2.76	ND
34	15	0.49	10.59	5.93	4.93	2.23
35	14	1.27	6.16	2.52	ND	ND

[a] These data have been selected from Willis *et al.* (1977). ND, Nondetectable.

initiation of viral DNA replication. Thus most of the late proteins are detectable even when viral DNA synthesis is prevented either by addition of cytosine arabinoside or naturally by infection of cells at the nonpermissive temperature with a DNA-negative *ts* mutant.

6.1.4b. Quantitative Control

The relative molar rates of synthesis of viral proteins have been determined and provide evidence for the existence of complex quantitative controls. Based on the time during the growth cycle when their rate of synthesis is maximum, FV3-specific proteins have been classified into three groups. Approximately one-half of the detectable viral proteins (termed "early" protein) were synthesized at maximum rate early in infection (1 or 2 hr after infection). Another class (termed "intermediate" proteins) reached their maximum rate of synthesis at 4 hr after infection (Table 4). Both early and intermediate proteins were synthesized in the presence of FPA. The late proteins were barely detectable at 2 hr after infection and reached the highest rate of synthesis late in infection (6 hr after infection). Additionally, late proteins were not synthesized if FPA was present throughout the growth cycle.

When viral DNA synthesis was inhibited or FPA was present starting at the beginning of infection, the reduction in the rates of early and intermediate protein synthesized normally seen did not occur. In cells infected with a temperature-sensitive mutant, *ts2436*, at nonpermissive temperature, late proteins were synthesized at a low rate even late in infection. These results suggest that the rate of synthesis of viral proteins is controlled by viral regulatory proteins.

There is a wide variation (as much as fiftyfold) in molar rate of synthesis of early and intermediate proteins at 1 hr after infection (Table 4). At this time, as mentioned earlier, all of the RNA species that are detected are synthesized at nearly equimolar rates. Apparently, therefore, there is a great variation in the translational efficiencies of mRNA for early and late proteins. Parenthetically, it should be mentioned that the half-life (about 5 hr) of various viral mRNAs does not differ significantly.

6.1.4c. Viral Regulatory Proteins

The necessity of a functional, early virus-induced protein for both late RNA and protein synthesis has already been established (Willis *et al.*, 1977). Recently, we have also examined the number of viral proteins involved in transcriptional and translational controls and when these viral regulatory proteins appear during the replication cycle. In these experiments, FPA was added at various times after infection, and RNAs and proteins made between 6.0 and 6.5 hr were examined. The rationale was that if a viral regulatory protein is synthesized before the time of addition of FPA, then RNA and protein synthesis would be regulated normally. However, if the regulatory protein is synthesized after the addition of FPA, then this protein may not function and RNA and protein synthesis patterns would be altered. FPA added at the beginning of infection locked RNA synthesis into the early pattern for at least 6.0 hr. The transition from early to late RNA synthesis occurred only when the addition of FPA was delayed by 1–1.5 hr, indicating that a viral protein normally synthesized within the first 1.5 hr of infection is required for late transcription. A corresponding experiment with viral protein synthesis showed that when FPA was present from the beginning of infection, late proteins were not synthesized. As with RNA, if the addition of FPA was delayed 1–1.5 hr after infection, late proteins were synthesized. Thus the appearance of late proteins was probably the consequence of qualitative changes in transcription.

   In contrast to normal infection, the rates of synthesis of early and intermediate proteins were not reduced when cells were exposed to FPA within 1.5 hr of infection. The rate of synthesis of early proteins was reduced only when addition of FPA was delayed by 2 hr or more, and the rate of synthesis of intermediate proteins was reduced only when FPA was added at 3–4 hr after infection. Willis *et al.* (1977) have shown that there is no significant decrease in the rate of synthesis of RNA species beyond 2 hr after infection. Therefore, reduction in the rates of early and intermediate protein synthesis must be at the posttranscriptional level. Furthermore, these data suggest that the protein involved in posttranscriptional control of early proteins is different from the one involved in the posttranscriptional control of intermediate proteins.

6.1.4d. Posttranslational Modification of Viral Proteins

   Two types of modification of viral proteins have been reported: rapid posttranslational cleavage, as seen in picornaviruses (Holland and Kiehn, 1968), and addition of prosthetic groups such as glycosylation, phosphorylation, and acetylation. Experimental evidence suggests that there is no rapid posttranslational cleavage of viral proteins in FV3-

infected cells (R. Goorha, D. Willis, and A. Granoff, unpublished observation). The conclusion is based on three kinds of experiments: (1) a short pulse (3 min) followed by a chase for 30, 60, 90, 120, 180, and 240 min, which failed to show cleavage of viral proteins, (2) inhibitors of proteolytic enzymes, such as tolyl-sulfonyl-phenylalanyl chloromethyl ketone (TPCK) and tolyl-sulfonyl-lyal chloromethyl ketone (TLCK), which did not affect the profile of viral proteins in gel electrophoresis, and (3) the presence of FPA (to block the activity of a phenylalanine requiring proteolytic enzyme), which also failed to affect the migrational characteristics of viral protein on gel electrophoresis. The absence of rapid translational cleavage is important from two points of view: (1) these results suggest that FV3 mRNAs are monocistronic, and (2) since in many DNA viruses, such as adenovirus and vaccinia virus, cleavage of viral proteins occurs during assembly of virions, these results also suggest that morphogenesis of FV3 is quite different from that of these two viruses. In preliminary experiments, we have failed to detect glycosylation of structural or nonstructural proteins in FV3 infected cells (R. Goorha and A. Granoff, unpublished observation). A similar situation is found with several iridescent ICDVs (Wagner et al., 1974; Krell and Lee, 1974). Similarly, the presence of glycoproteins could not be detected in purified FV3 virions. No information is available concerning the phosphorylation or other modification of FV3 proteins.

6.1.5. Correlation between Transcriptional and Posttranscriptional Controls

With FV3, the results clearly demonstrate the importance of posttranscriptional control in the switch off of early and intermediate protein synthesis—groups comprising at least two-thirds of all the detectable viral protein species. Willis et al. (1977) selected ten RNA species as the messengers for specific viral polypeptides by size and by coordinate temporal behavior in rates of synthesis (Table 5). Three viral RNAs that could potentially code for three late proteins were positively correlated, i.e., an increase in the rate of synthesis of a particular mRNA species was followed by an increased rate of synthesis of corresponding protein (Fig. 10). However, seven RNA species assigned to code for seven early and intermediate proteins did not show decreased rates of synthesis between 2 and 6 hr, even though the rate of synthesis of corresponding proteins showed a definite and significant decline during this

TABLE 5

Correlation of Frog Virus 3 Specific mRNAs and Proteins

ICP molecular weight[a] (×10^{-3})	Classification	RNA calculated molecular weight[b] (×10^{-3})	ICR molecular weight[b] (×10^{-3})	RNA synthesized in presence of FPA
68	Early	612	597	+
65	Early	585	577	+
47/45	Early	405, 423	425	+
36	Early	324	345	+
50	Intermediate	450	463	+
39/37	Intermediate	333, 351	358	+
18	Intermediate	162	169	+
62	Late	558	560	0
55	Late	495	534	0
19	Late	270	240, 235	0

[a] Molecular weights of proteins were determined by relative mobility compared with standards in SDS–polyacrylamide gels.

[b] Molecular weights of RNAs required to code for such proteins were calculated from an average amino acid molecular weight of 100 and that of 300 for nucleotides, with three nucleotides per amino acid. Observed molecular weight of RNAs (ICR) were determined by electrophoretic mobility in formamide–polyacrylamide gels. From Willis *et al.* (1977).

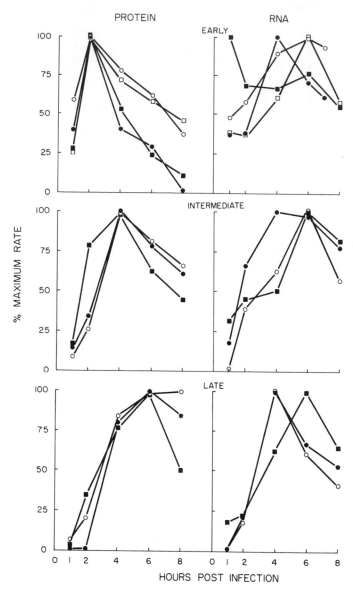

Fig. 10. Molar rate of synthesis of early, intermediate, and late FV3 RNAs and proteins. The values are expressed as percentage of the maximum molar rate of synthesis. Identical symbols are used for the polypeptide and its presumptive mRNA. Early proteins: ICP 68, ●; ICP 65, ○; ICP 47/45, ■; ICP 36, □. Early RNAs: ICR 597, ●; ICR 577, ○; ICR 425, ■; ICR 332, □. Intermediate proteins: ICP 50, ●; ICP 39/37, ○; ICP 18, ■. Intermediate RNAs: ICR 463, ●; ICR 358, ○; ICR 169, ■. Late proteins: ICP 62, ●; ICP 55, ○; ICP 19, ■. Late RNAs: ICR 560, ●; ICR 534, ○; ICR 240/235, ■. From Willis *et al.* (1977).

period. Thus early RNAs not only were present late in infection but still were actively being synthesized, despite an apparent inability to be translated.

The only RNAs whose molar rates of synthesis declined with time were the high molecular weight species (817,000–947,000). However, the molar rates of synthesis of these RNA species were low, and a consistent pattern of synthesis during the infectious cycle was difficult to obtain. Nevertheless, these are the only RNA species which might be negatively controlled at the transcriptional level. Both at qualitative and quantitative levels there was a positive transcriptional control of most or all viral RNA species during the replication cycle of FV3. The molar rates of synthesis of several RNAs and proteins changed as the infectious cycle progressed. Thus the molar rate of synthesis of certain RNAs and proteins changed as much as twentyfold or more between 1 and 6 hr after infection. Furthermore, at any given time (with the exception of the first hour of infection for RNA synthesis) all RNAs and proteins were not synthesized in equimolar rates. In fact, there was as much as a fiftyfold or more difference in the most abundant and scarce species of RNAs and proteins at any given time. The existence of different abundance classes of viral RNAs has been suggested in herpesvirus (Frenkel and Roizman, 1972), adenovirus (Wold *et al.*, 1976), and the vaccinia virus (B. Moss, personal communication) infected cells. However, an analysis of the molar rates of synthesis of FV3 RNAs shows that there are no distinct classes, but there is a continuous spectrum of abundances of viral RNAs. We believe that a similar situation will be found to exist with other viruses when a detailed analysis, possible so far only with FV3, can be made. It is evident that quantitative controls on the rates of RNA and protein synthesis are performed by viral regulatory proteins in FV3-infected cells and that these quantitative controls are superimposed on top of qualitative controls.

The translational efficiencies of various FV3 messages are strikingly different since at 1 hr after infection viral RNAs are synthesized at almost equimolar rates, but the molar rate of synthesis of viral proteins at this time was different by fifty fold or more. The translational efficiency of early and intermediate messages was presumably further modulated by several viral regulatory proteins late in the infection. Apparently, such an extensive posttranscriptional control of FV3 gene expression becomes necessary because there is very little or no repression of viral RNA synthesis and viral RNAs are quite stable (half-life of approximately 5 hr, Goorha and Granoff, 1974b). Whether or not other ICDVs or eukaryotic viruses follow a similar strategy of control of gene expression remains to be established.

6.1.6. Viral Genome (DNA) Replication

Most information on DNA synthesis of ICDVs comes from studies of cells infected with FV3 and iridescent virus types 2 and 6. During a single growth cycle in infected FHM cells, FV3 DNA synthesis begins within 2 hr and the maximum rate of viral DNA synthesis occurs between 4 and 5 hr, declining rapidly thereafter (Goorha et al., 1978). In BHK cells, viral DNA synthesis continues for 12–17 hr after infection (Maes and Granoff, 1967; McAuslan and Smith, 1968; Kucera, 1970). Most of the replicating viral DNA has been found associated with the nuclear fraction after disruption of the infected cells into nuclear and cytoplasmic fractions (McAuslan and Smith, 1968; Kucera, 1970). The association of replicating viral DNA (DNase sensitive) was considered an artifact of the fractionation technique, since most of it could be removed by centrifugation through a sucrose solution. Viral DNA found in the cytoplasmic fraction was resistant to DNase action and was considered encapsidated. However, it has been recently reported that a considerable amount of newly synthesized viral DNA is found within the nuclei (Goorha et al., 1978). This observation and its significance will be discussed in the next section.

Viral DNA is encapsidated soon after its synthesis, and both viral RNA and protein synthesis are required for the encapsidation process (Purifoy et al., 1973). Viral DNA replication is initiated at 33°C, a temperature nonpermissive for production of infectious virus, but is not initiated at 34°C. However, if viral DNA synthesis is initiated at a permissive temperature (e.g., 28°C) and cells are shifted to 34°C, viral DNA synthesis continues at 34°C, indicating that replication is not sensitive at this temperature (Kucera, 1970). At 37°C, no viral DNA is synthesized even if initiated at permissive temperature. Viral DNA synthesized at nonpermissive temperature (33–34°C for wild type or 30°C for ts mutants) can be utilized for encapsidation and infectious virion production when infected cells are shifted to permissive temperature (Kucera, 1970; Purifoy et al., 1973). In normal infection there is a concomitant production of viral DNA and virus particles (McAuslan and Smith, 1968; Kucera, 1970), but all of the detectable proteins are synthesized in the absence of viral DNA replication (Goorha and

Granoff, 1974a; Willis *et al.*, 1977). However, virus particles are not assembled if there is no viral DNA synthesis (Tripier *et al.*, 1977). In iridescent virus-infected cells, viral DNA is synthesized before the virus particles can be detected (Kelly, 1972*a,b*).

Very little is known about the structure of replicating DNA or the mechanism of viral DNA replication in ICDV-infected cells. Preliminary results obtained on the mechanism of viral DNA replication in FV3-infected cells will be discussed in the next section. Increased DNA-dependent DNA polymerase and thymidine kinase activities have been found in cells infected with FV3 (Kucera and Granoff, 1969; Aubertin and Longchampt, 1974) or African swine fever virus (Polatnick and Hess, 1970, 1972). Iridescent virus-infected cells also show an increase in DNA polymerase activity (Kelly and Robertson, 1973). Although these virus-induced enzymes are reported to differ biochemically from host enzymes, there is no compelling genetic evidence to establish their viral origin.

6.2. Nuclear Requirement for ICDV Replication

A salient feature of the ICDV growth cycle, indeed a major characteristic for their classification, has been their cytoplasmic site of replication. However, it has been suggested that some members of the ICDV group, such as FV3 and carnation etched-ring virus, may involve the nucleus during replication (Rubio-Huertos *et al.*, 1972; Kelly, 1975). The evidence was based solely on detecting the presence of virus particles in some nuclei late in infection. However, egress from the cytoplasm to the nucleus could not be ruled out. The most extensive and unequivocal evidence for the requirement of a functional nucleus has come from studies with FV3 (Goorha *et al.*, 1977, 1978). In these studies FV3 did not initiate infection in enucleated or UV-irradiated cells, infectious virus was not produced, nor were virus-specific DNA and RNA synthesized.

It appears that the nucleus plays a major role in viral nucleic acid synthesis based on two lines of evidence, electron microscopic autoradiography data and biochemical data (Goorha *et al.*, 1978). These data were obtained under conditions where host DNA synthesis was inhibited by ΔFV3 (Fig. 11). The results of electron microscopic autoradiography showed that some 30% of viral DNA was synthesized in the nucleus (Fig. 12A,B and Table 6). The majority of the viral DNA was transported into the cytoplasm as determined by pulse-chase

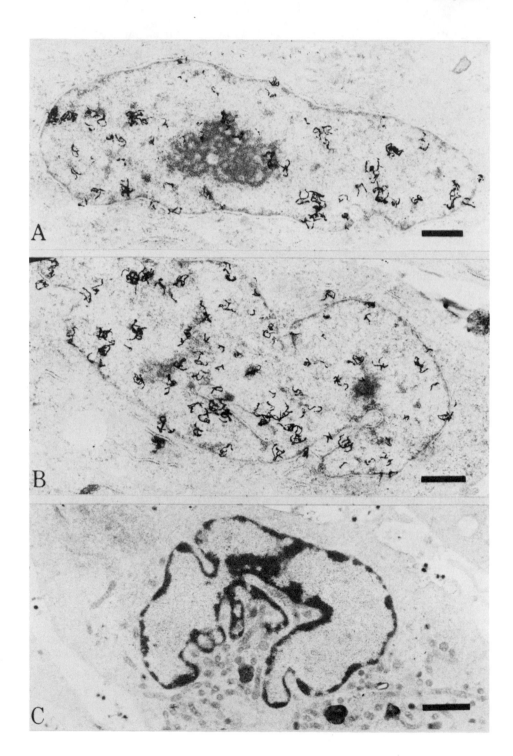

experiments (Fig. 12C and Table 6). Similar results were obtained when RNA synthesis was analyzed by the same technique.

The viral nature of the DNA and RNA found in the nucleus was confirmed by hybridization experiments. The DNA was further characterized by obtaining DNA from purified FV3-infected nuclei and from the cytoplasmic fractions of these cells. Analysis of the DNAs from the two compartments by centrifugation through alkaline sucrose gradients revealed that the nuclear DNA was approximately one-sixth the genome size of FV3 while cytoplasmic DNA was genome size or larger (Fig. 13). Pulse-chase experiments also indicated a precursor–product relationship between nuclear and cytoplasmic DNA. The size differences therefore suggested that subgenomic DNA fragments were synthesized in the nucleus and then transported to the cytoplasm, where they were completed into full genome size.

Two other lines of evidence also support the conclusion that viral DNA synthesis is initiated in the nucleus and that elongation, ligation, or maturation to genome size takes place in the cytoplasm. Cycloheximide inhibits the initiation of viral DNA replication by inhibiting viral protein synthesis (Kang *et al.*, 1971; Yu *et al.*, 1975). Addition of cycloheximide in cells synthesizing DNA results in the completion of already initiated chains, but the initiation of new rounds of replication is prevented. Interruption of viral DNA synthesis by cycloheximide in FV3-infected cells resulted in a greater inhibition of nuclear viral DNA synthesis than that of cytoplasmic viral DNA, indicating that the nucleus was the site of initiation of viral DNA replication. Corroborative data were obtained with a DNA-negative *ts* mutant defective in initiation of DNA replication (R. Goorha, unpublished observation); when DNA synthesis, initiated by the mutant at permissive temperature, was interrupted by shifting the infected cells to nonpermissive temperature, there was a preferential inhibition of viral nuclear DNA synthesis.

Although all of the data indicate that the nucleus is a site of FV3

←——————————————————————————————

Fig. 11. Electron microscopic autoradiographs of [³H]thymidine-labeled, uninfected cells. All sections in this and Fig. 12 were exposed to the autoradiographic emulsion for 2 months. A: Uninfected cells labeled for 15 min. The grains are associated with the nucleus. ×10,800. B: Uninfected cells labeled for 15 min and chased for 2 hr in the presence of cytosine arabinoside (10⁻³ M). The grains remain associated with the nucleus during the chase period. ×11,790. C: Cells exposed to ΔFV3 and labeled for 15 min. No grains are evident either over the nucleus or over the cytoplasm, indicating marked inhibition of host DNA synthesis. ×12,870. From Goorha *et al.* (1978). Reduced 17% for reproduction.

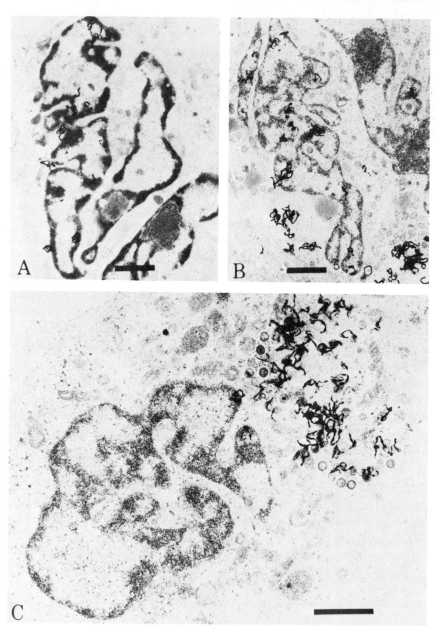

Fig. 12. Electron microscopic autoradiographs of DNA synthesis in FV3-infected cells. Cells received ΔFV3 prior to infection with active FV3. Labeling was with [³H]thymidine for 15 min at 3.5 hr after infection with active FV3. A,B: Labeling patterns in cells at the end of the pulse. In some cells the grains are seen exclusively in the nucleus (A) and in others the grains are evident in both nucleus and cytoplasm (B). A and B, ×11,700. C: Sample that was labeled similarly and then chased for 2 hr in the presence of 10^{-3} M cytosine arabinoside. The grains are now associated with a viral assembly site in the cytoplasm. ×22,280. From Goorha *et al.* (1978). Reduced 27% for reproduction.

TABLE 6

Grain Number and Distribution in [³H]Thymidine-Labeled Cells[a]

Inocula	Number of cells counted	Total number of grains	Number of grains in nucleus	Number of grains in cytoplasm
ΔFV3 + ΔFV3 (15-min pulse)	126	20	17	3
ΔFV3 + active FV3 (15-min pulse)	50	982	298	684
ΔFV3 + active FV3 (15-min pulse, 2-hr chase)	50	1065	35	1030

[a] Cells were exposed to ΔFV3 for 4 hr and then infected with active FV3 or ΔFV3 as control. Infected cells were labeled for 15 min with [³H]thymidine (25 μCi/ml) at 3.5 hr after infection with active FV3. The chase was performed in the presence of 10^{-3} M cytosine arabinoside.

DNA synthesis, they do not exclude the possibility of independent synthesis of viral DNA in the cytoplasm as well.

The presence of subgenomic size DNA in the nucleus may be interpreted in two ways: (1) part of the FV3 genome is synthesized in the nucleus which is transported to the cytoplasm, where genome synthesis is completed, or (2) the full genomic complement of FV3 is represented in subgenomic nuclear viral DNA. These fragments are transported to the cytoplasm where ligation to genomic size takes place. Preliminary experiments (D. Willis, R. Goorha, and A. Granoff, unpublished data) using restriction endonuclease fragments and the Southern blotting technique (Southern, 1975) indicate that subgenomic DNA fragments represent the full genomic complexity, thus favoring the second possibility.

The requirement of a nuclear function(s) for viral DNA replication may be either direct or indirect. The direct nuclear function might be utilization of host enzymatic machinery by FV3 for its genome replication; examples of indirect function would be uncoating of viral particles or requirement for viral primary transcription in the nucleus before viral DNA can be replicated. The dependence of FV3 on host machinery for its genome replication is probably only partial as viral protein synthesis is required for initiation of viral DNA synthesis (R. Goorha and A. Granoff, unpublished results).

The requirement of a nuclear function for replication of FV3 DNA is not unique among ICDVs. ASFV cannot replicate in enucleated cells and viral DNA is not synthesized in them (Ortin and Viñuela, 1977). Whether a nuclear requirement is a general feature of replication of other ICDVs remains to be established.

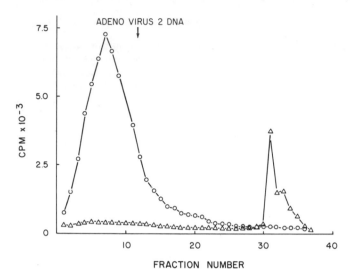

Fig. 13.   Alkaline sucrose gradient sedimentation profiles of DNA from FV3-infected cells. Infected cells were labeled with [³H]thymidine (10 μCi/ml) for 10 min at 3.5 hr after infection. Purified nuclear or cytoplasmic fractions were layered on top of alkaline sucrose gradients; after centrifugation, 1-ml fractions were collected, DNA was precipitated with 10% trichloroacetic acid, and radioactivity was determined. Sedimentation is from left to right. O——O, Nuclear fraction; Δ——Δ, cytoplasmic fraction. Arrow represents position of adenovirus 2 DNA; molecular weight 12×10^6; S = 34. From Goorha *et al.* (1978).

7.   CONCLUSIONS AND PROSPECTS FOR THE FUTURE

The studies reviewed in this chapter clearly demonstrate that the term "ICDV" encompasses radically different viruses having very little in common, particularly the plant viruses, whose size, composition, and structure differ strikingly from those of the rest of the group. The family Iridoviridae has been designated by the International Committee on Nomenclature of Viruses to include the large ICDVs of invertebrates and vertebrates (Fenner, 1976). Kelly and Robertson (1973) have pointed out that "Iridoviridae" gives undue weight to a feature which (1) is present only in the minority of members, (2) is a phenomenon not yet linked to any characteristic feature of structure or replication, and (3) even as a phenomenon is not unique to this group of viruses. However, because of common usage and for historical reasons it may be best to retain Iridoviridae as a family with a number of genera encompassing invertebrate and vertebrate viruses as members (Fenner, 1976). The plant ICDVs have tentatively been placed in the group Caulimovirus (Fenner, 1976).

Biochemical studies on the replication of ICDVs have been limited mainly to FV3, and the results suggest that its strategy of replication may be unique; the virus utilizes the host nucleus for nucleic acid synthesis, but virus assembly takes place in the cytoplasm. This mode of replication is therefore strikingly different from that of nuclear DNA viruses as well as the cytoplasmic DNA poxviruses. Nuclear DNA viruses utilize the nucleus not only for genome replication and transcription but also for morphogenesis and assembly of virions, thus necessitating the transport of viral proteins from the cytoplasm to the nucleus. The poxviruses apparently synthesize their nucleic acids in the cytoplasm, which is also a site for morphogenesis and assembly. It appears that FV3 replicates its DNA in the nucleus in fragments. However, the genome fragments are then transported into the cytoplasm, where they are ligated or elongated and then encapsidated. Thus this mode of replication may represent an evolutionary link between the replication strategies of cytoplasmic and nuclear DNA viruses. Detailed analysis of this intriguing mode of viral replication and the impact it may have on control of viral gene expression remain to be explored.

Resolution of FV3 RNAs into 47 species, a feat not yet accomplished in any other viral system, and their quantitation have greatly facilitated our understanding of complex qualitative and quantitative transcriptional controls. A quantitative analysis of viral RNAs and proteins has also demonstrated extensive control of viral gene expression at the posttranscriptional level. A detailed analysis of the control elements in FV3 gene expression, and possibly other ICDVs, is very likely to provide new insight into the control of gene expression in other animal viruses and their cells.

ACKNOWLEDGMENTS

The preparation of this chapter and of unpublished information from the authors' laboratories was supported by Research Grant CA 07055 from the National Cancer Institute, Grant GM 23638 from the Institute of General Medical Sciences, and Cancer Center Support (CORE) Grant CA 21765 from the National Cancer Institute, and by ALSAC.

We are indebted to Dr. David Kelly, Dr. N. J. Wrigley, and Dr. R. J. Shepherd for providing electron micrographs and gratefully acknowledge their contributions. We thank Dr. G. Murti for help in preparation of illustrations.

8. REFERENCES

Adldinger, K. K., Stone, S. S., Hess, W. R., and Bachrach, H. L., 1966, Extraction of infectious DNA from African swine fever virus, *Virology* **30**:570.

Almeida, J. D., Waterson, A. P., and Plowright, W., 1967, The morphological characteristics of African swine fever virus and its resemblance to *Tipula* iridescent virus, *Arch. Gesamte Virusforsch.* **20**:392.

Anderson, J. G., 1970, An iridescent virus infecting the mosquito *Aedes stimulans*, *J. Invert. Pathol.* **15**:219.

Armentrout, R. W., and McAuslan, B. R., 1974, RNA synthesis in cells infected with an icosahedral cytoplasmic deoxyvirus (frog virus 3), *J. Virol.* **13**:1083.

Aubertin, A. M., and Longchampt, M. O., 1974, Thymidine kinase induction in FV 3-infected mouse cells, *Virology* **58**:111.

Aubertin, A., Palese, P., Tan, K. B., Vilagines, R., and McAuslan, B. R., 1971, Proteins of a polyhedral cytoplasmic deoxyvirus. III. Structure of frog virus 3 and location of virus-associated adenosine triphosphate phosphohydrolase, *J. Virol.* **8**:643.

Aubertin, A., Hirth, C., Travo, C., Nonnenmacher, H., and Kirn, A., 1973, Preparation and properties of an inhibitory extract from frog virus 3 particles, *J. Virol.* **11**:694.

Aubertin, A. M., Anton, M., Bingen, A., Elharrar, M., and Kirn, A., 1977, Solubilised viral proteins produce fatal hepatitis in mice, *Nature (London)* **265**:456.

Bailey, L., Ball, B. V., and Woods, R. D., 1976, An iridovirus from bees, *J. Gen Virol.* **31**:459.

Balls, M., and Ruben, L. N., 1968, Lymphoid tumours in amphibia: A review, *Prog. Exp. Tumour Res.* **10**:238.

Batson, B. S., Johnston, M. R. L., Arnold, M. K., and Kelly, D. C., 1976, An iridescent virus from *Simulium* sp. (Diptera:Simuliidae) in Wales, *J. Invertebr. Pathol.* **27**:133.

Bellett, A. J. D., 1968, The iridescent virus group, *Adv. Virus Res.* **13**:225.

Ben-Porat, T., Stehn, B., and Kaplan, A. S., 1976, Fate of parental herpesvirus DNA, *Virology* **71**:412.

Bernard, G. W., Cooper, E. L., and Randell, M. L., 1969, Lamellar membrane encirculated viruses in erythrocytes of *Rana pipiens*, *J. Ultrastruct. Res.* **26**:8.

Bingen-Brendel, A., Tripier, F., and Kirn, A., 1971, L'étude morphologique sequentielle du development du FV 3 sur cellular BHK 21, *J. Microsc. (Oxford)* **11**:249.

Bird, F. T., 1961, The development of *Tipula* iridescent virus in the crane fly, *Tipula paludosa* Meig., and the waxmoth, *Galleria mellonella* L., *Can. J. Microbiol.* **7**:827.

Bird, F. T., 1962, On the development of *Tipula* iridescent virus particles, *Can. J. Microbiol.* **8**:533.

Black, D. N., and Brown, F., 1976, Purification and physicochemical characteristics of African swine fever virus, *J. Gen. Virol.* **32**:509.

Breese, S. S., and DeBoer, C. J., 1966, Electron microscope observations of African swine fever virus in tissue culture cells, *Virology* **28**:420.

Brunt, A. A., 1966, Partial purification, morphology, and serology of dahlia mosaic virus, *Virology* **28**:778.

Brunt, A. A., 1971, Dahlia mosaic virus, *Commonw. Mycol. Inst./Assoc. Appl. Biol. Descript. Plant Viruses*, No. 51.

Came, P. E., and Dardiri, A. H., 1969, Host specificity and serological disparity of African swine fever virus and amphibian polyhedral cytoplasmic viruses, *Proc. Soc. Exp. Biol. Med.* **130**:128.

Chapman, H. C., Peterson, J. J., Woodard, D. B., and Clark, T. B., 1968, New records of parasites of *Ceratopogonidae, Mosq. News* **28**:123.

Chapman, H. C., Clark, T. B., Anthony, D. W., and Glen, F. E., 1971, An iridescent virus from the larvae of *Corethralla brakelyi* (Diptera: Chaoboridae) in Louisiana, *J. Invertebr. Pathol.* **18**:284.

Christmas, J. Y., and Howse, H. D., 1970, The occurrence of lymphocystis in *Micropogon undulatus* and *Cynoscian arenius* from Mississippi estuaries, *Gulf Res. Rep.* **3**:131.

Clark, H. F., Brennan, J. C., Ziegel, R. F., and Karzon, D. T., 1968, Isolation and characterization of viruses from the kidneys of *Rana pipiens* with renal adeno-carcinoma before and after passage in the red eft (*Triturus viridescens*), *J. Virol.* **2**:629.

Clark, H. F., Gray, G., Fabian, F., Ziegel, R. F., and Karzon, D. T., 1969, Comparative studies of amphibian cytoplasmic virus strains isolated from the leopard frog, bullfrog, and newt, in: *Biology of Amphibian Tumors* (M. Mizell, ed.), Recent Results in Cancer Research, Springer-Verlag, Heidelberg.

Coggins, L., 1968, A modified hemadsorption-inhibition test for African swine fever virus, *Bull. Epizoot. Dis. Afr.* **16**:61.

Cunningham, J. C., and Tinsley, T. W., 1968, A serological comparison of some iridescent non-occluded insect viruses, *J. Gen. Virol.* **3**:1.

Darlington, R. W., Granoff, A., and Breeze, D. C., 1966, Viruses and renal carcinoma of *Rana pipiens*. II. Ultrastructural studies and sequential development of virus isolated from normal and tumor tissue, *Virology* **29**:149.

Day, M. F., and Mercer, E. H., 1964, Properties of an iridescent virus from the beetle *Sericesthis pruinosa, Aust. J. Biol. Sci.* **17**:892.

DeTray, D. E., 1963, African swine fever virus, *Adv. Vet. Sci.* **8**:299.

Elharrar, M., Hirth, C., Blanc, J., and Kirn, A., 1973, Pathogénie de l'hépatite toxique de la souris provoquée par le FV 3 (frog virus 3). Inhibition de la synthèse des macromolécules du foie, *Biochim. Biophys. Acta* **319**:91.

Elliott, R. M., Thelma, L., and Kelly, D. C., 1977, Serological relationships of an irridescent virus (type 25) recently isolated from *Tipula* sp. with two other iridescent viruses (types 2 and 22), *Virology* **81**:309.

Enjuanes, L., Carrascosa, A. L., and Viñuela, E., 1976, Isolation and properties of the DNA of African swine fever virus, *J. Gen. Virol.* **32**:479.

Enjuanes, L., Cubero, I., and Viñuela, E., 1977, Sensitivity of macrophages from different species to African swine fever (ASF) virus, *J. Gen. Virol.* **34**:455.

Federici, B. A. and Hazard, E. I., 1975, Iridovirus cytoplasmic polyhedrosis virus in the fresh water daphnid *Simocephalus expinosis, Nature* **254**:327.

Fenner, F., 1976, Classification and nomenclature of viruses: Second Report of International Committee on Taxonomy of Viruses, *Intervirology* **7**:1.

Fowler, M., and Robertson, J. S., 1971, Iridescent virus infection in field populations of *Wiseana cervinata* (Lepidoptera: Hepialidae) and *Witlesia* Sp. (Lepidoptera: Pyralidae) in New Zealand, *J. Invertebr. Pathol.* **19**:154.

Frenkel, N., and Roizman, B., 1972, RNA synthesis in cells infected with herpes simplex virus: Control of transcription and of RNA abundance, *Proc. Natl. Acad. Sci.* **69**:2654.

Gaby, N. S. and Kucera, L. S., 1974, DNA-dependent RNA polymerase activity associated with subviral particles of polyhedral cytoplasmic deoxyribovirus, *J. Virol.* **14**:231.

Ginsberg, H. S., 1969, Biochemistry of adenovirus infection, in: *The Biochemistry of Viruses* (H. B. Levy, ed.), pp. 329–413, Dekker, New York.

Glitz, D. O., Hills, G. J., and Rivers, C. F., 1968, A comparison of *Tipula* and *Sericesthis* iridescent viruses, *J. Gen. Virol.* **3**:209.

Goorha, R., and Granoff, A., 1974a, Macromolecular synthesis in cells infected by frog virus 3. I. Virus specific protein synthesis and its regulation, *Virology* **60**:237.

Goorha, R., and Granoff, A., 1974b, Macromolecular synthesis in cells infected by frog virus 3. II. Evidence for post-transcriptional control of a viral structural protein, *Virology* **60**:251.

Goorha, R., Naegele, R. F., Purifoy, D., and Granoff, A., 1975, Macromolecular synthesis in cells infected by frog virus 3. III. Virus-specific protein synthesis by temperature-sensitive mutants, *Virology* **66**:428.

Goorha, R., Willis, D. B., and Granoff, A., 1977, Macromolecular synthesis in cells infected by frog virus 3. VI. Frog virus 3 replication is dependent on the cell nucleus, *J. Virol.* **21**:802.

Goorha, R., Murti, G., Granoff, A., and Tirey, R., 1978, Macromolecular synthesis in cells infected by frog virus 3. VIII. The nucleus is a site of frog virus 3 DNA and RNA synthesis, *Virology* **84**:32.

Granoff, A., 1969, Viruses of Amphibia, *Curr. Top. Microbiol. Immunol.* **50**:107.

Granoff, A., Came, P. E., and Rafferty, K. A., 1965, The isolation and properties of viruses from *Rana pipiens:* Their possible relationship to the renal adenocarcinoma of the leopard frog, *Ann. N.Y. Acad. Sci.* **126**:237.

Granoff, A., Gravell, M., and Darlington, R. W., 1969, Studies on the viral etiology of the renal adenocarcinoma of *Rana pipiens* (Lucké tumor), in: *Biology of Amphibian Tumors.* (M. Mizell, ed.), Recent Results in Cancer Research, Springer-Verlag, Heidelberg.

Gravell, M., and Cromeans, T. L., 1971, Mechanisms involved in the nongenetic reactivation of frog polyhedral deoxyribovirus: Evidence for RNA polymerase in the virion, *Virology* **46**:39.

Gravell, M., and Granoff, A., 1970, Viruses and renal adenocarcinoma of *Rana pipiens*. IX. The influence of temperature and host cell on replication of frog polyhedral cytoplasmic deoxyribovirus, *Virology* **41**:596.

Gravell, M., and Naegele, R. F., 1970, Nongenetic reactivation of frog polyhedral cytoplasmic deoxyribovirus, *Virology* **40**:170.

Guir, M., Braunwald, J., and Kirn, A., 1970, Inhibition de la synthèse du DNA et des RNA cellulaires dans les cellules KB infectées avec le virus 3 de la grenouille (FV 3). *C. R. Acad. Sci.* **270**:2605.

Hasan, S., Croizier, G., Vago, C., and Duthoit, J.-L., 1970, Infection a virus irisant dans une population naturelle d'*Aedes detritus* Haliday en France, *Ann. Zool. Ecol. Anim.* **2**:295.

Hess, W. R., 1971, African swine fever virus, *Virol. Monogr.* **9**:1.

Holland, J. J., and Kiehn, E. D., 1968, Specific cleavage of viral proteins as steps in the synthesis and maturation of enteroviruses, *Proc. Natl. Acad. Sci. USA* **60**:1015.

Hollings, M., and Stone, O., 1969, Carnation viruses: Carnation etched ring. Report, *Glasshouse Crops Res. Inst. Annu. Rep.*, 1968, p. 162.

Houts, G. E., Gravell, M., and Darlington, R. W., 1970, Base composition and molecular weight of DNA from a frog polyhedral cytoplasmic deoxyribovirus, *Proc. Soc. Exp. Biol. Med.* **135**:232.

Houts, G. E ., Gravell, M., and Granoff, A., 1974, Electron microscopic observation of early events of frog virus 3 replication, *Virology* **58**:589.

Howse, H. D., and Christmas, J.Y., 1971, Observations on the ultrastructure of lymphocystis virus in the Atlantic croaker, *Micropogon undulatus* (Linnaeus), *Virology* **44**:211.

Hull, R., and Shepherd, R. J., 1977, The structure of cauliflower mosaic virus genome, *Virology* **79**:216.

Kalmakoff, J., and Robertson, J. S., 1970, Serological relationship of *Wiseana* iridescent virus to other iridescent viruses, *Proc. Univ. Otago Med. Sch.* **48**:16.

Kalmakoff, J., Moore, S., and Pottinger, R. P., 1972, An iridescent virus from grass grub *Costelytra zealandica:* Serological study, *J. Invertebr. Pathol.* **20**:70.

Kaminski, S., Clark, H. F., and Karzon, D. T., 1969, Comparative immune response to amphibian cytoplasmic viruses assayed by the complement fixation and gel immunodiffusion techniques, *J. Immunol.* **103**:260.

Kang, H. S., and McAuslan, B. R., 1972, Virus-associated nucleases: Location and properties of deoxyribonucleases and ribonucleases in purified frog virus 3, *J. Virol.* **10**:202.

Kang, H. S., Eshbach, T. B., White, D. A., and Levine, A. J., 1971, DNA replication in SV40-infected cells. IV. Two different requirements for protein synthesis during SV40 DNA replication, *J. Virol.* **7**:112.

Kates, J. R., and McAuslan, B. R., 1967a, Messenger RNA synthesis by a coated viral genome, *Proc. Natl. Acad. Sci. USA* **57**:314.

Kates, J. R., and McAuslan, B. R., 1967b, Poxvirus DNA-dependent RNA polymerase, *Proc. Natl. Acad. Sci. USA* **58**:134.

Kelly, D. C., 1972a, Patterns of nucleic acid synthesis in iridescent virus infected cells, *Monogr. Virol.* **6**:9.

Kelly, D. C., 1972b, The replication of some iridescent viruses in cell cultures, Ph.D. thesis, University of Oxford.

Kelly, D. C., 1975, Frog virus 3 replication; electron microscope observations on the sequence of infection in chick embryo fibroblasts, *J. Gen. Virol.* **26**:71.

Kelly, D. C., and Atkinson, M. A., 1975, Frog virus 3 replication: Electron microscope observations on the terminal stages of infection in chronically infected cell cultures, *J. Gen. Virol.* **28**:391.

Kelly, D. C., and Avery, R. J., 1974a, The DNA content of four small iridescent viruses: Genome size, redundancy and homology determined by renaturation kinetics, *Virology* **57**:425.

Kelly, D. C., and Avery, R. J., 1974b, Frog virus 3 deoxyribonucleic acid, *J. Gen. Virol.* **24**:339.

Kelly, D. C., and Robertson, J. S., 1973, Icosahedral cytoplasmic deoxyriboviruses, *J. Gen. Virol. (Suppl.)* **20**:17.

Kelly, D. C., and Tinsley, T. W., 1972, The proteins of iridescent virus types 2 and 6, *J. Invertebr. Pathol.* **19**:273.

Kelly, D. C., and Tinsley, T. W., 1973, RNA polymerase activity associated with particles of iridescent virus types 2 and 6, *J. Invertebr. Pathol.* **22**:199.

Kelly, D. C., and Tinsley, T. W., 1974, Iridescent virus replication: Patterns of nucleic acid synthesis in insect cells infected with iridescent virus types 2 and 6, *J. Invertebr. Pathol.* **24**:169.

Kelly, D. C., and Vance, D. E., 1973, The lipid content of two iridescent viruses, *J. Gen Virol.* **21**:417.

Kirn, A., Gut, J. P., Bingen, A., and Hirth, C., 1972, Acute hepatitis produced by frog virus 3 in mice, *Arch. Gesamte Virusforsch.* **36**:394.

Kitajima, E. W., Betty, J. A., and Costa, A. S., 1973, Strawberry veinbanding virus, a member of the cauliflower mosaic virus group, *J. Gen. Virol.* **20**:117.

Krell, P., and Lee, P. E., 1974, Polypeptides in *Tipula* iridescent virus (TIV) and in TIV-infected hemocytes of *Galleria mellonella* (L) larvae, *Virology* **60**:315.

Kucera, L., 1970, Effects of temperature on frog polyhedral cytoplasmic deoxyribovirus multiplication: Thermosensitivity of initiation, replication, encapsidation of viral DNA, *Virology* **42**:576.

Kucera, L. S., and Granoff, A., 1969, Induction and regulation of DNA nucleotidyl-transferase activity in fish cells infected with frog virus 3, *Virology* **37**:455.

Lehane, D. E., Clark, H. F., and Karzon, D. T., 1968, Antigenic relationships among frog viruses demonstrated by plaque reduction and neutralization kinetics tests, *Virology* **34**:590.

Lunger, P. D., and Came, P. E., 1966, Cytoplasmic viruses associated with Lucke tumors, *Virology* **30**:116.

Maes, R., and Granoff, A., 1967, Viruses and renal carcinoma of *Rana pipiens*. IV. Nucleic acid synthesis in frog virus 3-infected BHK 21/13 cells, *Virology* **33**:491.

Malmquist, W. A., and Hay, D., 1960, Hemadsorption and cytopathic effect produced by African swine fever virus in swine bone marrow and buffy coat cultures, *Am. J. Vet. Res.* **21**:104.

Matta, J. F., 1970, The characterization of a mosquito iridescent virus (MIV). II. Physico-chemical characterization, *J. Invertebr. Pathol.* **16**:157.

Matta, J. F., and Lowe, R. E., 1970, The characterization of a mosquito iridescent virus (MIV). Biological characteristics, infectivity, and pathology, *J. Invertebr. Pathol.* **6**:38.

Mattern, C. F. T., Diamond, L. S., and Daniel, W. A., 1972, Viruses of *Entamoeba histolytica*. II. Morphogenesis of the polyhedral particle (ABRM2→HK-9)→HB-301 and the filamentous agent (ABRM)₂→HK-9, *J. Virol.* **9**:342.

McAuslan, B. R., 1969, The biochemistry of poxvirus replication, in *The Biochemistry of Viruses* (H. B. Levy, ed.), pp. 361–413, Dekker, New York.

McAuslan, B. R., and Armentrout, R. W., 1974, The biochemistry of icosahedral cytoplasmic deoxyriboviruses, *Curr. Top. Microbiol. Immunol.* **68**:77.

McAuslan, B. R., and Smith, W., 1968, DNA synthesis in frog virus 3-infected mamalian cells, *J. Virol.* **2**:1006.

McIntosh, A. H., and Kimura, M., 1974, Replication of the insect *Chilo* iridescent virus in poikilothermic vertebrate cell line, *Intervirology* **4**:257.

Meagher, R. G., Shepherd, R. J., and Boyer, H. W., 1977, The structure of cauliflower mosaic virus. I. A restriction endonuclease map of cauliflower mosaic virus DNA, *Virology* **80**:362.

Midlige, F. H., and Malsberger, R. G., 1968, *In vitro* morphology and maturation of lymphocystis virus, *J. Virol.* **2**:830.

Monnier, C., and DeVauchelle, G., 1976, Enzyme activities associated with an invertebrate iridovirus: Nucleotide phosphohydrolase activity associated with iridescent virus type 6 (CIV), *J. Virol.* **19**:180.

Morris, O. N., 1970, Metabolic changes in diseased insects. III. Nucleic acid metabolism in *lipidoptera* infected by densonucleosis and *Tipula* iridescent virus, *J. Invertebr. Pathol.* **16**:180.

Morris, V. L., Spear, P. G., and Roizman, B., 1966, Some biophysical properties of frog viruses and their DNA, *Proc. Natl. Acad. Sci. USA* **56**:1155.

Moss, B., 1974, Reproduction of poxviruses, in: *Comprehensive Virology*, Vol. 3 (H. Fraenkel-Conrat and R. R. Wagner, eds.), pp. 405–474, Plenum, New York.

Naegele, R. F., and Granoff, A., 1971, Viruses and renal carcinoma of *Rana pipiens*. XI. Isolation of FV 3 temperature-sensitive mutants; complementation and genetic recombination, *Virology* **44**:286.

Ortin, J., and Viñuela, E., 1977, Requirement of cell nucleus for African swine fever virus replication in Vero cells, *J. Virol.* **21**:902.

Pickett-Heaps, J. D., 1972, A possible virus infection in green alga *Oedogonium*, *J. Phycol.* **8**:44.

Pirone, T. P., Pound, G. S., and Shepherd, R. J., 1961, Properties and serology of purified cauliflower mosaic virus, *Phytopathology* **51**:541.

Plowright, W., 1972, African swine fever virus and other large DNA viruses with cubic symmetry and cytoplasmic synthesis, in: *Proceedings of the Second International Congress for Virology*, p. 264, Karger, Basel.

Pogo, B. G. T., and Dales, S., 1971, Biogenesis of vaccinia: Separation of early stages from maturation by means of hydroxyurea, *Virology* **43**:144.

Polatnick, J., and Hess, W. R., 1970, Altered thymidine kinase activity in culture cells inoculated with African swine fever virus, *Am. J. Vet. Res.* **31**:1609.

Polatnick, J., and Hess, W. R., 1972, Increased DNA polymerase activity in African swine fever virus infected cells, *Arch. Gesamte Virusforsch.* **38**:383.

Purifoy, D., Naegele, R. F., and Granoff, A., 1973, Viruses and renal carcinoma of *Rana pipiens*. XIV. Temperature-sensitive mutants of frog virus 3 with defective encapsidation, *Virology* **54**:525.

Robertson, J. S., and Longworth, J. F., 1973, A comparison of iridescent virus types 1, 2, and 9, *J. Invertebr. Pathol.* **22**:219.

Rottman, F., Shatkin, A. J., and Perry, R. P., 1974, Sequences containing methylated nucleotides at the 5′ termini of messenger RNAs: Possible implications for processing, *Cell* **3**:197.

Rubio-Huertos, M., Castro, S., Fujisawa, I., and Matsui, C., 1972, Electron microscopy of the formation of carnation etched-ring virus intracellular inclusions, *J. Gen. Virol.* **15**:257.

Rungger, D., Rastelli, M., Braendle, E., and Malsberger, R. G., 1971, A virus-like particle associated with lesions in muscles of *Octopus vulgaris*, *J. Invertebr. Pathol.* **17**:72.

Russell, G. J., Follett, E. A. C., Subak-Sharpe, J. H., and Harrison, B. D., 1971, The double-stranded DNA of cauliflower mosaic virus, *J. Gen. Virol.* **11**:129.

Schnepf, E., Soeder, C. J., and Hegiwald, E., 1970, Polyhedral viruslike particles lysing the aquatic-phycomycete *Aphelidium* sp., a parasite of green alga *Scenedesmus armatus*, *Virology* **42**:482.

Shepherd, R. J., 1970, Cauliflower mosaic virus, *Commonw. Mycol. Assoc. Appl. Biol. Descript. Plant Viruses*, No. 24.

Shepherd, R. J., Wakeman, R. J., and Romano, R. R., 1968, DNA in cauliflower mosaic virus, *Virology* **36**:150.

Shepherd, R. J., Bruening, G. E., and Wakeman, R. J., 1970, Double-stranded DNA from cauliflower mosaic virus, *Virology* **41**:339.

Sigel, M. M., Lopez, D. M., Beasley, A. R., and Caliguri, L. A., 1971, Virus–cell interaction in lymphocystis disease of fish, in: *Viruses Affecting Man and Animals* (M. Sanders and M. Schaeffer, eds.), p. 124, Warren H. Green, St. Louis.

Silberstein, H., and August, J. T., 1973, Phosphorylation of animal virus proteins by a virion protein kinase, *J. Virol.* **12**:511.

Silberstein, H., and August J. T., 1976, Characterization of a virion protein kinase as a virus-specified enzyme, *J. Biol. Chem.* **251**:3185.

Silberstein, H, McAuslan, B. R., and August, J. T., 1972, Protein kinase and phosphate acceptor proteins of animal viruses, *Fed. Proc.* **31**:407.

Smith, K. M., 1958, A study of early stages of infection with *Tipula* iridescent virus, *Parasitology* **48**:459.

Smith, K. M., 1967, *Insect Virology*, Academic Press, New York.

Smith, K. M., and Hill, G. J., 1962, Replication and ultrastructure of insect viruses, in: *Proceedings of the Eleventh International Congress for Entomology*, Vol. 2, p. 823, Vienna.

Smith, W. R., and McAuslan, B. R., 1969, Biophysical properties of frog virus 3 and its DNA: Fate of radioactive virus in early stages of infection, *J. Virol.* **4**:332.

Southern, E. M., 1975, Detection of specific sequences among DNA fragments separated by gel electrophoresis, *J. Mol. Biol.* **98**:503.

Stebhens, W. E., and Johnston, M. R. L., 1966, The viral nature of *Pirhemocyton tarentole*, *J. Ultrastruct. Res.* **15**:543.

Stoltz, D. B., 1971, The structure of icosahedral cytoplasmic deoxyriboviruses, *J. Ultrastruct. Res.* **37**:219.

Stoltz, D. B., 1973, The structure of icosahedral cytoplasmic deoxyriboviruses. II. An alternative model, *J. Ultrastruct. Res.* **43**:58.

Stoltz, D. B., Hilsenhoff, W. L., and Stich, H. F., 1968, A virus disease in *Chironomus plumosus*, *J. Invertebr. Pathol.* **12**:118.

Tan, K. B., and McAuslan, B. R., 1971, Proteins of polyhedral cytoplasmic deoxyriboviruses. 1. The structural polypeptides of FV 3, *Virology* **45**:200.

Tan, K. B., and McAuslan, B. R., 1972, Binding of DNA-dependent DNA polymerase to poxvirus, *J. Virol.* **9**:70.

Tezuka, N., and Taniguchi, T., 1972, Structural proteins of cauliflower mosaic virus, *Virology* **48**:277.

Thomas, R. S., 1961, The chemical composition and particle weight of *Tipula iridescent virus*, *Virology* **14**:240.

Tinsley, T. W., Robertson, J. S., Rivers, C. F., and Service, M. W., 1971, An iridescent virus of *Aedes cantans* in Great Britain, *J. Invertebr. Pathol.* **18**:427.

Toth, R., and Wilce, R. T., 1972, Virus-like particles in marine alga *Chorda tomentosa*. Lynfbye (Phaeophyceae), J. Phycol. **8**:126.

Tripier, F. Braunwald, J., Markovic, L., and Kirn, A., 1977, Frog virus 3 morphogenesis: Effect of temperature and metabolic inhibitors, *J. Gen. Virol.* **37**:39.

Tweedell, K. S., and Granoff, A., 1968, Viruses and renal carcinoma of *Rana pipiens*. V. Effect of frog virus 3 on developing embryos and larvae, *J. Natl. Cancer Inst.* **40**:407.

Vago, C., Rioux, J.-A., Duthoit, J. L., and Dedet, J.-P., 1969, Infection spontanée a virus irisant dans une population d'*Aedes detritus* (Hal., 1933) des environs de Tunis, *Ann. Parasitol. Hum. Comp.* **44**:667.

Vilagines, R., and McAuslan, B. R., 1971, Proteins of polyhedral cytoplasmic deoxyribovirus. II. Nucleotide phosphohydrolase activity associated with frog virus 3, *J. Virol.* **7**:619.

Wagner, G. W., and Paschke, J. D., 1977, A comparison of the DNA of the "R" and "T" strains of mosquito iridescent virus, *Virology* **81**:298.

Wagner, G. W., Paschke, J. D., Campbell, W. R., and Webb, S. R., 1973, Biochemical and biophysical properties of two strains of mosquito iridescent virus, *Virology* **52**:72.

Wagner, G. W., Paschke, J. D., Campbell, W. R., and Webb, S. R., 1974, Proteins of two strains of mosquito iridescent virus, *Intervirology* **3**:97.

Walker, R., 1962, Fine structure of lymphocystis virus of fish, *Virology* **18**:503.

Walker, R., and Weissenberg, R., 1965, Conformity of light and electron microscopic studies on virus particle distribution in lymphocystis tumor cells of fish, *Ann. N.Y. Acad. Sci.* **126**:375.

Weiser, J., 1965, A new virus of mosquito larvae, *Bull. WHO* **33**:586.

Weiser, J., 1968, Iridescent virus from the blackfly *Simulium ornatum* Meigen in Czechoslovakia, *J. Invertebr. Pathol.* **12**:36.

Weissenberg, R., 1965, Fifty years of research on lymphocystis diseases of fishes (1914–1964), *Ann. N.Y. Acad. Sci.* **126**:362.

Willis, D., and Granoff, A., 1974, Lipid composition of frog virus 3, *Virology* **61**:256.

Willis, D., and Granoff, A., 1976a, Macromolecular synthesis in cells infected by frog virus 3. IV. Regulation of virus-specific RNA synthesis, *Virology* **70**:399.

Willis, D., and Granoff, A., 1976b, Macromolecular synthesis in cells infected by frog virus 3. V. The absence of polyadenylic acid in the majority of virus-specific RNA species, *Virology* **73**:543.

Willis, D. B., and Granoff, A., 1978, Macromolecular synthesis in cells infected by frog virus 3. IX. Two temporal classes of early viral RNA, *Virology* **86**:443.

Willis, D. B., Goorha, R., Miles, M., and Granoff, A., 1977, Macromolecular synthesis in cells infected by frog virus 3. VII. Transcriptional and post-transcriptional regulation of virus gene expression, *J. Virol.* **24**:326.

Wold, W. S. Green, M., Brackmann, K. H., Cartus, M. A., and Devine, C., 1976, Genome expression and mRNA maturation at late stages of productive adenovirus types 2 infection, *J. Virol.* **20**:465.

Wolf, K., Gravell, M., and Malsberger, R. G., 1966, Lymphocystis virus: Isolation and propagation in centrachid fish cell lines, *Science* **151**:1004.

Wolf, K., Bullock, G. L., Dunbar, C. E., and Quimby, M. C., 1968, Tadpole edema virus: a viscerotrophic pathogen for anuran amphibians, *J. Infect. Dis.* **118**:253.

Wrigley, N. G., 1969, An electron microscopic study of the structure of *Sericesthis* iridescent virus, *J. Gen. Virol.* **5**:123.

Wrigley, N. G., 1970, An electron microscope study of the structure of *Tipula* iridescent virus, *J. Gen. Virol.* **6**:169.

Xeros, N., 1964, Phagocytosis of virus in *Tipula paludosa* Meigen, *J. Insect Pathol.* **6**:225.

Yu, K., Kowalski, J., and Cheevers, W., 1975, DNA synthesis in polyoma virus infection. III. Mechanism of inhibition of viral DNA replication by cycloheximide, *J. Virol.* **15**:1409.

Zwillenberg, L. O., and Wolf, K., 1968, Ultrastructure of lymphocystis virus, *J. Virol.* **2**:393.

CHAPTER 7

Fish Viruses and Viral Infections

Philip E. McAllister

U.S. Fish and Wildlife Service
National Fish Health Research Laboratory
Kearneysville, West Virginia 25430

1. INTRODUCTION

The advent of fish cell and tissue culture in the mid-1950s provided the technical impetus for expanding fish virology beyond the confines of disease transmission studies. A variety of fish viruses and viruslike agents have now been recognized, and most are associated with pathological conditions. Not unexpectedly, research interests have focused on those fish viruses which impact most significantly on economic and aesthetic sensitivities. As a result, some of the fish viruses have been well characterized and classified into established viral taxonomic groupings while others have been only partly characterized or demonstrated solely by electron microscopy and their classification is tentative.

This chapter presents a comprehensive, systematic account of the biochemical, biophysical, and biological properties of the fish viruses and viruslike agents as well as an overview of the diseases with which they are associated.

2. FISH HERPESVIRIDAE

Five herpeslike viruses have been identified in fish. Three of the viruses—the channel catfish virus (CCV), herpesvirus salmonis, and the Nerka virus in Towada Lake, Akita and Aomori Prefecture (NeVTA)—have been isolated in cell culture, and some of their biochemical, biophysical, and morphological characteristics have been determined. Two additional herpesviruslike agents have been recognized in electron micrographs of diseased tissue: one from cyprinids with epithelioma papillosum and a second from turbot showing epithelial pathology. The agent from turbot has been tentatively designated "herpesvirus scophthalmi."

2.1. Biology of the Diseases

2.1.1. Channel Catfish Virus (CCV) Disease

Channel catfish, generally less than 4 months old, are affected by an acute hemorrhagic disease which results in high mortality (Fijan *et al.*, 1970; Wolf, 1973). The disease occurs throughout most of the southern half of the United States but has also been reported in Central America (McCraren, 1973; Plumb, 1977, 1971c). Essentially only the channel catfish (*Ictalurus punctatus* R.) is susceptible to natural infection; additional catfish species are susceptible to experimental infection (Plumb, 1977). Clinical signs of CCV disease develop within 6 days after infection in fish held at 25–30°C whereas lower temperatures promote a longer incubation period. Pathological changes occur in most organs and tissues, but the kidneys, liver, and digestive tract are the most extensively affected (Major *et al.*, 1975; Plumb *et al.*, 1974; Wolf *et al.*, 1972). The virus can be readily isolated from infected fry and fingerlings until the disappearance of clinical signs; the virus has yet to be recovered from suspected adult carriers (Plumb, 1971a,b,c). Channel catfish virus can be presumptively identified by correlating temperature and host and cell culture specificity; virus identification is confirmed by serum neutralization or fluorescent antibody assay.

2.1.2. Herpesvirus Salmonis: Nerka Virus in Towada Lake, Akita and Amori Prefecture (NeVTA)

Herpesvirus salmonis was isolated from adult rainbow trout (*Salmo gairdneri*) at the Winthrop, Washington, National Fish Hatchery in the United States (Wolf *et al.*, 1975a,b). A similar virus (NeVTA) was isolated independently in Japan from both fry and adult landlocked sockeye salmon (*Oncorhynchus nerka*) (Sano, 1976).

Epizootics may result in levels of mortality ranging from 50% to 100%. Clinical manifestations become apparent 30–45 days after experimental infection at temperatures below 14°C, but will be variable or absent at higher temperatures (Wolf, 1976). Pathological changes occur principally in the kidney hematopoietic tissue, the liver, and the pancreatic acinar cells. Herpesvirus salmonis has been recovered from the internal organs of moribund fry and fingerlings and from the sex products of ostensibly healthy adults. NeVTA has been isolated from similar specimens. Virus may be presumptively identified by correlating the low temperature required for virus replication with the distinctive syncytium formation in salmonid cell cultures. Virus identification is confirmed by serological reactivity in a neutralization or fluorescent antibody assay.

2.1.3. Herpesvirus Scophthalmi

Histological examination of moribund turbot (*Scophthalmus maximus* L.) from a Scottish fish farm revealed epithelial cell giantism in both the skin and gills (Buchanan and Madeley, 1978; Buchanan *et al.*, 1978; Richards and Buchanan, 1978). The giant cells varied from 45 to 130 μm in diameter and in most cases were multinucleate. Affected cells were examined by electron microscopy, and viruslike particles were evident in the cytoplasm and the nucleus. A survey of preserved specimens suggested that the condition is endemic in feral turbot. In hatchery populations manifestations of the disease were associated with physiological stress. Attempts to isolate the virus in cell culture have been unsuccessful.

2.1.4. Epithelioma Papillosum of Carp (Carp Pox)

Common carp (*Cyprinus carpio* L.) and several other species of cyprinids in Europe, Asia, and the Middle East are affected by a benign epidermal hyperplasia (Bauer *et al.*, 1969; Hines *et al.*, 1974; Schäperclaus, 1954; Wolf, 1966, 1973). Large areas of epidermis may become involved, but mortality does not result from the condition. The mechanism by which epithelioma papillosum is transmitted in nature is not known, and all attempts to experimentally transmit the disease have been unsuccessful. Electron micrographs reveal herpesviruslike particles associated with affected tissue, but as yet the virus has not been isolated (Schubert, 1964, 1966; Schubert and Meyer, 1960).

2.2. Biology of the Viruses

2.2.1. Morphology

Electron micrographs indicate that CCV, herpesvirus salmonis, NeVTA, herpesvirus scophthalmi, and the agent associated with epithelioma papillosum possess characteristic herpesvirus morphology (Buchanan and Madeley, 1978; Buchanan *et al.*, 1978; Plumb *et al.*, 1974; Schubert, 1964, 1966; Wolf and Darlington, 1971; Wolf *et al.*, 1978). The piscine herpesvirion is surrounded by an envelope of host cell origin and contains an icosahedral nucleocapsid composed of two morphologically distinct units, the outer capsid with 162 hollow, elongated capsomers and the inner core (Fig. 1). The middle and inner capsids found in other herpesviruses have not been distinguished. The dimensions of the herpesviruses detected in fish are indicated in Table 1. The

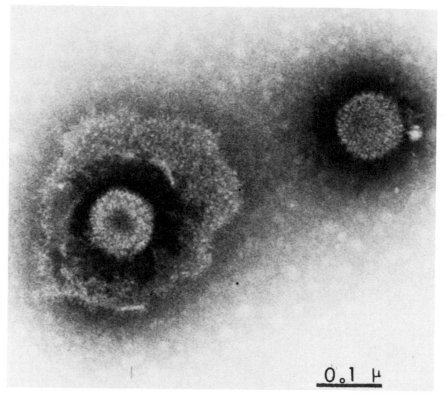

Fig. 1. Electron micrograph of released herpesvirus salmonis. Particle on the left retains some disrupted envelope material. From Wolf *et al.* (1978); reprinted with the permission of the American Society for Microbiology.

TABLE 1

Dimensions of Herpesviruses Detected in Fish

Virus	Virion dimensions (nm)		
	Enveloped particle	Outer capsid	Inner core
Channel catfish virus	175–200	95–105	40–50
Herpesvirus salmonis	~150	80–90	50–60
Nerka Virus Towada Lake, Akita and Aomori Prefecture	~230	nd[a]	nd[a]
Herpesvirus scophthalmi	200–220	85–100	25–30
Epithelioma papillosum–associated virus	140–150	~110	~50

[a] nd, Not determined.

apparent differences in the particle diameter of herpesvirus salmonis and NeVTA need to be critically examined.

2.2.2. Biological Properties

2.2.2a. Antigenicity

The piscine herpesviruses have been distinguished from the other fish viruses by serum neutralization, fluorescent antibody, and indirect hemagglutination assays. Potential group-specific antigens have not been investigated, nor has more than one serotype of any of the viruses been identified. The antigenic relationship between herpesvirus salmonis and NeVTA has not been determined—these two viruses may be very similar, if not identical.

Antisera to CCV have been prepared in channel catfish, but host immune response declines markedly unless repetitive booster inoculations are administered (Heartwell, 1975; Plumb, 1973). Survivors of a natural epizootic may show virus-neutralizing activity in their sera (Plumb, 1971*b*, 1973).

The immune response of salmonids following injection or infection with herpesvirus salmonis or NeVTA has not been determined.

2.2.2b. Stability

Both CCV and herpesvirus salmonis are moderately stable when suspended in cell culture medium supplemented with serum. Little loss of infectivity occurred when CCV was stored for 9 months at $-80°C$, and similar results occur with herpesvirus salmonis (Plumb, 1977; Wolf, 1973; Wolf *et al.*, 1978). At higher temperatures and in the absence of supplementary protein, infectivity declines rather rapidly—e.g., at 4°C herpesvirus salmonis titer decreased by 3 $\log_{10}$ units in 3 weeks while CCV titer decreased by $\sim 1 \log_{10}$ unit in 3 months.

Both viruses are inactivated by exposure to ether, chloroform, glycerol, sodium hypochlorite, acid (pH 3.0), and heat (60°C for 1 hr) (Fijan, 1968; Plumb, 1977; Wolf, 1973, 1976; Wolf *et al.*, 1978). Channel catfish virus is sensitive to multiple cycles of freezing and thawing and to drying, whereas herpesvirus salmonis appears stable to freezing and thawing.

2.2.3. Chemical Composition

2.2.3a. Viral Nucleic Acid

The nucleic acid of both CCV and herpesvirus salmonis was presumptively identified as DNA by 5-iodo-2-deoxyuridine inhibition of virus replication. Viral DNA was subsequently purified and partly characterized.

Channel catfish virus DNA sediments to a density of 1.715 g/cm^3 in CsCl and has a sedimentation coefficient of 53 S and a contour length of 44 μm (Dixon and Farber, 1977; Goodheart and Plummer, 1975; Wolf, 1973). The data indicate that the DNA has a molecular weight of 8.5×10^7 and a 56.1% G plus C content. Restriction endonuclease digestion studies suggest that the CCV genome is terminally redundant and unfragmented (Dixon and Farber, 1977).

Herpesvirus salmonis DNA bands at a density of 1.709 g/cm^3 in CsCl gradients, suggesting a G plus C content of 50% (Wolf *et al.*, 1976, 1978). No other physical or biochemical characteristics of the herpesvirus salmonis genome have been reported.

2.2.3b. Viral Protein

F. E. Farber and R. A. F. Dixon (personal communication) have detected 32 virus-specific proteins in CCV-infected cells by polyacrylamide gel electrophoresis. Sixteen of these proteins are structural components of the virion. Pulse-labeling showed three major classes of proteins are synthesized.

No analysis of herpesvirus salmonis structural proteins has been reported.

2.2.3c. Virion-Associated Lipid and Carbohydrate

Channel catfish virus and herpesvirus salmonis are inactivated by exposure to ether or chloroform, indicating that both virions contain lipid components essential for infectivity. F. E. Farber and R. A. F. Dixon (personal communication) have detected carbohydrate associated with CCV structural proteins and envelope lipid. No other chemical or structural characterization of lipid or carbohydrate has been reported for either virus.

2.2.4. Growth Cycle of Infectious Virus

Channel catfish virus replicates in cell culture at 10–30°C, with the optimum temperature being 25–30°C (Plumb, 1977; Wolf, 1973; Wolf and Darlington, 1971). In BB cells (see Table 2 for cell culture abbreviations), progeny virus first appears 4–6 hr after infection and increases exponentially for 7–11 hr, plateauing at about 20 hr after infection (Fig. 2). Virus titer reaches $\sim 10^7$ PFU/ml by 25–35 hr, but a significant amount of the progeny virions remain cell associated. Viral-induced syncytium formation may be evident as early as 2 hr after infection. Syncytia continue to enlarge, and intranuclear inclusions become evident. Lysis or sloughing of affected cells occurs by 19–24 hr after infection (Plumb *et al.*, 1974; Wolf, 1973; Wolf and Darlington, 1971; Wolf and Quimby, 1970a).

Herpesvirus salmonis replicates in cell culture at 5–10°C, with variable replication at 15°C (Wolf, 1976; Wolf *et al.*, 1976, 1978). Cell-associated progeny virions appear about 20 hr after infection and increase exponentially, plateauing 50–60 hr after infection. Released virions increase at a much slower rate, approaching a plateau about 100 hr after infection at a titer of $\sim 10^5$ PFU/ml. Cytopathic effects may become evident as early as 24 hr after infection, with syncytia and intranuclear inclusions developing by 48 hr after infection (Sano, 1976; Wolf, 1976; Wolf *et al.*, 1975b, 1978).

TABLE 2
Cell Culture Abbreviations Mentioned in Text

Abbreviation	Species of origin	Certified cell line[a]
A6	South African clawed toad	102
AS	Atlantic salmon	
BB	Brown bullhead	59
BF-2	Bluegill fry	91
BGL	Bluegill	
BHK-21	Syrian hamster	10
CAR	Goldfish	71
CCO	Channel catfish ovary	
CHSE-214	Chinook salmon embryo	
CSE	Coho salmon embryo	
EPC	Common carp hyperplasia	
FHM	Fathead minnow	42
FT	Bullfrog	41
GF	Bluestriped grunt	58
GL1	*Gekko gecko*	111
HeLa	Human	2
HEp-2	Human	23
IgH-2	Iguana	108
KB	Human	17
KF-1	Kokanee	
LBF-1	Largemouth bass	
MDCK	Canine	34
RTF-1	Rainbow trout fry	
RTG-2	Rainbow trout gonad	55
SK	Porcine	
SSE	Sockeye salmon embryo	
STE-137	Steelhead trout embryo	
SWT	Red swordtail	
TH-1	Box turtle	50
Vero	African green monkey	81
VH2	Russell's viper	140
VSW	Russell's viper	129
WI-38	Human	75
WISH	Human	25

[a] American Type Culture Collection, 1975.

2.2.5. Cell Culture Susceptibility

Two cell lines of ictalurid origin (BB and CCO) will support the replication of CCV. Numerous mammalian, avian, piscine, and reptilian cell lines have been tested; however, none will support the replication of CCV (Fijan *et al.*, 1970; Plumb, 1977; Wolf and Darlington, 1971).

Herpesvirus salmonis appears to replicate only in cells of salmonid origin. The cell lines RTG-2, RTF-1, CHSE-214, and KF-1 will support virus replication (Wolf *et al.*, 1978). The NeVTA isolate was propagated in RTG-2 cells (Sano, 1976).

3. FISH IRIDOVIRIDAE

Lymphocystis virus and the putative piscine erythrocytic necrosis (PEN) virus are tentatively classified in the icosahedral cytoplasmic deoxyribovirus (iridovirus) group. Lymphocystis virus has been isolated in cell culture and partly characterized. The virus of PEN has been observed in electron micrographs of affected erythrocytes, but not yet isolated in cell culture.

3.1. Biology of the Diseases

3.1.1. Lymphocystis

Lymphocystis occurs worldwide, and at least 97 species of teleosts belonging to 33 families are affected. The lesions develop principally on the body surface and may occur on the internal organs and tissues (Dukes and Lawler, 1975; Dunbar and Wolf, 1966; Russell, 1974). Lymphocystis is not lethal, and the lesions eventually heal (Lawler *et al.*, 1977; Mann, 1970). The disease can be transmitted experimentally

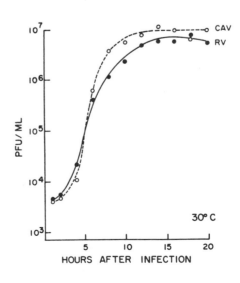

Fig. 2. Single-cycle growth curve of CCV in BB cells infected with MOI ≥ 25 PFU/cell and incubated at 30°C. CAV is cell-associated virus; RV is released virus. From Wolf and Darlington (1971); reprinted with the permission of the American Society for Microbiology.

by cohabitation, exposure to water containing virus, and by feeding, implantation, or injection of lesion, lesion homogenate, or infected cell culture fluid (Dunbar and Wolf, 1966; Rašín, 1927; Weissenberg, 1939, 1951; Wolf, 1962; Wolf *et al.*, 1966). Within a genus lymphocystis can be transmitted with relative ease, while transmission between families is difficult. The lymphocystis lesion is composed of grossly hypertrophied cells—increases in cell volume of 10^5-fold or more are not uncommon. The unique character of the lesion permits histological diagnosis of the disease (Dunbar and Wolf, 1966; Midlige and Malsberger, 1968; Nigrelli and Ruggieri, 1965).

3.1.2. Piscine Erythrocytic Necrosis (PEN): Viral Erythrocytic Necrosis

Piscine erythrocytic necrosis (PEN), also called viral erythrocytic necrosis (VEN), occurs in at least 13 genera of marine and anadromous fish (Evelyn and Traxler, 1978; Johnston and Davies, 1973; Laird and Bullock, 1969; Sherburne, 1977; Walker and Sherburne, 1977). Few clinical manifestations are associated with mild cases of the disease. Severely affected fish may show signs of anemia, but mortality due to PEN *per se* appears low. Pathological changes appear to occur only in erythrocytes. The irregular cellular and nuclear morphology as well as intracytoplasmic and intranuclear inclusions is discernible in a Giemsa- or Wright-stained blood film. The presence of virus is confirmed by electron microscopy. Although virus has not yet been isolated, the disease has been experimentally transmitted by injection of affected erythrocytes or of filtrates of homogenized kidneys and spleen (Evelyn and Traxler, 1978; B. L. Nicholson, personal communication).

3.2. Biology of the Viruses

3.2.1. Morphology

Electron micrographs of affected tissue and, with lymphocystis, also of infected cell cultures indicate that both lymphocystis virus and the virus of PEN possess the morphological characteristics of iridoviruses (Howse and Christmas, 1971; Reno *et al.*, 1978; Walker, 1962; Walker and Sherburne, 1977; Wolf *et al.*, 1966; Yamamoto *et al.*, 1976). The capsid has icosahedral symmetry with lamellar construction and is separated from the nucleoid by a translucent zone (Fig. 3). Electron

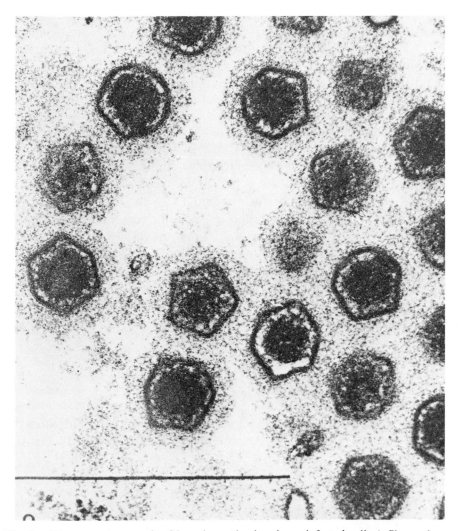

Fig. 3. Electron micrograph of lymphocystis virus in an infected cell. A fibrous layer surrounds the viral capsid. Bar is 1.0 μm. From Yamamoto *et al.* (1976); reprinted with the permission of the Journal of the Fisheries Research Board of Canada.

micrographs of purified lymphocystis virus suggest that the capsid is enveloped and that filaments extend from the vertices (Midlige and Malsberger, 1968; Zwillenberg and Wolf, 1968). Within infected cells, virions and putative developmental intermediates appear adjacent to an amorphous structure (viroplasm) which probably corresponds to the cytoplasmic inclusion seen by light microscopy. Both lymphocystis virus and the virus of PEN have been observed in several genera of fish, and, although overall morphological characteristics are consistent, the dimensions of both viruses vary considerably between genera (Table 3). This, in concert with the difficulty in transmitting the diseases between families, suggests that the viruses may have adapted to certain hosts and that strains or types of the viruses may occur.

3.2.2. Biological Properties

Lymphocystis virus is remarkably stable. Infectivity can be recovered from infected tissue dried for 15 years over P_2O_5 at 4°C or from lyophilized lesion homogenate held 13.5 years at 4°C. Infectivity was also recovered from lesion and lesion homogenates held 20 months at −20°C but not from lesions held 20 months in 50% glycerol at 4°C (Rašín, 1927; Wolf, 1962; Wolf et al., 1979).

The titer of lymphocystis virus suspended in cell culture medium decreased ∼10^2 $TCID_{50}$/ml in 74 weeks at −70°C and in 46 weeks at 4°C. The virus is inactivated by exposure to ether, heating (60°C for 1 min), and sonication, but is stable to freezing and thawing (Midlige, 1968; Wolf, 1962; Wolf et al., 1966).

3.2.3. Chemical Composition

Electron micrographs show complete and developing lymphocystis and PEN virions associated with a cytoplasmic inclusion. Cytochemical

TABLE 3
Dimensions of *Iridoviridae* Detected in Fish

Virus	Genus	Diameter of particle (nm)
Lymphocystis	*Bairdiella*	280–330
	Cichlosoma	180–260
	Lepomis	200–300
	Micropogon	240–260
	Pleuronectes	130–150
	Stizostedion	180–260
Piscine erythrocytic necrosis	*Blennius*	200–300
	Clupea	average 145
	Gadus	300–360
	Oncorhynchus	155–195

staining, thymidine uptake, and autoradiographic data indicate that the virus-induced cytoplasmic inclusion contains DNA (Midlige and Malsberger, 1968; Reno and Nicholson, 1978; Reno *et al.*, 1978; Walker, 1965; Walker and Sherburne, 1977). In addition, Midlige (1968) demonstrated that lymphocystis virus replication and inclusion formation were inhibited by exposing infected cell cultures to 5-fluoro-2-deoxyuridine. Based on these data, the nucleic acid of lymphocystis virus and the virus of PEN has been presumptively identified as DNA. No structural protein characterization has been reported for either virus. The sensitivity of lymphocystis virus infectivity to ether suggests the presence of essential lipid.

3.2.4. Growth Cycle of Infectious Virus

Lymphocystis virus replication and lesion formation have been monitored in experimentally infected bluegills (Fig. 4) (Dunbar and Wolf, 1966; Wolf and Carlson, 1965). Tissue-associated infectivity,

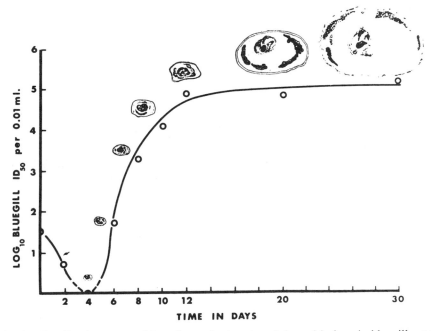

Fig. 4. Replication curve of lymphocystis virus in subdermal lesions in bluegills at 25 ± 1°C. Cell sketches are proportional to mean cell sizes, and they represent generalized developmental stages of lymphocystis cells in bluegills. From Wolf and Carlson (1965); reprinted with the permission of the New York Academy of Sciences.

ostensibly due to progeny virus, could be detected beginning at day 5
after infection and increased exponentially thereafter, plateauing ~ 12
days after infection. The development of the lymphocystis lesion
paralleled the virus replication curve. Midlige and Malsberger (1968)
found that lymphocystis virus in cell culture remained highly aggregated both intracellularly and when released, but estimated released
virus titer to be 10^6 TCID$_{50}$/ml.

3.2.4a. Cell Culture Susceptibility

Lymphocystis virus will replicate in BF-2, GF, LBF-1, blue striped
grunt kidney, and lane snapper fin cells, but not in BB, FHM, RTG-2,
or bluegill ovary cells (Beasley *et al.*, 1967; Lopez *et al.*, 1969; Midlige
and Malsberger, 1968; Wolf, 1962; Wolf and Quimby, 1973; Wolf *et
al.*, 1966; Zwillenberg and Wolf, 1968). Evelyn and Traxler (1978) have
attempted, albeit unsuccessfully, to cultivate the virus of PEN in
CHSE-214, FHM, RTG-2, and rainbow trout ovary cells. Reno and
Nicholson (1978) have maintained PEN-infected erythrocytes *in vitro*
for up to 2 weeks.

3.2.4b. Viral Macromolecular Synthesis

Fluorescent antibody staining indicates that lymphocystis virus
antigen accumulates in the cytoplasm by 16 hr after infection, and
autoradiographs show that DNA synthesis in cytoplasmic inclusions
occurs by 4–5 days after infection (Beasley *et al.*, 1967; Lopez *et al.*,
1968, 1969; Midlige, 1968). The antineoplastic drug 6-mercaptopurine
inhibits lymphocystis virus-specific macromolecular synthesis.

Reno and Nicholson (1978) monitored the uptake of nucleic acid
and protein precursors in PEN infected erythrocytes and reported an
eight- to tenfold increase in thymidine uptake and a significant incorporation of amino acids by day 6, but little difference in uridine uptake.

4. FISH REOVIRIDAE

Two viruses having biochemical, biophysical, and morphological
characteristics similar to those of a reovirus have been recovered from

fish. One, infectious pancreatic necrosis virus, was isolated in 1960 and continues to be a significant problem in salmonid husbandry. The second, golden shiner virus, was only recently isolated and its impact on the culturing of golden shiners (*Notemigonus crysoleucas*) is under study.

4.1. Biology of the Diseases

4.1.1. Infectious Pancreatic Necrosis

Infectious pancreatic necrosis (IPN) virus was first isolated from brook trout; subsequently, IPN and IPN-like viruses have been recovered worldwide from a variety of salmonid and nonsalmonid fishes as well as from marine invertebrates (Ahne, 1977; Bellet, 1969; Hill, 1976; Ljungberg and Jørgensen, 1973; MacKelvie and Artsob, 1969; McMichael *et al.*, 1973; Munro and Duncan, 1977; Parisot *et al.*, 1963; Sano, 1973, 1976; Sonstegard *et al.*, 1972; Underwood *et al.*, 1977; Wolf and Pettijohn, 1970; Wolf *et al.*, 1960). Mortality is generally high in salmonids less than 6 months of age, but survivors may become lifelong carriers. A variety of external and internal clinical manifestations become evident during the course of the disease, but none distinguishes IPN from other salmonid virus diseases (Parisot *et al.*, 1965; Wolf, 1966, 1972; Yasutake, 1970; Yasutake *et al.*, 1965). Pathological changes occur in the pancreatic, renal, and hepatic tissues and in the intestinal mucosa, but none is IPN specific (Kudo *et al.*, 1973; McKnight and Roberts, 1976; Yasutake, 1970). Horizontal transmission occurs via virus shed with urine, feces, and sex products, and vertical transmission is suspected (Bullock *et al.*, 1976; Desautels and MacKelvie, 1975; Wolf *et al.*, 1968; Seeley *et al.*, 1977). The disease can be transmitted experimentally by injection, feeding, and cohabitation. The virus is recovered from internal organs with greater frequency than from feces, sex products, or peritoneal washings, and the probability of recovering the virus is enhanced if the fish are physiologically stressed (Billi and Wolf, 1969; Frantsi and Savan, 1971; Wolf *et al.*, 1968; Yamamoto, 1974, 1975a,b). The distinctive plaque morphology of IPN virus in RTG-2 cells (Fig. 5) aids in presumptive identification; neutralization, fluorescent antibody, or complement-fixation assays are used for confirmation (Finlay and Hill, 1975; Jørgensen and

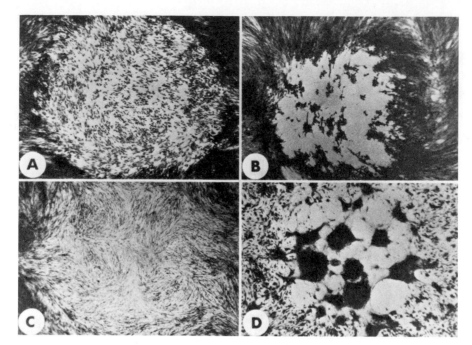

Fig. 5. Comparative plaque characteristics of four fish viruses. A,B,C: Plaques in RTG-2 cells. D: Plaque in BB cells. A: Viral hemorrhagic septicemia virus. B: Infectious hematopoietic necrosis virus. C: Infectious pancreatic necrosis virus. D: Channel catfish virus. From Wolf and Quimby (1973); reprinted with the permission of the American Society for Microbiology.

Meyling, 1972; Lientz and Springer, 1973; Tu et al., 1974; Wolf and Quimby, 1973).

4.1.2. Golden Shiner Virus (GSV) Disease

The golden shiner virus (GSV) disease was only recently recognized, but appears to be widely distributed throughout the southeastern and midwestern regions of the United States (A. J. Mitchell, personal communication; J. A. Plumb, personal communication). Throughout the summer and early fall sexually mature golden shiners 5–6 months of age, suffer chronic mortality characterized both externally and internally by profuse hemorrhaging. No histopathological observations have been reported, and little is known of the biology of the disease. Experimentally, the disease has been transmitted by intraperiotineal injection of cell-culture-grown virus.

4.2. Biology of the Viruses

4.2.1. Morphology

4.2.1a. Infectious Virions

Electron micrographs of negatively stained and thin-sectioned IPN virus (Fig. 6) show that the virion is an unenveloped icosahedron 55–74 nm in diameter; little variation in particle diameter has been observed among the various serotypes (Cerini and Malsberger, 1965; Chang *et al.*, 1978; Cohen and Scherrer, 1972; Cohen *et al.*, 1973; Kelly and Loh, 1972; Macdonald and Yamamoto, 1977*a*; Moss and Gravell, 1969). The morphological characteristics of IPN virus are consistent with those of a reovirus, with the exception that IPN virus has a single capsid and reoviruses have a double capsid. The single capsid of IPN virus is composed of 180 structural subunits shared by 92 pentagonal and hexagonal capsomers. Measurement of the hydrophobic diameter by laser quasielastic light-scattering spectroscopy (LQELS) indicates

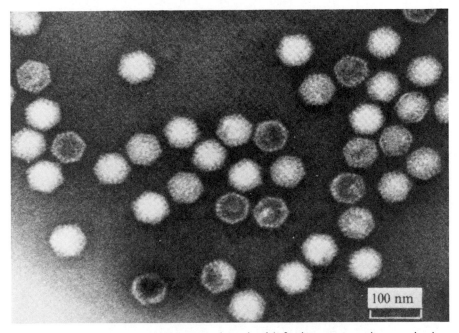

100 nm

Fig. 6. Electron micrograph of negatively stained infectious pancreatic necrosis virus. From Cohen *et al.* (1973); reprinted with the permission of Cambridge University Press.

that IPN virus has a more rigid capsid than a reovirus (Dobos *et al.*, 1977).

Subviral structures resembling empty capsids and virus cores have been observed in electron micrographs. The corelike particles have not been isolated, but the empty capsids have been separated from intact virions by CsCl density gradient centrifugation. The intact virion sediments to a density of 1.33 g/cm³ and the empty capsid to 1.29 g/cm³.

Electron micrographs of golden shiner virus-infected cells show icosahedral virus particles 61–82 nm in diameter in intracytoplasmic accumulations.

4.2.1b.   Defective Virions

Malsberger and Cerini (1963) were the first to describe the homologous interference of IPN virus replication. Subsequent studies by Macdonald and Yamamoto (1977*b*, 1978) and Nicholson and Dunn (1974) showed that autointerfering virus copurified with infectious virus, was sensitive to ultraviolet irradiation and freezing and thawing, and was neutralized by IPN virus-specific immune serum. Autointerfering particles have only recently been separated on CsCl density gradients and sediment to a density of 1.28 g/cm³ (Hedrick *et al.*, 1978).

4.2.2.   Biological Properties

4.2.2a.   Antigenicity

Both IPN virus and GSV are distinct from the other fish viruses. Six IPN virus serotypes have been identified by serum neutralization while three have been identified by complement fixation (Finlay and Hill, 1975; Lientz and Springer, 1973). Immunodiffusion and immunoelectrophoresis of IPN virus preparations revealed three antigenic components; no correlation has been made between these three antigens and virus structure (McMichael *et al.*, 1975). Eel virus— European (EVE), isolated in Japan, is antigenically related to IPN virus (Sano, 1976).

4.2.2b.   Genetic Considerations

Little is known concerning the genetics of IPN virus, but variant or mutant virus strains have been implicated in alterations of host range, plaque size, virulence, and sensitivity to neutralization by normal serum (Dorson *et al.*, 1975b; Frantsi and Savan, 1971; Jørgensen and Kehlet, 1971; Nicholson *et al.*, 1978; Scherrer, 1973; Scherrer and Cohen, 1975). Dorson *et al.* (1975b) reported that IPN virus strain 27/70 lost virulence when passaged in RTG-2 cells and that accompanying the loss in virulence was an increase in plaque size and sensitivity to normal trout serum. Nicholson *et al.*, (1978) and Scherrer and Cohen (1975) found that adaptation of virus grown in RTG-2 cells to growth in FHM cells selected for a large-plaque mutant. Scherrer and Cohen (1975) proposed that a high-frequency (10^{-4} to 10^{-5}) mutation altered the characteristics of the capsid, thereby affecting adsorption and penetration.

4.2.2c. Stability

Infectious pancreatic necrosis virus is, in general, quite stable. Infectivity whether associated with whole fish, tissue homogenates, or cell culture medium can be preserved for years by freezing at $-20°C$ or lower, storage at 4°C in 50% glycerol, or lyophilization; in addition, the virus may remain stable for months in freshwater or seawater at 4°C (MacKelvie and Desautels, 1975; Malsberger and Cerini, 1963; Tu *et al.*, 1975; Wolf *et al.*, 1969). Some IPN virus isolates are sensitive to a single freeze-thaw cycle or require acidic conditions for storage (Wolf and Quimby, 1971).

Infectious pancreatic necrosis virus is rapidly inactivated by exposure to chlorine, iodophor, and ultraviolet irradiation and progressively inactivated by exposure to extremes of pH (pH 2.0 or 9.0), formalin, drying, or heating at 60°C (Amend, 1976; Amend and Pietsch, 1972; Bullock *et al.*, 1976; Desautels and MacKelvie, 1975; Eskildsen and Jørgensen, 1974; Jorgensen, 1973a; MacKelvie and Desautels, 1975). Infectivity is not affected by ether, chloroform, or glycerol.

Few details are known concerning GSV stability. The virus is unaffected by ether and only partly inactivated by heating at 60°C for 90 min (J. A. Plumb, personal communication).

4.2.3. Chemical Composition

The IPN virion has a molecular weight of 55×10^6 and a sedimentation coefficient of 435 S. The virion mass is composed of 8.7%

RNA and 91.3% protein. Biochemical and biophysical characterization of the virus has been limited essentially to strain VR-299.

4.2.3a. Viral Nucleic Acid

Malsberger and Cerini (1965) and Argot (1969) concluded that the nucleic acid of IPN virus was RNA from enhanced uridine uptake in infected cells, unabated virus replication in the presence of halogenated deoxyuridines, and a positive orcinol test with extracted viral nucleic acid. Early attempts to characterize the viral nucleic acid as single- or double-stranded and segmented or unsegmented resulted in conflicting interpretations (Argot, 1969; Argot and Malsberger, 1972; Kelly and Loh, 1972; Nicholson, 1971a). Subsequent reports established that IPN virus contains two segments of double-stranded RNA (Fig. 7) (Cohen et al., 1973; Dobos, 1976; Macdonald and Yamamoto, 1977a). The biochemical and biophysical characteristics of IPN virion RNA (Table 4) differ significantly from those described for reoviruses, suggesting that IPN and IPN-like viruses may represent a new taxonomic grouping of double-stranded RNA viruses.

The nucleic acid of GSV was presumptively identified as double-stranded RNA by the use of metabolic inhibitors and cytochemical staining (J. A. Plumb, personal communication). No other characteristics have been determined.

4.2.3b. Viral Proteins

Three classes of IPN virus structural proteins have been identified by polyacrylamide gel electrophoresis. Using the Greek letter notation proposed by Dobos (1977), the viral proteins have been designated according to their relative migration into high (α), intermediate (β), and low (γ) molecular weight classes (Table 5). Different numbers of proteins have been resolved. Chang et al. (1978) and Cohen et al. (1973) reported three proteins, Loh et al. (1974) seven, and Dobos and Rowe (1977) and Dobos et al. (1977) four (Fig. 8). These differences may represent artifacts generated by preparation, storage, or dimerization (Dobos and Rowe, 1977). The distribution, structure–function relationships, and characteristics of the proteins are poorly defined. Dobos et al. (1977) found only β class protein associated with capsid preparations and surmised that α and γ class proteins are internal components.

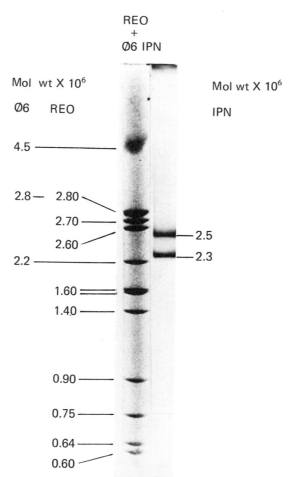

Fig. 7. Polyacrylamide gel electrophoresis of ^{32}P-labeled IPN virus RNA together with unlabeled reovirus RNA and φ6 phage RNA. The left column shows the stained marker RNA bands; the right column is an autoradiograph of the same gel. From Dobos (1976); reprinted with the permission of Information Retrieval Limited.

4.2.4. Growth Cycle of Infectious Virions

The kinetics of IPN virus replication have been monitored in a variety of cell lines, and the results are typified by those of Malsberger and Cerini (1963, 1965) illustrated in Fig. 9. Cell-associated virus became evident ~4 hr after infection and increased in an exponential manner for the next 7 hr. Released virus could be detected ~7 hr after infection and increased exponentially for the next 9 hr. Released and cell-associated virus reached a similar plateau ~16 hr after infection.

TABLE 4

Biochemical and Biophysical Characteristics of IPN Virion RNA

Conformation:	Two segments of double-stranded RNA
Molecular weight:	2.3×10^6 and 2.5×10^6
Sedimentation coefficient:	Native—15 S, RNase resistant
	Denatured—24 S, RNase sensitive
Density (Cs_2SO_4):	1.60–1.615 g/cm^3
Melting point (T_m):	85–89°C
Contour length:	$0.92 \pm 0.07 \mu$m
Base composition:	23.5% A; 23.5% U; 27.0% G; 26.0% C

Immunofluorescent microscopy by Piper *et al.* (1973) and Tu *et al.* (1974) revealed the accumulation of virus-specific antigen in the cytoplasm as early as 3–4 hr after infection.

Infectious pancreatic necrosis virus replicates well at 10–26°C, poorly at 4°C, and not at all at 30°C. Virus replication is suppressed if infected cells are exposed to actinomycin D or ultraviolet irradiation within 2 hr after infection, but there is no effect if the cells are exposed later in the infectious cycle (Dobos, 1977; Kelly and Loh, 1975; Nicholson, 1971b).

Golden shiner virus replicates well at 25–30°C, and focal cytopathic effects become evident in 24 hr. Little else is known concerning the replication cycle of the virus.

TABLE 5

Molecular Weights of IPN Virus-Specific Polypeptides[a]

Protein designation	Molecular weight	
	Infected cell	Virion
α	90,000	90,000
β_1	59,000	
β_2	58,000	
β_3	57,000	57,000
γ_1	29,000	29,000
γ_{1A}	28,000	28,000
γ_2	27,000	
γ_3	25,000	

[a] Adapted from Dobos and Rowe (1977); reprinted with the permission of the American Society for Microbiology.

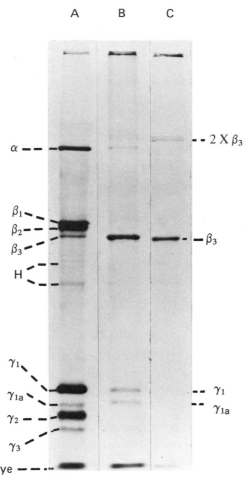

Fig. 8. Autoradiograph of labeled polypeptides of (A) IPN virus-infected RTG-2 cells UV-irradiated at 2 hr after infection and labeled for 4 hr at 6 hr after infection, (B) labeled purified IPN virus, and (C) labeled IPN virus capsid preparation dissolved before electrophoresis in hot sodium dodecylsulfate without mercaptoethanol. H, Host-cell-specific proteins. Dimer of B_3 is represented by the symbol $2 \times B_3$. Adapted from Dobos and Rowe (1977); reprinted with the permission of the American Society for Microbiology.

4.2.4a. Cell Culture Susceptibility

Infectious pancreatic necrosis virus replicates to a titer of about 10^8–10^9 PFU/ml. The RTG-2 cell line has been extensively used in IPN virus studies, but AS, BB, BF-2, CHSE-214, FHM, GF, STE-137, and SWT cells provide comparable yields. The virus will not replicate in FT, primary embryonic seahorse, or any of 11 mammalian cell lines

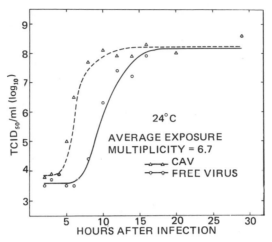

Fig. 9. Single-cycle growth curve of IPN virus in RTG-2 cells infected at a MOI of 6.7 $TCID_{50}$/cell and incubated at 24°C. Δ, Cell-associated virus (CAV); O, released virus. From Malsberger and Cerini (1965); reprinted with the permission of the New York Academy of Sciences.

tested (Moewus-Kobb, 1965; Wolf, 1966; Wolf *et al.*, 1960). The omaka cell line yields only low titers of virus (Lee and Loh, 1975). Some IPN virus strains appear to have restricted cell culture host range (Jørgensen and Grauballe, 1971; Jørgensen and Kehlet, 1971; Scherrer and Cohen, 1975).

Golden shiner virus replicates well in FHM cells. Brown bullhead, CCO, and RTG-2 cells were tested for susceptibility to infection and no CPE was observed; however, supernatant fluids were not assayed for progeny virus (J. A. Plumb, personal communication).

4.2.4b. Viral Protein Synthesis

Eight IPN virus-specific proteins have been detected in infected cells and designated as high (α), intermediate (β_1, β_2, β_3) and low (γ_1, γ_{1A}, γ_2, γ_3) molecular weight protein classes (Fig. 8 and Table 5) (Dobos, 1977; Dobos and Rowe, 1977). Only four of these proteins (α, β_3, γ_1, γ_{1A}) have been detected as structural components of the virion. All eight proteins are evident throughout the virus replication cycle; however, only four (α, β_1, γ_1, γ_2) are primary gene products, and their aggregate molecular weight (205,000) complements the estimated coding capacity of the viral genome (266,000). The primary gene products are processed intracellularly, with the β_1 protein as the precursor of β_2

and β_3 and γ_1 and γ_2 yielding γ_{1A} and γ_3, respectively. The peptide maps of the cleavage products are virtually identical to those of the parental primary gene products. Dobos and Rowe (1977) suggest that the precursor proteins are synthesized from different cistrons, but only genome-length 24 S viral mRNA has been identified (Alayse et al., 1975).

4.2.4c.   Viral Nucleic Acid Synthesis

An RNA-dependent RNA polymerase is associated with the IPN virion (Cohen, 1975). Enzyme activity in vitro requires all four ribonucleoside triphosphates and Mg^{2+}. Activity diminishes if the virion is treated with chymotrypsin (100 $\mu g/ml$) or Triton X-100 (0.1%), if the reaction mixture contains NaCl (100 mM) or KCl (150 mM), or if Mn^{2+} is substituted for Mg^{2+}. The in vitro reaction was not affected by actinomycin D (10 $\mu g/ml$) or rifampicin (10 $\mu g/ml$). Cohen (1975) monitored polymerase activity at temperatures from 10°C to 52°C. Uridine triphosphate incorporation at 39°C and 52°C was the most rapid but plateaued in 20 min; at 24°C and 29°C continued linear incorporation was observed but at about half the rate observed at 39°C and 52°C. At 20°C and below, the reaction rate was much reduced. Sensitivity to ribonuclease indicated that the RNA synthesized in vitro was single-stranded, but no other characteristics have been determined.

Alayse et al. (1975) isolated 14–15 S and 23–24 S virus-specific RNA from infected cells. The 14–15 S RNA showed nuclease sensitivity and sedimentation characteristics consistent with newly synthesized double-stranded virion RNA. Whether one or both segments of virion RNA were recovered was not determined. The 23–24 S RNA was single-stranded and separable into four peaks by polyacrylamide gel electrophoresis. Alayse et al. (1975) suggested that the 23–24 S RNA was viral messenger RNA, but no hybridization assays were performed. They also proposed that viral transcription began within 30 min and replication within 1 hr after virus infection.

4.2.5.   Cellular Response to Virus Infection

Inhibition of host cell macromolecular synthesis, development of persistently infected cells, and induction of interferon synthesis are effects of IPN virus infection.

Cellular DNA synthesis is inhibited 65–85% by 7–10 hr after virus infection (Argot, 1969; Argot and Malsberger, 1972; Kelly and Loh, 1975; Lothrop and Nicholson, 1974; Nicholson, 1971a). Initiation of DNA synthesis rather than elongation is affected, with maximal inhibition occurring in middle to late S phase. Studies using irradiated virus suggest that a functional viral genome is required for inhibition (Lothrop and Nicholson, 1974). Reports detailing the effect of infection on cellular protein synthesis are conflicting. Argot (1969) reported inhibition of cellular protein synthesis in BF-2 cells, while Dobos (1977) and Nicholson (1971a) observed no such effect in RTG-2 cells.

Nearly all cells in a population are killed by virus infection; however, those that survive maintain their normal growth characteristics but continue to release low levels of infectious virus consistent with a persistently infected or carrier culture (Hedrick et al., 1978; Beasley et al., 1965, 1966).

Infection with IPN virus also induces the synthesis of interferon, at least in FHM and RTG-2 cells (Scherer et al., 1974; de Sena and Rio, 1975). The interferon has broad antifish virus activity but is somewhat cell culture specific.

5. FISH RHABDOVIRIDAE

As many as six antigenically distinct rhabdoviruses have been isolated from fish. These are infectious hematopoietic necrosis virus, viral hemorrhagic septicemia virus (Egtved virus), spring viremia of carp virus (rhabdovirus carpio), pike fry rhabdovirus, eel virus— American, and a rhabdovirus of European eel. Two additional rhabdovirus isolations have been reported, swim bladder inflammation virus and grass carp rhabdovirus, but investigations have shown that the isolates are antigenically indistinguishable from spring viremia of carp virus and pike fry rhabdovirus, respectively.

5.1. Biology of the Diseases

5.1.1. Infectious Hematopoietic Necrosis

The sockeye salmon virus disease, Sacramento River chinook disease, and infectious hematopoietic necrosis were originally considered to be separate diseases (Amend et al., 1969; Ross et al., 1960; Wingfield et al., 1969). However, because of the similarity in their clinical and histopathological manifestations and because of the very close biochemical, biophysical, antigenic, and morphological relationships among the virus isolates, the single designation infectious hematopoietic necrosis (IHN) is now used as the collective descriptor (Amend *et al.*, 1973; McCain *et al.*, 1971).

Infectious hematopoietic necrosis occurs in a variety of salmonid species and is endemic to the Pacific Northwest of North American (Amend *et al.*, 1973; Grischkowsky and Amend, 1976; Parisot *et al.*, 1965). The disease has occurred in other parts of the world, but ultimately all outbreaks have been traced to materials originating in North America (Holway and Smith, 1973; Plumb, 1972; Sano, 1976; Sano *et al.*, 1977b). Generally, fish 3 weeks to 6 months old are affected, and the epizootic potential appears greatest at temperatures of 10–12°C (P. E. McAllister, unpublished data). At 18°C mortality is reduced, but the development of the carrier state is not necessarily prevented (Amend, 1970, 1976; P. E. McAllister, unpublished data). Affected fish may show a variety of clinical signs, but none of these alterations in appearance or behavior is IHN specific (Parisot *et al.*, 1965; Yasutake, 1970). Histopathological changes occur in the kidneys, spleen, pancreas, and liver. Necroses of the granular cells of the laminar propria, stratum compactum, and stratum granulosum of the alimentary tract are distinguishing pathological characteristics of IHN (Yasutake, 1970; Yasutake *et al.*, 1965). Horizontal transmission occurs as the result of virus shed with feces, urine, or sex products. Surface contamination of eggs rather than true vertical contamination seems to occur as eggs can be effectively disinfected in an iodophor bath (Amend and Pietsch, 1972). Virus can be recovered from homogenates of whole fish or internal organs and from the sex products of spawning carrier fish. The IHN virus can be presumptively identified by plaque morphology (Fig. 5) (Wolf and Quimby, 1973). Neutralization and fluorescent antibody assays have been used to confirm the identity of the virus (Hill *et al.*, 1975; McAllister *et al.*, 1974a,b; McCain *et al.*, 1971).

5.1.2.   Viral Hemorrhagic Septicemia

Viral hemorrhagic septicemia (VHS) is a disease principally of the rainbow trout (*Salmo gairdneri*) and to date has been diagnosed only in Europe. Several salmonid and nonsalmonid species have been experimentally infected, and natural outbreaks have been suspected in nonsalmonid species (Ahne et al., 1976; Ghittino, 1965, 1968, 1973; Ord et al., 1976; Pfitzner, 1966; Rasmussen, 1965; Reichenbach-Klinke, 1959). A broad range of clinical manifestations may be associated with VHS infection (Ghittino, 1973; Yasutake, 1970), and, based on the differences in the severity of the clinical signs, Ghittino (1973) described three stages of VHS—acute, chronic, and nervous or latent. Histopathological changes also vary considerably and, if present, occur in the liver, kidneys, spleen, and muscle (Ghittino, 1965, 1973; Hofmann, 1971; Yasutake, 1970; Yasutake and Rasmussen, 1968). Unfortunately, none of the clinical or histopathological manifestations is VHS specific. Viral hemorrhagic septicemia can be transmitted horizontally to fish of any age, and survivors of infection may become carriers. The virus is shed at spawning and becomes a readily dissipated surface contaminant of the egg (Jørgensen, 1970, 1973b). The virus can be recovered from homogenates of whole fish and internal organs and from sex products. The plaque morphology of VHS virus (Fig. 5) provides a presumptive identification which must be confirmed by a neutralization, fluorescent antibody, complement-fixation, or immune precipitation assay (Jørgensen, 1968, 1973c, 1974; Jørgenson and Meyling, 1972; McAllister et al., 1974a; Meier and Jørgensen, 1975; Pfeil and Wiedemann, 1977).

5.1.3. Spring Viremia of Carp

Spring viremia of carp (SVC) disease has been identified in most countries of Eastern and Western Europe (W. Ahne, personal communication; Fijan, 1973, 1976). A variety of cyprinid species are naturally susceptible to infection and, experimentally, the host range has been extended to noncyprinid species and to the fly *Drosophila melanogaster* (Bachmann and Ahne, 1974; Bussereau et al., 1975; Fijan, 1976; Fijan et al., 1971; de Kinkelin et al., 1973; Rudikov et al., 1975). An extensive array of clinical and histopathological manifestations have been described by Fijan (1972), Fijan et al. (1971), Negele (1977), Rudikov et al. (1975), and Varović and Fijan (1973), but none is unique to spring viremia. Fish of any age are susceptible to infection, and, although infection ostensibly occurs by water-borne virus, the mode of transmission is poorly understood (Fijan, 1972, 1976). Seasonal outbreaks occur at temperatures of 11–22°C; 16–17°C is the optimal temperature for the disease (Fijan, 1976; Fijan et al., 1971). The virus can be isolated from most organs and tissues, and neutralization, immune precipitation, and indirect hemagglutination assays are used to identify the virus (Ahne and Wolf, 1977; Fijan, 1972; Fijan *et al.*, 1971; Hill *et al.* 1975; Sulimanovic, 1973).

5.1.4. Pike Fry Rhabdovirus Disease

The northern pike (*Esox lucius*) is the only fish presently known to be susceptible to the pike fry rhabdovirus (PFR) disease, and the disease is known to occur only in Western Europe (Bootsma, 1971, 1976). Clerx and Horzinek (1978) reported that a rhabdovirus isolated from diseased grass carp (*Ctenopharyngodon idella*) (Ahne, 1975) is antigenically indistinguishable from PFR. No studies have been reported to clarify the natural host range of the virus, which may not be totally restricted to fish since Bussereau *et al.* (1975) reported that the virus will replicate in *Drosophila melanogaster*. Pike fry rhabdovirus disease occurs in northern pike fry and fingerlings up to 6 cm in length, and susceptibility decreases with age. Bootsma (1971, 1976) has described a hemorrhagic and a hydrocephalus form of clinical pathology. A variety of nonspecific changes may occur in the appearance and behavior of infected fish. Histopathological changes consistently occur in the kidneys but are variable in the liver, heart, pancreas, gastrointestinal tract, and muscle (Bootsma, 1971, 1976; Bootsma and Van Vorstenbosch, 1973). Outbreaks of the disease occur at temperatures of 10–20°C. The virus has been recovered from the tissues of affected young but has yet to be isolated from prespawning or spawning adults. The virus is identified by serum neutralization assay.

5.1.5. Eel Rhabdovirus Diseases

Two rhabdoviruses have been isolated from eels imported to Japan, but as yet little is known concerning the diseases caused by the viruses (McAllister *et al.*, 1977; Sano, 1976; Sano *et al.*, 1977a). No disease outbreaks have been reported in the countries of origin.

The population of American eels (*Anguilla rostrata*) from Cuba was being reared at 20–27°C when heavy mortality occurred. Clinical manifestations were limited to external hemorrhaging, but histopathological changes were evident in the branchial vessels, skeletal muscle, and kidneys.

In contrast, the population of European eels (*Anguilla anguilla*) from France showed no clinical or histopathological manifestations or mortality, although a virus was isolated.

5.2. Biology of the Viruses

5.2.1. Morphology

5.2.1a. Infectious Virions

All of the fish rhabdovirus isolates possess characteristic animal rhabdovirus morphology—one end of the virus particle is planar, the other hemispherical (Fig. 10). In thin-section preparations IHN and VHS virions measure ~185 nm in length and ~65 nm in diameter while SVC and PFR virions measure ~160 nm in length and ~70 nm in diameter. Negatively stained preparations show more varied dimensions, reflecting apparently differential structural stability—IHN and VHS virions appear to be rather fragile whereas SVC, PFR, and the eel rhabodviruses appear more structurally durable. Only negatively

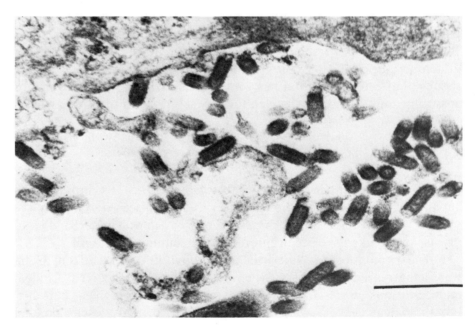

Fig. 10.   Electron micrograph of CHSE-214 cells infected with IHN virus. Bar is 500 nm. From McAllister and Pilcher (1974); reprinted with the permission of the Society for Experimental Biology and Medicine.

stained preparations have been used to determine the dimensions of eel virus—American (143 nm × 68 nm), the rhabdovirus of European eel (172 nm × 92 nm), the grass carp rhabdovirus (GRV) isolate (120 nm × 70 nm), and the swim bladder inflammation (SBI) isolate (110 nm × 65 nm).

The virion envelope is acquired as the nucleocapsid buds from the cell surface or into cytoplasmic vacuoles, and peplomers averaging 8 nm in length are arrayed over the envelope surface. Degradation of the virion envelope by detergent or enzyme treatment releases the helical nucleocapsid.

5.2.1b. Defective Virions

Truncated, autointerfering virions have been demonstrated in preparations of IHN, SVC, and PFR viruses, but not VHS virus. Electron microscopic examination of cells infected with IHN virus at a high multiplicity (MOI) revealed a trimodal length distribution of progeny virions (McAllister and Pilcher, 1974). While infections B virions (~188 nm in length) were evident in low MOI preparations, defective LT (~118 nm) and T (~81 nm) virions predominated in cells infected at a high MOI. The infectious and defective particles were separable by density gradient centrifugation. Clark and Soriano (1974), Hill *et al.* (1975), and de Kinkelin and Le Berre (1974*b*) reported the isolation of defective SVC virions, and noted that with SVC virus autointerference occurs with some cell lines but not others. de Kinkelin *et al.* (1974) isolated truncated virions 70–80 nm in length from PFR-infected cells.

5.2.2. Biological Properties

5.2.2a. Antigenicity

Neutralization assays indicate that IHN,VHS, SVC, and PFR viruses are antigenically distinct from each other and from the other fish viruses. McCain *et al.* (1974) demonstrated that the IHN virus isolates (IHNV, OSV, and SRCV) are very closely related. In contrast, two and possibly three VHS serotypes have been described (Le Berre *et al.*, 1977; Jørgensen, 1972; de Kinkelin and Le Berre, 1977). The SVC virus and SBI isolate are antigenically indistinguishable, as are PFR and the GRV isolate (Bachmann and Ahne, 1974; Clerx and Horzinek, 1978; Hill *et al.*, 1975; de Kinkelin and Le Berre, 1974*b*). Limited neutralization assays have been performed with the two eel rhabdoviruses. Comparative complement-fixation assays indicate that the nucleocapsid protein of SVC virus is unrelated to that of the mammalian rhabdoviruses, vesicular stomatitis virus, rabies virus, Lagos bat virus, or Mokola virus (Sokol *et al.*, 1974).

5.2.2b. Genetic Considerations

The virulence of IHN and VHS viruses, but not SVC virus, decreases after cell culture passage (Fryer *et al.*, 1976; Jensen, 1965; Jørgensen, 1971, 1973*b*, 1976). There is hope that a stable genetic marker will be found associated with virulence which could be used to identify isolates for vaccine production. However, attempts to correlate alterations in virus replication and virulence with genetic determinants have not been described. P. Roy (personal communication) has isolated an array of SVC virus temperature-sensitive mutants, but they are not yet characterized.

5.2.2c. Hemagglutination

The hemagglutinating potential of the fish viruses has not been adequately assessed. The IHN virion hemagglutinates goose erythrocytes; however, restrictive conditions of pH and ionic strength are required to demonstrate the reaction (P. E. McAllister, unpublished data; Wagner, 1975).

5.2.2d. Stability

The fish rhabdoviruses are moderately stable under a variety of storage conditions. Infectivity can be preserved for years at $-20°C$ or lower in cell culture medium supplemented with 2–10% serum; the viruses can also be preserved by lyophilization. As the temperature increases, the rate of inactivation becomes significant; for example, IHN virus titer decreases 3 $\log_{10}$ in 4–5 months at 4°C. Comparable reductions in virus titers occur with the other fish rhabdoviruses. In the presence of supplemental protein, the viruses are stable to multiple cycles of freezing and thawing.

The fish rhabdoviruses are inactivated by exposure to ether, chloroform, formalin, glycerol, sodium hypochlorite, organic iodophors, extremes of pH (below pH 4 or above pH 10), and heating (60°C for 15 min).

5.2.3. Chemical Composition

The essential molecular components of rhabdovirus structure—RNA, protein, lipid, and carbohydrate—have been recognized for all the fish rhabdoviruses, but only rudimentary chemical characteristics are known. The viruses can be readily concentrated and purified, but the virus yield in cell culture varies from 10^7 PFU/ml for IHN and VHS viruses to 10^8–10^9 PFU/ml for SVC and PFR viruses (Hill *et al.*, 1975; Lenoir and de Kinkelin, 1975; McAllister and Wagner, 1975). The viruses sediment to a density of 1.14–1.16 g/cm^3 in sucrose gradients (de Kinkelin, 1972, 1973; de Kinkelin *et al.*, 1974; Lenoir, 1973; McCain *et al.*, 1974).

5.2.3a. Viral Nucleic Acid

Data from metabolic inhibitor, uridine uptake, and nuclease digestion studies indicate that the fish rhabdoviruses contain a single-stranded, nonsegmented RNA genome (Campbell and Wolf, 1969; Fijan *et al.*, 1971; McAllister *et al.*, 1974b; McCain *et al.*, 1974; Wingfield and Chan, 1970; Wingfield *et al.*, 1969; Zwillenberg *et al.*, 1965). Some biochemical and biophysical characteristics of the viral nucleic acid are indicated in Table 6. In addition, Roy and Clewley (1978a) reported that SVC viral RNA has an unblocked 5′-terminal pppAp and that the "fingerprint" of a T1 ribonuclease digest indicates a nucleotide complexity comparable to that of mammalian rhabdoviruses.

5.2.3b. Viral Proteins

All the fish rhabdoviruses examined are composed of five virus-specific structural proteins, but their polyacrylamide gel electrophoretic profiles vary, paralleling the diversity observed with mammalian rhabodviruses (Wagner, 1975). The profiles of IHN and VHS viruses (Fig. 11) are nearly identical and resemble the rabies virus type, while the profiles of SVC and PFR viruses (Fig. 12) resemble the vesicular stomatitis virus type. Comparative molecular weight data are shown in Table 7.

TABLE 6

Characteristics of Fish Rhabdovirus Viral RNA

Virus	Sedimentation coefficient (S)	Molecular weight	Density (g/cm³)	Base composition (%)			
				A	U	G	C
IHN[a]	38–40	nd[e]	1.59	22.5	27.7	24.2	25.4
VHS[b]	38–40	nd	1.69	23.6	14.5	32.6	29.3
SVC[c]	38–40	3.8×10^6	nd	nd	nd	nd	nd
PFR[d]	38–40	4.0×10^6	1.65	24.9	32.4	20.2	22.5

[a] Hill *et al.* (1975), McAllister and Wagner (1977), McCain *et al.* (1974).
[b] Hill *et al.* (1975), McAllister and Wagner (1977), Robin and Rodrigue (1977).
[c] Hill *et al.* (1975), Bishop and Smith (1977).
[d] Clerx *et al.* (1975), Hill *et al.* (1975), Roy *et al.* (1975).
[e] Not determined.

Rudimentary details of viral protein structure-function relationships have been reported. The virions contain a single glycoprotein (G) which can be reaily solubilized by nonionic detergent in low ionic strength buffer; additional viral proteins are solubilized at higher ionic strength (Lenoir and de Kinkelin, 1975; McAllister and Wagner, 1975; Roy and Clewley, 1978b; Roy *et al.*, 1975). Proteolytic enzyme treatment removes the G protein, and electron micrographs of enzyme-treated virus show virus particles denuded of peplomers. Isolated IHN and VHS virus nucleocapsids contain only the L and N proteins and viral RNA, whereas SVC and PFR virus nucleocapsids contain the L, N, and NS proteins and viral RNA. The endogenous viral RNA polymerase activity attests to the functional association of the

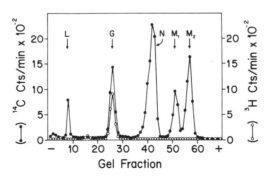

Fig. 11.   Electropherogram of polypeptides of IHN virus grown in the presence of [³H]glucosamine and ¹⁴C-labeled amino acids. The arrows indicate the L, G, N, M₁, and M₂ proteins. From McAllister and Wagner (1975); reprinted with the permission of the American Society for Microbiology.

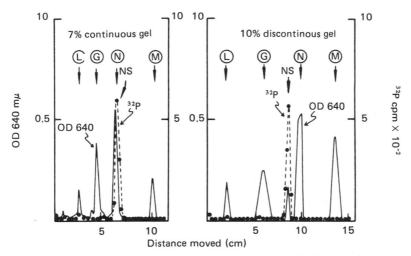

Fig. 12. Pike fry rhabdovirus proteins resolved by continuous and discontinuous polyacrylamide gel electrophoresis. Gels were stained and scanned at 640 nm; the distribution of ^{32}P incorporated into viral protein was determined. The relative positions of L, G, N, NS, and M proteins are indicated. From Roy *et al.* (1975); reprinted with the permission of the American Society for Microbiology.

TABLE 7

Representative Molecular Weights of Fish Rhabdovirus Structural Proteins

Virus	Protein molecular weight $\times 10^{-3}$							Reference
	L	G	N	NS	M	M_1	M_2	
IHN	>150	88	55	—	—	40	35	Hill *et al.* (1975)[a]
	190	80	38	—	—	25	19	Lenoir and de Kinkelin (1975)[b]
	157	72	40	—	—	25	20	McAllister and Wagner (1975)[a]
VHS	>150	88	62	—	—	38	33	Hill *et al.* (1975)[a]
	190	80	38	—	—	25	19	Lenoir and de Kinkelin (1975)[b]
	157	74	41	—	—	21.5	19	McAllister and Wagner (1975)[a]
SVC	>150	82	52	44	23	—	—	Hill *et al.* (1975)[a]
	>150	70	40	nd[c]	19	—	—	Lenoir (1973)[a]
	190	80	42	50	21	—	—	Lenoir and de Kinkelin (1975)[b]
	160	85	45	27[d]	21	—	—	Roy and Clewley (1978)[a,b]
	nd[c]	88	52	43	23	—	—	Sokol *et al.* (1974)[a]
PFR	>150	80	55	nd[c]	21	—	—	Hill *et al.* (1975)[a]
	190	80	42	50	21	—	—	Lenoir and de Kinkelin (1975)[b]
	160	85	45	na[e]	21	—	—	Roy *et al.* (1975)[a,b]

[a] Continuous polyacrylamide gel system.
[b] Discontinuous polyacrylamide gel system.
[c] nd, Protein not detected.
[d] Protein molecular weight for discontinuous polyacrylamide gel system: NS = 50,000.
[e] Protein detected but no molecular weight assigned.

nucleocapsid proteins and the virion RNA. The relationship of the M protein of SVC and PFR viruses and the M_1 and M_2 proteins of IHN and VHS viruses to the envelope and the nucleocapsid is unclear. Lenoir and de Kinkelin (1975) suggest that the M_1 protein may be closely associated with the nucleocapsid. The number of viral phosphoproteins varies—in IHN virus the N and M_1 proteins are phosphorylated, in VHS virus the N protein, in SVC virus the NS protein and an unidentified protein which migrates in the N protein region, and in PFR the NS protein is the sole virion phosphoprotein (McAllister and Wagner, 1975; Roy and Clewley, 1978b; Roy et al., 1975). A protein kinase is also associated with the fish rhabdoviruses and, as in mammalian rhabdoviruses, appears to be of cellular origin.

5.2.3c. Virion-Associated Lipid and Carbohydrate

The fish rhabdoviruses are inactivated by exposure to ether and chloroform, indicating the presence of virus-associated lipid essential for infectivity. Glucosamine incorporation studies indicate that carbohydrate is associated with the G protein and with viral envelope lipid. Characterization of the lipid and carbohydrate composition has not been reported, but the membrane microviscosity studies of Moore et al. (1976) suggest that specific host lipids are selected to form the viral envelope.

5.2.4. Growth Cycle of Infectious Virus

Infectious hematopoietic necrosis virus replicates in cell culture at temperatures from 4°C to 20°C; the optimal temperature range is 13–18°C. A single-cycle growth curve for IHN virus is illustrated in Fig. 13 (McAllister et al., 1974b). Cell associated progeny virus could be detected at 4 hr after infection. Total virus titer increased exponentially, reaching a plateau by 20 hr after infection, and released virus reached a similar plateau between 48 and 72 hr after infection. The virus yield is 10–50 PFU/cell. Virus-specific products accumulate in the cell cytoplasm and could be detected as early as 2 hr after infection by fluorescent antibody staining.

The optimum temperature for VHS virus replication is 14–15°C; virus yield is reduced at 6°C and only slight replication occurs above 20°C. In a single-cycle growth study, FHM cells were infected at a

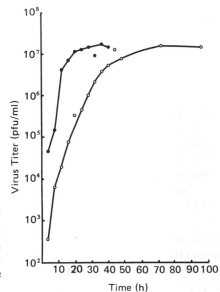

Fig. 13. Single-cycle growth curve of IHN virus in CHSE-214 cells infected at a MOI of ~4 PFU/cell and incubated at 18°C. ●, Total virus; O, released virus. From McAllister *et al.* (1974*b*); reprinted with the permission of Springer-Verlag.

MOI of 2 PFU/cell and incubated at 14°C (de Kinkelin, 1973). Total virus increased exponentially beginning 8 hr after infection and reached a plateau about 20 hr after infection. The virus yield is 25–100 PFU/cell.

Spring viremia of carp virus replicates at temperatures of 4–32°C. The optimum temperature varies with the cell line (Bachman and Ahne, 1973; Clark and Soriano, 1974; Fijan, 1972; de Kinkelin and Le Berre, 1974*b*). Clark and Soriano (1974) suggest that a temperature-dependent host cell factor may be required for virus replication. In FHM cells infected at a MOI of 5 PFU/cell and incubated at 21°C, total virus increased in an exponential manner beginning 4–5 hr after infection, plateauing 10–12 hr after infection (de Kinkelin and Le Berre, 1974*b*). Released virus plateaued about 22 hr after infection. The virus yield is 50–150 PFU/cell.

Pike fry rhabdovirus replicates at temperatures of 10–31°C, with the optimal range being 21–28°C. In FHM cells infected at a MOI of 5 PFU/cell and incubated at 21°C, the exponential increase in total virus began about 4 hr after infection and plateaued about 12 hr after infection. The virus yield varies from 50 to 1500 PFU/cell (de Kinkelin *et al.*, 1974).

The eel virus—American replicates at 29°C and the rhabdovirus of European eel at 15°C (Sano, 1976; Sano *et al.*, 1977*a*).

5.2.4a. Cell Culture Susceptibility

Replication of IHN and VHS viruses has been reported in a variety of piscine cell lines, most notably CHSE-214, FHM, RTG-2, and STE-137 (Ghittino, 1973; McAllister *et al.*, 1974*a,b*; McCain *et al.*, 1971; Nims *et al.*, 1970; Pfitzner, 1966, Wingfield *et al.*, 1970; Wolf and Quimby, 1973; Zwillenberg *et al.*, 1968). The viruses have also been cultivated in mammalian and reptilian cells, but virus yield is reduced compared to the yield in piscine cells (Clark and Soriano, 1974).

Spring viremia of carp virus replicates well in BB, BF-2, EPC, and FHM cells and a variety of other cells of piscine origin (Bachmann and Ahne, 1974; Fijan *et al.*, 1971; de Kinkelin and Le Berre, 1974*b*). The virus also replicates in a variety of avian, mammalian, and reptilian cell lines (Bachmann and Ahne, 1974; Clark and Soriano, 1974).

Pike fry rhabdovirus replicates in piscine (BB, EPC, FHM, and RTG-2) and mammalian (BHK-21) cell lines (Hill *et al.*, 1975; de Kinkelin *et al.*, 1974; Roy *et al.*, 1975).

Replication of the two eel rhabdoviruses has been monitored only in a piscine (RTG-2) cell line (Sano, 1976; Sano *et al.*, 1977*a*).

5.2.4b. Viral Protein Synthesis

Although the structural proteins of the fish rhabdoviruses are well defined, the monitoring of their synthesis *in vivo* has not been reported. As occurs with the mammalian rhabdoviruses (Wagner, 1975), it is likely that each viral peptide is translated from a single monocistronic messenger RNA.

5.2.4c. Viral Nucleic Acid Synthesis

In Vitro: An endogenous RNA-dependent transcriptase is associated with IHN, VHS, SVC, and PFR virions (McAllister and Wagner, 1977; Roy and Clewley, 1978*a*; Roy *et al.*, 1975). For optimal expression of enzyme activity *in vitro*, all four ribonucleoside triphosphates, a nonionic detergent, a reducing agent, and monovalent (Na^+ or K^+) and divalent (Mg^{2+}) cations are required. The IHN virus transcriptase does not show a strict reducing agent requirement, and in both the IHN and VHS virus transcriptase assay Mn^{2+} (1 mM) can effectively substitute for Mg^{2+} (5 mM), yielding 92% and 60% of the

optimal Mg^{2+} activity; Mn^{2+} will not substitute for Mg^{2+} in the SVC
and PFR virus assay systems. The SVC virus transcriptase is stimulated by the addition of S-adenosyl-L-methionine (0.5–1.0 mM). The
optimal temperature for *in vitro* activity is ~18°C for IHN virus,
~15°C for VHS virus, 20–25°C for SVC virus, and ~20°C for PFR.

The RNA synthesized *in vitro* is sensitive to ribonuclease and
hybridizes completely with the parental virion RNA. Analysis in sucrose gradients and polyacrylamide gels reveals the accumulation of
10–17 S IHN and VHS virus-specific species (Fig. 14) and 11–20 S
PFR-specific species. Roy (1976) reported that both capped and
methylated and uncapped and unmethylated SVC virus transcripts were
synthesized *in vitro* but none was polyadenylated.

In Vivo: Infectious hematopoietic necrosis virus-specific RNA
synthesis in infected CHSE-214 cells increased exponentially for 17
hr after infection, paralleling the single-cycle virus growth curve
(McAllister *et al.*, 1974*b*). McAllister and Wagner (1977) purified and
fractionated the IHN virus-specific RNA, and the polyadenylated
species were analyzed on sucrose gradients and polyacrylamide gels
and by hybridization to IHN virion RNA. A 28 S species showed
considerable self-annealing, and its significance is unclear. The 12–17 S
species showed 72% homology to IHN virion RNA and represented
newly synthesized virus-specific messenger RNA. Whether all viral
messenger species are polyadenylated is unknown.

Roy and Clewley (1978*a*) monitored the synthesis of SVC virus-
specific RNA in infected BHK-21 and FHM cells, and Roy *et al.*

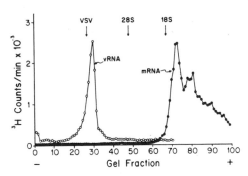

Fig. 14. Analysis of IHN virion RNA (vRNA) and *in vitro* IHN virus transcripts
(mRNA) by polyacrylamide gel electrophoresis with marker vesicular stomatitis (VSV)
virion RNA and 28 S plus 18 S ribosomal RNA (arrows). From McAllister and
Wagner (1977); reprinted with the permission of the American Society for
Microbiology.

(1975) monitored the synthesis of PFR-specific RNA in infected FHM cells. In both studies, complementary RNA species were identified but not characterized.

5.2.5.   Cell Culture Response to Virus Infection

5.2.5a.   Molecular Cytopathology

Cells infected with the fish rhabdoviruses generally manifest severe cytopathic effects, attesting to the lethal effect of virus infection. However, detailed studies of the effects of infection on host cell DNA, RNA, and protein synthesis have not been reported. A comparison of total RNA synthesis in IHN virus-infected and uninfected CHSE-214 cells suggests that host cell RNA synthesis is inhibited by virus infection (P. E. McAllister, unpublished data). De Kinkelin and Le Berre (1974b) noted that uridine incorporation in SVC virus-infected FHM cells was reduced by 60–70% in the first hour after infection, and de Kinkelin et al. (1974) reported that PFR infection inhibited FHM cell RNA synthesis.

5.2.5b.   Interferon Response

Infectious hematopoietic necrosis and VHS viruses induce interferon synthesis in cell culture and in infected fish, and replication of the viruses in inhibited by exogenously supplied interferon (Dorson and de Kinkelin, 1974; Dorson et al., 1975a; de Kinkelin, 1973; de Kinkelin and Le Berre, 1974a, 1977; de Kinkelin and Dorson, 1973; de Kinkelin et al., 1977; Sena and Rio, 1975). In contrast, SVC and PFR viruses elicit no interferon response, and virus replication is not sensitive to exogenously supplied interferon (de Kinkelin and Le Berre, 1974b; de Kinkelin et al., 1974).

6.   FISH RETROVIRIDAE

Several proliferative lesions occurring in fish are considered to be caused by retrovirus infections (Table 8). Viral etiology has been proposed based on electron micrographs which reveal retroviruslike particles in association with affected tissue, but as yet none of the

TABLE 8

Diseases of Putative Retrovirus Etiology and Dimensions of Viruslike Particles Associated with Diseased Tissue

Disease	Dimensions of C-type viruslike particles		Reference
	Diameter of particle (nm)	Diameter of nucleoid (nm)	
Atlantic salmon fibrosarcoma	~120	~90	Duncan (1978)
Esox lymphosarcoma (*Esox* sarcoma)	~100	~50	Papas *et al.* (1976), Winqvist *et al.* (1973)
Esox epidermal hyperplasia	120–150	65–80	Sonstegard (1976), Winqvist *et al.* (1968)
Walleye dermal sarcoma	~135	~75	Walker (1961, 1969*a*)
Walleye epidermal hyperplasia	~80	na[a]	Walker (1969*a*), Yamamoto *et al.* (1976)
White sucker epidermal papilloma	~100	na[a]	Sonstegard (1977*a,b*)

[a] na, No dimension assigned.

viruses has been isolated in cell culture. Some of the tumors have been experimentally transmitted.

6.1. Biology of the Diseases

6.1.1. Atlantic Salmon Fibrosarcoma

A tumor classified as a leiomyosarcoma was detected at an incidence of 4.6% in dead and moribound 1- and 2-year-old Atlantic salmon (*Salmo salar*) in Scotland (McKnight, 1978). There were no external manifestations of tumor development, but internally multiple nodules 5–30 mm in diameter were evident on the swim bladder. There was no evidence of invasion or metastasis. Attempts to experimentally transmit the tumor have been unsuccessful.

6.1.2. *Esox* Lymphosarcoma (*Esox* Sarcoma)

Esox lymphosarcoma and sarcoma were previously considered separate neoplastic conditions, but it has been recognized that the conditions are not significantly different (Ljungberg, 1976; O. Ljungberg, personal communication). Lymphosarcoma occurs in northern pike (*Esox lucius*) and muskellunge (*Esox masquinongy*) at an incidence approaching 21% (Mulcahy, 1963, 1976; Sonstegard, 1975, 1976). The nodular lesions develop in the subepidermal connective tissue and generally metastasize to the muscle and eventually the internal organs; lymphosarcoma usually causes death. The condition is described as a stem cell lymphoreticular neoplasm. The undifferentiated neoplastic hemocytoblasts contain cytoplasmic cylindroid lamella–particle complexes (Fig. 15) and nucleoid bodies which, at least morphologically, are similar to structures evident in several types of human lymphoma and leukemia (Dawe *et al.*, 1976). Lymphosarcoma has been experimentally transmitted by injection of filtered (0.22 μm) tumor homogenate, implantation of neoplastic tissue, and cohabitation (Bown *et al.*, 1976; Mulcahy and O'Leary, 1970; Schlumberger, 1957; Sonstegard, 1976). Tumorigenesis appears to be affected by water temperature (Papas *et al.*, 1976; Sonstegard, 1976).

6.1.3. *Esox* Epidermal Hyperplasia

Hyperplastic epidermal lesions 5–10 mm in diameter and 1–3 mm thick have been observed in northern pike and muskellunge in Canada and northern pike in Sweden at an incidence approaching 6% (Ljungberg, 1976; Sonstegard, 1976; Winqvist *et al.*, 1968). The lesions show no evidence of invasion or metastasis and appear to be composed of cells derived from the middle epidermis. The effect of the lesion on the host is unknown, and no transmission studies have been reported.

6.1.4. Walleye Dermal Sarcoma

Walleyes (*Stizostedion vitreum vitreum*) in the United States and Canada may show single or multiple dermal nodules about 10 mm in diameter (Walker, 1958, 1961, 1969a; Yamamoto *et al.*, 1976). These sarcomas occur at an incidence approaching 10% and are confined to the skin. The tumors have been observed in fish concurrently infected with lymphocystis and and epidermal hyperplasia and appear to occur with higher frequency in the young and in females. The effect of the tumor on the host is unknown, and no transmission studies have been reported.

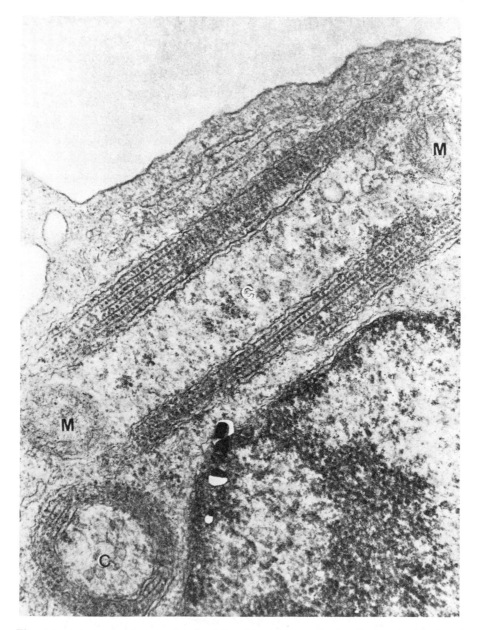

Fig. 15. Electron micrograph of a pike lymphoma cell showing longitudinal and transverse sections of cylindroid bodies. Note mitochondria (M) at either end of central cytoplasmic core (C). From Dawe *et al.* (1976); reprinted with the permission of S. Karger, AG, Basel.

6.1.5. Walleye Epidermal Hyperplasia

Epidermal hyperplastic lesions occur in walleyes in Lake Oneida, New York, at an incidence approaching 10% (Walker, 1969a,b). The lesions are several centimeters in diameter and about 0.5 mm thick. There is no evidence of invasion or metastasis, and, in fact, there is little histological difference between the normal and hyperplastic epidermis except the pronounced cellular proliferation and infiltration into layers above the basal strata. The lesions have been observed in fish with lymphocystis and dermal sarcoma. No attempts to experimentally transmit the disease have been reported.

6.1.6. White Sucker Epidermal Papilloma

Benign epidermal papillomatous growths occur on the white sucker (*Catostomus commersoni*) in the United States and Canada (Sonstegard, 1977a,b). Single or multiple proliferations begin to appear in 4-year-old fish; the size of the tumor and its incidence increase with age. Tumor incidence may approach 51% in heavily polluted waters, but may be only 0.7% or less in unpolluted waters. Sonstegard suggest that environmental toxicants may affect tumorigenesis by triggering expression of a virus. Attempts to experimentally transmit the papilloma have been unsuccessful.

6.2. Evidence of Putative Virus

Type C retroviruslike particles (Fig. 16) have been observed in intercellular spaces, within cytoplasmic vesicles, and budding from cytoplasmic membranes of cells from the various proliferative lesions. The dimensions of the particles are indicated in Table 8. RNA-dependent DNA polymerase (reverse transcriptase) activity, a hallmark of the retrovirus group, has been detected in cell-free particulate fractions derived from *Esox* lymphosarcoma and white sucker epidermal papilloma tissue (Papas *et al.*, 1976, 1977; Sonstegard, 1977b). The activity was recovered from a virus-containing fraction which sedimented to a density of 1.15–1.16 g/cm^3 in a sucrose gradient. Attempts to demonstrate cell transformation in primary and establish fish cell lines inoculated with cell-free tumor extracts have been unsuccessful, as have attempts to induce virogenesis in cultured neoplastic cells (Mulcahy, 1976; Mulcahy *et al.*, 1970; Sonstegard, 1976, 1977b).

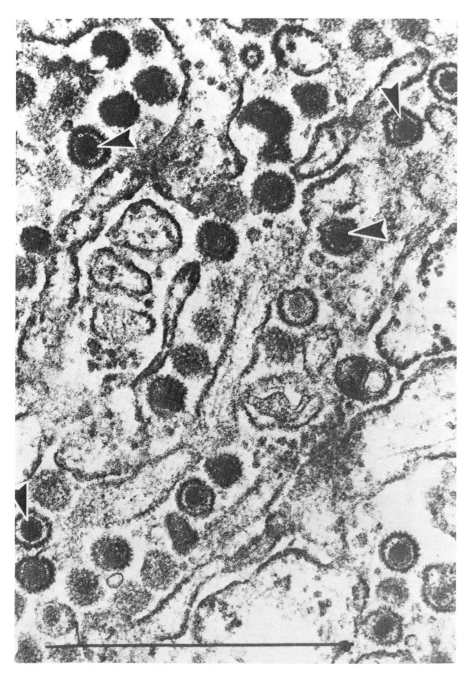

Fig. 16. Electron micrograph of viruslike particles in walleye dermal sarcoma cell. Arrows indicate the inner core of the particles. Spicules are evident on the envelope. Bar is 1 μm. From Yamamoto *et al.* (1976); reprinted with the permission of the Journal of the Fisheries Research Board of Canada.

7. UNCLASSIFIED AND PUTATIVE FISH VIRUSES ASSOCIATED WITH NEOPLASIA

7.1.   Stomatopapilloma of Eel–Associated Viruses

European eels (*Anguilla anguilla*) are affected by a benign epidermal neoplasm known as stomatopapilloma or "cauliflower disease" (Deys, 1976; Koops and Mann, 1966). The etiology of the condition is unknown, but both environmental toxicants and viral infections have been indicted. As many as three putative viruses have been isolated from eels with the disease (McAllister *et al*., 1977).

7.1.1.   Biology of the Disease

The disease occurs only in Europe, and in some areas the incidence approaches 40%.The single or multiple nodular proliferations occur usually about the mouth and head, and, while the growth are not lethal *per se*, they may impede feeding and thereby cause starvation (Fig 17). Pathological changes are confined to the epidermis. The normal, well-differentiated epidermal structure is replaced by undifferentiated cells which rarely invade beyond the basal layer or metastasize (Deys, 1976; Koops *et al*., 1970; Schmid, 1969). The optimum temperature for tumor growth is 15–22°C. Attempts to experimentally transmit the tumor using lesion homogenates, blood from affected eels, infected cell

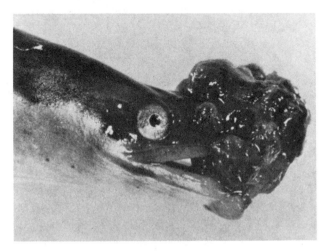

Fig. 17.   Head of an eel with stomatopapilloma. From Koops *et al*. (1970); reprinted with the permission of the American Fisheries Society.

culture fluid, or tumor implants have been unsuccessful (Deys, 1969; Koops *et al.*, 1970; Schwanz-Pfitzner, 1976). Peters and Wilke (1972) and Peters and Peters (1970) reported that the proliferations could be chemically induced. Various chemical treatments ostensibley promote cellular redifferentiation, thereby causing regression, destruction, and sloughing of the tumor (Peters, 1970; Peters and Peters, 1970; Peters *et al.*, 1972a,b).

7.1.2. Biology of the Viruses

Pfitzner and Schubert (1969) reported the isolation of a virus from the blood of eels with stomatopapilloma. Electron microscopic examination of infected RTG-2 cells revealed aggregates of polyhedral particles ~55 nm in diameter (Fig. 18), ostensibly of nuclear origin (Pfitzner, 1969, 1973; Schubert, 1969). The particles were not observed in tumor tissue. The virus replicated in RTG-2 cells and caused lysis of the cells at 16–22°C. Schwanz-Pfitzner (1976) designated the virus "eel Virus (Berlin)" and tentatively assigned it to the papovavirus group.

Wolf and Quimby (1970b, 1973) also isolated a small polyhedral virus, but their isolation was made from homogenates of tumors and internal organs. The isolate was designated "EV-1." Virus-infected RTG-2 cells showed massive syncytium formation with pyknotic necrotic foci. The virus has not been characterized. Nagabayashi and Wolf (1979) isolated an additional virus, designated "EV-2," from the tumor and internal organ homogenates. EV-2 replicates only in FHM cells. Electron micrographs of infected cells and puified virus preparations reveal pleomorphic virus particles 80–140 nm in diameter (Fig. 19). Peplomers ~10 nm in length radiate from the surface of the virion. The virion sediments to a density of 1.19 g/cm³ in sucrose, and the viral nucleic acid has been presumptively identified as RNA. EV-2 replicates in the cytoplasm, but replication is inhibited by actinomycin D added within 2 hr after infection. the virus agglutinates chicken and sheep erythrocytes and is inactivated by exposure to ether or chloroform, acid (pH 3.0), and heat (50°C for 10 min). Nagabayashi and Wolf (1979) tentatively classified EV-2 in the orthomyxovirus group.

7.2. Brown Bullhead Papilloma–Associated Virus

Oral papillomas have been observed on brown bullheads (*Ictalurus nebulosus*) taken from Caanan Lake, Long Island, New York (Edwards

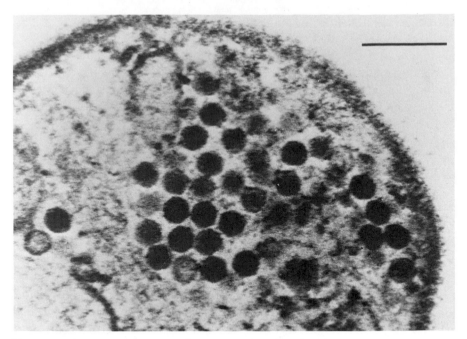

Fig. 18. Electron micrograph of RTG-2 cells infected with blood from an eel with stomatopapilloma. Intracytoplasmic virus particles are ~55 nm in diameter. Electron micrograph kindly provided by G. Schubert. From McAllister *et al.* (1977); reprinted with the permission of the New York Academy of Sciences.

et al., 1977). The tumors were composed of abnormal epidermal cells and showed no evidence of invasiveness or metastasis. The significance of the tumor on the survival of the host has not been determined.

Examination of the neoplastic tissue by electron microscopy revealed spheroidal viruslike particles ~50 nm in diameter. Edwards *et al.* (1977) reported that the pathological changes in the nucleus and the perinuclear accumulations of the viruslike particles were indicative of nuclear virogenesis and suggested that the virus resembled a papovavirus. As yet not virus has been isolated from affected fish, nor has the tumor been experimentally transmitted.

7.3. Atlantic Salmon Papilloma–Associated Virus

Carlisle and Roberts (1977), Ljungberg (1963), Wirén (1971), and Wolf (1966) described the occurrence of a benign epidermal papilloma in the Atlantic salmon in Europe and the United States. In hatchery-reared fish the incidence may approach 55%. The smooth to nodular proliferations are 2–5 mm thick and up to 4 cm in diameter. Single or multiple lesions may occur on any exterior body surface; they eventually slough, and the tissues heal. The papilloma is composed of atypical middle epidermal cells.

Electron microscopic examination of affected tissue reveals, albeit infrequently, intracytoplasmic and extracellular viruslike particles 125–150 nm in diameter, with a centrally placed, electron-dense nucleoid (Carlisle, 1976, 1977; Wirén, 1971). The etiological significance of these putative viruslike particles is unknown; attempts to isolate the virus and to experimentally transmit the tumor have been unsuccessful.

7.4. Pleuronectid Epidermal Papilloma–Associated Virus

Single or multiple benign epidermal papillomas may occur in several species of European and North American flatfishes (Pleuronectiformes) (Cooper and Keller, 1969; Nigrelli *et al.*, 1965; Wellings *et al.*, 1965, 1976). Tumor incidence is significant only on the Pacific Coast of North America and may approach 50% in some populations. Several types of lesions are evident during tumor development (Cooper and Keller, 1969; Miller and Wellings, 1971; Nigrelli *et al.*, 1965; Wellings, 1970; Wellings *et al.*, 1964, 1965, 1976). The earliest lesion is the angioepithelial nodule, which matures usually to the epithelial papilloma or, less frequently, to an angioepithelial polyp. The lesion types

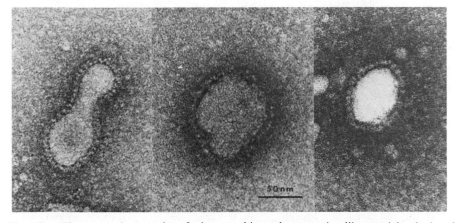

Fig. 19.   Electron micrographs of pleomorphic orthomyxoviruslike particles isolated from tissue homogenates from eels with stomatopapilloma. From McAllister *et al.* (1977); reprinted with the permission of the New York Academy of Sciences.

are differentiated by their appearance and by the amount of vascu-
larized connective tissue vs. hyperplastic epidermal tissue. All three
lesions contain unique, pathognomonic tumor cells, "X-cells," which
Wellings et al. (1976) contend are transformed. The tumors show some
invasiveness but no metastasis.

Viruslike particles and a potential virogenic structure (Fig. 20)
have been observed in the tumor-specific X-cells (Brooks et al., 1969;
Wellings et al., 1965, 1976). An ostensibly enveloped particle ~45 nm
in diameter containing a centrally placed, electron-dense nucleoid ~6
nm in diameter was often found in association with an amorphous,
electron-dense structure ~150 nm in diameter. Wellings et al. (1965,
1976) suggested that the 150-nm structure might be the site for the
genesis of the 45-nm particle or might be a developmental stage of a
second viruslike particle (granular body) 160–200 nm in diameter
containing numerous electron-dense granules. Attempts to recover virus
particles from tumor cell homogenates, to induce CPE or cell
transformation in normal pleuronectid cell cultures with papilloma

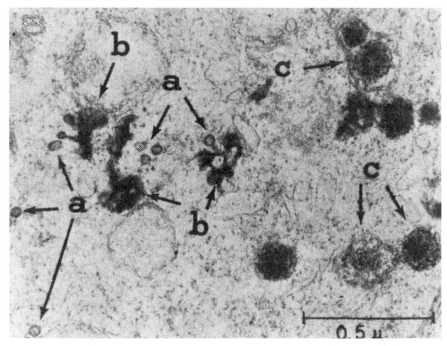

Fig. 20. Electron micrograph of an epithelial cell of a flathead sole epidermal
papilloma: viruslike particles (a), homogeneous bodies (b), and granular bodies (c).
From Wellings and Chuinard (1964); reprinted with the permission of the American
Association for the Advancement of Science, Copyright 1964.

cells, or to transmit the tumor by injection of tumor cells or tumor homogenates have been unsuccessful.

8. UNCLASSIFIED AND PUTATIVE FISH VIRUSES

8.1. Bluegill Virus

A virus was isolated from bluegills (*Lepomis macrochirus*) held at the Leetown National Fish Hatchery in West Virginia (Hoffman *et al.*, 1969). Later attempts to reisolate the virus from the Leetown population were unsuccessful, as were attempts to detect the virus in other feral bluegill populations (Beckwith, 1974, 1975). Beckwith (1974) and Hoffman *et al.* (1969) could detect no pathology associated with infection and were unable to induce pathological changes by experimental infection.

8.1.1. Morphology

Spheroidal virus particles were evident in electron micrographs of infected BF-2 cells; the particles were present in cytoplasmic vacuoles and extracellular arrays and budding from cellular membranes. Hoffman *et al.* (1969) reported that the bluegill virus was 70–80 nm in diameter, was rather uniform in electron density, and resembled a myxovirus. Beckwith (1974, 1975), however, reported that the virus was pleomorphic, varying from 80 to 250 nm in diameter, and contained electron-dense granules $\sim$20 nm in diameter. Beckwith suggested that the bluegill virus resembled an arenavirus or an atypical paramyxovirus. Membrane filtration studies indicated a particle diameter of 75–220 nm (Beckwith, 1974, 1975).

8.1.2. Biological Properties

The bluegill virus can be stored for months at $-70°C$ in cell culture medium supplemented with 10% serum with little loss of infectivity. At higher temperatures the virus is unstable, e.g., at 24°C infectivity decreased by $\sim10^4$ $TCID_{50}$/ml in 8 days. The virus is inactivated by exposure to ether, acid (pH 3.0), or ultraviolet light. Neither hemagglutination nor neuraminidase activities are detectable in virus preparations. No antigenic relationships were detected in serological assays using antisera against two orthomyxoviruses, a paramyxovirus, an atypical paramyxovirus, and an arenavirus (Beckwith, 1974, 1975).

8.1.3. Chemical Composition

The chemical composition of the bluegill virus is poorly defined. Cytochemical staining and uridine uptake studies suggest that the viral genome contains single-stranded RNA, and the sensitivity to ether indicates that the virus contains lipid essential to infectivity (Beckwith, 1974, 1975). Viral structural proteins have not been characterized, nor has the potential association of carbohydrate with the mature virion been assessed.

8.1.4. Growth of Infectious Virus

The bluegill virus replicates only in cell lines of piscine origin and attains a titer of $\sim 10^6$ $TCID_{50}/ml$. The BF-2 cell line is commonly used, and the virus reportedly replicates in LBF-1, BGL, RTG-2, and AS cell lines (Beckwith, 1974, 1975; Hoffman *et al.*, 1969; Nicholson and Byrne, 1973; Wolf and Quimby, 1973). A single-cycle growth curve at 21°C indicates that released virus appears about 10 hr after infection and approaches a plateau about 40 hr after infection. The temperature range over which the virus will replicate has not been established.

Beckwith (1974, 1975) monitored the time course of viral protein and nucleic acid synthesis in BF-2 cells. Protein synthesis essential to virus replication occurred by 8 hr after infection and RNA synthesis by 8–12 hr after infection. Virus replication was not affected by actinomycin D (5 $\mu g/ml$) but was significantly inhibited by cycloheximide (5 $\mu g/ml$) and 6-azauridine (5 $\mu g/ml$).

8.2. Grunt Fin Agent

Clem *et al.* (1961) developed a marine fish cell line from fin tissue of the bluestriped grunt (*Haemulon sciurus*). At the 65th passage, a single necrotic focus appeared which ultimately involved the entire monolayer. Clem *et al.* (1965) isolated an infectious cytopathogenic agent that replicated only in living cells and possessed many of the other essential properties of a virus. The isolate remains inadequately characterized and is designated the "grunt fin agent" (GFA).

Attempts to transmit GFA have been unsuccessful. Adult, juvenile, and fingerling bluestriped grunts, newborn mice, and embryonated chicken eggs have been experimentally infected; the agent persisted at the site of inoculation for several days, but no pathological changes were induced, nor was there evidence of GFA replication in any organ or tissue (Clem *et al.*, 1965; Wellings, 1970).

8.2.1. Morphology

Electron micrographs of partially purified GFA preparations occasionally contain ellipsoidal particles with a centrally placed, electron-dense nucleoid. The particles are 120–140 nm in diameter on the long axis and ~100 nm in diameter on the short axis. The calculated particle diameter from membrane filtration experiments is 100–150 nm (Clem *et al.*, 1965).

8.2.2. Biological Properties

Grunt fin agent infectivity can be preserved for extended periods by freezing at −65°C or below; at temperatures of 20°C and above, GFA is decidedly thermolabile. Infectivity is inactivated by exposure to ether and heat (45°C for 15 min) but is stable to cycles of freezing and thawing. Grunt fin agent does not agglutinate human, guinea pig, or fish erythrocytes and is only weakly antigenic in bluestriped grunts and rabbits (Clem *et al.*, 1965).

8.2.3. Chemical Composition

The biochemical characterization of GFA is virtually nil. the replication of GFA is not affected by halogenated deoxyuridines, suggesting that, if GFA is a virus, its genome presumptively contains RNA. The sensitivity to ether indicates that GFA contains lipid essential to infectivity (Clem *et al.*, 1965).

8.2.4. Growth Cycle of GFA

Grunt fin agent replicates well in cell lines derived from the bluestriped grunt, the lane snapper (*Lutjanus synagris*), and the goldfish

(*Carassius auratus*) and attains a titer of $\sim 10^6$ TCID$_{50}$/ml (Clem *et al.*, 1965). Some of an infected cell population will survive and become carriers. The carrier state is mediated by an interferonlike substance (Beasley and Sigel, 1968; Beasley *et al.*, 1965, 1966; Sigel *et al.*, 1968).

Single-cycle growth curve at 20°C in GF cells indicates that released infectivity becomes evident about 12 hr after infection and increases exponentially, reaching a plateau about 18 hr after infection (Clem *et al.*, 1965). The temperature range of GFA replication has not been determined.

8.3. Ulcerative Dermal Necrosis–Associated Virus

Atlantic salmon (*Salmo salar*), sea trout (*Salmo trutta trutta*), and brown trout (*Salmo trutta lacustris*) in Europe are affected by a degenerative condition called ulcerative dermal necrosis (UDN) (Roberts, 1972). Ulcerative dermal necrosis has been recognized since the middle 1800s, but there is no reliable assessment of incidence. The disease occurs only in adult fish and is characterized by degeneration of the cranial epidermis. The affected tissue sloughs, leaving an ulcerous lesion which, in advanced stages, shows secondary invasion by bacteria and fungi. Fish with mild lesions may survive. The disease has been experimentally transmitted by cohabitation and by inoculation with membrane-filtered lesion homogenates, but the etiology is unknown (Roberts, 1972). Bacterial and fungal agents are associated with the lesions, and changes in endocrine organ function have been implicated as a predisposing factor. Viral etiology has also been proposed, but no virus has been isolated.

Lounatmaa and Janatuinen (1978) examined lesion tissue from Atlantic salmon affected by UDN-like disease. Electron micrographs revealed cytoplasmic concentrations of viruslike particles. The particles appeared to be unenveloped icosahedra 30–33 nm in diameter and were detected only in diseased fish. The significance of the viruslike particles is unknown.

8.4. Gill Necrosis of Carp–Associated Virus

Carp in Europe and Russia are affected by a disease called gill necrosis. The etiology of the disease is uncertain, but a virus has been suspected. Attempts to experimentally transmit gill necrosis in carps have yielded equivocal results, and some studies suggest that water quality and physiological stress may be associated with outbreaks of the disease.

Popkova and Shchelkunov (1978) reported the recovery of a virus from affected carp. The agent was isolated in FHM cells infected with homogenates of gills and kidneys and incubated at 28°C. The cells showed enlarged nuclei containing one or more inclusions 1.4–5.6 nm in diameter. The virulence of the agent decreased with cell culture passage. Electron micrographs revealed hexagonal virus particles 200–216 nm in diameter in the cell culture medium.

ACKNOWLEDGMENTS

I am grateful to B. R. Griffin, B. C. Lidgerding, S. F. Snieszko, K. E. Wolf, and P. H. Eschmeyer for their critical review of the manuscript. Preprints and other materials and personal communications of results were unselfishly contributed by J. P. M. Clerx, P. Dobos, F. E. Farber, R. D. Macdonald, B. L. Nicholson, J. A. Plumb, P. Roy, G. Schubert, G. S. Traxler, and K. E. Wolf. I also thank B. D. Lawson for typing the manuscript, H. M. Stuckey for the photography, and M. C. Quimby for assistance in proofreading the manuscript. The encouragement of the National Fish Health Research Laboratory staff was much appreciated.

9. REFERENCES

Ahne, W., 1975, A rhabdovirus isolated from grass carp (*Ctenopharyngodon idella* Val.), *Arch. Virol.* **48**:181.

Ahne, W., 1977, Some properties of an IPN-virus isolated from pike (*Esox lucius*), *Bull. Office Int. Epiz.* **87**:417.

Ahne, W., and Wolf, K. E., 1977, Spring viremia of carp, *U.S. Fish Wildlife Service Fish Disease Leaflet 51*, 11 pp.

Ahne, W., Negele, R. D., and Ollenschläger, B., 1976, Vergleichende Infektions-versuche mit Egtved-viren (Stamm F1) by Regenbogenforellen (*Salmo gairdneri*) und Goldforellen (*Salmo aguabonita*), *Berl. Muench. Tieraerztl. Wochenschr.* **89**:161.

Alayse, A. M., Cohen, J., and Scherrer, R., 1975, Étude de la synthèse des arn viraux dans les cellules FHM et RTG-2 infectées par le virus de la nécrose pancréatique infectieuse (NPI), *Ann. Microbiol. (Paris)*. **126B**:471.

Amend, D. F., 1970, Control of infectious hematopoietic necrosis virus disease by elevating the water temperature, *J. Fish. Res. Board Can.* **27**:265.

Amend, D. F., 1976, Prevention and control of viral diseases of salmonids, *J. Fish. Res. Board Can.* **33**:1059.

Amend, D. F., and Pietsch, J. P., 1972, Virucidal activity of two iodophors to salmonid viruses, *J. Fish. Res. Board Can.* **29**:61.

Amend, D. F., Yasutake, W. T., and Mead, R. W., 1969, A hematopoietic virus disease of rainbow trout and sockeye salmon, *Trans. Am. Fish. Soc.* **98**:796.

Amend, D. F., Yasutake, W. T., Fryer, J. L., Pilcher, K. S., and Wingfield, W. H., 1973, Infectious hematopoietic necrosis (IHN), in: *Symposium on the Major Communicable Fish Diseases in Europe and Their Control* (W. A. Dill, ed.), pp. 80–98, EIFAC (European Inland Fisheries Advisory Committee) Tech. Paper 17, Suppl. 2.

Argot, J. E., 1969, Infectious pancreatic necrosis virus intracellular replication, Ph.D. dissertation, Lehigh University, 120 pp., Bethlehem, Pa.

Argot, J., and Malsberger, R. G., 1972, Intracellular replication of infectious pancreatic necrosis virus, *Can. J. Microbiol.* **18**:865.

Bachmann, P. A., and Ahne, W., 1973, Isolation and characterization of agent causing swim bladder inflammation in carp, *Nature (London)* **244**:235.

Bachmann, P. A., and Ahne, W., 1974, Biological properties and identification of the agent causing swim bladder inflammation in carp, *Arch. Gesamte Virusforsch.* **44**:261.

Bauer, O. N., Musselius, V. A., and Strelkov, Yu. A., 1969, Diseases of pond fishes, Izdatel'stvo "Kolos," translated from Russian, *Israel Program for Scientific Translations*, 220 pp., Jerusalem, 1973, TT-72-50070.

Beasley, A. R., and Sigel, M. M., 1968, Interferon production in cold-blooded vertebrates, *In Vitro* **3**:154.

Beasley, A. R., Sigel, M. M., and Clem, L. W., 1965, Virus-carrier cell cultures from a marine fish, *Abstr. Bacteriol. Proc. Am. Soc. Microbiol.* **1965**:99.

Beasley, A. R., Sigel, M. M., and Clem, L. W., 1966, Latent infection in marine fish cell tissue cultures, *Proc. Soc. Exp. Biol. Med.* **121**:1169.

Beasley, A. R., Sigel, M. M., and Lopez, D. M., n.d. (ca. 1967), Virological and related problems in marine animals, *Final Report Contract NONR 4008(05)*, not published.

Beckwith, D. G., 1974, Characterization and intracellular replication of the bluegill virus, Ph.D. Dissertation, Lehigh University, 160 pp., Bethlehem, Pa.

Beckwith, D. G., 1975, Characterization and intracellular replication of the bluegill virus, *Fish Health News* **4**(2): 10.

Bellet, R., 1969, La nécrose pancréatique virale (I.P.N.), *Pisciculture Fr.* **18**:15.

Billi, J. L., and Wolf, K., 1969, Quantitative comparison of peritoneal washes and feces for detecting infectious pancreatic necrosis (IPN) virus in carrier brook trout, *J. Fish. Res. Board Can.* **26**:1459.

Bishop, D. H. L., and Smith, M. S., 1977, Rhabdoviruses, in: *Molecular Biology of Animal Viruses*, Vol. I (D. Nayak, ed.), pp. 167–280, Dekker, New York.

Bootsma, R., 1971, Hydrocephalus and red-disease in pike fry *Esox lucius* L., *J. Fish Biol.* **3**:417.

Bootsma, R., 1976, Studies on two infectious diseases of cultured freshwater fish, rhabdovirus disease of pike fry, *Esox lucius* L., columnaris disease of carp, *Cyprinus carpio* L., Ph.D. dissertation, State University of Utrecht, 41 pp., Netherlands.

Bootsma, R., and Van Vorstenbosch, C. J. A. H. V., 1973, Detection of a bullet-shaped virus in kidney sections of pike fry (*Esox lucius* L.) with red-disease, *Neth. J. Vet. Sci.* **98**:86.

Brooks, R. E., McArn, G. E., and Wellings, S. R., 1969, Ultrastructural observations on an unidentified cell type found in epidermal tumors of flounders, *J. Natl. Cancer Inst.* **43**:97.

Brown, E. R., Sinclair, T. F., Keith, L., Hazdra, J. J., Callaghan, O. H., and Inch, W. R., 1976, Lymphoma in *Esox lucius* (northern pike): Viral and environmental interactions, *Proc. Am. Assoc. Cancer Res. Abstr.* **17**:2.

Buchanan, J. S., and Madeley, C. R., 1978, Studies on *Herpesvirus scophthalmi* infection of turbot *Scophthalmus maximus* L. ultrastructural observations, *J. Fish Dis.* **1**:283.

Buchanan, J. S., Richards, R. H., Sommerville, C., and Madeley, C. R., 1978, A herpes-type virus from turbot (*Scophthalmus maximus* L.), *Vet. Rec.* **102**:527.

Bullock, G. L., Rucker, R. R., Amend, D., Wolf, K., and Stuckey, H. M., 1976, Infectious pancreatic necrosis: Transmission with iodine-treated and nontreated eggs of brook trout (*Salvelinus fontinalis*), *J. Fish. Res. Board Can.* **33**:1197.

Bussereau, F., Kinkelin, P. de, and Le Berre, M., 1975, Infectivity of fish rhabdoviruses for *Drosophila melanogaster*, *Ann. Microbiol.* (*Paris*). **126**:389.

Campbell, J. B., and Wolf, K., 1969, Plaque assay and some characteristics of Egtved virus (virus of viral hemorrhagic septicemia of rainbow trout), *Can. J. Microbiol.* **15**:635.

Carlisle, J. C., 1976, A study of epithelioma in the Atlantic salmon (*S. salar*), in: *Wildlife Diseases* (L. A. Page, ed.), pp. 443–444, Plenum, New York.

Carlisle, J. C., 1977, An epidermal papilloma of the Atlantic salmon. II. Ultrastructure and etiology, *J. Wildl. Dis.* **13**:235.

Carlisle, J. C., and Roberts, R. J., 1977, An epidermal papilloma of the Atlantic salmon. I. Epizootiology, pathology and immunology, *J. Wildl. Dis.* **13**:230.

Cerini, C. P., and Malsberger, R. G., 1965, Morphology of infectious pancreatric [*sic*] necrosis virus, *Ann. N.Y. Acad. Sci.* **126**:315.

Chang, N., Macdonald, R. D., and Yamamoto, T., 1978, Purification of infectious pancreatic necrosis (IPN) virus and comparison of polypeptide composition of different isolates, *Can. J. Microbiol.* **24**:19.

Clark, H. F., and Soriano, E. Z., 1974, Fish rhabdovirus replication in non-piscine cell culture: New system for the study of rhabdovirus-cell interaction in which the virus and cell have different temperature optima, *Infec. Immun.* **10**:180.

Clem, L. W., Moewus, L., and Sigel, M. M., 1961, Studies with cells from marine fish in tissue culture, *Proc. Soc. Exp. Biol. Med.* **108**:762.

Clem, L. W., Sigel, M. M., and Friis, R. R., 1965, An orphan virus isolated in marine fish cell tissue culture, *Ann. N.Y. Acad. Sci.* **126**:343.

Clerx, J. P. M., and Horzinek, M. C., 1978, Comparative protein analysis of non-salmonid fish rhabdoviruses, *J. Gen. Virol.* **40**:287.

Clerx, J. P. M., van der Zeijst, B. A. M., and Horzinek, M. C., 1975, Some physicochemical properties of pike fry rhabdovirus RNA, *J. Gen. Virol.* **29**:133.

Cohen, J., 1975, Ribonucleic acid polymerase activity in purified infectious pancreatic necrosis virus of trout, *Biochem. Biophys. Res. Commun.* **62**:689.

Cohen, J., and Scherrer, R., 1972, Structure de la capside du virus de la nécrose pancréatique infectieuse (NPI) de la truite, *C. R. Acad. Sci. Paris*, **274**:1222.

Cohen, J., Poinsard, A., and Scherrer, R., 1973, Physico-chemical and morphological features of infectious pancreatic necrosis virus, *J. Gen. Virol.* **21**:485.

Cooper, R. C., and Keller, C. A., 1969, Epizootiology of papillomas in English sole, *Parophrys vetulus*, *Natl. Cancer Inst. Monogr.* **31**:173.

Dawe, C. J., Banfield, W. G., Sonstegard, R., Lee, C. W., and Michelitch, H. J., 1976, Cylindroid lamella-particle complexes and nucleoid intracytoplasmic bodies in lymphoma cells of northern pike (*Esox lucius*), *Prog. Exp. Tumor Res.* **20**:166.

de Kinkelin, P., 1972, Le virus d'Egtved. II. Purification, *Ann. Rch. Vet.* **3**:199.

de Kinkelin, P., 1973, *In vitro* properties of the Egtved virus, in: *Symposium on the Major Communicable Fish Diseases in Europe and their Control* (W. A. Dill, ed.), pp. 28–33, EIFAC (European Inland Fisheries Advisory Committee) Tech. Paper 17, Suppl. 2.

de Kinkelin, P., and Dorson, M., 1973, Interferon production in rainbow trout (*Salmo gairdneri*) experimentally infected with Egtved virus, *J. Gen. Virol.* **19**:125.

de Kinkelin, P., and Le Berre, M., 1974a, Nécrose hématopoïétique infectieuse des salmonidés: Production d'interferon circulant induite après l'infection expérimentale de la truite arc-en-ciel (*Salmo gairdneri*), *C. R. Acad. Sci. Paris* **279(D)**:445.

de Kinkelin, P., and Le Berre, M., 1974b, Rhabdovirus des Poissons. II. Propriétés in vitro du virus de la virémie printanière de la carpe, *Ann. Microbiol. (Paris)* **125A**:113.

de Kinkelin, P., and Le Berre, M., 1977, Isolement d'un rhabdovirus pathogène de la truite fario (*Salmo trutta*, L., 1766), *C. R. Acad. Sci. Paris* **284(D)**:101.

de Kinkelin, P., Galimard, B., and Bootsma, R., 1973, Isolation and identification of the causative agent of "red disease" of pike (*Esox lucius* L. 1766), *Nature (London)* **241**:465.

de Kinkelin, P., Le Berre, M., and Lenoir, G., 1974, Rhabdovirus des poissons. I. Propriétés in vitro du virus de la maladie rouge de l'alevin de brochet, *Ann. Microbiol. (Paris)* **125**:93.

de Kinkelin, P., Baudouy, A.-M., and Le Berre, M., 1977, Reaction de la truite fario (*Salmo trutta*, L. 1766) et arc-en-ciel (*Salmo gairdneri* Richardson, 1836) a l'infection par un nouveau rhabdovirus, *C. R. Acad. Sci. Paris* **284(D)**:401.

Desautels, D., and MacKelvie, R. M., 1975, Practical aspects of survival and destruction of infectious pancreatic necrosis virus, *J. Fish. Res. Board Can.* **32**:523.

de Sena, J., and Rio, G. J., 1975, Partial purification and characterization of RTG-2 fish cell interferon, *Infect. Immun.* **11**:815.

Deys, B. F., 1969, Papillomas in the Atlantic eel, *Anguilla vulgaris*, *Natl. Cancer Inst. Monogr.* **31**:187.

Deys, B. F., 1976, Atlantic eels and cauliflower disease (*Orocutaneous papillomatosis*), *Prog. Exp. Tumor Res.* **20**:94.

Dixon, R. A. F., and Farber, F. E., 1977, Macromolecular characterization of channel catfish herpesvirus (CCV), *Abstr. Annu. Meeting Am. Soc. Microbiol.* **1977**:314.

Dobos, P., 1976, Size and structure of the genome of infectious pancreatic necrosis, *Nucleic Acids Res.* **3**:1903.

Dobos, P., 1977, Virus-specific protein synthesis in cells infected by infectious pancreatic necrosis virus, *J. Virol.* **21**:242.

Dobos, P., and Rowe, D., 1977, Peptide map comparison of infectious pancreatic necrosis virus-specific polypeptides, *J. Virol.* **24**:805.

Dobos, P., Hallett, R., Kells, D. T. C., Sorensen, O., and Rowe, D., 1977, Biophysical studies of infectious pancreatic necrosis virus, *J. Virol.* **22**:150.

Dorson, M., and de Kinkelin, P., 1974, Mortalité et production d'interféron circulant chez la truite arc-en-ciel après infection expérimentale avec le virus d'Egtved: Influence de la température, *Ann. Rech. Vet.* **5**:365.

Dorson, M., Barde, A., and de Kinkelin, P., 1975a, Egtved virus induced rainbow trout serum interferon: Some physiochemical properties, *Ann. Microbiol. (Paris)* **126B**:485.

Dorson, M., de Kinkelin, P., and Torchy, C., 1975*b*, Virus de la nécrose pancréatique infectieuse: Acquisition de la sensibilitée au facteur neutralisant du sérum de truite après passages successifs en culture cellulaire, *C. R. Acad. Sci. Paris* **281**:1435.

Dukes, T. W., and Lawler, A. R., 1975, The ocular lesions of naturally occurring lymphocystis in fish, *Can. J. Comp. Med.* **39**:406.

Dunbar, C. E., and Wolf, K., 1966, The cytological course of experimental lymphocystis in the bluegill, *J. Infect. Dis.* **116**:466.

Duncan, I. B., 1978, Evidence for an oncovirus in swimbladder fibrosarcoma of Atlantic salmon *Salmo salar* L., *J. Fish Dis.* **1**:127.

Edwards, M. R., Samsonoff, W. A., and Kuzia, E. J., 1977, Papilloma-like viruses from catfish, *Fish Health News* **6**:94–95.

Eskildsen, U. K., and Jørgensen, P. E. V., 1974, Jodophorer som desinfektionsmiddel i dambrugene, *Ferskvandsfiskeribladet*, 72, Argang Nr. 12, n.p.

Evelyn, T. P. T., and Traxler, G. S., 1978, Viral erythrocytic necrosis: Natural occurrence in Pacific salmon and experimental transmission, *J. Fish. Res. Board Can.* **35**:903.

Fijan, N., 1968, Progress report on acute mortality of channel catfish fingerlings caused by a virus, *Bull. Office Int. Epiz.* **69**:1167.

Fijan, N. N., 1972, Infectious dropsy in carp—A disease complex, *Symp. Zool. Soc. London* **30**:39.

Fijan, N., 1973, Spring viremia of carp (SVC)—A review, in: *Symposium on the Major Communicable Fish Diseases in Europe and their Control* (W. A. Dill, ed.), pp. 119–123, EIFAC (European Inland Fisheries Advisory Committee) Tech. Paper 17, Supp.. 2.

Fijan, N., 1976, Diseases of cyprinids in Europe, *Fish Pathol.* **10**:129.

Fijan, N. N., Wellborn, T. L., Jr., and Naftel, J. P., 1970, An acute viral disease of channel catfish, *U. S. Fish Wildl. Serv. Tech. Paper*, No. 43, 11 pp.

Fijan, N., Petrinec, Z., Sulimanovic, D., and Zwillenberg, L. O., 1971, Isolation of the viral causative agent from the acute form of infectious dropsy of carp, *Vet. Arh.* **41**:125.

Finlay, J., and Hill, B. J., 1975, The use of the complement fixation test for rapid typing of infectious pancreatic necrosis virus, *Aquaculture* **3**:305.

Frantsi, C., and Savan, M., 1971, Infectious pancreatic necrosis virus—temperature and age factors in mortality, *J. Wild. Dis.* **7**:249.

Fryer, J. L., Rohovec, J. S., Tebbit, G. L., McMichael, J. S., and Pilcher, K. S., 1976, Vaccination for control of infectious diseases in Pacific salmon, *Fish Pathol.* **10**:155.

Ghittino, P., 1965, Viral hemorrhagic septicemia (VHS) in rainbow trout in Italy, *Ann. N.Y. Acad. Sci.* **126**:468.

Ghittino, P., 1968, Grave enzoozia di setticemia emorragica virale in trote fario di allevamento (*Salmo trutta*), *Riv. Ital. Piscic. Ittiop.* **3**:17.

Ghittino, P., 1973, Viral hemorrhagic septicemia (VHS), in: *Symposium on the Major Communicable Fish Diseases in Europe and their Control* (W. A. Dill, ed.), pp. 4–11, EIFAC (European Inland Fisheries Advisory Committee) Tech. Paper 17, Suppl. 2.

Goodheart, C. R., and Plummer, G., 1975, The densities of herpesviral DNAs, *Prog. Med. Virol.* **19**:324.

Grischkowsky, R. S., and Amend, D. F., 1976, Infectious hematopoietic necrosis virus: Prevalence in certain Alaskan sockeye salmon, *Oncorhynchus nerka, J. Fish. Res. Board Can.* **33**:186.

Heartwell, C. M., III, 1975, Immune response and antibody characterization of the channel catfish (*Ictalurus punctatus*) to a naturally pathogenic bacterium and virus, *U.S. Wildl. Serv. Tech. Paper*, No. 85, 34 pp.

Hedrick, R. P., Leong, J. C., and Fryer, J. L., 1978, Persistent infections in salmonid fish cells with infectious pancreatic necrosis virus (IPNV), *J. Fish Dis.* **1**:297.

Hill, B. J., 1976, Molluscan viruses: Their occurrence, culture, and relationships, in: *Proc. Int. Colloq. Invertebr. Pathol.* **1**:25.

Hill, B. J., Underwood, B. O., Smale, C. J., and Brown, F., 1975, Physico-chemical and serological characterization of five rhabdoviruses infecting fish, *J. Gen. Virol.* **27**:369.

Hines, R. S., Wohlfarth, G. W., Moav, R., and Hulata, G., 1974, Genetic differences in susceptibility to two diseases among strains of the common carp, *Aquaculture* **3(1974)**:187.

Hoffman, G. L., Dunbar, C. E., Wolf, K., and Zwillenberg, L. O., 1969, Epitheliocystis, a new infectious disease of the bluegill (*Lepomis macrochirus*), *J. Microbiol. Serol.* **35(2)**:146.

Hofmann, W., 1971, Zur diagnostischen Bedeutung der Einschlusskörperchen bei der hämorrhagischen Virussepptikämie (HVS) der Forellen, *Dtsch. Tieraerztl. Wochenschr.* **1**:14.

Holway, J. E., and Smith, C. E., 1973, Infectious hematopoietic necrosis of rainbow trout in Montana: A case report, *J. Wildl. Dis.* **9**:287.

Howse, H. D., and Christmas, J. Y., 1971, Observations on the ultrastructure of lymphocystis virus in the Atlantic croaker, *Micropogon undulatus* (Linneaus), *Virology* **44**:211.

Jensen, M. H., 1965, Research on the virus of Egtved disease, *Ann. N.Y. Acad. Sci.* **126**:422.

Johnston, M. R. L., and Davies, A. J., 1973, A *Pirhemocyton*-like parasite of the blenny, *Blennius pholis* L. (Teleostei: Blenniidae) and its relationship to *Immanoplasma* (Neumann, 1909), *Int. J. Parasitol.* **3**:235.

Jørgensen, P. E. V., 1968, Serological identification of Egtved virus (virus of viral haemorrhagic septicaemia of rainbow trout) a preliminary report, *Bull. Office Int. Epiz.* **69**:985.

Jørgensen, P. E. V., 1970, The survival of viral hemorrhagic septicemia (VHS) virus associated with trout eggs, *Riv. Ital. Piscic. Ittiop.* **5**:13.

Jørgensen, P. E. V., 1971, Egtved virus: Demonstration of neutralizing antibodies in serum from artificially infected rainbow trout (*Salmo gairdneri*), *J. Fish. Res. Board Can.* **28**:875.

Jørgensen, P. E. V., 1972, Egtved virus: Antigenic variation in 76 virus isolates examined in neutralization tests and by means of the fluorescent antibody technique, *Symp. Zool. Soc. London* **30**:333.

Jørgensen, P. E. V., 1973a, Inactivation of IPN and Egtved virus, *Riv. Ital. Piscic. Ittiop.* **8**:107.

Jørgensen, P. E. V, 1973b, Artificial transmission of viral haemorrhagic septicaemia (VHS) of rainbow trout, *Riv. Ital. Piscic. Ittiop.* **8**:101.

Jørgensen, P. E. V., 1973c, Diagnostic methods and serological studies on the virus of viral hemorrhagic septicemia (VHS), in: *Symposium on the Major Communicable Fish Diseases in Europe and their Control* (W. A. Dill, ed.), pp. 34–36, EIFAC (European Inland Fisheries Advisory Committee) Tech. Paper 17, Suppl. 2.

Jørgensen, P. E. V., 1974, Indirect fluorescent antibody techniques for demonstration of trout viruses and corresponding antibody, *Acta Vet. Scand.* **15**:198.

Jørgensen, P. E. V., 1976, Partial resistance of rainbow trout (*Salmo gairdneri*) to viral haemorrhagic septicaemia (VHS) following exposure to non-virulent Egtved virus, *Nord. Veterinarmed.* **28**:570.

Jørgensen, P. V., and Grauballe, P. C., 1971, Problems in the serological typing of IPN virus, *Acta Vet. Scand.* **12**:145.

Jørgensen, P. E. V., and Kehlet, N. P., 1971, Infectious pancreatic necrosis (IPN) viruses in Danish rainbow trout. Their serological and pathogenic properties, *Nord. Veterinarmed.* **23**:568.

Jørgensen, P. E. V., and Meyling, A., 1972, Egtved virus: Demonstration of virus antigen by the fluorescent antibody technique in tissues of rainbow trout affected by viral haemorrhagic septicaemia and in cell cultures infected with Egtved virus, *Arch. Gesamte Virusforsch.* **36**:115.

Kelly, R. K., and Loh, P. C., 1972, Electron microscopical and biochemical characterization of infectious pancreatic necrosis virus, *J. Virol.* **10**:824.

Kelly, R. K., and Loh, P. C., 1975, Replication of IPN virus: A cytochemical and biochemical study in SWT cells (38611), *Proc. Soc. Exp. Biol. Med.* **148**:688.

Koops, H., and Mann, H., 1966, The cauliflower disease of eels in Germany, *Bull. Office Int. Epiz.* **65**:991.

Koops, H., Mann, H., Pfitzner, I., Schmid, O. J., and Schubert, G., 1970, The cauliflower disease of eels, in: *A Symposium on Diseases of Fishes and Shellfishes* (S. F. Snieszko, ed.), pp. 291–295, Am. Fisheries Soc. Spec. Publ. 5.

Kudo, S., Kurosawa, D., Kunimine, I., Nobusawa, K., and Kobayashi, S., 1973, Electron microscopic observations of the pancreas and liver in the fingerling rainbow trout with symptoms of IPN, *Jpn. J. Ichthyol.* **20**:163.

Laird, M., and Bullock, W. L., 1969, Marine fish haematozoa from New Brunswick and New England, *J. Fish. Res. Board Can.* **26**:1075.

Lawler, A. R., Ogle, J. T., and Donnes, C., 1977, *Dascyllus* spp.: New hosts for lymphocystis and a list of recent hosts, *J. Wildl. Dis.* **13**:307.

Le Berre, M., de Kinkelin, P., and Metzger, A., 1977, Identification sérologique des rhabdovirus des salmonidés, *Bull. Office Int. Epiz.* **87**:391.

Lee, M. H., and Loh, P. C., 1975, Some properties of an established fish cell line from the marine fish, *Caranx mate* (Omaka), *Proc. Soc. Exp. Biol. Med.* **150**:40.

Lenoir, G., 1973, Structural proteins of spring viremia virus of carp, *Biochem. Biophys. Res. Commun.* **51**:895.

Lenoir, G., and de Kinkelin, P., 1975, Fish rhabdoviruses: Comparative study of protein structure, *J. Virol.* **16**:259.

Lientz, J. C., and Springer, J. E., 1973, Neutralization tests of infectious pancreatic necrosis virus with polyvalent antiserum, *J. Wildl. Dis.* **9**:120.

Ljungberg, O., 1963, Report on fish diseases and inspection of fish products in Sweden, *Bull. Office Int. Epiz.* **59**:111.

Ljungberg, O., 1976, Epizootiological and experimental studies of skin tumours in northern pike (*Esox lucius* L.) in the Baltic Sea, *Prog. Exp. Tumor Res.* **20**:156.

Ljungberg, O., and Jørgensen, P. E. V., 1973, Infectious pancreatic necrosis (IPN) of salmonids in Swedish fish farms, in: *Symposium on the Major Communicable Fish Diseases in Europe and their Control* (W. A. Dill, ed.), pp. 67–70, EIFAC (European Inland Fisheries Advisory Committee) Tech. Paper 17, Suppl. 2.

Loh, P. C., Lee, M. H., and Kelly, R. K., 1974, The polypeptides of infectious pancreatic necrosis virus, *J. Gen. Virol.* **22**:421.

Lopez, D. M., Beasley, A. R., Dietrich, L. S., and Sigel, M. M., 1968, Biochemical and morphological aspects of the early phase of lymphocystis infection in tissue culture, *Bacteriol. Proc.* **1968**:176.

Lopez, D. M., Sigel, M. M., Beasley, A. R., and Dietrich, L. S., 1969, Biochemical and morphologic studies of lymphocystis disease, *Natl. Cancer Inst. Monogr.* **31**:223.

Lothrop, D., and Nicholson, B. L., 1974, Inhibition of cellular DNA synthesis in cells infected with infectious pancreatic necrosis virus, *J. Virol.* **14**:485.

Lounatmaa, K., and Janatuinen, J., 1978, Electron microscopy of an ulcerative dermal necrosis (UDN)-like salmon disease in Finland, *J. Fish Dis.* **1**:369.

Macdonald, R. D., and Yamamoto, T., 1977a, The structure of infectious pancreatic necrosis virus RNA, *J. Gen. Virol.* **34**:235.

Macdonald, R. D., and Yamamoto, T., 1977b, Defective interfering particles as the basis of autointerference in infectious pancreatic necrosis virus, *Abstr. Annu. Meeting Am. Soc. Microbiol.*, New Orleans, May 8–13, p. 353.

Macdonald, R. D., and Yamamoto, T., 1978, Quantitative analysis of defective interfering particles in infectious pancreatic necrosis virus preparations, *Arch. Virol.* **57**:77–89.

MacKelvie, R. M., and Artsob, H., 1969, Infectious pancreatic necrosis virus in young salmonids of the Canadian Maritime Provinces, *J. Fish. Res. Board Can.* **26**:3259.

MacKelvie, R. M., and Desautels, D., 1975, Fish viruses—Survival and inactivation of infectious pancreatic necrosis virus, *J. Fish. Res. Board Can.* **32**:1267.

Major, R. D., McCraren, J. P., and Smith, C. E., 1975, Histopathological changes in channel catfish (*Ictalurus punctatus*) experimentally and naturally infected with channel catfish virus disease, *J. Fish. Res. Board Can.* **32**:563.

Malsberger, R. G., and Cerini, C. P., 1963, Characteristics of infectious pancreatic necrosis virus, *J. Bacteriol.* **86**:1283.

Malsberger, R. G., and Cerini, C. P., 1965, Multiplication of infectious pancreatic necrosis virus, *Ann. N.Y. Acad. Sci.* **126**:320.

Mann, H., 1970, Über den Befall der Plattfische der Nordsee mit Lymphocystis, *Ber. Dtsch. Wiss. Komm. Meeresforsch.* **21**:219.

McAllister, P. E., and Pilcher, K. S., 1974, Autointerference in infectious hematopoietic necrosis virus of salmonid fish, *Proc. Soc. Exp. Biol. Med.* **145**:840.

McAllister, P. E., and Wagner, R. R., 1975, Structural proteins of two salmonid rhabdoviruses, *J. Virol.* **15**:733.

McAllister, P. E., and Wagner, R. R., 1977, Virion RNA polymerases of two salmonid rhabdoviruses, *J. Virol.* **22**:839.

McAllister, P. E., Fryer, J. L., and Pilcher, K. S., 1974a, An antigenic comparison between infectious hematopoietic necrosis virus (OSV strain) and the virus of haemorrhagic septicaemia of rainbow trout (*Salmo gairdneri*) (Denmark strain) by cross neutralization, *J. Wildl. Dis.* **10**:101.

McAllister, P. E., Fryer, J. L., and Pilcher, K. S., 1974b, Further characterization of infectious hematopoietic necrosis virus of salmonid fish (Oregon strain), *Arch. Gesamte Virusforsch.* **44**:270.

McAllister, P. E., Nagabayashi, T., and Wolf, K., 1977, Viruses of eels with and without stomatopapillomas, *Ann. N.Y. Acad. Sci.* **298**:233.

McCain, B. B., Fryer, J. L., and Pilcher, K. S., 1971, Antigenic relationships in a group of three viruses of salmonid fish by cross neutralization, *Proc. Soc. Exp. Biol. Med.* **317**:1042.

McCain, B. B., Fryer, J. L., and Pilcher, K. S., 1974, Physicochemical properties of RNA of salmonid hematopoietic necrosis virus (Oregon strain), *Proc. Soc. Exp. Biol. Med.* **146**:630.

McCraren, J. P., 1973, The channel catfish virus, *Farm Pond Harvest* **7**:20.

McKnight, I. J., 1978, Sarcoma of the swim bladder of Atlantic salmon (*Salmo salar* L.), *Aquaculture* **13**(1978):55.

McKnight, I. J., and Roberts, R. J., 1976, The pathology of infectious pancreatic necrosis. I. The sequential histopathology of the naturally occurring condition, *Br. Vet. J.* **132**:76.

McMichael, J. S., Fryer, J. L., and Pilcher, K. S., 1973, Salmonid virus isolations in Oregon (U.S.A.), *Food Agr. Organ. Aquacult. Bull.* **5**:14.

McMichael, J., Fryer, J. L., and Pilcher, K. S., 1975, An antigenic comparison of three strains of infectious pancreatic necrosis virus of salmonid fishes, *Aquaculture* **6**:203.

Meier, W., and Jørgensen, P. E. V., 1975, A rapid and specific method for the diagnosis of viral haemorrhagic septicaemia (VHS) of rainbow trout, *Rev. Ital. Piscic. Ittiop.* **10**:11.

Midlige, F. H., 1968, Lymphocystis disease virus multiplication and morphology, Ph.D. dissertation, Lehigh University, 118 pp, Bethlehem, Pa.

Midlige, F. H., Jr., and Malsberger, R. G., 1968, *In vitro* morphology and maturation of lymphocystis virus, *J. Virol.* **2**:830.

Miller, B. S., and Wellings, S. R., 1971, Epizootiology of tumors on flathead sole (*Hippoglossoides elassodon*) in East Sound, Orcas Island, Washington, *Tr. Am. Fish. Soc.* **100**:247.

Moewus-Kobb, L, 1965, Studies with IPN virus in marine hosts, *Ann. N.Y. Acad. Sci.* **126**:328.

Moore, N. F., Barenholz, Y., McAllister, P. E., and Wagner, R. R., 1976, Comparative membrane microviscosity of fish and mammalian rhabdoviruses studied by fluorescence depolarization, *J. Virol.* **19**:275.

Moss, L. H., and Gravell, M., 1969, Ultrastructure and sequential development of infectious pancreatic necrosis virus, *J. Virol.* **3**:52.

Mulcahy, M. F., 1963, Lymphosarcoma in the pike, *Esox lucius* L., (Pisces; Esocidae) in Ireland, *Proc. R. Ir. Acad. Sect. B* **63**(7):103.

Mulcahy, M. F., 1976, Epizootiological studies of lymphomas in northern pike in Ireland, *Prog. Exp. Tumor Res.* **20**:129.

Mulcahy, M. F., and O'Leary, A., 1970, Cell-free transmission of lymphosarcoma in northern pike *Esox lucius* L. (Pisces; Esocidae), *Experientia* **26**:891.

Mulcahy, M. F., Winqvist, G., and Dawe, C. J., 1970, The neoplastic cell type in lymphoreticular neoplasms of the northern pike, *Esox lucius* L., *Cancer Res.* **30**:2712.

Munro, A. L. S., and Duncan, I. B., 1977, Current problems in the study of the biology of infectious pancreatic necrosis virus and the management of the disease it causes in cultivated salmonid fish, in: *Aquatic Microbiology* (F. A. Skinner and J. M. Shewan, eds.), pp. 325–337, Academic Press, New York.

Nagabayashi, T., and Wolf, K., 1979, Characterization of a virus isolated from eels (*Anguilla anguilla*) with stomatopapilloma, *J. Virol.* **30**:358.

Negele, R. D., 1977, Histopathological changes in some organs of experimentally infected carp fingerlings with *Rhabdovirus carpio*, *Bull. Office Int. Epiz.* **87**:449.

Nicholson, B. L., 1971a, Macromolecule synthesis in RTG-2 cells following infection with infectious pancreatic necrosis (IPN) virus, *J. Gen. Virol.* **13**:369.

Nicholson, B. L., 1971b, Effect of actinomycin D on the multiplication of the infectious pancreatic necrosis virus of trout, *Experientia* **27**:1362.

Nicholson, B. L., and Byrne, C., 1973, An established cell line from the Atlantic salmon (*Salmo salar*), *J. Fish. Res. Board Can.* **30**:913.

Nicholson, B. L., and Dunn, J., 1974, Homologous viral interference in trout and Atlantic salmon cell cultures infected with infectious pancreatic necrosis virus, *J. Virol.* **14**:180.

Nicholson, B. L., and Reno, P. W., 1978, Piscine erythrocytic necrosis (PEN) in marine fishes, *Proc. 3rd Biennial Fish Health Sect. 9th Annu. Midwest Fish Dis. Workshop* **1978**:47.

Nicholson, B., Thorne, W., and Janicki, C., 1978, A host range variant from isolates of infectious pancreatic necrosis virus (IPNV), *Abstr. Annu. Meet. Am. Soc. Microbiol.* **1978**:267.

Nigrelli, R. F., and Ruggieri, G. D., 1965, Studies on virus diseases of fishes. Spontaneous and experimentally induced cellular hypertrophy (lymphocystis disease) in fishes of the New York Aquarium, with a report of new cases and an annotated bibliography (1874–1965), *Zoologica* **50**:83.

Nigrelli, R. F., Ketchen, K. S., and Ruggieri, G. D., 1965, Studies on virus diseases of fishes: Epizootiology of epithelial tumors in the skin of flatfishes of the Pacific coast, with special reference to the sand sole (*Psettichthys melanosticus*) from northern Hecate Strait, British Columbia, Canada, *Zoologica* **50**:115.

Nims, L., Fryer, J. L., and Pilcher, K. S., 1970, Studies of replication of four selected viruses in two cell lines derived from salmonid fish, *Proc. Soc. Exp. Biol. Med.* **135**:6.

Ord, W. M., Le Berre, M., and de Kinkelin, P., 1976, Viral hemorrhagic septicemia: Comparative susceptibility of rainbow trout (*Salmo gairdneri*) and hybrids (*S. gairdneri X Oncorhynchus kisutch*) to experimental infection, *J. Fish. Res. Board Can.* **33**:1205.

Papas, T. S., Dahlberg, J. E., and Sonstegard, R. A., 1976, Type C virus in lymphosarcoma in northern pike (*Esox lucius*), *Nature (London)* **261**:506.

Papas, T. S., Pry, T. W., Schafer, M. P., and Sonstegard, R. A., 1977, Presence of DNA polymerase in lymphosarcoma in northern pike (*Esox lucius*), *Cancer Res.* **37**:3214.

Parisot, T. J., Yasutake, W. T., and Bressler, V., 1963, A new geographic and host record for infectious pancreatic necrosis, *Tr. Am. Fish. Soc.* **92**:63.

Parisot, T. J., Yasutake, W. T., and Klontz, G. W., 1965, Virus diseases of the Salmonidae in western United States. I. Etiology and epizootiology, *Ann. N.Y. Acad. Sci.* **126**:502.

Peters, N., 1970, Abstossung von Tumoren unter Einwirkung von anorganischem Diphosphat, *Experientia* **26**:1135.

Peters, N., and Peters, G., 1970, Tumorgenese, ein Energieproblem der Zelle? Untersuchungen an Papillomen des europäischen Aals, *Anguilla anguilla* (L), *Arch. Fischereiwiss.* **21**:238.

Peters, N., and Wilke, H., 1972, Proliferation der Fischepidermis nach der Einwirkung von Inhibitoren des glykolytischen Energiestoffwechsels, *Experientia* **28**:315.

Peters, N., Fröhlich, K. H., and Bresching, G., 1972*a*, Experimentelle Reversion von Tumorzellen *in vivo*, *Experientia* **28**:319.

Peters, N., Peters, G., and Bresching, G., 1972*b*, Redifferenzierung und Wachstumshemmung von epidermalen Tumoren des europäischen Aals unter Einwirkung von Chininsulfat, *Arch. Fischereiwiss.* **23**:47.

Pfeil, V. C., and Wiedemann, H., 1977, Virusnachweis durch indirekte Immunofluoreszenz und Virusanzüchtung bei experimentell erzeugter viraler haemorrhagischer Septikämie (VHS) der Regenbogenforelle (*Salmo gairdneri*), *Dtsch. Tieraerztl. Wochenschr.* **84**:152.

Pfitzner, I., 1966, Beitrag zur Ätiologie der "haemorrhagischen Virusseptikaemie der Regenbogenforellen," *Zentralbl. Bakteriol. Parasitend. Infectionskr. Hyg.* **201**:306.

Pfitzner, I., 1969, Zur Ätiologie der Blumenkohlkrankheit der Aale, *Arch. Fischereiwiss.* **20**:24.

Pfitzner, I., 1973, Untersuchungen zur Klärung der Ätiologie der "Blumenkohlkrankheit der Aale" und zum Einfluss dieses Tumors auf Ernährung und Wachstum, *Verh. Int. Ver. Limnol.* **18**:1666.

Pfitzner, I., and Schubert, G., 1969, Ein virus aus dem Blut mit Blumenkohlkrankheit behafteter Aale, *Z. Naturforsch.* **24b**:790a–790b.

Piper, D., Nicholson, B. L., and Dunn, J., 1973, Immunofluorescent study of the replication of infectious pancreatic necrosis virus in trout and Atlantic salmon cell cultures, *Infect. Immun.* **8**:249.

Plumb, J. A., 1971*a*, Tissue distribution of channel catfish virus, *J. Wildl. Dis.* **7**:213.

Plumb, J. A., 1971*b*, Channel catfish virus research at Auburn University, *Auburn Univ. Agr. Exp. Stn., Prog. Rep. Ser. 95*, 3 pp.

Plumb, J. A., 1971*c*, Channel catfish virus disease in southern United States, *Proc. Annu. Conf. Southeast. Assoc. Game Fish Comm.* **25**:489.

Plumb, J. A., 1972, A virus-caused epizootic of rainbow trout (*Salmo gairdneri*) in Minnesota, *Tr. Am. Fish. Soc.* **101**:121.

Plumb, J. A., 1973, Neutralization of channel catfish virus by serum of channel catfish, *J. Wildl. Dis.* **9**:324.

Plumb, J. A., 1977, Channel catfish virus disease, *U.S. Fish Wildl. Serv. Fish Dis. Leaflet 52*, 8 pp.

Plumb, J. A., Gaines, J. L., Mora, E. C., and Bradley, G. G., 1974, Histopathology and electron microscopy of channel catfish virus in infected channel catfish, *Ictalurus punctatus* (Rafinesque), *J. Fish Biol.* **6**:661.

Popkova, T. I., and Shchelkunov, I. S., 1978, Vedelenie virusa ot karpoy, bol'nykh zhabernym nekrozom, *VNIIPRKH Rybn. Khoz.* **4**:34.

Rašín, K., 1927, Prispevek k pathogenesi *Lymphocystis johnstonei* Woodcock. I., *Biol. Spisy Vysokė Skoly Zverolek. Brno CSR* **6**(2):11.

Rasmussen, C. J., 1965, A biological study of the Egtved disease (INUL), *Ann. N.Y. Acad. Sci.* **126**:427.

Reichenbach-Klinke, H., 1959, Fischkrankheiten in Bayern in den Jahren 1957 und 1958, *Allg. Fischwirtschaftsztg.* **84**:226.

Reno, P., and Nicholson, B. L., 1978, The replication of piscine erythrocytic necrosis (PEN) virus in erythrocytes of the Atlantic cod (*Gadus morhua*) maintained *in vitro*, *29th Annu. Meet. of the Tissue Culture Assoc.*, p. 385.

Reno, P. W., Philippon-Fried, M., Nicholson, B. L., and Sherburne, S. W., 1978, Ultrastructural studies of piscine erythrocytic necrosis (PEN) in Atlantic herring (*Clupea harengus harengus*), *J. Fish. Res. Board Can.* **35**:148.

Richards, R. H., and Buchanan, J. S., 1978, Studies on *Herpesvirus scophthalmi* infection of turbot *Scophthalmus maximus* (L.): Histopathological observations, *J. Fish Dis.* **1**:251.

Roberts, R. J., 1972, Ulcerative dermal necrosis (UDN) of salmon (*Salmo salar* L.), *Symp. Zool. Soc. London* **30**:53.

Robin, J., and Rodrigue, A., 1977, Purification and biochemical properties of Egtved viral RNA, *Can. J. Microbiol.* **23**:1489.

Ross, A. J., Pelnar, J., and Rucker, R. R., 1960, A virus-like disease of chinook salmon, *Tr. Am. Fish. Soc.* **89**:160.

Roy, P., 1976, The transcription process of the RNA polymerase of spring viremia of carp virus, *Fed. Proc.* **35**:812.

Roy, P., and Clewley, J. P., 1978a, Spring viremia of carp virus RNA and virion-associated transcriptase activity, *J. Virol.* **25**:912.

Roy, P., and Clewley, J. P., 1978b, Phosphoproteins of spring viremia of carp virus and other rhabdoviruses, in: *Negative Strand Viruses* (R. D. Barry and B. W. J. Mahy, eds.), pp 117–125, Academic Press, New York.

Roy, P., Clark, H. F., Madore, H. P., and Bishop, D. H. L., 1975, RNA polymerase associated with virions of pike fry rhabdovirus, *J. Virol.* **15**:338.

Rudikov, N. I., Grishchenko, L. I., and Lobuncov, K. A., 1975, Vesennaja virusnaja boleznej ryb, *Byull. Vses. Inst. Eksp. Vet.* **20**:16.

Russell, P. H., 1974, Lymphocystis in wild plaice *Pleuronectes platessa* (L.), and flounder *Platichthys flesus* (L.) in British coastal waters: A histopathological and serological study, *J. Fish Biol.* **6**:771.

Sano, T., 1973, The current preventive approach to infectious pancreatic necrosis (IPN) in Japan, in: *Symposium on the Major Communicable Fish Diseases in Europe and Their Control* (W. A. Dill, ed.), pp. 71–75, EIFAC (European Inland Fisheries Advisory Committee) Tech. Paper 17, Suppl. 2.

Sano, T., 1976, Viral diseases of cultured fishes in Japan, *Fish Pathol.* **10**:221.

Sano, T., Nishimura, T., Okamoto, N., and Fukuda, H., 1977a, Studies on viral diseases of Japanese fishes. VII. A rhabdovirus isolated from European eel, *Anguilla anguilla*, *Bull. Jpn. Soc. Sci. Fish.* **43**:491.

Sano, T., Nishimura, T., Okamoto, N., Yamazaki, T., Hanada, H., and Watanabe, Y., 1977b, Studies on viral diseases of Japanese fisheries. VI. Infectious hematopoietic necrosis (IHN) of salmonids in the mainland of Japan, *J. Tokyo Univ. Fish.* **63**:81.

Schäperclaus, W., 1954, *Fischkrankheiten*, 708 pp, Akad. Verlag, Berlin.

Scherrer, R., 1973, Infectious pancreatic necrosis (IPN) of Salmonidae, in: *Symposium on the Major Communicable Fish Diseases in Europe and their Control* (W. A. Dill, ed.), pp. 51–58, EIFAC (European Inland Fisheries Advisory Committee) Tech. Paper 17, Suppl. 2.

Scherrer, R., and Cohen, J., 1975, Studies on infectious pancreatic necrosis virus interactions with RTG-2 and FHM cells: Selection of a variant virus-type in FHM cells, *J. Gen. Virol.* **28**:9.

Scherrer, R., Bic, E., and Cohen, J., 1974, Le virus de la nécrose pancréatique infectieuse: Étude de la réplication et de l'induction de la synthèse d'interféron en fonction de l'hote et de la température, *Ann. Microbiol.* (*Inst. Pasteur*) **125A**:455.

Schlumberger, H. G., 1957, Tumors characteristic for certain animal species: A review, *Cancer Res.* **17**:823.

Schmid, O. J., 1969, Beitrag zur Histologie und Ätiologie der Blumenkohlkrankheit der Aale, *Arch. Fischereiwiss.* **20**:16.

Schubert, G. von, 1964, Elektronenmikroskopische Untersuchungen zur Pockenkrankheit des Karpfens, *Z. Naturforsch.* **19b**:675.

Schubert, G. H., 1966, The infective agent in carp pox, *Bull. Office Int. Epiz.* **65**:1011.

Schubert, G., 1969, Elektronenmikroskopische Untersuchungen an der Haut mit Blumenkohlkrankheit behaftetes Aale, *Arch. Fischereiwiss.* **20**:36.

Schubert, G., and Meyer, G., 1960, Licht- und elektronenmikroskopische Untersuchungen zur Pockenkrankheit des Karpfens, *Zool. Anz. Suppl.* **23**:472.

Schwanz-Pfitzner, I., 1976, Further studies of eel virus (Berlin) isolated from the blood of eels (*Anguilla anguilla*) with skin papilloma, *Prog. Exp. Tumor Res.* **20**:101.

Seeley, R. J., Perlmutter, A., and Seeley, V. A., 1977, Inheritance and longevity of infectious pancreatic necrosis virus in the zebra fish, *Brachydanio rerio* (Hamilton-Buchanan), *Appl. Environ. Microbiol.* **34**:50.

Sherburne, S. W., 1977, Occurrence of piscine erythrocytic necrosis (PEN) in the blood of the anadromous alewife, *Alosa pseudoharnegus*, from Maine coastal streams, *J. Fish. Res. Board Can.* **34**:281.

Sigel, M. M., Russell, W. J., Jensen, J. A., and Beasley, A. R., 1968, Natural immunity in marine fishes, *Bull, Office Int. Epiz.* **69**:1349.

Sokol, F., Clark, H. F., Wiktor, T. J., McFalls, M. L., Bishop, D. H. L., and Obijeski, J. F., 1974, Structural phosphoproteins associated with ten rhabdoviruses, *J. Gen. Virol.* **24**:433.

Sonstegard, R., 1975, Lymphosarcoma in muskellunge (*Esox masquinongy*), in: *The Pathology of Fishes* (W. E. Ribelin and G. Migaki, eds.), pp. 907–924, University of Wisonsin Press, Madison.

Sonstegard, R. A., 1976, Studies of the etiology and epizootiology of lymphosarcoma in *Esox* (*Esox lucius* L. and *Esox masquinongy*), *Prog. Exp. Tumor Res.* **20**:141.

Sonstegard, R. A., 1977a, The potential utility of fishes as indicator organisms for environmental carcinogens, in: *Wastewater Renovation and Reuse* (F. M. D'Itri, ed.), pp. 561–577, Dekker, New York.

Sonstegard, R. A., 1977b, Environmental carcinogenesis studies in fishes of the Great Lakes of North America, *Ann. N.Y. Acad. Sci.* **298**:261.

Sonstegard, R. A., McDermott, L. A., and Sonstegard, K. S., 1972, Isolation of infectious pancreatic necrosis virus from white suckers (*Catastomus* [*sic*] *commersoni*), *Nature* (*London*) **236**:174.

Sulimanovic, D., 1973, Immunity of carp to *Rhabdovirus carpio* and determination of antibodies by indirect hemagglutination, *Vet. Arh.* **43**:153.

Tu, K.-C., Spendlove, R. S., and Goede, R. W., 1974, Immunofluorescent cell assay of infectious pancreatic necrosis virus, *Appl. Microbiol.* **27**:593.

Tu, K., Spendlove, R. S., and Goede, R. W., 1975, Effect of temperature on survival and growth of infectious pancreatic necrosis virus, *Infect. Immun.* **11**:1409.

Underwood, B. O., Smale, C. J., Brown, F., and Hill, B. J., 1977, Relationship of a virus from *Tellina tenuis* to infectious pancreatic necrosis virus, *J. Gen. Virol.* **36**:93.

Varović, K., and Fijan, N., 1973, Osjetljivost šarana prema *Rhabdovirus carpio* pri raznim načinima inokulacije, *Vet. Arh.* **43**:271.

Wagner, R. R., 1975, Reproduction of rhabdoviruses, in: *Comprehensive Virology*, Vol. 4 (H. Fraenkel-Conrat and R. R. Wagner, eds.), pp. 1–93, Plenum, New York.

Walker, R., 1958, Lymphocystis warts and skin tumors of walleyed pike, *Rensselaer Rev. Grad. Stud.* **14:**1.

Walker, R., 1961, Fine structure of a virus tumor of fish, *Am. Zool.* **1:**395.

Walker, R., 1962, Fine structure of lymphocystis virus of fish, *Virology* **18:**503.

Walker, R., 1965, Viral DNA and cytoplasmic RNA in lymphocystis cells of fish, *Ann. N.Y. Acad. Sci.* **126:**386.

Walker, R., 1969a, Virus associated with epidermal hyperplasia in fish, *Natl. Cancer Inst. Monogr.* **31:**195.

Walker, R., 1969b, Epidermal hyperplasia in fish: Two types without visible virus, *Natl. Cancer Inst. Monogr.* **31:**209.

Walker, R., and Sherburne, S. W., 1977, Piscine erythrocytic necrosis virus in Atlantic cod, *Gadus morhua*, and other fish: Ultrastructure and distribution, *J. Fish. Res. Board Can.* **34:**1188.

Weissenberg, R., 1939, Studies on virus diseases of fish. III. Morphological and experimental observations on the lymphocystis disease of the pike perch, *Stizostedion vitreum*, *Zoologica* **24:**245.

Weissenberg, R., 1951, Experimental lymphocystis infection of the killifish *Fundulus heteroclitus* with emulsion of lymphocystis tumors of the perch *Stizostedion vitreum*, *Anat. Rec.* **111:**582.

Wellings, S. R., 1970, Biology of some virus diseases of marine fish, in: *A Symposium on Diseases of Fishes and Shellfishes* (S. F. Snieszko, ed.), pp. 296–306, Am. Fisheries Soc. Spec. Publ. 5.

Wellings, S. R., and Chuinard, R. G., 1964, Epidermal papillomas with virus-like particles in flathead sole, *Hippoglossoides elassodon*, *Science* **146:**932.

Wellings, S. R., Chuinard, R. G., Gourley, R. T., and Cooper, R. A., 1964, Epidermal papillomas in the flathead sole, *Hippoglossoides elassodon*, with notes on the occurrence of similar neoplasms in other pleuronectids, *J. Natl. Cancer Inst.* **33:**991.

Wellings, S. R., Chuinard, R. G., and Bens, M., 1965, A comparative study of skin neoplasms in four species of pleuronectid fishes, *Ann. N.Y. Acad. Sci.* **126:**479.

Wellings, S. R., McCain, B. B., and Miller, B. S., 1976, Epidermal papillomas in Pleuronectidae of Puget Sound, Washington, *Prog. Exp. Tumor Res.* **20:**55.

Wingfield, W. H., and Chan, L. D., 1970, Studies on the Sacramento River chinook disease and its causative agent, in: *A Symposium on Diseases of Fishes and Shellfishes* (S. F. Snieszko, ed.), pp. 307–318, Am. Fisheries Soc. Spec. Publ. 5.

Wingfield, W. H., Fryer, J. L., and Pilcher, K. S., 1969, Properties of the sockeye salmon virus (Oregon strain), *Proc. Soc. Exp. Biol. Med.* **130:**1055.

Wingfield, W. H., Nims, L., Fryer, J. L., and Pilcher, K. S., 1970, Species specificity of the sockeye salmon virus (Oregon strain) and its cytopathic effects in salmonid cell lines, in: *A Symposium on Diseases of Fishes and Shellfishes* (S. F. Snieszko, ed.), pp. 319–326, Am. Fisheries Soc. Spec. Publ. 5.

Winqvist, G., Ljungberg, O., and Hellstroem, B., 1968, Skin tumours of northern pike (*Esox lucius* L.). II. Viral particles in epidermal proliferations, *Bull. Office Int. Epiz.* **69:**1023.

Winqvist, G., Ljungberg, O., and Ivarsson, B., 1973, Electron microscopy of sarcoma of the northern pike (*Esox lucius* L.), *Bibl. Haematol.* **39:**26.

Wirén, B., 1971, Vårtsjuka hos lax (*Salmo salar* L.) histologiska studier över epidermala papillom hos odlad lax, *Swed. Salmon Res. Inst. Rep. LFI MEDD*, 7/1971, 4 pp.

Wolf, K., 1962, Experimental propagation of lymphocystis disease of fishes, *Virology* **18:**249.

Wolf, K., 1966, The fish viruses, in: *Advances in Virus Research*, Vol. 12 (K. M. Smith and M. A. Lauffer, eds.), pp. 35–101, Academic Press, New York.

Wolf, K., 1972, Advances in fish virology: A review 1966–1971, *Symp. Zool. Soc. London* **30:**305.

Wolf, K., 1973, Herpesviruses of lower vertebrates, in: *The Herpesviruses* (A. S. Kaplan, ed.), pp. 495–520, Academic Press, New York.

Wolf, K., 1976, Fish viral diseases in North America, 1971–75, and recent research of the Eastern Fish Disease Laboratory, U.S.A., *Fish Pathol.* **10:**135.

Wolf, K., and Carlson, C. P., 1965, Multiplication of lymphocystis virus in the bluegill (*Lepomis macrochirus*), *Ann. N.Y. Acad. Sci.* **126:**414.

Wolf, K., and Darlington, R. W., 1971, Channel catfish virus: A new herpesvirus of ictalurid fish, *J. Virol.* **8:**525.

Wolf, K., and Pettijohn, L. L., 1970, Infectious pancreatic necrosis virus isolated from coho salmon fingerlings, *Prog. Fish Cult.* **32:**17.

Wolf, K., and Quimby, M. C., 1970a, Channel catfish virus (CCV), in: *Progress in Sport Fishery Research 1969* (Resource Publ. 88), pp. 52–54, U.S. Fish Wildlife Service, Washington, D.C.

Wolf, K., and Quimby, M. C., 1970b, Virology of eel stomatopapilloma, in: *Progress in Sport Fishery Research 1970* (Resource Publ. 106), pp. 94–95, U.S. Fish Wildlife Service, Washington, D.C.

Wolf, K., and Quimby, M. C., 1971, Salmonid viruses: Infectious pancreatic necrosis virus. Morphology, pathology, and serology of first European isolations, *Arch. Gesamte Virusforsch.* **34:**144.

Wolf, K., and Quimby, M. C., 1973, Fish viruses: Buffers and methods for plaquing eight agents under normal atmosphere, *Appl. Microbiol.* **25:**659.

Wolf, K., Snieszko, S. F., Dunbar, C. E., and Pyle, E., 1960, Virus nature of infectious pancreatic necrosis in trout, *Proc. Soc. Exp. Biol. Med.* **104:**105.

Wolf, K., Gravell, M., and Malsberger, R. G., 1966, Lymphocystis virus: Isolation and propagation in centrarchid fish cell lines, *Science* **151:**1004.

Wolf, K., Quimby, M. C., Carlson, C. P., and Bullock, G. L., 1968, Infectious pancreatic necrosis: Selection of virus-free stock from a population of carrier trout, *J. Fish. Res. Board Can.* **25:**383.

Wolf, K., Quimby, M. C., and Carlson, C. P., 1969, Infectious pancreatic necrosis virus: lyophilization and subsequent stability in storage at 4 C, *Appl. Microbiol.* **17:**623.

Wolf, K., Herman, R. L., and Carlson, C. P., 1972, Fish viruses: Histopathologic changes associated with experimental channel catfish virus disease, *J. Fish. Res. Board Can.* **29:**149.

Wolf, K., Sano, T., and Kimura, T., 1975a, Herpesvirus disease of salmonids, *U.S. Fish Wildlife Serv. Fish Disease Leaflet 44*, 8 pp.

Wolf, K., Herman, R. L., Darlington, R. W., and Taylor, W. G., 1975b, Salmonid viruses: Effects of *Herpesvirus salmonis* in rainbow trout fry, *Fish Health News* **4(3):**8.

Wolf, K., Darlington, R. W., Nagabayashi, T., and Quimby, M. C., 1976, *Herpesvirus salmonis:* Characterization of a new pathogen from rainbow trout (*Salmo gairdneri*), *Abstr. Annu. Meet. Am. Soc. Microbiol.* **1976**:235.

Wolf, K., Darlington, R. W., Taylor, W. G., Quimby, M. C., and Nagabayashi, T., 1978, *Herpesvirus salmonis*: Characterization of a new pathogen of rainbow trout, *J. Virol.* **27**:659.

Wolf, K. E., Quimby, M. C., Carlson, C. P., and Owens, W. J., 1979, Lymphocystis virus: Infectivity of lesion preparations stored after lyophilization or simple desiccation, *J. Fish Dis.* **2**:259.

Yamamoto, T., 1974, Infectious pancreatic necrosis virus occurrence at a hatchery in Alberta, *J. Fish. Res. Board Can.* **31**:397.

Yamamoto, T., 1975*a*, Frequency of detection and survival of infectious pancreatic necrosis virus in a carrier population of brook trout (*Salvelinus fontinalis*) in a lake, *J. Fish. Res. Board Can.* **32**:568.

Yamamoto, T., 1975*b*, Infectious pancreatic necrosis (IPN) virus carriers and antibody production in a population of rainbow trout (*Salmo gairdneri*), *Can. J. Microbiol.* **21**:1343.

Yamamoto, T., Macdonald, R. D., Gillespie, D. C., and Kelly, R. K., 1976, Viruses associated with lymphocystis disease and dermal sarcoma of walleye (*Stizostedion vitreum vitreum*), *J. Fish. Res. Board Can.* **33**:2408.

Yasutake, W. T., 1970, Comparative histopathology of epizootic salmonid virus diseases, in: *A Symposium on Diseases of Fishes and Shellfishes* (S. F. Snieszko, ed.), pp. 341–350, Am. Fisheries Soc. Spec. Publ. 5.

Yasutake, W. T., and Rasmussen, C. J., 1968, Histopathogenesis of experimentally induced viral hemorrhagic septicemia in fingerling rainbow trout (*Salmo gairdneri*), *Bull. Office Int. Epiz.* **69**:977.

Yasutake, W. T., Parisot, T. J., and Klontz, G. W., 1965, Virus diseases of the Salmonidae in western United States. II. Aspects of pathogenesis, *Ann. N.Y. Acad. Sci.* **126**:520.

Zwillenberg, L. O., and Wolf, K., 1968, Ultrastructure of lymphocystis virus, *J. Virol.* **2**:393.

Zwillenberg, L. O., Jensen, M. H., and Zwillenberg, H. H. L., 1965, Electron microscopy of the virus of viral haemorrhagic septicaemia of rainbow trout (Egtved virus), *Arch. Gesamte Virusforsch.* **17**:1.

Zwillenberg, L. O., Pfitzner, I., and Zwillenberg, H. H. L., 1968, Infektionsversuche mit Egtved-virus an Zellkulturen und Individuen der Schleie (*Tinca vulgaris* Cuv.) sowie an anderen Fischarten, *Zentralbl. Bakteriol. Parasitenkd. Abt. I. Orig.* **208**:218.

CHAPTER 8

Viruses of Human Hepatitis A and B

William S. Robinson

Department of Medicine
Stanford University School of Medicine
Stanford, California 94305

1. INTRODUCTION: RECOGNITION OF HEPATITIS VIRUSES

Viral hepatitis is one of the diseases earliest recognized by man to be infectious. Hippocrates described infectious icterus more than 2000 years ago, and epidemic jaundice has been widely recognized since the Middle Ages. Hepatitis has occurred frequently in military and civilian populations during wars, and it sometimes approached the importance of plague and cholera as a cause of pandemics in Europe in past centuries. Apart from recognition of their contagious nature, little was known about the infectious agents until well into the present century.

Hepatitis agents were shown to have a size consistent with that of viruses in the 1940s (Havens, 1945*b*; Neefe *et al.*, 1946; McCollum, 1952), and the existence of more than one agent associated with the viral hepatitis syndrome was appreciated from studies of natural infections and experimental transmission studies in human volunteers (Neefe *et al.*, 1946; Voegt, 1942; MacCallum and Bradley, 1944; Havens *et al.*, 1944; Paul *et al.*, 1945; Ward *et al.*, 1958; Krugman *et al.*, 1962, 1967; Krugman and Giles, 1970). At least two agents designated infectious hepatitis (or hepatitis A) virus (HAV) and serum hepatitis (or hepatitis B) virus (HBV), were distinguished by differences in incubation period, by antigenic differences demonstrated in cross-protection transmission studies, by the regular presence of HAV and never HBV in feces of infected patients (HBV was regularly found in the blood), by the common occurrence of persistant infection with chronic carriage of HBV in the blood (never observed with HAV), and by the ability to prevent hepatitis A but not hepatitis B with immune serum globulin. Fecal–oral or contact transmission was associated with the sporadic and epidemic patterns of HAV infection, and HBV appeared to be transmitted percutaneously by blood and blood products, resulting in different epidemiological features.

Compared to the progress made with other viruses pathogenic for man, little further progress was made in understanding the nature of hepatitis viruses and their control until the last decade. In large part this was due to the failure to infect convenient experimental animals or tissue culture cells, so assays for infectious virus were possible only by transmission to human volunteers and more recently to a few additional primates.

The finding of a specific viral antigen for hepatitis B in blood in the 1960s (Blumberg et al., 1967; Okachi and Murakami, 1968; Prince, 1968), the transmission of HBV to chimpanzees (Barker et al., 1973), the successful infection of marmosets with HAV (Holmes et al., 1969, 1971), and the finding of viral antigen by immune electron microscopy in feces of patients after infection with HAV (Feinstone et al., 1973) led to the development of methods for detecting the infectious viruses, viral antigens, and viral antibodies. These developments permitted further characterization of both agents and led to a more complete understanding of the courses of infection and the epidemiology of both viruses.

The clinical distinctions between hepatitis A and hepatitis B were found not to be so clear as previously believed. Hepatitis B virus (HBV) is now known to be commonly transmitted by routes other than overt percutaneous ones, previously thought to be the exclusive manner of transmission. It is now clear that HAV and HBV are completely unrelated viruses and are quite different in structure. Although both infect liver cells primarily, there are significant biological differences. HBV is a DNA virus with a unique structure, and it does not fit into any of the recognized groups of viruses. However, a virus has been identified recently in eastern woodchucks which appears to have physical and biological characteristics simlar to those of HBV (Summer et al., 1978). It crossreacts immunologically only weakly with HBV. Thus HBV may be a member of a larger group of viruses, and members of the group may be widespread in nature.

HAV, on the other hand, appears to be a small RNA virus (Picornavirus) and should be classified as an enterovirus along with the coxsackie, ECHO, and polio viruses. Only HBV causes chronic or persistent infection, manifested by circulation in the blood of high concentrations of viral antigen in the form of defective or incomplete virus as well as infectious virus. This is a unique form of virus infection for man, occurs much more frequently than previously believed, and is associated with a variety of clinical syndromes, including hepatocellular carcinoma, which are not associated with HAV infection. Both viruses appear to naturally infect only man.

The use of specific serological tests to identify infections with HAV and HBV has led more recently to recognition of hepatitis following blood transfusions that is not caused by hepatitis A or B virus, or by other recognized viruses which may cause hepatitis, such as cytomegalovirus and Epstein-Barr virus (Feinstone *et al.*, 1975; Knodell *et al.*, 1975; Alter *et al.*, 1978). This indicates the existence of one or more additional agents which cause clinical hepatitis in man. Such agents have been transmitted to chimpanzees (Alter *et al.*, 1978).

2. HEPATITIS B VIRUS (HBV)

2.1. Infectious HBV

HBV has been shown to experimentally infect chimpanzees, gibbons, orangutans, and possibly rhesus monkeys (Barker *et al.*, 1975*b*) as well as man, although man appears to be the only host in nature. Other experimental animals have not been shown to be infected, and no reproducible infection of tissue culture cells has been reported. The concentration of infectious virus in the blood of chronically infected patients has been found to be quite high in some studies. Infection of human volunteers or chimpanzees has resulted from 1 ml inoculation of serum from carriers diluted 10^{-7} (Barker and Murray, 1972) and 10^{-8} (Robinson *et al.*, unpublished results). The agent has been shown to retain infectivity for humans when stored in serum at 30–32°C for 6 months (Redeker *et al.*, 1968) and frozen at -20°C for 15 years. All infectivity for human volunteers is not lost at 60°C for up to 4 hr (Murray and Diefenback, 1953) but is lost at 60°C for 10 hr when in albumin (Gellis *et al.*, 1948), although not completely in whole serum (Soulier *et al.*, 1972). Infectivity in serum was destroyed at 98°C for 1 min (Krugman *et al.*, 1970) or 20 min (Wewalka, 1953). Infectivity has also been destroyed by dry heat at 160°C for 1 hr (Salaman *et al.*, 1944).

2.2. Hepatitis B Surface Antigen

Australia antigen was discovered by Blumberg *et al.* (1965) while studying serum proteins, and it was not immediately recognized to be a viral antigen. Its eventual association with acute hepatitis B (Blumberg *et al.*, 1967; Okachi and Murakami, 1968; Prince, 1968) led to renaming it first hepatitis-associated antigen (HAAg) and then hepatitis B surface antigen (HB$_s$Ag). Since then there has been much progress in understanding the nature of this antigen and of hepatitis B virus (HBV).

Several particulate structures in serum are known to carry HB$_s$Ag determinants on their surfaces (see Figs. 1–3), and the antigen has not

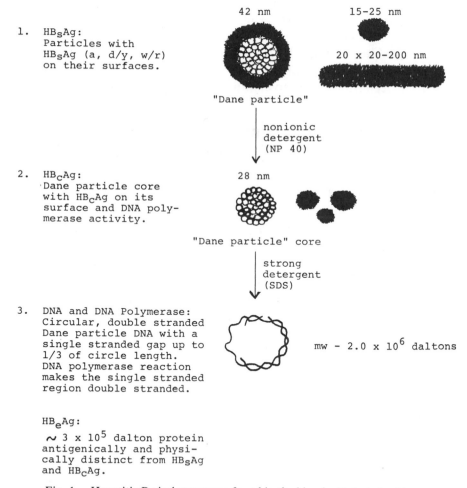

1. HB$_s$Ag:
    Particles with
    HB$_s$Ag (a, d/y, w/r)
    on their surfaces.

42 nm

15-25 nm

20 x 20-200 nm

"Dane particle"

nonionic
detergent
(NP 40)

2. HB$_c$Ag:
    Dane particle core
    with HB$_c$Ag on its
    surface and DNA poly-
    merase activity.

28 nm

"Dane particle" core

strong
detergent
(SDS)

3. DNA and DNA Polymerase:
    Circular, double stranded
    Dane particle DNA with a
    single stranded gap up to
    1/3 of circle length.
    DNA polymerase reaction
    makes the single stranded
    region double stranded.

mw – 2.0 x 10^6 daltons

HB$_e$Ag:
~ 3 x 10^5 dalton protein
antigenically and physi-
cally distinct from HB$_s$Ag
and HB$_c$Ag.

Fig. 1.   Hepatitis B viral structures found in the blood of infected subjects.

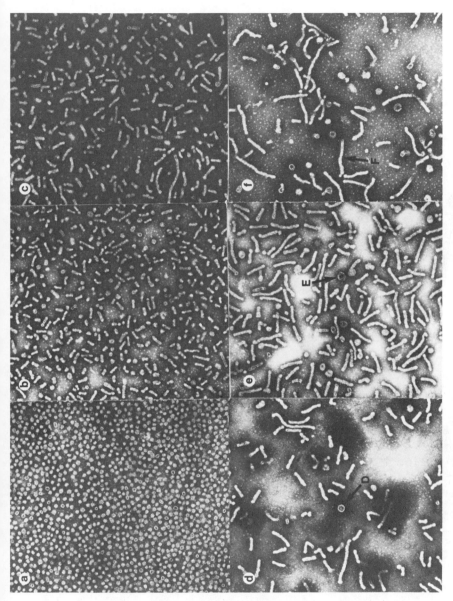

Fig. 2.   Electron micrographs of HB$_s$Ag forms from serum after sedimentation in a sucrose density gradient and examination of individual gradient fractions. Numerous small spherical particles, Dane particles with electron-dense centers (D), Dane particles with empty centers (E), and filamentous forms (F) can be seen. Modified from Gerin (Fractions *1* 1, 1976).

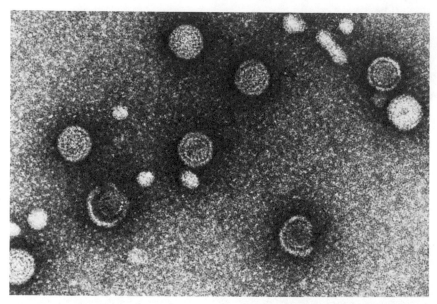

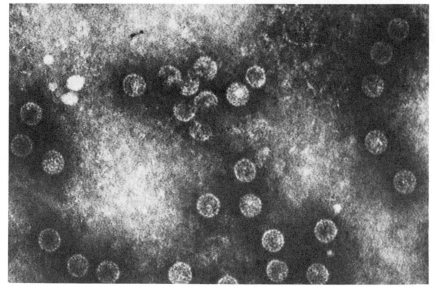

Fig. 3.   Electron micrographs of intact Dane particles (right) and Dane particle cores after Dane particle disruption with detergent (left). Kindly provided by June Almeida.

been found in a nonparticulate or low molecular weight form in serum (Alter and Blumberg, 1966; LeBouvier and McCollum, 1970). It is well established that the surface of the HB$_s$Ag-bearing particles is antigenically complex. At least five antigenic specificities may be present on HB$_s$Ag particles. A group-specific determinant (a) is shared by all HB$_s$Ag preparations, and two pairs of subtype determinants (d,y and w,r) which are for the most part mutually exclusive and thus usually behave as alleles have been demonstrated (LeBouvier, 1971; Bancroft *et al.*, 1972). Antigenic heterogeneity of the group-specific a and type-specific w determinants also appears to exist (Gibson, 1976). The eight HB$_s$Ag subtypes ayw$_1$, ayw$_2$, ayw$_3$, ayw$_4$, ayr, adw$_2$, adw$_4$, and adr have been identified. They have been very useful epidemiological markers. Isolated and usually single cases from the Far East with unusual combinations of HB$_s$Ag subtype determinants, such as awr, adwr, adyw, adyr, and adywr, have been reported. The subtype determinants in these cases are found on the same particles, suggesting that phenotypic mixing has occurred or unusual genetic recombinants have formed during mixed infections.

Evidence suggests that HB$_s$Ag is a virus-specified antigen. HB$_s$Ag appears in the blood early after infection with HBV (Shulman, 1971), and an antibody response to this antigen is associated with immunity (Trepo and Prince, 1976). Immunization with highly purified HB$_s$Ag particles results in protection against HBV infection (Purcell and Gerin, 1975) as does administration of γ-globulin with a high titer of antibody against HB$_s$Ag (anti-HB$_s$) (Grady *et al.*, 1975; Prince *et al.*, 1975; Redeker *et al.*, 1975; Seef *et al.*, 1975). The antigenic subtype found in secondary cases of hepatitis B virus infection is regularly the same as the subtype of the index case or the original source used in experimental infections (Le Bouvier, 1972; Mosley *et al.*, 1972), indicating that the subtype determinants are specified by the viral genome and not by the host. Other serological and epidemiological data are also consistent with HB$_s$Ag being a viral antigen (Shulman, 1971).

2.3. Hepatitis B Virion and Its DNA

The HB$_s$Ag form with the most complex structure and uniform appearance is the Dane particle (Dane *et al.*, 1970). It has an overall diameter of 42 nm (Dane *et al.*, 1970), HB$_s$Ag on its surface (Dane *et al.*, 1970; Almeida *et al.*, 1971), a lipid-containing outer layer or envelope (Robinson and Lutwick, 1976*b*), and an electron-dense 28-nm internal core or nucleocapsid (Dane *et al.*, 1970; Alameida *et al.*, 1971). Dane particles are illustrated in Figs. 1 and 3. Although there is no direct demonstration that the Dane particle is infectious, several properties suggest that it is HBV: (1) its surface antigen (HB$_s$Ag) is the viral antigen which induces protective antibody (anti-HB$_s$) (Purcell and Gerin, 1975); (2) its internal core or nucleocapsid contains a unique antigen, HB$_c$Ag (Almeida *et al.*, 1971), which is probably virus specified; (3) its size (Dane *et al.*, 1970) is consistent with estimates of the size of infectious HBV determined by ultrafiltration (McCollum, 1952); (4) its concentration in most sera (10^5–10^9 particles/ml) (Almeida, 1972) is consistent with titrations of infectivity in serum (Barker and Murray, 1972); (5) its concentration in sera appears to correlate with the probability that patients will transmit infection to contacts (Alter *et al.*, 1976; Okada *et al.*, 1976); (6) purified and concentrated preparations of Dane particles have been shown to be infectious at higher dilutions than previously shown for unfractionated HB$_s$g-positive serum (Thomssen *et al.*, 1977); (7) it is the only viral antigen form known to contain nucleic acid (DNA) (Robinson and Lutwick, 1976*b*); and (8) DNA reassociation experiments have shown that Dane particle DNA base sequences are present only in the DNA and RNA of infected liver and not in uninfected liver, and these sequences appear to be covalently attached to high molecular weight DNA (Lutwick and Robinson, 1977), as are other viral DNAs when integrated into chromosomal DNA (Sambrook *et al.*, 1968).

Unique properties of the hepatitis B virus include its ultrastructure, its antigenic composition, the size and structure of the small circular DNA within its core, and the presence of the DNA polymerase activity in the core (Robinson and Lutwick, 1976*b*).

In 1971 Hirschman *et al.* described small amounts of DNA polymerase activity in crude pellets obtained by high-speed centrifugation of three HB$_s$Ag-positive sera, and they postulated that the endogenous template was RNA because of results suggesting the reaction to be interrupted by RNase treatment of the enzyme preparation. Kaplan *et al.* (1973) found DNA polymerase activity in high-speed pellets from eight of eight HB$_s$Ag carriers with high concentrations of Dane particles in their serum. They found that the enzyme activity sedimented with Dane particles and with Dane particle cores after NP-40 treatment of Dane particles. Robinson and Greenman (1974) found that the enzyme-containing particles were specifically immunoprecipitated by anti-HB$_s$ and not anti-HB$_c$ before NP-40 treatment and by anti-HB$_c$ and not anti-HB$_s$ after NP-40 treatment, which removes the outer HB$_s$Ag layer of Dane particles and releases the inner core. These findings were consistent with the presence of DNA polymerase activity in the core of Dane particles or hepatitis B virions. Kaplan *et al.* (1973) showed that the DNA reaction product had a sedimentation coefficient of 15 S. The reaction was inhibited by actinomycin D and daunomycin, suggesting that the endogenous template was DNA, not RNA. The enzyme, the template, and the reaction product appeared to be internal components of the HBV core since DNase (and RNase) would not digest the template or the DNA product before disruption of cores and the enzyme failed to accept a wide variety of added polynucleotides which are accepted as primer/templates by other DNA polymerases.

Robinson *et al.* (1974) demonstrated that small circular DNA molecules could be isolated from purified Dane particles before or after a DNA polymerase reaction. Radioactive DNA reaction product sedimented with the circular molecules, indicating that these molecules and not RNA serve as the template for the DNA polymerases reaction. The circular molecules appeared to be double stranded, with a mean length of 0.78 μm, corresponding to approximately 1.6×10^6 daltons or 2300 nucleotide pairs (np) before a DNA polymerase reaction. No superhelical molecules were observed. Since Dane particles appear to be hepatitis B virions, the circular DNA from Dane particles is considered to be viral DNA. The thermal transition curve and buoyant density of DNA molecules made radioactive in a Dane particle DNA polymerase reaction were consistent with a cytosine plus guanosine content of 48–49%.

Several observations suggest that the circular DNA molecules from Dane particles contain a large single-stranded region of different length in different molecules and that the DNA polymerase reaction closes the single-stranded gaps. Summers *et al.* (1975) first proposed the existence of a single-stranded region in Dane particle DNA molecules because avain myeloblastasis virus (AMV) DNA polymerase, which contains no exonuclease activity and thus cannot introduce radioactive nucleotides into preexisting double-stranded DNA, successfully used Dane particle DNA as a template for DNA synthesis, presumably using a single-stranded part of the molecule. Because the endogenous DNA polymerase activity in Dane particles introduced radioactive nucleotides into the same restriction endonuclease *Hae*III-generated DNA fragments as did the AMV DNA polymerase, it was concluded that the endogenous enzyme used the same single-stranded regions as a template.

Hruska *et al.* (1977) showed that the electron microscopic length of the circular DNA molecules from Dane particles increased by an average of 23% when DNA was spread in formamide, which extends single-stranded regions compared with the length under aqueous spreading conditions, which do not extend such regions. This suggested that the circular DNA molecules contain single-stranded regions averaging one-fourth the length of the circle. After a Dane particle–DNA polymerase reaction, the mean circle length (aqueous spreading) increased by 27% and the length distribution became more homogeneous. This suggested that single-stranded regions of variable length were closed during the endogenous DNA polymerase reaction. Most of the circular molecules must have participated in the DNA polymerase reaction because the mean length of the population of molecules increased and the length distribution was greatly narrowed. The mean length of the DNA after an endogenous DNA polymerase reaction was 1.06 μm, corresponding to a molecular weight of approximately 2.1×10^6 or 3150 np for double-stranded DNA. No superhelical forms were observed in DNA after a DNA polymerase reaction, as none was before.

Landers *et al.* (1977) showed that DNA extracted from Dane particles before a DNA polymerase reaction and detected on polyacrylamide gels by ethidium bromide staining was electrophoretically heterogeneous. Treatment with the single-strand-specific endonuclease S1 produced double-stranded linear DNA molecules ranging in length from 1700 to 2800 np, indicating the presence of a nick or single-stranded region susceptible to the enzyme. After an endogenous DNA polymerase reaction, the S1-resistant double-stranded length was increased by 15–45% (average 25%) and made more homogeneous. The mean length of the elongated molecules was 3200 np. This length estimate is in good agreement with that determined by electron microscopy as described above. When the DNA was analyzed by endonuclease *Hae*III digestion, certain double-stranded DNA fragments increased in amount or first appeared only after an endogenous DNA polymerase reaction. These results are consistent with the existence of a single-stranded region of between 15% and 45% of the circle length in different DNA molecules and closure of the single-stranded gap during the endogenous DNA polymerase reaction.

Although the single-stranded gap appears to be closed by the endogenous DNA polymerase reaction, the ends of the open strand do not appear to be joined to make closed circular DNA. The circular molecules after the DNA polymerase reaction as before have a nuclease S1-sensitive site (Landers *et al.*, 1977), and no closed circular DNA has been detected by alkaline sucrose gradient sedimentation or equilibrium centrifugation in CsCl density gradients containing ethidium bromide (Robinson and Lutwick, 1976*a*).

The amount of DNA synthesis during the endogenous Dane particle DNA polymerase reaction has also been determined in two other ways. Lutwick and Robinson (1977) showed that the $C_0t_{1/2}$ value for the reassociation of the DNA synthesized in an endogenous Dane particle DNA polymerase reaction corresponded to an amount of unique DNA equivalent to about one-fourth of the circle length. This figure agrees with the amount of new DNA synthesis estimated by electron microscopic length change and change in electrophoretic mobility as described above.

Hruska and Robinson (unpublished results) carried out a Dane particle–DNA polymerase reaction with BrdUTP in place or TTP, isolated the DNA, denatured it by heating in dimethylsulfoxide, and separated DNA strands containing BrdU from light DNA by equilibrium centrifugation in CsCl density gradients. The buoyant density of the heavy DNA indicated that approximately one-third of each strand was new DNA (calculated as though 25% was BrdUMP), in good agreement with the other estimates of the amount of new DNA synthesis. The separated DNA fractions were also tested for ability to reassociate into double-stranded DNA to determine whether new DNA was synthesized on one or both strands of Dane particle DNA. None of the DNA in the heavy DNA component could be shown to reassociate into double-stranded DNA until DNA from the light component (or unfractionated Dane particle DNA) was mixed with it. This suggests that the new DNA synthesized in an endogenous Dane particle–DNA polymerase reaction consists of molecules without complementary base sequences indicating that they all represent the same strand of the Dane particle DNA.

In order to identify the primer for DNA synthesis in the endogenous Dane particle reaction, Robinson and Lutwick (1976a) examined the sedimentation of the Dane particle DNA in alkaline sucrose gradients after very short reaction times (average chain growth of five to ten nucleotides). They found that the DNA product was attached to a molecule with the sedimentation coefficient (11 S) corresponding to that of a linear DNA strand of approximately 1900 nucleotides mean length (Studier, 1965). This is near the length of the double-stranded region of the circular molecule before a DNA polymerase reaction (1700–2800 np by gel electrophoresis and an average of 2300 np by electron microscopy as described above), suggesting that the 3' end of the short strand of the circular DNA molecule serves as the primer for the reaction. No evidence for smaller oligodeoxynucleotides or an RNA primer was found. Thus it appears that Dane particle or HBV DNA consists of a long strand (a) of 3200 nucleotides in all molecules and a short strand (b) which varies in length between 1700 and 2800 nucleotides in different molecules.

Endogenous Dane particle DNA synthesis appears to be initiated at multiple sites over a large portion of the molecule. After very short reaction times (5 sec or 10 min) with a chain growth rate of five to ten nucleotides per minute under the conditions of low nucleotide concentration used, Landers *et al.* (1977) found that radioactive nucleotides were incorporated into endonuclease *Hae*III fragments with sizes totaling 1600 np. This is one-half the length of the circular Dane particle DNA molecule. After an extensive reaction (3–4 hr with high nucleotide concentrations) the same *Hae*III-generated fragments were heavily labeled. The wide distribution of sites for initiation of DNA synthesis indicates that the 3′ end of the short strand (b) occurs in different molecules at different sites within one-half of the molecule. This half of the molecule is between the single endonuclease *Eco*RI cleavage site in the DNA and the 5′ end of the short strand (Siddiqui *et al.*, 1979), as shown in Fig. 4. The 5′ end is at a unique site approximately 1600 np clockwise from the *Eco*RI site in the DNA of HBV/adw$_2$ oriented as shown in Fig. 4 and is the point at which endogenous DNA synthesis is terminated after the short strand has been fully elongated to 3200 nucleotides.

The long DNA strand (a) also contains a nick first postulated by Summers *et al.* (1975). This nick is at a unique site approximately 1860 np clockwise from the *Eco*RI site in the DNA of HBV/adw$_2$ oriented as shown in Fig. 4 (Siddiqui *et al.*, 1979). Thus a base-paired region of approximately 260 np exists between the 5′ end of the short strand and the nick in the long strand. This region can be selectively denatured by heating to convert circular molecules to linear forms (Sattler *et al.*, 1979). Such heat-generated linear molecules can be recircularized by incubating under appropriate annealing conditions. Reaction of heat linear molecules with nuclease S1 or avian myeloblastosis virus reverse transcriptase abolishes their ability to recircularize by respectively removing or making double-stranded the single-stranded ends. Figure 4 shows the locations of the unique physical features of the DNA within a map of restriction endonuclease cleavage sites for the DNA of HBV/adw$_2$.

DNA with a single-stranded region which is made double stranded by an endogenous DNA polymerase activity as found in HBV has not been described for other viruses. These features may be involved in DNA replication or integration into host DNA, but further work is needed to establish their role. Without a susceptible tissue culture

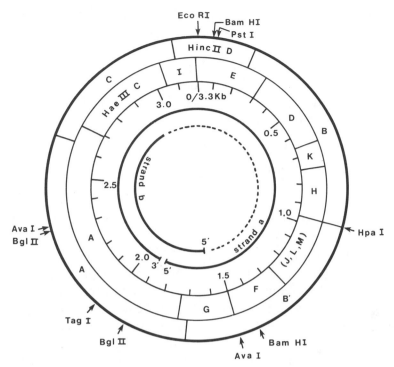

Fig. 4. Map of HBV DNA (HB_sAg subtype adw_2) (3.3 Kb) including cleavage sites for several restriction endonucleases and the locations of the nick in strand *a*, the 5' end of strand *b*, and the single-stranded region of the DNA. The 3' end of strand *b* in different molecules occurs at different sites within the region shown by the dotted line. The single-stranded region lies between the 3' and 5' ends of strand *b* and thus is of different length in different molecules.

system for this virus, however, investigation of these questions will be difficult.

Comparison of restriction endonuclease cleavage fragments of DNAs from viruses of different HB_sAg subtypes by gel electrophoresis has revealed both consistent differences among subtypes adw_2, ayw_3, and $adrq+$, and occasional differences within different viruses of the same subtype (Siddiqui *et al.*, 1979). The subtype differences indicate significant sequence differences in the DNAs of HBV of different subtypes and support the concept that this is viral DNA.

The DNA of HBV/adw_2 from a single HB_sAg carrier has recently been cloned in *E. coli* K12 using the unique *Eco*RI endonuclease cleavage site to introduce the viral DNA into an *Eco*RI cleavage site within the chloramphenicol resistance gene of the pACYC184 plasmid vector (Sninsky *et al.*, 1979). Restriction endonuclease analysis and hybridization studies indicated that the entire HBV DNA had been cloned. Examination of the restriction endonuclease fragments of the DNA from 20 different clones revealed no evidence of nucleotide sequence heterogeneity, a possibility suggested by previous findings with DNA from a single patient (Robinson, 1977). The sum of the sizes of the restriction fragments of cloned DNA was 3300 np in agreement with the size of DNA from HBV.

2.4. Incomplete Hepatitis B Viral Forms

The most numerous HB_sAg forms in the blood are small spherical particles with diameters between 16 and 25 nm ("22-nm particles") present in concentrations as high as 10^{13} particles/ml or more, and filamentous forms with diameters around 22 nm and variable lengths up to 1000 nm (Robinson and Lutwick, 1976b). Both are illustrated in Figs. 1 and 2. These forms consist of protein, carbohydrate, and lipid, and no HB_cAg or nucleic acid has been found in them. They are considered to be incomplete viral coat particles. Preparations of 22-nm particles consistently appear to contain small amounts of serum protein components (Millman et al., 1971; Neurath et al., 1974; Burrell, 1975) that have not been removed by extensive purification. Whether these are minor intrinsic constituents of the particles, or alternatively only avidly bound to the particle surface, or just contaminating the preparation and copurifying with HB_sAg in some cases is not yet clear.

Seven major polypeptides with apparent molecular weights between 20,000 and 100,000 have been isolated from purified preparations of HB_sAg 22-nm particles of subtypes adw, ayw, and adr (Shih and Gerin, 1977). The only serum component present in large enough amounts in purified HB_sAg preparations to be detected by Coomasie blue staining on SDS gels is apparantly human serum albumin, which comigrates as a separate polypeptide with one of the virus-specific polypeptides (Shih and Gerin, unpublished results). Two of the virus-specific polypeptides appear to be glycopeptides. Interestingly, several of the polypeptides which have been isolated and studied appear to contain the same group- and type-specific antigenic determinants (Gerin, 1974; Dreesman et al., 1975; Shih and Gerin, 1975; Gold et al., 1976), suggesting that the polypeptides are not unique but must share at least some amino acid sequences. Any subtype determinant is found only in polypeptides from HB_sAg particles of the same subtype.

Recent evidence suggests that the two major components (22,000 and 28,000 daltons, designated P22 and P28, respectively) may consist of identical polypeptide chains since they have identical sequences for 19 amino acid residues at the amino terminus and the same three residues at the carboxy terminus (Peterson *et al.*, 1978). The component with higher apparent molecular weight (P28) thus may differ from the smaller (P22) only by the presence of carbohydrate.

Since polypeptides not containing carbohydrate induce anti-HB$_s$, it is clear that the virus-specified antigenic determinants are contained in polypeptide rather than in carbohydrate of the glycoproteins. It is also clear that both group- and type-specific determinants reside on the same polypeptide. Thus polypeptides of different HB$_s$Ag subtypes may contain a region of constant amino acid sequence specifying the group-specific determinant a and a variable region specifying the type-specific determinant d or y. Multiple polypeptides of different apparent size, all of which contain the same antigenic determinants, have not been described for other viruses.

The amino acid compositions of P22 and P28 from HB$_s$Ag subtypes adw and awy are essentially indistinguishable (Peterson *et al.*, 1978). Amino acid sequence studies have revealed the following sequence from the amino terminus of P22 of HB$_s$Ag/ayw (Peterson *et al.*, 1978):

Met-Glu-Asn-Ile-Thr-Ser-Gly-Phe-Len-Gly-Pro-Leu-
Leu-Val-Ser-Gly-Ala-Gly-Phe----------Val-Tyr-Ile

The amino-terminal sequence for nine residues and the single carboxy-terminal residue (isoleucine) for P22's of HB$_s$Ag subtypes ayw and adw have been shown to be identical (Peterson *et al.*, 1977, 1978). Any sequence differences in the P22 of these subtypes must therefore exist in other regions of the polypeptides.

The above findings suggest that the amount of unique amino acid sequence specified by the HBV genome in HB$_s$Ag particles is probably significantly less than the sum of the sizes of the individual peptides isolated by SDS-gel electrophoresis. The minimum amount of unique amino acid sequence for the protein bearing the known HB$_s$Ag determinants is the amount in the smallest polypeptide shown to contain all the determinants (i.e., 22,000 daltons). How the different-sized polypeptides arise and their exact amino acid sequence relationship will require further study including sequence analysis.

2.5. Hepatitis B Core Antigen (HB$_c$Ag)

HB$_c$Ag is found in the blood only as an internal component of Dane particles as described above. Dane particle cores are illustrated in

Figs. 1 and 3. No free HB$_c$Ag has been detected in serum. HB$_c$Ag-bearing particles with the electron microscopic appearance of Dane particle cores have been isolated from homogenates of HBV-infected liver (Hoofnagle *et al.*, 1973). Such particles have been shown to contain DNA polymerase activity like that of Dane particles (Robinson and Lutwick, 1976*a*). However, most HB$_c$Ag particles from infected liver tissue appear to be empty and little or no DNA can be recovered. Similarly, Dane particles and Dane particle cores which do not manifest endogenous DNA polymerase activity and which band at a lower buoyant density in CsCl than particles with DNA polymerase activity have been found in the blood of some HB$_s$Ag carriers (Budkowska *et al.*, 1977; Hruska and Robinson, 1977), and these appear to be empty particles without DNA. Particles with the morphology of Dane particle cores have been seen in the nuclei of hepatocytes in electron micrographs of thin sections of HBV-infected liver (Almeida *et al.*, 1970; Caramia *et al.*, 1972; Huang, 1971). HB$_c$Ag is considered to be a virus-specified antigen because it has been found only during hepatitis B virus infection, there is an early and brisk antibody response to HB$_c$Ag during infection (Krugman *et al.*, 1974), and it is an internal component of one of the HB$_s$Ag forms, Dane particles (Almeida *et al.*, 1971).

Recent evidence indicates that highly purified Dane particle cores and liver-derived HB$_c$Ag particles contain a single predominant polypeptide of 17,000 (Budkowska *et al.*, 1977) or 19,000 daltons (Hruska and Robinson, 1977) in different studies. Smaller amounts of higher molecular weight polypeptides have also been found. The antigenic specificity of these polypeptides is not well defined, although recent evidence suggests that the 19,000 dalton polypeptide reacts with antibody to the hepatitis e antigen (anti-HB$_e$) as described in the following section.

Although the antigenic specificities of HB$_c$Ag from different sources have not been carefully compared, no antigenic heterogeneity or variation has been described.

2.6. Hepatitis B$_e$ Antigen (HB$_e$Ag)

The e antigen, discovered and named in 1972 (Magnius and Espmark, 1972), is physically and antigenically distinct from HB$_s$Ag and HB$_c$Ag (Nordenfeld and Kjellen, 1975). It is thought to exist in serum as a large protein with a size of approximately 300,000 daltons (Magnius, 1975), and it can be dissociated into smaller polypeptides

(Takahashi *et al.*, 1978). However, it has proven difficult to purify, and it is not well characterized chemically. HB$_e$Ag occurs exclusively in HB$_s$Ag-positive sera (Magnius *et al.*, 1975), and an antibody response to HB$_e$Ag is sometimes detected following HBV infection, suggesting that it may be an HBV-specified antigen. Recent evidence indicates that HB$_e$Ag is a complex of antigens, and more than one component is frequently detected by agar gel diffusion in the serum of a single patient (Williams and LeBouvier, 1976).

An intriguing feature of HB$_e$Ag is its common occurrence in sera of chronic HB$_s$Ag carriers with high concentrations of Dane particles (Alter *et al.*, 1976; Neilsen *et al.*, 1974). When detected by immunodiffusion, its presence thus correlates (as do Dane particles) with a propensity for transmission of infection to patient contacts (Alter *et al.*, 1976; Okada *et al.*, 1976; Grady *et al.*, 1976). Their regular occurrence together suggests that HB$_e$Ag and Dane particles (and HBV) may be related in some direct way, although a physical relationship has not been clearly established. A recent report indicates that HB$_e$Ag can be detected in Dane particle core preparations after treatment with sodium dodecylsulfate (SDS) and the HB$_e$Ag reactivity appears to correspond to the major polypeptide of core particles after dissociation with detergent (Takahashi *et al.*, 1979). This suggests that the polypeptides of Dane particle cores manifest different antigenic reactivity before (HB$_c$Ag) and after (HB$_e$Ag) detergent treatment. This report has not yet been confirmed, and more work will be required to finally establish the nature of this antigen.

2.7. Synthesis of HBV Antigens in Infected Liver

Immunofluorescent staining of tissue sections for viral antigens suggests that hepatocytes are the only cell type infected with HBV during persistent infection. No viral antigen synthesis has been detected in other tissues or cell types. During the acute phase of HBV infection, almost all hepatocytes appear to be infected. A variable number of hepatocytes contain detectable viral antigen at any given time during persistent infection. Liver tissue from persistently infected humans and chimpanzees has revealed different patterns of viral antigen synthesis in different cells. Immunofluorescent staining of liver sections for HB$_s$Ag and HB$_c$Ag has shown that most infected cells synthesize only HB$_s$Ag (in the cytoplasm), fewer cells synthesize only HB$_c$Ag (in the nucleus), and even fewer cells appear to synthesize both HB$_s$Ag and HB$_c$Ag

(Barker *et al.*, 1973; Gudat *et al.*, 1975; Ray *et al.*, 1976). The number of infected cells detected by immunofluorescence during persistent infection can vary from less than 1% to virtually 100% of hepatocytes in the liver, and the relative number synthesizing only HB_sAg, only HB_cAg, or both antigens varies widely in individual patients (Barker *et al.*, 1973; Ray *et al.*, 1976). In the liver of some chronic carriers, only cells synthesizing exclusively HB_sAg can be found (Barker *et al.*, 1973; Ray *et al.*, 1976).

In all chronic carriers producing relatively high concentrations of Dane particles, significant numbers of cells synthesizing HB_cAg can be found in the liver (Smith and Robinson, unpublished results). The observation that the number of cells synthesizing HB_sAg almost always exceeds the number synthesizing HB_cAg in most infected livers correlates with the fact that 22-nm spherical and filamentous HB_sAg forms greatly outnumber Dane particles in sera of most infected patients. The dramatic differences in the pattern of viral antigen synthesis in individual cells of chronically infected liver indicate that different viral genes are expressed in different cells, a phenomenon not described for tissues infected with other viruses.

2.8. Current Estimate of the Number of HBV Genes and the Total Virus-Specified Polypeptide

The size of the hepatitis B viral genome and the number of genes are not certain at this time, although as described above several probable viral gene products have been identified. The proteins containing HB_sAg, HB_cAg, and HB_eAg reactivity and that in Dane particles with DNA polymerase activity are probably all specified by viral genes. The total amount of unique virus-specified polypeptide is not known at this time, but a minimum estimate would include the smallest amount of unique polypeptide sequence containing all known HB_sAg determinants (which appears to be 22,000 daltons) and the polypeptides of HB_cAg particles (that is, at least a 19,000 dalton polypeptide). Additional polypeptide may or may not be required for HB_eAg since the 19,000 dalton polypeptide of HB_cAg particles as described above may contain the HB_eAg specificity. Additional virus-specific polypeptides may also exist in HB_cAg particles, including one or more necessary for the DNA polymerase activity. Although the polypeptide with DNA polymerase activity has not been characterized or shown to be virus coded, nucleic acid polymerases of several other viruses are known to be specified by the viral genome.

3. COURSE OF HBV INFECTION

3.1. Self-Limited HBV Infection

HB$_s$Ag is usually the first viral marker to appear in the blood after HBV infection. The presence of this antigen is considered to be synonymous with infection. HB$_s$Ag can usually be detected by complement fixation 6–12 weeks after exposure to HBV (Shulman, 1971), as shown in Fig. 5, but can be detected as early as 3 weeks in some patients when very sensitive assays are used (Hoofnagle *et al.*, 1978). Evidence of hepatitis usually follows in an average of 4 weeks (usual range 1–7 weeks). In self-limited infections, HB$_s$Ag usually remains detectable in the blood for 1–6 weeks (Shulman, 1971), although it may persist for up to 20 weeks (Hoofnagle *et al.*, 1978). Patients who remain HB$_s$Ag positive less than 7 weeks rarely appear to develop symptomatic hepatitis. The severity of hepatitis has been roughly correlated with the duration of HB$_s$Ag positivity in patients with self-limited experimental infections (Hoofnagle *et al.*, 1978). As symptoms and jaundice clear, the HB$_s$Ag titer usually falls, and HB$_s$Ag becomes undetectable in most symptomatic patients several weeks after resolution of hepatitis.

Dane particles detected by their DNA polymerase activity appear in the blood of most patients soon after the appearance of HB$_s$Ag, rise to high concentrations during the late incubation period of hepatitis B,

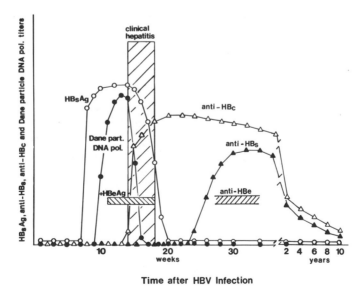

Fig. 5. Hepatitis B viral markers in the blood during the course of self-limited HBV infection.

and fall with the onset of hepatic disease (Kaplan *et al.*, 1974; Krugman *et al.*, 1974), as shown in Fig. 5.

Limited studies suggest that HB_eAg may be another regular and early marker of HBV infection (Magnius *et al.*, 1975; Talbot *et al.*, 1977) as depicted in Fig. 5.

A marker of infection which appears in virtually all patients and before the onset of hepatic injury in most is anti-HB_c, the antibody directed against the internal antigen of HBV. Anti-HB_c can usually be detected 3–5 weeks after the appearance of HB_sAg in the blood and before the onset of clinically apparent hepatitis (Krugman *et al.*, 1974; Hoofnagle *et al.*, 1978), as shown in Fig. 5. Anti-HB_c titers usually rise during the period of HB_sAg positivity, level off, and eventually fall after HB_sAg becomes undetectable. The highest titers of anti-HB_c appear in the patients with the longest period of HB_sAg positivity. Anti-HB_c titers fall three- to fourfold in the first year following acute infection and then more slowly (Hansson, 1977). Anti-HB_c can still be detected by immunoelectroosmophoresis 5–6 years after acute infection in most patients (Hansson, 1977). The good correlation between the prevalence of anti-HB_c detected by immunoelectroosmophoresis (Hansson, 1976) or RIA (Hoofnagle *et al.*, 1978) and anti-HB_s detected by RIA indicates that the two antibodies persist for a similar time after acute infection.

Antibody to HB_sAg (anti-HB_s) has been shown to appear during antigenemia and before the onset of clinically apparent hepatitis in the 10–20% of patients who develop arthritis and rash associated with immune complex formation (Gocke, 1975). In most patients with self-limited HBV infection, however, anti-HB_s can be detected only after HB_sAg disappears from the blood (Shulman, 1971; Krugman *et al.*, 1974; Lander *et al.*, 1970, 1972), as illustrated in Fig. 5. Anti-HB_s cannot be detected even by the most sensitive tests in many patients immediately after HB_sAg disappears. There is a time interval of up to several months between the disappearance of detectable HB_sAg and the appearance of anti-HB_s in approximately one-half of patients with self-limited infections (Krugman *et al.*, 1974; Hoofnagle *et al.*, 1978). In approximately 10% of patients with transient antigenemia, anti-HB_s never appears when tested for by the most sensitive assays (Hoofnagle *et al.*, 1978). In patients with measurable anti-HB_s responses, the antibody titer rises slowly during recovery and may still be rising 6–12 months after disappearance of HB_sAg (Krugman *et al.*, 1974; Hoofnagle *et al.*, 1978). In contrast to the anti-HB_c response, the highest titers of anti-HB_s appear in those with the shortest period of antigenemia (Hoofnagle *et al.*, 1978). This antibody may persist for years after HBV infection and is associated with protection against reinfection (Purcell and Gerin, 1975; Krugman and Giles, 1973; Barker *et al.*, 1975*a*).

The antibody response to HB_eAg has not been well studied in self-limited HBV infections. Limited studies have shown that after the disappearance of HB_eAg, anti-HB_e detected by immunodiffusion appears in 10–20% of individuals convalescing from acute hepatitis B (Eleftheriou *et al.*, 1975; Smith *et al.*, 1976).

3.2. Persistent HBV Infection

Patients who remain HB_sAg positive for 20 weeks or longer are very likely to remain positive indefinitely and be designated chronic HB_sAg carriers. Approximately 10% of adults hospitalized with acute hepatitis in one study (Redeker, 1975) and 5% adults after experimental infection in another (Hoofnagle *et al.*, 1978) became persistently infected. Several factors, including low infecting virus dose, mild or inapparent initial hepatitis, and very young age, appear to favor development of persitent infection. Prolonged infection appears to be the rule for chronic carriers, and one carrier has been documented to have remained HB_sAg positive for 20 years (Zuckerman and Taylor, 1969). Spontaneous termination of the carrier state, although unusual, can occur at any time (Redeker, 1975). No precise information about the duration of the carrier state for any population is available. Most HB_sAg in the serum of chronic carriers as well as patients with acute hepatitis B is in the form of 20-nm particles (Alter and Blumberg, 1966), and tests for the antigen essentially detect that form. The titer of HB_sAg appears to be relatively constant during persistent infection, although enough fluctuation may occur so that HB_sAg falls below the level of detection and then reappears in some carriers with low HB_sAg titers (Hoofnagle *et al.*, 1978; Edgington and Chisari, 1975).

Although commonly undetectable or present in low concentrations in chronic HB_sAg carriers, high concentrations of Dane particles persist in 5–10% of carriers, and the high level may remain for years (Robinson, 1975), as illustrated in Fig. 6. A spontaneous fall in Dane particle levels occurs in such patients infrequently (Robinson, unpublished results).

HB_eAg has been detected by immunodiffusion in 10–40% of HB_sAg carriers in different studies and anti-HB_e in a similar number

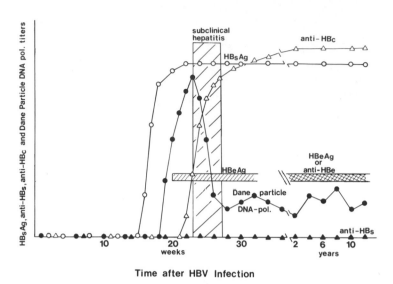

Time after HBV Infection

Fig. 6. Hepatitis B viral markers in the blood during the course of HBV infection which becomes persistent.

(Eleftheriou *et al.*, 1975; Smith *et al.*, 1976: Neilsen *et al.*, 1974; Fay *et al.*, 1977).

Anti-HB$_c$ is present in all persistently infected patients (Hoofnagle *et al.*, 1975, 1978), as shown in Fig. 6. The titers of anti-HB$_c$ are significantly higher during persistent infection than in most self-limted infections or in convalescence (Hoofnagle *et al.*, 1978).

Anti-HB$_s$ has been detected as a complex with HB$_s$Ag in most persistently infected patients (Edgington and Chisari, 1975), although free anti-HB$_s$ is not detected by standard assays because HB$_s$Ag is in excess. Anti-HB$_s$ is clearly present in HB$_s$Ag-positive individuals with syndromes associated with immune complex formation (Gocke, 1975). It is not known whether the anti-HB$_s$ response is quantitatively diminished during persistent infection, although the regular presence of this antibody and anti-HB$_c$ would suggest that immunological tolerance does not account for persistent infection.

4. DISEASE ASSOCIATED WITH HBV INFECTION

4.1. Acute and Chronic Hepatitis B

A wide spectrum of hepatic and extrahepatic disease may be associated with acute and persistent HBV infections. Acute viral hepatitis results in direct hepatocellular injury, and the histopathology of acute hepatitis B is indistinguishable from that of acute hepatitis A (Peters, 1975). Acute viral hepatitis may vary in severity from very mild changes in the liver and no symptoms to fulminant hepatitis with extensive hepatocellular necrosis leading to death.

Chronic HBV infection may be associated with a histologically normal liver and normal liver functions. More often, the syndrome of chronic persistent hepatitis (CPH) occurs; it is not associated with progressive liver disease, although mild histological and liver function abnormalities are present. Chronic HBV infection may also be associated with chronic active hepatitis (CAH), which can progress to cirrhosis. In one series of 429 patients hospitalized with acute hepatitis B, 10% became persitent HB_sAg carriers and of these 70% had chronic persistent hepatitis and 30% chronic active hepatitis (Redeker, 1975).

The mechanisms of hepatic injury in acute and chronic hepatitis B are not well understood. Because many self-limited as well as persistent infections are not associated with significant hepatic injury, it is possible that HBV does not cause cytopathic effects when replicating in hepatic cells. Many investigators believe that the liver injury of acute and chronic hepatitis B may be mediated for the most part by the immune response (Chisari *et al.*, 1978). Although some evidence supports this view, more work is needed to establish it.

4.2. Hepatocellular Carcinoma

In areas of the world where HB_sAg carrier rates are very high, as many as 80% of patients with hepatocellular carcinoma have HB_sAg in their blood (Szmuness, 1978) and most have postnecrotic cirrhosis. This suggests the possibility that in some cases hepatocellular carcinoma may be causally related to HBV infection. The association is not so great in the United States (Szmuness, 1978), where the frequency of HBV infection is much less and hepatocellular carcinoma occurs most often in the setting of alcoholic liver disease.

4.3. Other Disease Syndromes Associated with HBV Infection

Several disease syndromes with extrahepatic manifestations have been associated with HBV infection, and in some cases there is evidence suggesting that HB_sAg–anti-HB_s complexes may play an important role in disease pathogenesis (Gocke, 1975, 1978). In the serum sickness-like syndrome consisting of rash, urticaria, arthralgias, and sometimes acute arthritis which occurs in 10–20% of patients during the incubation period of acute hepatitis B, HB_sAg–antibody complexes and low levels of complement components have been regularly observed in serum, synovial fluid, and synovial membranes from involved joints (Schumacher and Gall, 1974; Wands *et al.*, 1975).

Thirty to forty percent of patients with biopsy-proven polyarteritis nodosa have persistent HBV infection (Gocke, 1975). Among all HB_sAg carriers this syndrome occurs infrequently (1 in 500 in a recent series, Redeker, 1975). These patients have low serum complement levels and circulating HB_sAg–anti-HB_s complexes. Immune complexes and complement components have also been regularly detected in diseased vessels by immunofluorescent staining (Gocke *et al.*, 1971; Fye *et al.*, 1977).

Several well-studied cases of a membranous glomerulonephritis associated with chronic active hepatitis and persistent HBV infection have been reported (Gocke, 1975). Immune complex deposits have been observed along the subepithelial surface of glomerular basement membranes by electron microscopy, and nodular depositis of HB_sAg, immune globulin, and C3 in glomeruli have been demonstrated by immunofluorescent staining in these cases (Combes *et al.*, 1971; Kohler *et al.*, 1974; Knieser *et al.*, 1974; Ozawa *et al.*, 1976; McIntosh *et al.*, 1976).

Infantile papular acrodermatitis has been found to be associated with persistent HBV infection with a high frequency in Mediterranean countries (Gianotti, 1973) and Japan (Ishimaru *et al.*, 1976). In one series of 19 patients with essential mixed cryoglobulinemia, cryoprecipitates were shown to contain HB_sAg in six cases and anti-HB_s in 11 (Levo *et al.*, 1977), suggesting that some cases of cryoglobulinemia may be related to HBV infection. Further studies are needed to clarify the pathogenesis of these syndromes and determine whether HB_sAg–antibody complexes or HBV infection in some other way plays an important role.

5. EPIDEMIOLOGY OF HBV

5.1. Total Viral Hepatitis in the United States

Between 50,000 and 60,000 cases per year of acute viral hepatitis have been reported to the Center for Disease Control (1977*a,b*) in recent years. These figures probably greatly underestimate the true incidence of infection with hepatitis viruses because 5–10 times as many subclinical as clinically apparent infections probably occur (Szmuness *et al.*, 1973; Barker and Murray, 1971; Schober *et al.*, 1972). Correction for significant underreporting has permitted an estimation that more than 300,000 clinically apparent cases of acute viral hepatitis occur each year in the United States (Hoff *et al.*, 1973).

Before the availability of specific testing for hepatitis B, the mortality from posttransfusion hepatitis was between 5% and 10% in most studies. Most of these cases were undoubtedly hepatitis B. The mortality of hepatitis B acquired by other routes of transmission is probably significantly lower. For all acute viral hepatitis cases reported to the CDC in the years 1973–1975 the fatality rates were about 1%.

5.2. HBV Infections in the United States

In 1975, 51% of all reported viral hepatitis patients in the United States who were tested were HB_sAg positive (Center for Disease Control, 1977*a,b*). The incidence of HBV infections estimated by frequency of HB_sAg and/or anti-HB_s positives differs significantly in different populations within the United States. Different socioeconomic groups clearly have different risks for infection. The frequency of anti-HB_s was found to be 44%, 18%, and 10% for people over age 30 in New York City sections of Harlem, Staten Island, and Park Avenue, respectively (Cherubin *et al.*, 1972). High infection rates have been found in percutaneous drug abusers, patients frequently receiving blood products, hemodialysis patients, laboratory personnel working with human sera, some institutionalized populations such as children and the mentally retarded, prostitutes, and homosexual populations.

5.3. HBV Infections in Other Parts of the World

The epidemiology of HBV infections in Western European countries is similar to that in the United States but differs significantly in underdeveloped and tropical areas of the world. Infection occurs at very early ages and by adulthood virtually all have acquired anti-HB_s in tropical Africa, Southeast Asia, and Oceania.

5.4. Persistent HBV Infection

Persistent or chronic HBV infection (usually designated the HB_sAg carrier state) is one of the most common persistent viral infections in man. It has been estimated that more than 170 million people in the world today are persistently infected with HBV (Szmuness, 1975).

Patients HB$_s$Ag positive for more than 6 months following acute hepatitis B are considered to be chronic carriers, although a small number of patients become HB$_s$Ag negative after this time. Infrequently, long-established carriers become HB$_s$Ag negative (Redeker, 1975) having apparently cleared the virus. However, most remain infected for many years (Zuckerman and Taylor, 1969), and infection for life is probably the rule. Good data for the duration of the carrier state, however, are not available for any population.

The HB$_s$Ag carrier rate varies over a wide range from 0.01% to 20% in different populations. To a great extent the incidence of the HB$_s$Ag carrier state in populations is related to the incidence of primary infection, but clearly there are also host and viral factors which appear to increase the risk for developing persistent infection. These may become quite important in determining the carrier rates for some epidemiological groups. A possible genetic predisposition for persistent infection has been suggested by family studies in which the chronic carrier state appears to cluster in families and segregate as an autosomal recessive trait (Blumberg et al., 1969; Grossman et al., 1975). An association between persistent infection and certain HLA types has also been reported (Hillis et al., 1977). Other studies have failed to confirm either of these findings (Stevens and Beasley, 1976; Patterson et al., 1977), and the question of a genetic predisposition remains unsettled.

The severity of initial disease and age also appear to influence the probability for developing persistent infection. Persistent infection occurs more frequently after initial anicteric hepatitis compared with initial icteric disease (Barker and Murray, 1972; Krugman, 1972). Survivors of fulminant hepatitis rarely become persistently infected, and HB$_s$Ag carriers frequently give no history of recognized acute hepatitis (Redeker, 1975). Approximately 10% of adults hospitalized with acute hepatitis B in this country have been shown to become chronically infected (Redeker, 1975). In contrast, persistent infection almost invariably follows acute neonatal hepatitis B, which is usually anicteric (Schweitzer et al., 1973). The HB$_s$Ag carrier state appears to be most common in the age group around 15–19 years, and the frequency in males is several times that in females in this age group (Mosley, 1972; Blumberg, 1972).

Anecdotal cases suggest that immunosuppression may be associated with milder initial hepatitis B and more frequent persistent infection than in immunological normals. Persistent HBV infection also appears to be more common in patients with certain diseases such as Down's syndrome, lepromatous leprosy, and chronic lymphocytic leukemia than in the general population (Blumberg, 1972). Although the mechanism by which each of the above leads to persistent infection is not clear, a common mechanism could be a modified or inadequate immune response so that the virus is not eliminated, as it is after most acute infections.

The infecting dose of HBV has also been clearly shown to correlate with the probability of developing persistent infection. Experimental infections with different dilutions of infectious serum have shown that lower doses of virus result more often in long incubation periods, mild initial disease, and subsequent chronic infection than do larger virus doses (Barker and Murray, 1972).

There is no evidence that hepatitis B virus strains (e.g., HB_sAg subtypes) have different virulence or propensity for persistent infection.

There are great differences in HB_sAg carrier rates in different populations in this country and different areas of the world. In most parts of the United States less than 0.1% of volunteer blood donors have been found to be HB_sAg positive (Shulman, 1971), and almost all of these are chronic HB_sAg carriers. The carrier rate in paid donors is usually closer to 1%. Among certain populations such as percutaneous drug abusers, patients in some hemodialysis centers, and certain homosexual populations, the carrier rate may be 1–5% (Szmuness *et al.*, 1975). These high rates are probably due to the frequent exposure to virus experienced by these groups. The carrier rates in most Western European countries are similar to those in the United States (Shulman, 1971). In areas of the world such as many countries in Africa, Asia, and Oceania, carrier rates may approach 20% of the population (Shulman, 1971; Blumberg, 1972). Not only may the increased rates in some underdeveloped countries be related to poor sanitary conditions and increased exposure at very early ages, but also there could be differences in predisposition for chronic infection on a genetic, nutritional, or other basis in different populations. Transmission of virus from persistently infected mothers to newborn infants who then usually develop persistent infection appears to be a significant means by which high carrier rates are maintained in some populations. The common occurrence of neonatal infection in some populations and the large number of carriers in the world suggest that it may be difficult to completely eliminate HBV by vaccination programs.

5.5. HBV Transmission

Blood and blood products are the best-documented vehicles of HBV infection. HB_sAg has also been found in feces, urine, bile, sweat, tears, saliva, semen, breast milk, vaginal secretions, cerebrospinal fluid, synovial fluid, and cord blood. Only serum (Barker and Murray, 1972), saliva (Alter *et al.*, 1977), and semen (Alter *et al.*, 1977) have actually been shown to contain infectious HBV in experimental transmission studies. Consistent with the presence of HBV in human saliva is the report of transmission by a human bite (Center for Disease Control, 1974). More than 50 attempts to transmit HBV to human volunteers using feces from experimentally infected subjects have been unsuccessful (Havens, 1946*b*; MacCallum, 1951; Neefe *et al.*, 1945), suggesting that infectious HBV probably enters feces infrequently in the absence of gastrointestinal bleeding. Other body fluids have not been tested for infectious virus. Often the concentrations of HB_sAg are low in fluids other than serum, if detected at all. Antigen can sometimes be demonstrated only after concentration. If infectious virus is present in such fluids, its concentration may also be lower than that in serum. Infrequently infectious HBV has been found in blood without detectable HB_sAg, so that the failure to detect antigen does not exclude the presence of infectious virus.

All natural routes of HBV transmission and their relative importance may not be recognized at this time. Direct percutaneous inoculation of virus by needles can occur with contaminated blood or blood products, hemodialysis, tatooing, ear piercing, acupuncture, drug abuse, or accidental needle sticks by hospital personnel. HBV is also transmitted by routes other than these overt parenteral ones. Infectious material contacting open skin breaks or mucous membranes such as the eye can also result in infection.

In areas of the world where HBV infection rates are much higher than in the United States and the opportunity for virus transmission by overt parenteral routes is less, other routes of transmission must be common. Crowded or close living conditions, such as occur among family members of the same household and among institutionalized children, favor transmission. The exact route of transmission in such circumstances is not clear. The failure to find infectious virus in feces as described above would suggest that fecal–oral transmission is probably not a common route. Infection after oral intake of infectious material has, however, been clearly shown (Krugman and Giles, 1970). It may be that infection does not occur via the intestinal tract in these cases but through small breaks postulated to regularly exist in the oral mucosa. When infectious material was placed directly in the stomachs of two susceptible chimpanzees it failed to result in infection, but after their gums had been lightly brushed with a tooth brush they were infected with an oral spray of infectious material (Center for Disease Control, 1977a,b).

Evidence consistent with an intestinal phase of HBV infection is the occurrence of appreciable levels of anti-HB_s IgA in feces of patients convalescing from hepatitis B (Ogra, 1973). HB_sAg and HB_cAg have not been detected by immunofluorescence in cells of any tissue except liver, however, and further investigation is needed to establish whether intestinal or other mucosal surfaces actually contain cells susceptible to infection by HBV.

Persistent viremia is a favorable condition for virus transmission by blood-feeding insects. Although some populations of wild mosquitoes and bedbugs caught in Africa (Prince et al., 1972; Brotman et al., 1973; Willis et al., 1977) and the United States (Dick et al., 1974) have been shown to contain HB_sAg, there has been no direct demonstration of transmission to man by insect vectors. HBV is not known to infect insects as do arboviruses, so that passive transfer would be required.

Because HBV is quite stable, transmission by way of environmental surfaces which may contact mucous membranes or open skin breaks such as tooth brushes, baby bottles, toys, eating utensils, or razors (Gocke, 1974; Pattison et al., 1974) or hospital equipment such as respirators or endoscopes (Morris et al., 1975; McDonald and Silverstein, 1975) can be expected. Food and water appear to be unusual sources of virus for human HBV infections. HB_sAg has been detected in clams from costal waters into which untreated sewage drained (Mahoney et al., 1974). Despite this finding, published outbreaks of shellfish-associated hepatitis have been non-type B.

Transmission between heterosexual as well as male homosexual partners appears to occur commonly (Szmuness et al., 1975; Wright, 1975), but whether the route of transmission is venereal or nonvenereal is not proven. The demonstration of infectious virus in semen and saliva of infected patients (Alter et al., 1977) supports the possibility of venereal transmission.

Neonatal transmission from chronic carrier mothers (Okada et al., 1976) and mothers with acute hepatitis B in the third trimester or first 2 months postpartum (Schweitzer et al., 1973) has been clearly documented, although whether the mechanism involves infection at delivery or infection after delivery via maternal milk or other routes has not been shown. In these cases cord blood has been shown to be HB$_s$Ag negative, suggesting that transplacental infection is not common if it occurs. Increased rates of abortion, stillbirth, or developmental anomalies have not been reported in association with maternal HBV infection.

Health care personnel have been shown to be at greater risk for HBV infection than the general population (Lewis *et al.*, 1973; Mosley *et al.*, 1975; Maynard, 1978), undoubtedly because of their more frequent exposure to infected patients. The specific routes of transmission from patients to medical and dental workers is not known, although it appears that the greater the direct exposure to blood and serum—e.g., as by surgeons (Maynard, 1978; Rosenberg *et al.*, 1973) and workers in renal dialysis units (Maynard, 1978)—the greater the frequency of HBV infection.

The presence of significant Dane particle concentrations and HB$_e$Ag detected by immunodiffusion in the blood has recently been shown to correlate with transmission of infection from carrier mothers to neonates (Okada *et al.*, 1976), from carriers to health care personnel accidentally inoculated with contaminated needles (Alter *et al.*, 1976; Grady *et al.*, 1976), and from carrier health care personnel to patient contacts (Smith and Robinson, unpublished results). The regular appearance of Dane particles in high concentrations in the serum of patients during the late incubation period of acute hepatitis B (Kaplan *et al.*, 1974; Krugman *et al.*, 1974) suggests that this may be a time when patients are highly infectious, as appear to be the few chronic HB$_s$Ag carriers with high Dane particle levels in their blood. The very frequent transmission of infection from mothers with acute hepatitis B during the third trimester of pregnancy or the first 2 months postpartum (Schweitzer *et al.*, 1973) is consistent with this possibility.

6. HEPATITIS A VIRUS (HAV)

6.1. Infectious HAV

HAV, like HBV, has a very restricted host range. In addition to humans, HAV has been shown to experimentally infect several species of South American *Sanguinus* marmoset (tamaran) monkeys and chimpanzees. *S. fuscicollis*, *S. nigricollis* (white-lipped marmoset), and *S. oedipus* (cotton-topped marmoset) infection was first clearly shown by Deinhardt and co-workers (Holmes *et al.*, 1969, 1971) in studies using

control and virus-containing specimens under code. Marmoset susceptibility has been confirmed and extended the more more susceptible *S.
mystax* (white-mustached marmoset) (Hillis, 1968; Lorenz *et al.*, 1970;
Mascoli, 1973; Provost *et al.*, 1973). Human convalescent serum has
been shown to neutralize the infectivity for marmosets (Provost *et al.*,
1973; Holmes *et al.*, 1973). *S. labiatus* (known also as *Jacchus
rufiventer* or *Markina labiata*) and *S. mystax* are the most susceptible
species to HAV infection, *S. nigricollis* and *S. fusciocollis* are intermediate, and *S. oedipus* is among the most resistant species. Serial
passage of HAV in marmosets results in adaptation, with shortening of
incubation period. Prolonged passage in rufiventer marmosets has
yielded virus which infects 100% of these animals with an incubation
period of only 7 days (Provost *et al.*, 1977). High titers of HAV were
found in liver tissue. Marmoset infection results in mild illness with histological and biochemical changes similar to those in man.

A hepatitis-A-like illness was observed in the 1960s in animal
caretakers after close exposure to chimpanzees (Hillis, 1961, 1963;
Mosley *et al.*, 1967), suggesting that HAV might infect that species.
Following the development of assays for hepatitis A antigen (HAAg)
and antibody to HAAg (anti-HA), experimental transmission of HAV
to chimpanzees by oral and parenteral routes was demonstrated (Maynard *et al.*, Dienstag *et al.*, 1975*b*). The hepatitis following HAV infection of chimpanzees is extremely mild. Attempts to infect other primates
as well as lower animal species have not been clearly successful to date
(Dienstag *et al.*, 1978*a*).

Although extensive efforts over many years failed to demonstrate
infection of tissue culture cells with HAV from human sources, a recent
report indicates successful infection of fetal marmoset liver explants
and fetal rhesus monkey kidney cells in culture with the marmoset-
adapted CR326 strain of HAV (Provost and Hilleman, 1979). This
important advance should lead to much greater understanding of the
nature of the virus and its replication, and enhance the prospects for
vaccine development.

Infectious HAV has been shown to pass through a Seitz filter
which retains bacteria (Neefe *et al.*, 1946), indicating that the agent has
a size smaller than that of bacteria. No more precise sizing of the
infectious agent has been reported.

Limited information is available on the stability of HAV to
chemical and physical agents. HAV infectivity for human volunteers
was destroyed by boiling for 20 min (Wewalka, 1953) and by exposure
to 160°C dry heat for 60 min (Salaman *et al.*, 1944), but has survived

60°C for 1 hr (Provost *et al.*, 1973). Infectivity of HAV in water was also destroyed by chlorination, and the concentration required depended on the organic content of the water (Neefe *et al.*, 1947). HAV has also been inactivated by ultraviolet irradiation and formalin but not by ether or acid (pH 3 for 3 hr) (Provost *et al.*, 1973). The virus is stable during storage at 4°C and −20°C.

6.2. Hepatitis A Antigen (HAAg) Forms in Feces, Liver, and Bile

In 1973 Feinstone *et al.* described viruslike particles in the feces of patients experimentally infected with HAV. The particles were immunoprecipitated by serum from patients in the convalescent phase but not the acute phase of hepatitis A, interpreted to indicate the appearance of antibody directed against these particles during the illness. The particles were considered to be hepatitis A viral antigen forms. Similar particles were observed during natural infections, and their presence in feces were associated in time with the illness. The particles were uniform in size and appearance, being spherical structures 27 nm in diameter (Fig. 7). Both full and empty particles were observed. Similar particles were observed in liver, bile, and serum of HAV-infected *Sanguinus mystax* (Provost *et al.*, 1975). Most HAAg particles purified from infected human feces (Moritsugu *et al.*, 1976; Siegl and Frosner, 1978*a*) and chimpanzee feces (Bradley *et al.*, 1975; Schulman *et al.*, 1976) and from marmoset liver (Provost *et al.*, 1975) have been demonstrated to have a buoyant density in CsCl of approximately 1.34 g/ml. Empty particles banded at density 1.29–1.30 g/ml (Siegl and Frosner 1978*a*; Schulman *et al.*,1976; Feinstone *et al.*, 1974; Bradley *et al.*, 1977*a*). Another less well-defined component of HAAg has been found in the density range 1.38–1.44 g/ml (Moritsugu *et al.*, 1976; Bradley *et al.*, 1977*a*). This component is variable in amount in different preparations. The sedimentation coefficient of full particles has been shown to be 160 S (Siegl and Frosner, 1978*a*). The size and appearance in electron micrographs, the buoyant density, and the sedimentation coefficient are similar to those of poliovirus (Siegl and Frosner, 1978*a*).

Biochemical characterization of HAAg particles has been greatly impaired by the very limited amounts of material available from any source. Coulepais *et al.* (1978) analyzed the polypeptides of 27-nm HAAg particles purified from the feces of HAV-infected patients. Three polypeptides with approximate molecular weights of 34,000,

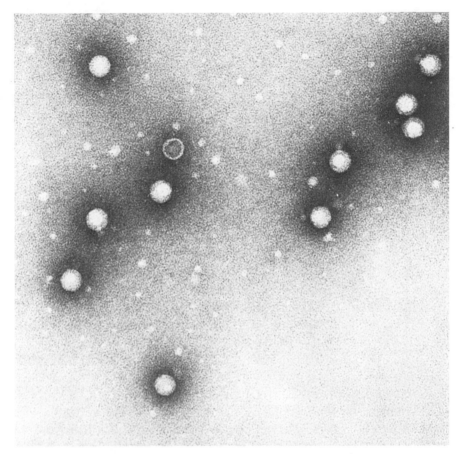

Fig. 7. Electron micrograph (196,000×) of HAV particles highly purified from human feces and stained with 1% phosphotungstic acid. Kindly provided by John L. Gerin.

25,500, and 23,000 were detected by Coomasie blue staining after electrophoresis in polyacrylamide gels containing sodium dodecylsulfate (SDS). Gerin and colleagues (Feinstone *et al.*, 1978) observed similar peptides detected by radiolabeling purified HAAg particles with I^{125}. In addition, a 59,000 dalton polypeptide and a polypeptide of approximately 7000–9000 daltons were observed. The smallest three polypeptides are near the sizes of polypeptides VP1, VP2, and VP3 of poliovirus (Maizel *et al.*, 1967). The 59,000 dalton polypeptide, however, is larger than polio VP0, which is an uncleaved precursor of VP2 and VP4 (Maizel and Summers, 1968). More work will be required to resolve the differences found in these two studies and more completely characterize the polypeptides of HAAg particles.

Studies of the nucleic acid in HAAg particles have been even more difficult than polypeptide characterization. HAAg particles have been reported to emit orange-red color when stained with acridine range, suggesting the presence of single-stranded nucleic acid, and infectivity appeared to be partially inactivated by RNase treatment (Provost et al., 1975).

In more recent studies, HAAg particles were disrupted with urea and formamide on electron microscope grids and structures resembling single-stranded nucleic acid were observed (Siegl and Frosner, 1978b). Alkali eliminated these molecules but not ϕ174 DNA, suggesting that HAAg preparations contain RNA. Molecular lengths from 0.5 to 3.5 μm and two length distribution peaks around 1.2 and 1.7 μm were observed for HAAg nucleic acid compared with 0.5–3.0 μm range and peaks of 1.2 and 2.3 μm for poliovirus RNA used as a control. Thus significant poliovirus RNA breakage occurred in these experiments, and it is not possible to draw conclusions about the precise length of the RNA extracted from the HAAg preparation. Gerin and colleagues (Feinstone et al., 1978) have confirmed these findings and found that the nucleic acid extracted from HAAg particle preparations was susceptible to RNase and not DNase.

Thus HAAg particles from feces and liver tissue have many characteristics of enteroviruses such as poliovirus and these particles undoubtedly represent hepatitis A virions.

Although no reports of careful comparison of the antigenic specificity of HAAg from different sources have appeared, there is no suggestion of antigenic heterogeneity or variation at this time. Protection of individuals by passive immunization in areas of the world different from the source of immune serum globulin used (Woodson and Clinton, 1969; Conrad, 1971) indicates that HAV is antigenically similar in different parts of the world.

6.3. Viral Antigen Synthesis in Infected Liver

Direct immunofluorescent staining of liver tissue of experimentally infected chimpanzees (Mathiesen et al., 1977) and marmosets (Mathiesen et al., 1978) has shown specific staining in a finely granular pattern in the cytoplasm and not in the nucleus of hepatocytes. Positive cells were distributed diffusely throughout the liver. Other tissues including small and large bowel mucosa failed to reveal evidence of viral antigen synthesis. Thus, no evidence of an intestinal phase of replication was found after infection by parenteral inoculation. Whether oral infection may result in gastrointestinal tract infection remains to be determined.

The cytoplasmic localization of HAAg by immunofluorescence is consistent with the finding of 27-nm particles (indistinguishable from those in feces) in vesicles within hepatocyte cytoplasm of experimentally infected chimpanzees by electron microscopy (Schulman *et al.*, 1976). Similar particles have been observed in bile (Schulman *et al.*, 1976; Bradley *et al.*, 1976).

The cytoplasmic location of HAAg is consistent with the cellular site of synthesis of other small RNA viruses such as polio (Franklin and Rosner, 1962; Franklin and Baltimore, 1962; Dales *et al.*, 1965).

7. COURSE OF HAV INFECTION

Only limited studies on the sequence of viral events early in HAV infection in man have been done, because specific serological testing was not available in the 1940s and 1950s when studies of experimental infection of human subjects were done. Recent chimpanzee and marmoset models of HAV infection have permitted more extensive studies of early events. Although infection in both animal models appears to be similar to that in man and the sequence of events is probably the same, the actual time course of infection may not be the same in each host.

In the chimpanzee, the first evidence of infection is the appearance of HAAg detected by immunofluorescent staining in liver 1–2 weeks after infection (Mathiesen *et al.*, 1977). (Fig. 8). At this time 27-nm-virus-like particles can be observed in vesicles within hepatocyte cytoplasm by electron microscopy (Schulman *et al.*, 1976). In the marmoset, antigen has been observed in the liver as early as 1 week after infection (Provost *et al.*, 1977). Within a few days, HAAg can be detected in feces (Mathiesen *et al.*, 1977; Bradley *et al.*, 1976) and bile (Schulman *et al.*, 1976; Bradley *et al.*, 1976) by immune electron microscopy (IEM) and radioimmunoassay (RIA) in these animals. In experimentally infected humans, HAAg has been detected in feces several days before and usually has reached a maximum amount about the time of the first liver function abnormality (Dienstag *et al.*, 1975*a*; Rakela and Mosley, 1977; Flehmig *et al.*, 1977). Bile may be the source of fecal HAAg since antigen has not been detected in bowel mucosa after parenteral inoculation of chimpanzees or marmosets (Mathiesen

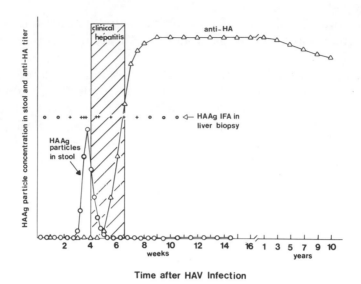

Fig. 8.   Hepatitis A viral markers in blood, liver, and feces during the course of HAV infection.

et al., 1977, 1978). Whether bowel mucosa is infected after oral inoculation is unknown. Antigenemia has been detected before the onset of disease (Mathiesen *et al.*, 1978), but its onset and duration are not well defined.

In most studies fecal HAAg excretion detected by IEM has appeared to end before the peak serum glutamic-oxalic transminase activity (SGOT) (Dienstag *et al.*, 1975*a*; Rakela and Mosley, 1977; Flehmig *et al.*, 1977; Hopkins and Scott, 1976). In general, the studies of fecal HAAg are consistent with the studies of fecal infectivity described in Section 10.

Viral antigen can be detected by IFA in liver longer than by RIA in blood or feces. HAAg has been found in chimpanzee liver for 4–5 weeks total, and low levels were regularly present even after liver functions had returned to normal (Mathieson *et al.*, 1977).

Anti-HA detected by immune adherence hemagglutination (IAHA) rises in titer following acute hepatitis A to a maxium in around 10–16 weeks (Krugman *et al.*, 1975; Rakela *et al.*, 1977). The immunoglobulin class containing most of the anti-HA in acute phase sera (between onset of symptoms and peak of icterus) is IgM and in convalescent sera it is IgG (Bradley *et al.*, 1977*b*). Anti-HA can be detected for many years following most infections.

8. IMMUNITY TO HAV

HAV infection appears to result in solid immunity, and reinfections, if they occur, must be unusual. Experimental transmission of infectious hepatitis virus (Neefe *et al.*, 1946; Havens, 1945*a*) or serologically documented HAV (Krugman *et al.*, 1967) to human volunteers and subsequent rechallenge has shown resistance to reinfection by the same virus and no resistance to serum hepatitis virus (Neefe *et al.*, 1946; Havens, 1945*a*), or serologically documented HBV (Krugman *et al.*, 1967). Studies of multiple episodes of apparent viral hepatitis by natural routes of transmission have not found individuals with more than a single episode of HAV infection, although HAV infection can follow HBV and *vice versa* (Karvountzis *et al.*, 1975; Mosley, 1975*b*; Mosely *et al.*, 1977). These studies indicate that homologous immunity develops with first infections with HAV and no apparent heterologous immunity to HBV infection results.

9. DISEASE ASSOCIATED WITH HAV INFECTION

The histopathological changes in liver during acute hepatitis A are indistinguishable from those during acute hepatitis B. The mechanism of hepatic injury in acute hepatitis A is unknown. Because very limited amounts of HAAg have been available, the specific cellular immune response during HAV infection and its role in hepatic injury have not been studied.

No cases of chronic hepatitis following serologically documented HAV infection have been described.

10. EPIDEMIOLOGY OF HAV INFECTIONS

The epidemiologies of HAV and HBV differ because of significant differences in their biological behavior. Persistent infection with continuous viremia as occurs with HBV does not occur with HAV. Thus transmission by blood via parenteral routes, which is common for HBV, almost never occurs with HAV. No form of persistent infection has been documented for HAV and no animal or other reservoir is known, so this virus must be maintained in a population by serial transmission from acute cases to susceptibles. In isolated populations of limited size, HAV has actually been found to disappear after an epi-

demic which followed its introduction from outside and then reappear
years later when again brought in from outside (Maynard, 1963). This
behavior in small isolated populations is similar to that of measles,
mumps, rubella, and poliomyelitis viruses (Black *et al.*, 1974), which do
not commonly cause persistent infection in man and for which no
reservoir outside of man is known.

The most important mode of spread of HAV is by person-to-
person contact via the fecal–oral route. These and other features of
HAV determine its behavior in populations, which has been summarized by Mosley (1975*a*) to include (1) a cyclic tendency with an epidemic surge after a sufficient number of susceptibles have accumulated,
(2) age-specific attack rates that are highest among children of primary
or nursery school age, (3) a distinctive seasonal cycle, (4) higher attack
rates in rural than in urban communities, (5) high secondary attack
rates among household members, giving familial aggregations, (6) a
reduction in incidence among exposed persons promptly given small
doses of almost any normal immunoglobulin preparation, and (7) a
consistently low case fatality rate.

10.1. Incidence of HAV Infection

The number of hepatitis cases in the United States which are type
A specifically is not precisely known because of the difficulty in carrying out extensive epidemiological studies and surveillance due to a
general scarcity of reagents needed for HAV serological testing. It is
clear, however, that the highest incidence is usually among children and
adolescents in highly endemic areas as well as in many epidemics
(Davis and Hanlon, 1946), that males and females appear to be equally
susceptible (Dienstag *et al.*, 1978*b*), and that the highest incidence in
the United States in past years has occurred during autumn and winter.

Several studies have revealed great differences in incidence of anti-
HA in the populations of different areas of the world (Dienstag *et al.*,
1978*b*; Szmuness *et al.*, 1977). The highest rates of HAV infection are
in economically developing countries where housing and sanitation are
poor. In such areas antibody appears at very early ages and most infections at these ages appear to be subclinical and anicteric (Villarejos *et
al.*, 1976). In a representative study, by adulthood more than 90% of
the population in a developing country was found to have antibody,
compared with around 20% in the United States (Villarejos *et al.*,
1976).

In the United States a correlation between socioeconomic status and the presence of antibody to HAAg has been shown and is similar to findings with HBV. Lower socioeconomic groups have a higher incidence of anti-HA than upper socioeconomic groups (Szmuness *et al.*, 1976). Rates of HAV infection are particularly high in circumstances where there is group living under crowded conditions such as in schools, military institutions, prisons, and custodial facilities (Dienstag *et al.*, 1978*b*). A detailed review of seroepidemiological studies employing HAV-specific testing has recently been published (Dienstag *et al.*, 1978*b*).

Experimental transmission studies have clearly demonstrated that HAV infections may be associated with subclinical and anicteric hepatitis (Krugman *et al.*, 1962), and most natural infections are probably associated with subclinical disease. Serological testing has shown that 30–50% of adult populations in the United States have been infected with HAV, although only 3–5% of adults can recall an illness suggesting or documented to be hepatitis (Dienstag *et al.*, 1978*b*). In general, HAV infections appear to result in milder illness than HBV infections. HAV infection is a relatively infrequent cause of fulminant hepatitis (Rakela *et al.*, 1975). The mortality of HAV infections is not well established but must be very low. There is no evidence that chronic liver disease ever follows HAV infection.

10.2. Routes of HAV Transmission

10.2.1. Fecal–Oral Transmission of HAV

The most common manner of HAV transmission is clearly through close person-to-person contact, probably almost always by the fecal–oral route. HAV has been shown to infect humans when given by mouth (Krugman *et al.*, 1962; Havens *et al.*, 1944; Giles *et al.*, 1964; Boggs *et al.*, 1970; Findlay and Willcox, 1945). Infectivity of feces in the preicteric and icteric phases of hepatitis A after experimental and natural infections of man has also been shown on many occasions using transmission to both human subjects and susceptible animals to detect virus (Krugman *et al.*, 1959, 1962; Havens *et al.*, 1944; Deinhardt *et al.*, 1975; Havens, 1946*b*; Neefe *et al.*, 1945). No infectivity has been found 4 weeks or more before, or 19 days or more after, the onset of jaundice. These figures probably define the outside limits for virus shedding in most infected patients.

The period when HAAg particles can be detected by immune electron microscopy or radioimmunoassay in feces of infected patients (see Section 7) is consistent with the data on fecal infectivity. The greatest numbers of HAAg particles have been found in the late incubation period and at the time of onset of symptoms (Dienstag *et al.*, 1975*a*; Frosner *et al.*, 1977; Rakela and Mosley, 1977; Flehmig *et al.*, 1977; Hopkins and Scott, 1976). Excetion of particles in most studies has appeared to end before the peak of serum transaminase activity or the onset of jaundice.

Epidemiological data on spread of HAV in households (Rakela and Mosley, 1977; Knight *et al.*, 1954) and institutions (Ward *et al.*, 1958; Batten *et al.*, 1963) and after transmission from primary cases via drinking water (Mosley and Smithers, 1957) or food (Leger *et al.*, 1975; Dull *et al.*, 1963; Denes *et al.*, 1977) indicate that most secondary cases occur approximately one incubation period after onset of symptoms in the index case, suggesting that patients are most infectious in the late incubation period or about the time symptoms begin.

10.2.2. Nonfecal Sources of HAV in Contact Transmission

There is little evidence for important sources of virus other than feces to account for contact transmission. Respiratory secretions contain infectious HAV infrequently (MacCallum and Bradley, 1944) if at all (Havens, 1946*a*; Neefe and Stokes, 1945), and transmission by contact or aerosol via such secretions would be an unlikely event. Urine collected just before or at the time on onset of jaundice appears to contain low levels of infectious HAV in only a few patients (Giles *et al.*, 1964; Findlay and Willcox, 1945; Havens, 1946*a*; MacCallum and Bradley, 1944; Neefe and Stokes, 1945), and it seems unlikely that urine is commonly involved in infections in contact transmission in the community.

Epidemiological evidence suggests that venereal transmission is not common. Serological evidence of past HAV infection in populations with high numbers of sexual contacts such as homosexuals has not been found to exceed that in controls such as blood donors (Szmuness *et al.*, 1976) and persons applying for marriage licenses (Mosley, 1978).

No cases of intrauterine infection with HAV have been reported.

10.2.3. Viremia and Percutaneous HAV Transmission

Transient viremia has been documented after HAV infection. Percutaneous transfer of blood or serum, however, appears to be a very infrequent route of transmission. Data on the period when infectious virus is present in the blood are less complete than for fecal virus, and virus has been found in blood only during the latter half of the incubation period (Krugman *et al.*, 1962; Giles *et al.*, 1964; Boggs *et al.*, 1970; Havens, 1946a; Barker *et al.*, 1977; Francis *et al.*, 1946). The time when viremia is terminated in most patients is not well established, and the period of viremia may vary in different patients. Because the data on infectivity in blood and on antigenemia are quite limited, more investigation with improved methods will be needed to conclusively establish the frequency, duration, and precise time limits of viremia in HAV infections in man. Consistent with the infectivity data in man is the period of antigenemia in experimentally infected chimpanzees, which has been found to be transient and exclusively during the late incubation period of hepatitis A.

Because the incubation period of hepatitis A and the period of viremia are much shorter than for hepatitis B, and persistent infection does not occur, the period for potential percutaneous transmission of HAV from asymptomatic patients is much less than for HBV. Epidemiological evidence is consistent with this. Multiply transfused children have been found to have a much higher frequency of anti-HB$_s$ than nontransfused populations, but the frequency of anti-HA has been found to be the same (Stevens *et al.*, 1978). Patients and staff of hemodialysis centers have been found to have no higher incidence of anti-HA (unlike anti-HB$_s$) than expected for non-dialysis-associated groups of similar demography (Szmuness *et al.*, 1977). Recent studies of posttransfusion hepatitis have failed to reveal cases of hepatitis A by specific serological testing (Feinstone *et al.*, 1975; Knodell *et al.*, 1975; Alter *et al.*, 1975; Dienstag *et al.*, 1977). Thus, although percutaneous transmission of HAV is theoretically possible, except for experimental transmission it has not been demonstrated to occur and it probably plays an insignificant role in infections in the community.

10.2.4. Other Modes of HAV Transmission

Besides spread of HAV by close personal contact, water and food clearly been documented vehicles for transmission of hepatitis A virus. Although private water supplies contaminated with sewage have most often been the reported sources of water-borne disease (Bryan *et al.*, 1974; Rindge *et al.*, 1962; Tucker *et al.*, 1954), public water systems have also been implicated (Mosley *et al.*, 1959; Poskauzer and Beadenkoph, 1961; Morse *et al.*, 1972). Numerous examples of epidemic and endemic hepatitis A have been associated with ingestion of raw shellfish contaminated with sewage (Ross, 1956; Mason and McLean, 1962; Dougherty and Altman, 1962; Ruddy *et al.*, 1969; Koff and Sear, 1967; Portnoy *et al.*, 1975; Dienstag *et al.*, 1976*b*; MacKowiak *et al.*, 1976). Milk-borne hepatitis A has been described (Murphy *et al.*, 1946; Raska *et al.*, 1966) and thought to be caused by contaminated water used to wash milk containers and equipment. Transmission via other food and drink has been reported on numerous occasions (Read *et al.*, 1946; Ballance, 1954; Joseph *et al.*, 1965; Philip *et al.*, 1973; Levy *et al.*, 1975; Meyers *et al.*, 1975; Dienstag *et al.*, 1975*c*; Schoenbaum *et al.*, 1976; Barker *et al.*, 1977; Eisenstein *et al.*, 1963), and in some instances a food handler with hepatitis A has been implicated as the source (Read *et al.*, 1946; Joseph *et al.*, 1965; Philip *et al.*, 1973; Levy *et al.*, 1975; Meyers *et al.*, 1975).

Many cases of hepatitis following contact with chimpanzees and a few other nonhuman primates have been reported (Hillis, 1961; Davenport *et al.*, 1966; Mosley *et al.*, 1967; Ruddy *et al.*, 1967; Friedmann *et al.*, 1971). Such cases have been confirmed serologically to be type A hepatitis (Dienstag *et al.*, 1976*a*). Animals in captivity with previous contact with man have been involved. The animals in these cases were probably first infected by contact with man rather than being infected in the wild. The infection is associated with subclinical illness in nonhuman primates.

Much of the epidemiological, experimental transmission, and serological evidence concerning HAV transmission has recently been reviewed in detail by Mosley (1978).

11. REFERENCES

Almeida, J. D., 1972, Individual morphological variation seen in Australia antigen positive sera, *Am. J. Dis. Child.* **123**:303.

Almeida, J. D., Waterson, A. P., Trowell, J. M., and Neal, G., 1970, The findings of virus-like particles in two Australia-antigen-positive human livers, *Microbios* **2**:145.

Almeida, J. D., Rubenstein, D., and Stott, J. E., 1971, New antigen–antibody system in Australia-antigen-positive hepatitis, *Lancet* **2**:1225.

Alter, H. J., and Blumberg, B. S., 1966, Further studies on a "new" human isoprecipitin system (Australia antigen), *Blood* **27**:297.

Alter, H. J., Purcell, R. H., Holland, P. V., Feinstone, S. M., Morrow, A. G., and Moritsugu Y., 1975, Clinical and serological analysis of transfusion-associated hepatitis, *Lancet* **2**:838.

Alter, H. J., Seeff, L. B., Kaplan P. M., McAuliffe, V. J., Wright, E. C., Gerin, G. L., Purcell, R. H., Holland, P. V., and Zimmerman, H. J., 1976, Type B hepatitis:

The infectivity of blood positive for e antigen and DNA polymerase after accidental needlestick exposure, *New Engl. J. Med.* **295**:909.

Alter, H. J., Purcell, R. H., Gerin, J. L., London, W. T., Kaplan, P. M., McAuliffe, V. J., Wagner, J., and Holland, P. V., 1977, Transmission of hepatitis B to chimpanzees by hepatitis B surface antigen-positive saliva and semen, *Infect. Immun.* **16**:928.

Alter, H. J., Purcell, R. H., Feinstone, S. M., Holland, P. V., and Morrow, A. G., 1978, Non A/non B hepatitis: A review and interium report of an ongoing prospective study, in: *Viral Hepatitis: A Contemporary Assessment of Etiology, Epidemiology, Pathogenesis and Prevention* (G. N. Vyas, S. N. Cohen, and R. Schmid, eds.), p. 358, Franklin Institute Press, Philadelphia.

Ballance, G. A., 1954, Epidemic of infective hepatitis in an Oxford college, *Br. Med. J.* **1**:1071.

Bancroft, W. H., Mundon, F. K., and Russell, P. K., 1972, Detection of additional antigenic determinants of hepatitis B antigen, *J. Immunol.* **109**:842.

Barker, L. F., and Murray, R., 1971, Acquisition of hepatitis associated antigen: Clinical features in young adults, *J. Am. Med. Assoc.* **216**:1970.

Barker, L. F., and Murray, R., 1972, Relationship of virus dose to incubation time of clinical hepatitis and time of appearance of hepatitis associated antigen, *Am. J. Med. Sci.* **263**:27.

Barker, L. F., Chisari, F. V., McGrath, P. P., Dalgard, D. W., Kirschstein, R. L., Almeida, J. W., Edgington, T. S., Sharp, D. G., and Peterson, M. R., 1973, Transmission of type B viral hepatitis to chimpanzees, *J. Infect. Dis.* **127**:648.

Barker, L. F., Maynard J. E., Purcell, R. H., Hoofnagle, J. H., Berquist, K. R., London, W. T., Gerety, R. J., and Krushak, D. H., 1975*a*, Hepatitis B virus infection in chimpanzees: Titration of subtypes, *J. Infect. Dis.* **132**:451.

Barker, L. F., Maynard J. E., Purcell R. H., Hoofnagle, J. H., Berquist, K. R., and London, W. T., 1975*b*, Viral hepatitis, type B, in experimental animals. *Am. J. Med. Sci.* **170**:189.

Barker, L. F., Dienstag, J. L., Lorenz, D. E., Purcell, R. H., Wong, D. C., Feinstone, S. M., Peterson, M. R., and Rosen, M. W., 1977, Serologic and animal inoculation studies of a communal outbreak of viral hepatitis, type A., *Am. J. Med. Sci.* **274**:247.

Batten, P. L., Runte, V. E., and Skinner, H. G., 1963, Infectious hepatitis: Infectiousness during the presymptomatic phase of the disease. *Am. J. Hyg.* **77**:129.

Black, F. L., Hierholzer, W. J., Pinheire, F., Evans, A. S., Woodall, J. P., Opton, E. M., Emmons, J. E., West, B. S., Edsall, G., Downs, W. G., and Wallace, G. D., 1974, Evidence for persistence of infectious agents in isolated human populations, *Am. J. Epidemiol.* **100**:230.

Blumberg, B. S., 1972, Australia antigen: The history of its discovery with comments on genetic and family aspects, in *Hepatitis and Blood Transfusion* (G. H. Vyas, H. A. Perkins, and R. Schmid, eds.), p. 63, Grune and Stratton, New York.

Blumberg, B. S., Alter, H. J., and Visnich, S., 1965, A "new" antigen in leukemia sera, *J. Am. Med. Assoc.* **191**:541.

Blumberg, B. S., Gerstley, B. J. S., London, W. T., and Sutnick, A. I., 1967, A serum antigen (Australia antigen) in Down's syndrome, leukemia and hepatitis, *Ann. Intern. Med.* **66**:924.

Blumberg, B. S., Friedlander, J. S., Sutnick, A. I., and London, W. T., 1969, Hepatitis and Australia antigen: Autosomal recessive inheritance of susceptibility to infection in humans, *Proc. Natl. Acad. Sci. USA* **62**:1108.

Boggs, J. D., Melnick, J. L., Conrad, M. E., and Felsher, B. F., 1970, Viral hepatitis—Clinical and tissue culture studies, *J. Am. Med. Assoc.* **214**:1041.

Bradley, D. W., Hornbeck, C. L., Graville, C. R., Cook, E. H., and Maynard, J. E., 1975, CsCl banding of hepatitis A-associated virus-like particles, *J. Infect. Dis.* **131**:304.

Bradley, D. W. Hollinger, F. B., Hornbeck, C. L., and Maynard, J. E., 1976, Isolation and characterization of hepatitis A virus, *Am. J. Clin. Pathol.* **65**:876.

Bradley, D. W., Gravelle, C. R., Cook, E. H., Fields, R. M., and Maynard, J. E., 1977*a*, Cyclic excretion of hepatitis A virus in experimentally infected chimpanzees, *J. Med. Virol.* **1**:113.

Bradley, D. W., Maynard, J. E., Hindman, S. H., Hornbeck, C. L., Fields, H. A., McCaustl, K. A., and Cook, E. H., 1977*b*, Serodiagnosis of viral hepatitis A: Detection of acute-phase immunoglobulin M anti-hepatitis A virus by radioimmunoassay, *J. Clin. Microbiol.* **5**:521.

Brotman, B., Prince, A. M., and Godfrey, H. K., 1973, Role of arthropods in transmission of hepatitis B virus in the tropics, *Lancet* **1**:1305.

Bryan, J. A., Lehmann, J. D., Stetiady, I. F., and Hatch, M. H., 1974, An outbreak of hepatitis A associated with recreational lake water, *Am. J. Epidemiol.* **99**:145.

Budkowska, A., Shih, J. W., and Gerin, J. L., 1977, Immunochemistry and polypeptide composition of hepatitis B core antigen (HBcAg), *J. Immunol.* **118**:1300.

Burrell, C. J., 1975, Host components in hepatitis B antigen, *J. Gen. Virol.* **27**:117.

Caramia, F., DeBac C., and Ricci, G., 1972, Virus-like particles within hepatocytes of Australia antigen carriers, *Am. J. Dis. Child.* **123**:309.

Center for Disease Control, 1974, Hepatitis transmitted by a human bite, *Morbidity and Mortality Weekly Report 23*, 24.

Center for Disease Control, 1977*a*, *Hepatitis Surveillance Report No. 39*.

Center for Disease Control, 1977*b*, *Hepatitis Surveillance Report No. 41*.

Cherubin, E. C., Purcell, R. H., Lander, J. J., McGinn, T. G., and Cone, L. A., 1972, Acquisition of antibody to hepatitis B antigen in three socioeconomically different medical populations, *Lancet* **2**:149.

Chisari, F. V., Edgington, T. S., Routenberg, J. A., and Anderson, D. S., 1978, Cellular immune reactivity in hepatitis B Virus induced liver disease in: *Viral Hepatitis: A Contemporary Assessment* (G. N. Vyas, S. N. Cohen, and R. Schmid, eds.), p. 245, Philadelphia, Franklin Institute Press.

Combes, B. Stastny, P. Shorey, J., Eigenbrodt, E. H., Barbera, A., Hull, A. R., and Carter, N. W., 1971, Glomerulophritis with deposition of Australia antigen-antibody complexes in glomerular basement membrane, *Lancet* **2**:234.

Conrad, M. E., 1971, Prophylactic gamma globulin for prevention of endemic hepatitis: Effects of U.S. gamma globulin upon incidence of viral hepatitis and other infectious diseases in U.S. soldiers abroad, *Arch. Intern. Med.* **128**:723.

Coulepais, A. G., Locarnini, S. A., Ferris, A. A., Lehman, N. I., and Gust, I. D., 1978, The polypeptides of hepatitis A virus, *Intervirology* **10**:24.

Dales, S., Eggers, H. J., Tamm, I., and Palade, G. E., 1965, Electron microscopic study of the formation of poliovirus, *Virology* **26**:379.

Dane, D. S., Cameron, C. H., and Briggs, M., 1970, Virus-like particles in serum of patients with Australia-antigen-associated hepatitis, *Lancet* **1**:695.

Davenport, F. M., Hennessy, A. V., Christopher, N., and Smith, C. K., 1966, A common source multihousehold outbreak of chimpanzee-associated hepatitis in humans, *Am. J. Epidemiol.* **83**:146.

Davis, D. J., and Hanlon, R. C., 1946, Epidemic infectious hepatitis in a small Iowa community, *Am. J. Hyg.* **43**:314.

Deinhardt, F., Peterson, D., Cross, G, Wolfe, L., and Holmes, A. W., 1975, Hepatitis in marmosets, *Am. J. Med. Sci.* **270**:73.

Denes, A. E., Smith, J. L., Hindman, S. H., Fleissner, M. L., Judelsohn, R., Englender, S. J., Tilson, H., and Maynard, J. E., 1977, Food borne hepatitis A infection: A report of two urban restaurant-associated outbreaks, *Am. J. Epidemiol.* **105**:156.

Dick, S. J., Tamborrow, C. H., and Leevy, C. M., 1974, Hepatitis B antigen in urban caught mosquitos, *J. Am. Med. Assoc.* **229**:1627.

Dienstag, J. L., Feinstone, S. M., Kapikian, A. Z., and Purcell, R. H., 1975*a*, Faecal shedding of hepatitis-A antigen, *Lancet* **1**:765.

Dienstag, J. L., Feinstone, S. M., and Purcell, R. H., 1975*b*, Experimental infection of chimpanzees with hepatitis A virus, *J. Infect. Dis.* **132**:532.

Dienstag, J. L. Routenberg, J. A., Purcell, R. H., Hooper, R. R., and Harrison, W. O., 1975*c*, Food-handler-associated outbreak of hepatitis type A—An immune electron microscopic study, *Ann. Intern. Med.* **83**:647.

Dienstag, J. L., Davenport, F. M., McCollum, R. W., Hennessy, A. V., Klatskin, G., and Purcell, R. H., 1976*a*, Non-human primate associated viral hepatitis type A: Serologic evidence of hepatitis A virus infection, *J. Am. Med. Assoc.* **236**:462.

Dienstag, J. L., Gust, I. D., Lucas, C. R., Wong, D. C., and Purcell, R. H., 1976*b*, Mussel-associated viral hepatitis type A: Serological confirmation, *Lancet* **1**:561.

Dienstag, J. L., Feinstone, S. M., Purcell, R. H., Wong, P. C., Alter, H. J., and Holland, P. V., 1977, Non A, non B post-transfusion hepatitis, *Lancet* **1**:560.

Dienstag, J. L., Mathiesen, J. R., and Purcell, H. H., 1978*a*, Test methods and animal models for hepatitis A virus infection, in: *Viral Hepatitis: A Contemporary Assessment of Etiology, Epidemiology, Pathogenesis and Prevention* (G. N. Vyas, S. N. Cohen, and R. Schmid, eds.), p. 13, Franklin Institute Press, Philadelphia.

Dienstag, J. L., Szmunness, W., Stevens, C. E., and Purcell, R. H., 1978*b*, Hepatitis A virus infection: New insights from seroepidemiologic studies, *J. Infect. Dis.* **137**:328.

Dreseman, G. L., Chairez, R., Suarez, M., Hollinger, F. B., Courtney, R. J., and Melnick, J. L., 1975, Production of antibody to individual polypeptides derived from purified hepatitis B surface antigen, *J. Virol.* **16**:508.

Dull, H. B., Doege, T. C., and Mosley, J. W., 1963, An outbreak of infections hepatitis associated with a school cafeteria, *South. Med. J.* **56**:475.

Edgington, T. S., and Chisari, F. V., 1975, Immunological aspects of hepatitis B virus infection, *Am. J. Med. Sci.* **270**:213.

Eisenstein, A. B., Aach, R. D., Jacobsohn, W., and Goldman, A., 1963, An epidemic of infectious hepatitis in a general hospital: Probable transmission by contaminated orange juice, *J. Am. Med. Assoc.* **183**:171.

Eleftheriou, N., Heathcoate, J., Thomas, H. C., and Sherlock, S., 1975, Incidence and clinical significance of e antigen and antibody in acute and chronic liver disease, *Lancet* **2**:1171.

Fay, O., Tanno, H., Ronocoroni, M., Edwards, V. M., Mosley, J. W., and Redeker, A.

G., 1977, Prognostic implications of the e antigen of hepatitis B virus, *J. Am. Med. Assoc.* **238**:2501.

Feinstone, S. M., Kapikian, A. Z., and Purcell, R. H., 1973, Hepatitis A: Detection by immune electron microscopy of a virus-like antigen associated with acute illness, *Science* **182**:1026.

Feinstone, S. M., Kapikian, A. Z., Gerin, J. L., and Purcell, R. H., 1974, Buoyant density of the hepatitis A virus-like particle in cesium chloride, *J. Virol.* **13**:1412.

Feinstone, S. M., Kapikian, A. Z., Purcell, R. H., Alter, H. J., and Holland, P. V., 1975, Transfusion associated hepatitis not due to viral hepatitis type A or B., *New Engl. J. Med.* **282**:767.

Feinstone, S. M., Moritsugu Y, Shih, J. W. K., Gerin, J. L., and Purcell, R. H., 1978, Characterization of hepatitis A virus, in: *Viral Hepatitis: A Contemporary Assessment of Etiology, Epidemiology, Pathogenesis and Prevention* (G. N. Vyas, S. N. Cohen, and R. Schmid, eds.), p. 41, Franklin Institute Press, Philadelphia.

Findlay, G. M., and Willcox, R. R., 1945, Transmission of infective hepatitis by faeces and virus, *Lancet* **1**:212.

Flehmig, B., Frank, H., Frosner, G. G., and Gerth, H. J., 1977, Hepatitis A-virus particles in stools of patients from a natural hepatitis outbreak in Germany, *Med. Microb. Immunol.* **163**:209.

Francis, T., Jr., Frisch, A. W., and Quilligan, J. J., Jr., 1946, Demonstration of infectious hepatitis virus in presymptomatic period after transfer by transfusion, *Proc. Soc. Exp. Biol. Med.* **61**:276.

Franklin, R. M., and Baltimore, D., 1962, Patterns of macromolecular synthesis in normal and virus-infected mammalian cells, *Cold Spring Harbor Symp. Quant. Biol.* **27**:175.

Franklin, R. M., and Rosner, Jr., 1962, Localization of RNA synthesis in mengovirus infected L cells, *Biochim. Biophys. Acta* **55**:240.

Friedmann, C. T. H., Dinnes, M. R., Bernstein, J. F., and Heinbred, G. A., 1971, Chimpanzee-associated infectious hepatitis among personnel at an animal hospital, *J. Am. Vet. Med. Assoc.* **159**:541.

Frosner, G. G., Overby, L. R., Flehmig, B., Gerth, H. J., Haas, H., Decker, R. H., Ling, C. M., Zuckerman, A. J., and Frozner, H. R., 1977, Seroepidemiological investigation of patients and family contacts in an epidemic of hepatitis A, *J. Med. Virol.* **1**:163.

Fye, K. H., Becker, M. J., Theofilopoulos, A. N., Moutsopo., H., Feldman, J. L., and Talal, M., 1977, Immune complexes in hepatitis B antigen associated polyarteritis nodosa: Detection by antibody dependent cell mediated cytotoxicity in the Raji cell assay, *Am. J. Med.* **62**:783.

Gellis, S. S., Neefe, J. R., Stokes, J., Jr., Strong, L. E., Janeway, C. A., and Scatchard, G., 1948, Chemical, clinical and immunological studies on the products of human plasma fractionation. XXXVI. Inactivation of the virus of homologous serum hepatitis in solutions of normal human serum albumin by means of heat, *J. Clin. Invest.* **27**:239.

Gerin, G. L., 1974, Structure of hepatitis B antigen (HBsAg), in: *Mechanisms of Virus Disease* (W. S. Robinson and C. R. Fox, eds.), pp. 215–224, Benjamin, Menlo Park, Calif.

Gianotti, F., 1973, Papular acrodermatitis of childhood: An Australia antigen disease, *Arch. Dis. Child.* **48**:794.

Gibson, P. E., 1976, Quantitative analysis of the major subdeterminants of hepatitis B surface antigen, *J. Infect. Dis*. **134**:540.

Giles, J. P., Liebhaber, H., Krugman, S., and Lattimer, C., 1964, Early viremia and viruria in fectious hepatitis, *Virology* **24**:107.

Gocke, D. J., 1974, Type B hepatitis—Good news and bad news, *New Engl. J. Med*. **291**:1409.

Gocke, D. J., 1975, Extrahepatic manifestation of viral hepatitis, *Am. J. Med. Sci*. **270**:49.

Gocke, D. J., 1978, Immune complex phenomena associated with hepatitis, in: *Viral Hepatitis: A Contemporary Assessment* (G. N. Vyas, S. N. Cohen, and R. Schmid eds.), p. 227, Franklin Institute Press, Philadelphia.

Gocke, D. J., Hsu, K., Morgan, C., Bombardi, S., Lockshin, M., and Christia, C. L., 1971, Vasculitis in association with Australia antigen, *J. Exp. Med*. **134**:330.

Gold, J. W. N., Shin, J. W., Purcell, R. H., and Gerin, J. L., 1976, Characterization of antibodies to the structural polypeptides of HBsAg: Evidence for subtype-specific determinants, *J. Immunol*. **117**:1404.

Grady, C. F., and Multicenter Study Group, 1975, Hepatitis B immune globulin: Prevention of hepatitis from accidental exposure among medical personnel, *New Engl. J. Med*. **293**:1067.

Grady, G. F., and U.S. National Heart and Lung Institute Collaborative Study Group, 1976, Relation of e antigen to infectivity of HB_sAg-positive inoculations among medical personnel, *Lancet* **2**:492.

Grossman, R. A., Benenson, M. W., Scott, R. M., Snitbhan, R., Top, F. H., and Pantuwat, S., 1975, An epidemiologic study of hepatitis B virus in Bangkok, Thailand, *Am. J. Epidemiol*. **101**:144.

Gudat, F., Bianchi, O., Sonnabend, W., Thiel, G., and Aenishae, W., 1975, Pattern of core and surface expression of liver tissue reflects state of specific immune response in hepatitis B, *Lab. Invest*. **32**:1.

Hansson, B. G., 1976, Age and sex-related distribution of antibodies to hepatitis B surface and core antigens in a Swedish population, *Acta Pathol. Microbiol. Scand. Sect. B* **84**:342.

Hansson, B. G., 1977, Persistence of antibody to hepatitis B core antigen, *J. Clin. Microbiol*. **6**:209.

Havens, W. P., 1945a, Experiment in cross immunity between infectious and homologous serum jaundice, *Proc. Soc. Exp. Biol. Med*. **59**:148.

Havens, W. P., 1945b, Properties of the etiologic agent of infectious hepatitis, *Proc. Soc. Exp. Biol. Med*. **58**:203.

Havens, W. P., 1946a, Period of infectivity of patients with experimentally induced infectious hepatitis, *J. Exp. Med*. **83**:251.

Havens, W. P., 1946b, Period of infectivity of patients with homologous serum jaundice and routes of infection in this disease, *J. Exp. Med*. **83**:441.

Havens, W. P., Ward, R., Drill, V. A., and Paul, J. R., 1944, Experimental production of hepatitis by feeding icterogenic materials, *Proc. Soc. Exp. Biol*. **57**:206.

Hillis, W. D., 1961, An outbreak of infectious hepatitis among chimpanzee handlers at a United States Air Force Base, *Am. J. Hyg*. **73**:316.

Hillis, W. D., 1963, Viral hepatitis associated with sub-human primates, *Transfusion*, **3**:445.

Hillis, W. D., 1968, Viral hepatitis: An unconquered foe, *Milit. Med*. **133**:343.

Hillis, W. D., Hillis, A., Bias, W. B., and Walker, W. G., 1977, Associations of hepatitis B surface antigenemia with HLA locus B specificities, *New Engl. J. Med.* **296**:1310.

Hirschman, S. Z., Vernace, S. J., and Schaffner, F., 1971, DNA polymerase in preparations containing Australia antigen, *Lancet* **1**:1099.

Hoff, R. S., Chalmers, T. C., Culhane, P. O., and Iber, F. L., 1973, Underreporting of viral hepatitis, *Gasteroenterology* **64**:1194.

Holmes, A. W., Wolfe, L., Rosenblate, H., and Deinhardt, F., 1969, Hepatitis in marmosets: Induction of disease with coded specimens from a human volunteer study, *Science* **164**:816.

Holmes, A. W., Wolfe, L., Deinhardt, F., and Conrad, M., 1971, Transmission of human hepatitis to marmosets: Further coded studies, *J. Infect. Dis.* **124**:520.

Holmes, A. W., Deinhardt, F., Wolfe, G., Froesner, G., Peterson, D., and Castro, B., 1973, Specific neutralization of human hepatitis A in marmoset monkeys, *Nature (London)* **243**:419.

Hoofnagle, J. H., Gerety, R. J., and Barker, L. F., 1973, Antibody to hepatitis V virus core in man, *Lancet* **2**:869.

Hoofnagle, J. H., Gerety, R. J., and Barker, L. F., 1975, Antibody to hepatitis B core antigen, *Am. J. Med. Sci.* **270**:179.

Hoofnagle, J. H., Seeff, L. B., Bales, Z. B., Gerety, R. J, and Tabor, E., 1978, Serologic responses in type B hepatitis, in: *Viral Hepatitis: A Contemporary Assessment* (G. N. Vyas, S. N. Cohen, and R. Schmid, eds.), p. 219, Franklin Institute Press, Philadelphia.

Hopkins, R., and Scott, T. G., 1976, Hepatitis A antigen in Edenburgh, *Lancet* **2**:206.

Hruska, J. F., and Robinson, W. S., 1977, The proteins of hepatitis B Dane particle cores, *J. Med. Virol.* **1**:119.

Hruska, J. F., Clayton, D. A., Rubenstein, J. L. R., and Robinson, W. S., 1977, Structure of hepatitis B Dane particle DNA before and after the Dane particle DNA polymerase reaction, *J. Virol.* **21**:666.

Huang, S. N., 1971, Hepatitis-associated antigen hepatitis, *Am. J. Pathol.* **64**:483.

Ishimaru, Y., Ishimaru, H., Toda, G., Baba, K., and Mayumi, M., 1976, An epidemic of infantile papular acrodermatitis in Japan associated with hepatitis B surface antigen subtype ayw, *Lancet* **1**:707.

Joseph, P. R., Miller, J. D., and Henderson, D. A., 1965, An outbreak of hepatitis traced to food contamination, *New Engl. J. Med.* **273**:188.

Kaplan, P. M., Greenman, R. L., Gerin, J. L., Purcell, R. H., and Robinson, W. S., 1973, DNA polymerase associated with human hepatitis B antigen, *J. Virol.* **12**:995.

Kaplan, P. M., Gerin, J. L., and Alter, H. J., 1974, Hepatitis B-specific DNA polymerase activity during post-transfusion hepatitis, *Nature (London)* **249**:762.

Karvountzis, G. G., Mosley, J. W., and Redeker, A. G., 1975, Serologic characterization of patients with two episodes of acute viral hepatitis, *Am. J. Med.* **58**:815.

Knieser, M. R., Jenis, E. H., Lowenthal, D. T., Bancroft, W. H., Burns, W., and Shalhoub, R., 1974, Pathogenesis of renal disease associated with viral hepatitis, *Arch Pathol.* **97**:193.

Knight, V., Drake, M. E., Belden, E. A., Franklin, B. J., Romer, M., and Copple, O., 1954, Characteristics of spread of infectious hepatitis in schools and households in an epidemic in a rural area, *Am. J. Hyg.* **59**:1.

Knodell, R. G., Conrad, M. E., Dienstag, J. L., and Bell, C. J., 1975, Etiologic spectrum of post transfusion hepatitis, *Gastroenterology* **69**:1278.

Koff, R. S., and Sear, H. S., 1967, Internal temperature of steamed clams: Viral hepatitis in a group of Boston hospitals. III. Importance of exposure to shell fish in a non epidemic period, *New Engl. J. Med.* **276**:737.

Kohler, P. F., Cronin, R. E., and Hammon, W. S., 1974, Chronic membranous glomerulonephritis caused by hepatitis B antigen–antibody immune complexes, *Ann. Intern. Med.* **81**:488.

Krugman, S., 1972, Hepatitis B immune globulin, in: *Hepatitis and Blood Transfusion* (G. N. Vyas, H. A. Perkins, and R. Schmid, eds.), p. 349, Grune and Stratton, New York.

Krugman, S., and Giles, J. P., 1970, Viral hepatitis: New light on an old disease, *J. Am. Med. Assoc.* **212**:1019.

Krugman, S., and Giles, J. P., 1973, Viral hepatitis type B (MS-2 strain): Further observations on natural history and prevention, *New Engl. J. Med.* **288**:755.

Krugman, S., Ward, R., Giles, J. P., Bodansky, O., and Jacobs, A. M., 1959, Infectious hepatitis: Detection of virus during incubation and in clinically inapparent infection, *New Engl. J. Med.* **261**:729.

Krugman, S., Ward, R., and Giles, J. P., 1962, The natural history of infectious hepatitis, *Am. J. Med.* **32**:717.

Krugman, S., Giles, J. P., and Hammond, J., 1967, Infectious hepatitis: Evidence for two distinctive clinical, epidemiological, and immunological types of infection, *J. Am. Med. Assoc.* **200**:365.

Krugman, S., Giles, J. P., and Hammond, J., 1970, Hepatitis virus: Effect of heat on infectivity and antigenicity of the MS-1 and MS-2 strains, *J. Infect. Dis.* **122**:432.

Krugman, S., Hoofnagle, J. H., Gerety, R. J., Kaplan, P. M., and Gerin, J. L., 1974, Hepatitis, type B: DNA polymerase activity and antibody to hepatitis B core antigen, *New Engl. J. Med.* **290**:1331.

Krugman, S., Friedman, H., and Lattimer, C., 1975, Viral hepatitis type A: Identification by specific complement fixation and immune adherence tests, *New Engl. J. Med.* **292**:1141.

Lander, J. J., Giles, J. P., Purcell, R. H., and Krugman, S., 1970, Viral hepatitis type B (MS-2 strain): Detection of antibody after primary infection, *New Engl. J. Med.* **283**:303.

Lander, J. J., Holland, P. V., Alter, H. J., Chanock, R. M., and Purcell, R. H., 1972, Antibody to hepatitis B associated antigen: Frequency and pattern of response detected by radioimmunoprecipitation, *J. Am. Med. Assoc.* **220**:1079.

Landers, T., Greenberg, H. B., and Robinson, W. S., 1977, Structure of hepatitis B Dane particle DNA and nature of the endogenous DNA polymerase reaction, *J. Virol.* **23**:368.

LeBouvier, G. L., 1971, The heterogeneity of Australia antigen, *J. Infect. Dis.* **123**:671.

LeBouvier, G, 1972, Sero analysis by immunodiffusion: The subtypes of type B hepatitis virus, in: *Hepatitis and Blood Transfusions* (G. N. Vyas, A. Perkins, and R. Schmid, eds.), p. 97, Grune and Stratton, New York.

LeBouvier, G. L., and McCollum, R. W., 1970, Australia (hepatitis associated) antigen: Physiochemical and immunological characteristics, *Adv. Virus Res.* **16**:357.

Leger, R. T., Boyer, K. M., Pattison, C. P., and Maynard, J. E., 1975, Hepatitis A: Report of the common-source outbreak with recovery of a possible etiologic agent. I. Epidemiologic studies, *J. Infect. Dis.* **131**:163.

Levo, Y., Gorevic, P. D., Kassab, H. J., Zuckerfr., D., and Franklin, E., 1977, Association between hepatitis B virus and essential mixed cyroglobulinemia, *J. Engl. J. Med.* **296**:1501.

Levy, B. S., Fontaine, R. E., Smith, C. A., Brinda, J., Hirman, G., Nelson, D. B., Johnson, P. M., and Larson, O., 1975, A large food-borne outbreak of hepatitis A—Possible transmission by oropharyngeal secretions, *J. Am. Med. Assoc.* **234**:289.

Lewis, T. L., Alter, H. J., Chalmers, T. C., Holland, P. V., Purcell, R. H., Alling, D. W., Young, D., Frenkel, L. D., Lee, S. L., and Lamson, M. E., 1973, A comparison of the frequency of hepatitis B antigen and antibody in hospital and non-hospital personnel, *New Engl. J. Med.* **289**:647.

Lorenz, D., Barker, L., Stevens, D., Peterson, M., and Kirsohst, R., 1970, Hepatitis in the marmoset, *Sanguinus mystax*, *Proc. Soc. Biol. Med.* **135**:348.

Lutwick, L. I., and Robinson, W. S., 1977, DNA synthesized in the hepatitis B Dane particle DNA polymerase reaction, *J. Virol.* **21**:96.

MacCallum, F. O., 1951, Infective hepatitis: Studies in East Anglia during the period 1943–47, *Medical Research Council Special Report Series No. 273*, HMSO, London.

MacCallum, F. O., and Bradley, W. H., 1944, Transmission of infective hepatitis to human volunteers, *Lancet* **2**:228.

Mackowiak, P. A., Caraway, C. T., and Portnoy, B. L., 1976, Oyster-associated hepatitis: Lessons from the Louisiana experience, *Am. J. Epidemiol.* **103**:181.

Magnius, L. O., 1975, Characterization of a new antigen–antibody system associated with hepatitis B, *Clin. Exp. Immunol.* **20**:209.

Magnius, L. O., and Espmark, J. A., 1972, New specificities of Australia antigen and the possible identification of hepatitis carriers, *J. Immunol.* **109**:1017.

Magnius, L. O., Lindhold M., Lundin, P., and Iwarson, S., 1975, Clinical significance of a new antigen-antibody system in long-term carriers of hepatitis B surface antigen, *J. Am. Med. Assoc.* **231**:356.

Mahoney, P., Fleischner, G., Millman, I., Blumberg, B., and Arias, M., 1974, Australia antigen: Detection and transmission in shell fish, *Science* **183**:80.

Maizel, J. V., and Summers, D. F., 1968, Evidence of large precursor proteins in poliovirus synthesis, *Proc. Natl. Acad. USA* **59**:966.

Maizel, J. V., Phillips, B. A., and Summers, D. F., 1967, Composition of artificially produced and naturally occurring empty capsids of polio virus type 1, *Virology* **32**:692.

Mascoli, D. C., Ittensoh, O. L., Villarejos, V. M., Arguedas, J. A., Provost, P. J., and Hilleman, M. R., 1973, Recovery of hepatitis agents in the marmoset from human cases occurring in Costa Rica, *Proc. Soc. Exp. Biol. Med.* **142**:276.

Mason, J. O., and McLean, W. R., 1962, Infectious hepatitis traced to the consumption of raw oysters, *Am. J. Hyg.* **75**:90.

Mathiesen, L. R., Feinstone, S. M., Purcell, R. H., and Wagner, J. A., 1977, Detection of hepatitis A antigen by immunofluorescence, *Infect. Immun.* **18**:524.

Mathiesen, L. R., Drucker, J., Lorenz, D., Wagner, J., Gerety, R. J., and Purcell, R. H., 1978, Localization of hepatitis A antigen in marmoset organs during acute infection with hepatitis A virus, *J. Infect. Dis.* **183**:369.

Maynard, J. E., 1963, Infectious hepatitis at Fort Yukon, Alaska—Report of an outbreak, 1960–61, *Am. J. Pub. Health* **53**:31.

Maynard, J. E., 1978, Viral hepatitis as an occupational hazard in the health care profession, in: *Viral Hepatitis: A Contemporary Assessment* (G. N. Vyas, S. N. Cohen, and R. Schmid, eds.), p. 321, Franklin Institute Press, Philadelphia.

Maynard, J. E., Bradley, D. W., Gravelle, C. R., Ebert, J. W., and Krushak, D. H., 1975, Preliminary studies of hepatitis A in chimpanzees, *J. Infect. Dis.* **131**:194.

McCollum, R. W., 1952, The size of serum hepatitis virus, *Proc. Soc. Exp. Biol. Med.* **81**:157.

McDonald, G. B., and Silverstein, F. E., 1975, Can gastrointestinal endoscopy transmit hepatitis B to patients? *Gastroint. Endosc.* **22**:168.

McIntosh, R. M., Koss, M. N., and Gocke, D. J., 1976, The nature and incidence of cryoproteins in hepatitis B antigen (HB$_s$Ag) positive patients, *Q. J. Med.* **45**:23.

Meyers, J. D., Rom, F. J., Tihen, W. S., and Bryan, J. A., 1975, Food-borne hepatitis A in a general hospital—Epidemiologic study of an outbreak attributed to sandwiches, *J. Am. Med. Assoc.* **231**:1049.

Millman, I, Hutanen, H., Merino, F., Bayer, M. E., and Blumberg, B. S., 1971, Australia antigen: Physical and chemical properties, *Res. Commun. Chem. Pathol. Pharmacol.* **2**:667.

Moritsugu, Y., Dienstag, J. L., Valdesuso, J., Wong, D. C., Wagner, J., Routebe, J. A., and Purchell, R. H., 1976, Purification of hepatitis A antigen from feces and detection of antigen and antibody by immune adherance hemagglutination, *Infect. Immun.* **13**:898.

Morris, I. M., Cattle, D. S., and Smits, B. J., 1975, Endoscopy and transmission of hepatitis B, *Lancet* **2**:1152.

Morse, L. J., Bryan, J. A., Hurley, J. P., Murphy, J. F., O'Brian, T. F., and Wacker, W. E. C., 1972, The Holy Cross football team hepatitis outbreak, *J. Am. Med. Assoc.* **219**:706.

Mosley, J. W., 1972, Epidemiologic implications of changing trends in type A and type B hepatitis, in: *Hepatitis and Blood Transfusion* (G. N. Vyas, H. S. Perkins, and R. Schmid, eds.), p. 349, Grune and Stratton, New York.

Mosley, J. W., 1975a, The epidemiology of viral hepatitis: An overview, *Am. J. Med. Sci.* **270**:253.

Mosley, J. W., 1975b, Hepatitis types B and non B: Epidemiologic background, *J. Am. Med. Assoc.* **233**:967.

Mosley, J. W., 1978, Epidemiology of HAV Infection, in: *Viral Hepatitis: A Contemporary Assessment of Etiology, Pathogenesis and Prevention* (G. N. Vyas, S. N. Cohen, and R. Schmid, eds.), p. 85, Franklin Institute Press, Philadelphia.

Mosley, J. W., and Smithers, W. W., 1957, Infectious hepatitis: Report of an outbreak probably caused by drinking water, *New Engl. J. Med.* **257**:590.

Mosley, J. W., Schrack, W. D., Jr., Densham, T. W., and Matter, L. D., 1959, Infectious hepatitis in Clearfield County, Pennsylvania. I. A probable water-borne epidemic, *Am. J. Med.* **26**:555.

Mosley, J. W., Reinhardt, H. P., and Hassler, F. R., 1967, Chimpanzee-associated hepatitis: An outbreak in Oklahoma, *J. Am. Med. Assoc.* **199**:695.

Mosley, J. W., Edwards, V. M., Meihaus, J. E., and Redeker, A. G., 1972, Subdeterminants d and y of hepatitis B antigen as epidemiologic markers, *Am. J. Epidemiol.* **95**:529.

Mosley, J. W., Edwards, V. M., Casey, B. S., Redeker, A. G., and White, E., 1975, Hepatitis virus infection in dentists, *New Engl. J. Med.* **293**:730.

Mosley, J. W., Redeker, A. G., Feinstone, S. M., and Purcell, R. H., 1977, Multiple hepatitis viruses in multiple attacks of acute viral hepatitis, *New Engl. J. Med.* **296**:75.

Murphy, W. J., Petrie, L. M., and Work, S. D., 1946, Outbreak of infectious hepatitis, apparently milk-borne, *Am. J. Publ. Health* **36**:169.

Murray, R., and Diefenback, W. C., 1953, Effect of heat on the agent of homologous serum hepatitis, *Proc. Soc. Exp. Biol. Med.* **84**:230.

Neefe, J. R., and Stokes, J., Jr., 1945, An epidemic of infectious hepatitis apparently due to a water-borne agent, *J. Am. Med. Assoc.* **128**:1063.

Neefe, J. R., Stokes, J., Jr., and Reinhold, J. G., 1945, Oral administration to volunteers of feces from patients with homologous serum hepatitis and infectious (epidemic) hepatitis, *Am. J. Med. Sci.* **210**:29.

Neefe, J. R., Gellis, S. S., and Stokes, J., Jr., 1946, Homologous serum hepatitis and infectious (epidemic) hepatitis: Studies in volunteers bearing on immunological and other characteristics of the etiological agents, *Am. J. Med.* **1**:3.

Neefe, J. R., Baty, J. B., Reinhold, J. L., and Stokes, J., Jr., 1947, Inactivation of the virus of infectious hepatitis in a drinking water, *Am. J. Public Health* **37**:365.

Neilsen, J. O., Dietrichson, O., and Juhl, E., 1974, Incidence and meaning of the "e" determinant among hepatitis B antigen positive patients with acute and chronic liver diseases, *Lancet* **2**:913.

Neurath, A. R., Prince, A. M., and Lippin, A., 1974, Hepatitis B antigen: Antigenic sites related to human serum proteins revealed by affinity chromatography, *Proc. Natl. Acad. Sci. USA* **71**:2663.

Nordenfeld, E., and Kjellen, E., 1975, Dane particles, DNA polymerase and e antigen in two different categories of hepatitis B antigen carriers, *Interviology* **5**:225.

Ogra, P. L., 1973, Immunologic aspects of hepatitis associated antigen and antibody in body fluids, *J. Immunol.* **110**:1197.

Okachi, D., and Murakami, S., 1968, Observations on Australia antigen in Japanese, *Vox Sang* **15**:374.

Okada, K., Kamiyama, I., Inomata, M., Imai, M., Miyakawa, I., and Mayumi, M., 1976, e antigen and anti-e in the serum of asymptomatic carrier methods as indicators of positive and negative transmission of hepatitis B virus to their infants, *New Engl. J. Med.* **294**:746.

Ozawa, T., Levisohn, P., Orsini, E., and McIntosh, R. M., 1976, Acute immune complex disease associated with hepatitis, *Arch. Pathol. Lab. Med.* **100**:484.

Patterson, M. J., Hourani, M. R., and Mayor, G. H., 1977, HLA antigens and hepatitis B virus, *New Engl. J. Med.* **297**:1124.

Pattison, C. P., Boyer, K. M., Maynard, J. E., and Kelly, P. C., 1974, Epidemic hepatitis in a clinical laboratory: Possible association with computer card handling, *J. Am. Med. Assoc.* **230**:854.

Paul, J. R., Havens, W. P., Sabin, A. B., and Philip, C. B., 1945, Transmission experiments in serum jaundice and infectious hepatitis, *J. Am. Med. Assoc.* **138**:911.

Peters, R. L., 1975, Viral hepatitis: A pathologic spectrum, *Am. J. Med. Sci.* **270**:17.

Peterson, D. L., Roberts, T. M., and Vyas, G. N., 1977, Partial amino acid sequence of two major component polypeptides of hepatitis B surface antigen, *Proc. Natl. Acad. Sci. USA* **74**:1530.

Peterson, D. L., Chien, D. Y., Vyas, G. N., Nitecki, D., and Bond, H. E., 1978, Characterization of polypeptides of HBsAg for the proposed "UC vaccine" for hepatitis B, in *Viral Hepatitis: A Contemporary Assessment* (G. N. Vyas, S. N. Cohen, and R. Schmid, eds.), p. 569, Franklin Institute Press, Philadelphia.

Philip, J. R., Hamilton, T. P., Albert, T. J., Stone, R. S., and Pait, C. F., 1973, Infectious hepatitis outbreak with mai tai as the vehicle of transmission, *Am. J. Epidemiol.* **97**:50.

Portnoy, B. L., Mackowiak, P. A., Caraway, C. T., Walker, J. A., McKinley, T. W., and Klein, C. A., 1975, Oyster-associated hepatitis—Failure of shellfish certification program to prevent outbreaks, *J. Am. Med. Assoc.* **233**:1065.

Poskanzer, D. C., and Beadenkoph, W. G., 1961, Water-borne infectious hepatitis epidemic from a chlorinated municipal supply, *Pub. Health Rep.* **76**:745.

Prince, A. M., 1968, An antigen detected in the blood during the incubation period of serum hepatitis, *Proc. Natl. Acad. Sci. USA* **60**:814.

Prince, A. M., Metselaar, D., Kafuko, G. W., Mukwaya, L. G., Ling, C. M., and Overby, L. R., 1972, Hepatitis B antigen in wild caught mosquitos in Africa, *Lancet* **2**:247.

Prince, A. M., Szmuness, W., Mann, M. K., Vyas, G. N., Grady, G. F., Shapiro, F. L., Suki, W. N., Friendman, E. A., and Stenzel, K. H., 1975, Hepatitis B "immune" globulin: Effectiveness in prevention of dialysis-associated hepatitis, *New Engl. J. Med.* **293**:1063.

Provost, P. J., and Hilleman, M. R., 1979, Propogation of human hepatitis A virus in cell culture *in vitro*, *Proc. Soc. Exp. Biol. Med.* **160**:213.

Provost, P. J., Ittensohn, O. L., Villarejos, V. M., Arguedas, G., and Hilleman, M. R., 1973, Etiologic relationship of marmoset-propagated CR 326 hepatitis A virus to hepatitis in man, *Proc. Soc. Exp. Biol. Med.* **142**:1257.

Provost, P. J., Wolanski, B. S., Miller, W. J., Ittensohn, O. L., McAleer, W. J., and Hilleman, M. R., 1975, Physical, chemical, and morphologic dimensions of human hepatitis A virus strain CR 326 (38578), *Proc. Soc. Exp. Biol. Med.* **148**: 532.

Provost, P. J., Villarejos, V. M., and Hilleman, M. R., 1977, Suitability of the rufiventer marmoset as a host animal for human hepatitis A virus, *Proc. Soc. Exp. Biol. Med.* **155**:283.

Purcell, R. H., and Gerin, J. L., 1975, Hepatitis B subunit vaccine: A preliminary report of safety and efficacy tests in chimpanzees, *Am. J. Med. Sci.* **270**:395.

Rakela, J., and Mosley, J. W., 1977, Fecal excretion of hepatitis A virus in humans, *J. Infect. Dis.* **135**:933.

Rakela, J., Mosley, J. W., and Redeker, A. G., 1975, The role of hepatitis A virus in fulminant viral hepatitis, *Gastroenterology* **69**:854.

Rakela, J., Stevenson, D., Edwards, V., Gordon, I., and Mosley, J. W., 1977, Antibodies to hepatitis A virus: Patterns by two procedures, *J. Clin Microbiol.* **5**:110.

Raska, K., Helch, J., Jezek, Z., Kubelka, Z., Litov, M., Novak, K., Radkousky, J., Sery, V., and Zikmund, V., 1966, A milk-borne infectious hepatitis epidemic, *J. Hyg. Epidemiol. Microb. Immunol.* **10**:413.

Ray, M. G., Desmet, V. J., Bradburne, A. F., Desmyter, J., Fevery, J., and Degroote, J., 1976, Distribution patterns of hepatitis B surface antigen (HB$_s$Ag) in the liver of hepatitis patients, *Gastroenterology* **71**:462.

Read, M. R., Bancroft, H., Doull, J. A., and Parker, R. F., 1946, Infectious hepatitis—Presumably food-borne outbreak, *Am. J. Publ. Health* **36**:367.

Redeker, A. G., 1975, Viral hepatitis: Clinical aspects, *Am. J. Med. Sci.* **270**:9.

Redeker, A. G., Hopkins, C. E., Jackson, B., and Peck, P., 1968, A controlled study of
    the safety of pooled plasma stored in the liquid state at 30–32°C for 6 months,
    Transfusion **8**:60.
Redeker, A. G., Mosley, J. W. Gocke, D. J., McKee, A. P., and Pollack, W., 1975,
    Hepatitis B immune globulin as a prophylactic measure for spouses exposed to
    acute type B hepatitis, *New Engl. J. Med.* **293**:1055.
Rindge, M. E., Mason, J. O., and Elsea, W. R., 1962, Infectious hepatitis: Report of an
    outbreak in a small Connecticut school, due to water-borne transmission, *J. Am.
    Med. Assoc.* **180**:33.
Robinson, W. S., 1975, DNA and DNA polymerase in the core of the Dane particle of
    hepatitis B, *Am. J. Med. Sci.* **270**:151.
Robinson, W. S., 1977, The genome of hepatitis B virus, *Annu. Rev. Microbiol.* **31**:357.
Robinson, W. S., and Greenman, R. L., 1974, DNA polymerase in the core of the
    human hepatitis B virus candidate, *J. Virol.* **13**:1231.
Robinson, W. S., and Lutwick, L. I., 1976a, Hepatitis B virus: A cause of persistent
    virus infection in man, in: Animal Virology (A. Huang and C. F. Fox, eds.), p.
    787, Academic Press, New York.
Robinson, W. S., and Lutwick, L. I., 1976b, The virus of hepatitis, type B, *New Engl.
    J. Med.* **295**:1168, 1232.
Robinson, W. S., Clayton, D. A., and Greenman, R. L., 1974, DNA of a human
    hepatitis B virus candidate, *J. Virol.* **14**:384.
Roos, B., 1956, Hepatitis epidemic conveyed by oysters, *Svenska Läker* **53**:989.
Rosenberg, J. L., Jones, D. P., Lipitz, L. R., and Kirsner, J. B., 1973, Viral hepatitis:
    An occupational hazard to surgeons, *J. Am. Med. Assoc.* **223**:295.
Ruddy, S. J., Mosley, J. W., and Held, J. R., 1967, Chimpanzee-associated viral hepa-
    titis in 1963, *Am. J. Epidemiol.* **86**:634.
Ruddy, S. J., Johnson, R. F., Mosley, J. W., Atwater, J. B., Rossitti, M. A., and Hart,
    J. C., 1969, An epidemic of clam-associated hepatitis, *J. Am. Med. Assoc.*
    208:649.
Salaman, M. H., Williams, D. I., King, A. J., and Nicol, C. S., 1944, Prevention of
    jaundice resulting from antisyphilitic treatment, *Lancet* **2**:7.
Sambrook, J., Westphal, H., and Srimivasan, R. P., 1968, The integrated state of viral
    DNA in SV 40 transformed cells, *Proc. Natl. Acad. Sci. USA* **60**:1288.
Sattler, F., and Robinson, W. S., 1979, Hepatitis B viral DNA molecules have cohesive
    ends, submitted for publication.
Schober, A., Thomssen, R., Kaboth U., and Worch, R., 1972, Inapparent infections of
    the course of an epidemic of Australia-SH antigen positive hepatitis, *Am. J. Dis.
    Child.* **123**:404.
Schoenbaum, S. C., Baker, O., and Jezek, Z., 1976, Common-source epidemic hepatitis
    due to glazed and iced pastries, *Am. J. Epidemiol.* **104**:74.
Schulman, A. N., Dienstag, J. L., Jackson, D. R., Hoofnagle, J. H., Gerety, R. J., Pur-
    cell, R. H., and Barker, L. F., 1976, Hepatitis A antigen particles in liver, bile, and
    stool of chimpanzees, *J. Infect. Dis.* **134**:80.
Schumacher, H. R., and Gall, E. P., 1974, Arthritis in acute hepatitis and chronic
    active hepatitis: Pathology of the synovial membrane with evidence for the
    presence of Australia antigen in synovial membranes, *Am. J. Med.* **57**:655.
Schweitzer, I. L., Dunn, A., Peters, R., and Spears, R. L., 1973, Viral hepatitis in
    neonates and infants, *Am. J. Med.* **55**:762.
Seef, L. B., Zimmerman, H. J., Wright, E. C., Finkelst, J. D., Greenlee, H. B.,

Hamilton, J., Leevy, C. M., Tamburrow, C. H., Vlahcevi, Z., Zimmon, D. S., and Zimmerman, H. J., 1975, Efficacy of hepatitis B immune serum globulin after accidental exposure: Preliminary report of the Veterans Administration Cooperative Study, *Lancet* **2**:939.

Shih, J. W., and Gerin, J. L., 1975, Immunochemistry of hepatitis B surface antigen (HBsAg): Prevention and characterization of antibodies to the constituent polypeptides, *J. Immunol.* **115**:634.

Shih, J. W., and Gerin, J. L., 1977, Proteins of hepatitis B surface antigen, *J. Virol.* **21**:347.

Shulman, R. N., 1971, Hepatitis-associated antigen, *Am. J. Med.* **49**:669.

Siddiqui, A., Sattler, F., and Robinson, W. S., 1979, A restriction endonuclease map and location of unique physical features of the DNA of hepatitis B virus, subtype adw$_2$, *Proc. Natl. Acad. Sci. USA* (in press).

Siegl, G., and Frosner, G. G., 1978a, Characterization and classification of virus particles associated with hepatitis A. I. Size, density and semimentation, *J. Virol.* **26**:40.

Siegl, G., and Frosner, G. G., 1978b, Characterization and classification of virus particles associated with hepatitis A. II. Type and configuration of nucleic acid, *J. Virol.* **26**:48.

Smith, J. L., Murphy, B. L., Auslander, M. O., Maynard, J. E., Schalm S. S., Summersk, W. H., and Gitnick, G. L., 1976, Studies of the "e" antigen in acute and chronic hepatitis, *Gastroenterology* **71**:208.

Sninsky, J., Siddiqui, A., Robinson, W. S., and Cohen, S. N., 1979, Cloning and endonuclease mapping of the hepatitis B viral genome, *Nature (London)* **279**:346.

Soulier, J. P., Saltix, C., Courouce, A. M., Benamon, D., Amouch, P., and Drouet, J., 1972, Prevention of virus B hepatitis (SH virus), *Am. J. Dis. Child.* **123**:429.

Stevens, C. E., and Beasley, R. P., 1976, Lack of an autosomal recessive genetic influence in the vertical transmission of hepatitis B antigen, *Nature (London)* **260**:715.

Stevens, C. E., Silbert, J. A., Miller, D. R., Dienstag, J. L., Purcell, R. H., and Szmuness, W., 1978, Serologic evidence of hepatitis A and B virus infections in thalassemia patients: A retrospective study, *Transfusion* **18**:356.

Studier, F. W., 1965, Sedimentation studies of the size and shape of DNA, *J. Mol. Biol.* **11**:373.

Summers, J., O'Connell, A., and Millman, I., 1975, Genome of hepatitis B virus: Restriction enzyme cleavage and structure of DNA extracted from Dane particles, *Proc. Natl. Acad. Sci. USA* **72**:4597.

Summers, J., Smolec, J. M., and Snyder, R., 1978, A virus similar to human hepatitis B virus associated with hepatitis and hepatoma in woodchucks, *Proc. Natl. Acad. Sci. USA* **75**:4533.

Szmuness, W., 1975, Recent advances in the study of the epidemiology of hepatitis B, *Am. J. Pathol.* **81**:629.

Szmuness, W., 1978, Hepatocellular carcinoma and hepatitis B virus: Evidence for a causal association, *Prog. Med. Virol.* **24**:40.

Szmuness, W., Prince, A. M., Hirsch, R. L., and Brotman, B., 1973, Familial clustering of hepatitis B infection, *New Engl. J. Med.* **299**:1162.

Szmuness, W., Much, W. M., Prince, A. M., Hoofnagle, J. H., Cherubin, C. E., Harley, E. J., and Block, G. H., 1975, On the role of sexual behavior in the spread of hepatitis B infection, *Ann. Intern. Med.* **83**:489.

Szmuness, W., Dienstag, J. L., Purcell, R. H., Harley, E. J., Stevens, C. E., and Wong, D. C., 1976, Distribution of antibody to hepatitis A antigen in urban adult populations, *New Engl. J. Med.* **295**:755.

Szmuness, W., Dienstag, J. L., Purcell, R. H., Prince, A. M., Stevens, C. E., and Levine, R. W., 1977, Type A hepatitis and hemodialysis: A seroepidemiologic study in 15 U.S. centers, *Ann. Intern. Med.* **87**:8.

Takahashi, K., Imai, M., Miyakawa, S., Iwakiri, S., and Mayuini, M., 1978, Duality of hepatitis B e antigen in serum of persons infected with hepatitis B virus: Evidence for the non-identity of e antigen with immunoglobulins, *Proc. Natl. Acad. Sci. USA* **75**:1952.

Takahashi, K., Akahane Y., Gotanda, T., Mishiro, T., Imai, M., Miyakawa, Y., and Mayum, M., 1979, Demonstration of hepatitis B e antigen in the core of Dane particles, *J. Immunol.* **122**:275.

Talbot, E., Gerety, R. J., and Barker, L. F., 1977, Detection of e antigen during acute and chronic hepatitis B virus infection in chimpanzees, *J. Infect. Dis.* **136**:541.

Thomssen, R., Gerlich, W., Stamm, B., Bismas, R., Lorenz, P. R., Majer, M., Weinmann, E., Arnold, W., Hess, G., Wepler, W., and Klinge, O., 1977, Infectivity of purified hepatitis B virus particles, *New Engl. J. Med.* **296**:396.

Trepo, C. G., and Prince, A. M., 1976, Absence of complete homologous immunity in hepatitis B infection after massive exposure, *Ann. Intern. Med.* **85**:427.

Tucker, C. B., Owen, W. H., and Farrell, M. S., 1954, Outbreak of infectious hepatitis apparently transmitted through water, *South. Med. J.* **47**:732.

Villarejos, V. M., Provost, P. J., Ittensohn, O. L., McLean, A. A., and Hilleman, M. R., 1976, Seroepidemiologic investigations of human hepatitis caused by A, B, and a possible third virus, *Proc. Soc. Exp. Biol. Med.* **152**:525.

Voegt, H., 1942, Zur Aetiologie der Hepatitis epidemica, *Munch. Med. Wochenschr.* **89**:76.

Wands, J. R., Mann, E. A., and Isselbacher, K. J., 1975, The pathogenesis of arthritis associated with acute hepatitis B surface antigen positive hepatitis: Complement activation and characterization of circulating immune complexes, *J. Clin. Invest.* **55**:930.

Ward, R., Krugman, S., Giles, J. P., Jacobs, A. M., and Bodansky, O., 1958, Infectious hepatitis: Studies of its natural history and prevention, *New Engl. J. Med.* **258**:407.

Wewalka, F., 1953, Zur Epidemiologie des Ikterus bei der antisyphlitischen Behandlung, *Schweiz. Z. Allg. Pathol.* **16**:307.

Williams, A., and LeBouvier, G., 1976, Heterogeneity and thermolability of "e," *Bibl. Haematol. Basel* **42**:71.

Willis, W., London, W. T., Werner, B. G., Pourtagh, M., Larouze, B., Millman, I., Ogston, W., Diallo, S., and Blumberg, B. S., 1977, Hepatitis B virus in bedbugs from Senegal, *Lancet* **2**:217.

Woodson, R. D., and Clinton, J. J., 1969, Hepatitis prophylaxis abroad: Effectiveness of immune serum globulin in protecting Peace Corps volunteers, *J. Am. Med. Assoc.* **209**:1053.

Wright, R. A., 1975, Hepatitis B and HBsAg carrier: An outbreak related to sexual contact, *J. Am. Med. Assoc.* **232**:171.

Zuckerman, A. J., and Taylor, P. E., 1969, Persistence of the serum hepatitis (SH-Australia) antigen for many years, *Nature (London)* **223**:81.

Index

Abadina virus, 322, 327
Acado virus, 322
Acara virus, 2, 31–33
  antibody, 31
  in *Culex* sp., 31
  in *Nectomys* sp., 31
  in sentinel mouse, 31
Acridine orange dye, 269
Acrodermatitis, infantile papular, and
        persistent hepatitis B virus, 494
Actinomycin D, 80, 181, 211, 212, 214, 479
Adenitis due to corona virus
  lymphoid, 220–221
  salivary, 220–221
Aedes sp., 8, 11, 12, 16–21, 23–29, 39, 41, 45,
        50, 51, 308, 348
  A. aegypti, 222
  A. albopictus, 289, 308, 348
African horsesickness virus (AHSV), 285
  an arbovirus, 286
  in *Culicoides* sp., 287
  cytopathogenicity, 290
  host range in mammals, 327
    domesticated, 327
    wild, 327
  isolation from yolk sac of embryonated egg,
        288
  pathogenesis, 331
  primary insect orbivirus, 286
  serotype, 287
African swine fever virus, 348, 349
  protein, structural, 358
  replication absent in enucleated cells, 389
Aquacate virus, 53
AHSV, *see* African horsesickness virus
Aino virus
  in *Aedes* sp., 39
  in *Culex* sp. (1968), 38
  in cattle, 39

Akabane virus, 39
  in *Aedes* sp., 39
  in cattle, 39
  in *Culex* sp. (1961), 38
  in *Culicoides brevitaris*, 39
  in sheep, 39
Akodon azarae, 159
Alaskan fur seal, 251
Alphavirus, 17
Amantadine hydrochloride, 182
α-Amantin, 181
Amapari virus, 158, 159, 172
  in *Neacomys quianae*, 159
  in *Oryzomys goeldi*, 159
Anguilla anguilla, 429, 446
  A. rostrata, 429
Anhanga virus, 53
Anhembi virus, 10
Anopheles sp., 9–12, 25, 27, 29, 46, 47, 64, 66
  group A viruses, 2, 15–17
  group B viruses, 4, 17, 46–47
  group C viruses, 2, 16–19
Antibesis spp., 159
Apen virus, 17, 19
Arboviruses
  A group, 2, 5
  B group, 5
  C group, 2, 5
  categories recommended, 6–7
  International Catalogue of Arboviruses
        (1975), 1
Arenaviruses
  antigen, 170–172
  budding, 166
  cell culture, 178–182
  component, internal, 175–178
  defective, 182–184
  DNA intermediate, 181
  enzymes, virus-associated, 177–178

Arenaviruses (*cont.*)
  enzymes (*cont.*)
    RNA polymerase, RNA-dependent,
      177–178
    RNA transcriptase, 178
  growth cycle, 184
  history, 158–160
  interference, 182–184
  and interferon, 183
  maturation by budding, 166
  members, listed, 159
  morphology, 164–168
  nucleic acids, 172–175
  particle, 164
    defective, interfering, 182–184
  pathobiology, 160–164
  persistence in reservoir host, 184
  polypeptide, 168–170
    structural, listed, 169
  properties, physical, 164–168
  protein, 168–172
    antigen, 170–172
  replication in cell culture, 178–182
  ribonucleoprotein, 176–177
  ribosome, virus-associated, 175–176, 184
  RNA
    negative stranded, 181, 183
    polymerase, RNA-dependent, 177–179
    species, listed, 172–175
    transcriptase, 178, 181
  rodent host, typical, 160
  sensitivity
    to heat, 168
    to lipid solvents, 168
Argas sp., 47, 62, 66, 328
Argentine hemorrhagic fever, 157, 158, 163
Arumowot virus
  in *Culex* sp. (1963), 55
  in rodents (1971), 55
Astravirus, 253
Atlantic salmon fibrosarcoma due to
      retrovirus, 441
Atlantic salmon papilloma-associated virus,
      448–449
Avalon virus
  in herring gull (1976), 59
  in *Ixodes uriae* (1972), 59
  in puffin (1976), 59
Avian infectious bronchitis virus, 195
Avian myeloblastosis virus (AMV), DNA
      polymerase, 479
5-Azacytidine, 116, 118

Bahig virus, 45
  in bird, 42
  in tick, 42
Bakau virus, 4
  in *Argas abdussalami*, 47
  in *Culex* sp. (1956), 47
  in *Macaca* sp., 47
Balkan nephropathy, endemic, in humans, 228
Barmah Forest virus, 4, 61
Batai virus, 8, 10, 13, 46
Batama virus, 45
  in bird, 44
Belem Virus Laboratory (Brazil), 35
Belmont virus, in *Culex* sp. (1968), 63
Bertioga Beach, Sao Paulo, Brazil, 34
Bertioga virus, in sentinel mouse (1962), 34
Bhanja virus
  in domestic animals (1971), 63
  in *Haemaphysalis* sp. (1954), 63
  in human, laboratory-acquired (1975), 63
  in mouse brain, electron microscope
      photograph, 70
Bile and hepatitis A antigen, 502–504
Bimiti virus, in *Culex* sp. (1955), 34
Birao virus, 9
Blood donor and hepatitis, 497, 498
Bluegill virus, 451–452
  composition, chemical, 452
  growth, 452
  morphology, 451
  properties, biological, 451–452
Bluetongue virus of sheep (BTV), 285
  agar gel precipitin test, 321
  an arbovirus, 285
  bighorn sheep immunized against, 324
  capsid, 297, 312
  and cattle diseases, 326
  in chicken egg embryo, 287, 288
  complement fixation test, 320
  in *Culicoides* sp., 287
  in fibroblast of mouse, 309
  and goat diseases, 326
  hemagglutination, 321
  hydranencephaly, 330
  infection, 330
  in insect, 286
  interferon induction in mouse, 318
  in lamb, congenital malformation, 330
  in lamb kidney cell, 289
  morphology of surface, 293
  neutralization, 319
  pinocytosis, 309

Bluetongue virus of sheep (BTV) (*cont*.)
  plaque inhibition technique, 319
  polypeptide, 312, 313
  pseudoenvelope, 309
  purification, 321
  RNA
    double-stranded, 296, 298
    genome, 298
    molecular weight, 296
    sedimentation, 294
  sensitization of animal to, 325
  serotyping, 289, 319, 322, 323
  and sheep diseases, 326
  surface morphology, 293
  ts mutant, 316, 317
  vaccine, polyvalent, attenuated, 324
  virus factories in cytoplasm, 309
  in yolk sac, 288
Bobia virus. 36
Bolivian hemorrhagic fever, 157, 158, 163
Boöphilus sp., 59, 328
Boraceia virus
  in *Anopheles cruzii* (1962), 46
  in *Phoniomyia* sp. (1974), 46
  subtype of *Anopheles* group B virus, 47
Botambi virus
  in *Culex* sp. (1968), 37
Bromelin, 201
5-Bromo-2-deoxyuridine, 80
Brown bullhead papilloma-associated virus,
    447–448
Bryanston virus, 331
Bujaru virus, 53
Bunyavirus
  assembly, 113–114
  budding, 113–114
  buoyant density, 78
  carbohydrate, 79
  characteristics
    biological, 7–68
    serological, 7–68
  classification, serological, 2, 4
  complementation analysis, 123–124
  complement-fixation test, 5
    formula for calculating index, 123
  composition, 78–105
    chemical, 79
  defective interfering, 131
  density, buoyant, 78
  electron microscope photograph, 69–72, 74
  envelope, phospholipid of, 79, 80

Bunyavirus (*cont*.)
  genetics, 114–131
    growth curve, 114–116
    mutation
      induced, 116–118
      ts, 114–119
    recombination
      formula for calculating, 119
      heterologous, high-frequency, 125–130
      homologous, high-frequency, 119–123
  glycoprotein, 91–98
  hemagglutination inhibition test, 5
  hepatotropism, 73
  infectivity, 82–83
  interference, 131
  isolation, 5–68
  lipid, 79
  maturation in smooth endoplasmic
      reticulum, 75
    in Golgi apparatus, 75
  members listed, 4
  morphogenesis, 68–78
  morphology, 68–78
    electron density, 76–77
    shape, 77–78
    size, 77–78
  mutant
    double, 125
    induction of, 116–118
    isolation of spontaneous, 118
    ts, 114–121, 124–126
  neutralization test, 5
  nucleocapsid, 91–93, 98–100, 102–104
  particle
    diagram, 106
    protein molecules per particle, 100
    structure, hypothetical, 106
    weight, 78–79
  phospholipid envelope, 79, 80
  phosphoprotein, 98
  polypeptide, 108–110
    molecular weight, 94–95
  properties, 78–105
  protein, 91–100
    glycoprotein, external, 91–98
    large, 100
    molecular weight, listed, 94–95
    nucleocapsid, internal, 91–93, 98–100,
        102–104
    polypeptide, 108–110
    –RNA coding relationship, 100–102

Bunyavirus (*cont.*)
  protein (*cont.*)
    sulfated, 98
    synthesis, viral, 108–110
  recombination, genetic, 119–123, 125–130
    analysis with *ts* mutant, 120–121
  relationship of members, 5–68
  replication, 106–114
    adsorption, 106–107
    penetration, 106–107
    transcription
      primary, 107–108
      mRNA synthesis, early, 107–108
  RNA
    base ratio, 81–82
    closed, circular, noncovalent, 83–85
    density, 81–82
    electrophoresis, 86–88
    genome, 79–91
    length measurement, 85
    molecular weight, 90–91
      listed, 88
    oligonucleotide fingerprinting, 88–90
    polyacrylamide gel analysis, 86–88
    polymerase, 104–105
    protein coding relationship, 100–102
    replication, 110–111
    mRNA synthesis, amplified, 111–113
    S RNA codes for N protein, the proof,
      129–130
    sedimentation coefficient, 85–86
    species, 80
      per particle, 91
    terminus, 82
  structure, 68–106
  in tissue, 73–76
  transcription, secondary, 111–113
  weight of particle, 78–79
Bunyamwera group viruses, 1, 8–15
  antibody
    in chimpanzee, 9
    in domestic animals, 9
    in human, 9
  characteristics
    biological, 7–46
    serological, 7–46
  established (1960), 8
  hemagglutination-inhibition reaction, 13
  in mouse brain, electron microscope
      photograph, 69
  RNA sedimentation coefficient, 85–86
  transmission, experimental, 9
Bursal disease virus, 229
  infectious, 229

Bush Bush Forest, Eastern Trinidad, 31, 32
Bushbush virus, 2, 32, 33
  in *Culex* sp. (1959), 31
Buttonwillow virus, 43, 44
  in midges, 42
  in rabbit (1962), 42
Bwamba County, Uganda, 8, 16
Bwamba group viruses, 2, 16

Caanan Lake, Long Island, New York, 447
Cacao virus, 53
Cache Valley virus, 11–13
CAH, *see* Hepatitis, chronic active
Caimito virus, 53
Calf diarrhea coronavirus, 195
Calicivirus
  amino acids, 273–274
    listed, 274
  antigen, 253–255
  and arboviruses, criteria for distinguishing
      between the two groups, 276
  base composition of RNA and homology,
      271
  buoyant density, 267–268
  calculation of mass, 275
  capsid polypeptide, 262
  cell culture, 255–263
    cytopathology, 257–259
    of domestic cat, 256
    growth curve, 256
    host range, 256
    of lion kidney, 256
  cell infection, 260
  cup-shaped depressions on surface typical,
      264
  cytolysis, rapid, 256
  in cytoplasm, 255
  defective interfering, 275
  description, 264–276
    summary, 275–276
  diseases caused by, 250–253
  electron microscope photograph, 258, 265
  electrophoresis of RNA, on gel, 270
  end-group analysis of RNA, 271–272
  feline (FCV), 249, 252
    in cat, 252
    in cheetah, captive, 252
    in kitten, 252
    serotype, single, 254
    in urolithiasis, 252
    vaccine, commercial, 254
  and gastroenteritis, infantile, non-bacterial,
      252
  gel electrophoresis of RNA, 270

Calicivirus (*cont.*)
  genetics, 259
  history, 250
  host range, 256
  human, 252–253
  inactivation, 268–269
    photodynamic, 269
    thermal, 268
    by trypsin, 268
  infectivity of RNA, 270
    is sensitive to ribonuclease, 270
  insect viruses resembling, 276
  mass, 274–275
  members, 249
  model based on subunits, 266
  molecular weight of polypeptide, 272, 273
  morphology, 264–266
  natural history, 250–253
  protein, 272–274, 277
    amino acids, 273–274
      listed, 274
    peptides, 273–274
    polypeptides, 261, 272–274
      major, 272–274
      minor, 273–274
      in trimers, 266
    viral, in infected cell, 261–263
  purification, 264
  replication, 256
  RNA, 259–261
    base composition, listed, 271
    components, 260
    content, 269, 274
    end-group, 271–272
    extraction, 269–270
    gel electrophoresis, 270
    homology, 271
    infectivity, 270–271
    sedimentation, 270
    single-stranded, 259
    stability, 268–269
  in stool specimen, 252, 253
  structure, 264–266
    double shell, 264
    icosahedral, 266
    single shell, 264
  swine virus (*see also* San Miguel sea lion
    virus; vesicular exanthema of swine),
    249
California encephalitis virus, 2, 20–22
California group viruses, 2, 19–30
  hemagglutination-inhibition reaction, 22
  members listed, 22
  in mouse after intracerebral inoculation, 73

California sea lion (*see also* San Miguel sea
  lion virus), 251
Calomys callosus, natural host of Machupo
  virus, 159
Calovo virus, 8, 10
Caluromys sp., 17, 18
Cauliflower virus, 349, 353
Candiru virus, 53
Canine coronavirus, 195
Capim group viruses, 2, 30–34, 45
  in *Caluromys philander* (1958), 31
  complement fixation reaction, 33
  in *Culex* sp., 31
  hemagglutination-inhibition reaction, 32
  members listed, 2, 32–33
  neutralization reaction, 32
  in *Proechimys* sp., 31
  in sentinel mouse, 31
Caraparu virus, 17, 19
Carassius auratus, 454
Carnation etched-ring virus, 349, 361, 385
Carp pox virus, 403
  antigenicity, 405
  biology, 404–409
  carbohydrate, 407
  cell culture
    lines listed, 408
    susceptibility, 408–409
  composition, chemical, 406–407
  DNA, 406
  growth cycle, 407–408
  lipid, 407
  morphology, 404–405
  protein, 406–407
  stability, 405–406
Carp spring viremia virus, 428–429, 437–438
Catostomus commersoni, 444
Catu virus
  in *Cebus* sp., 34
  in human, 34
  in sentinel mouse, 34
Cauliflower mosaic virus
  DNA, 358
  electron microscope photograph, 362
  protein, structural, 358
Cebus sp., 17, 18
Central African Empire, 37, 41, 44, 55, 60
Central nervous system (CNS), and persistent
  demyelination, 231
Chagres virus
  in human (1960), 54
  in mouse brain, electron microscope
    photograph, 70
  in sandfly, 54

Changuinold virus, 287, 323
Channel catfish virus (CCV), 401–409
  antiserum available, 405
  cell culture
    growth curve in, 409
    replication, 407, 408
  disease is acute hemorrhagic, 402
  DNA, 406
  protein, 406
Chilibre virus, 53
Chilo iridescent virus (CIV), 348
  enzymes
    nucleotide phosphorylase, 359
    protein kinase, 359
Chimpanzee and hepatitis, 512
Chironomus virus, 354
Chittoor virus, 10
Cholera enterotoxin, 226
Cirrhosis, postnecrotic, 493
CIV, *see* Chilo iridescent virus
Clenopharyngodon idella, 429
Clo Mor virus, in *Ixodes uriae* (1973), 59
Colorado tick fever virus, 287, 323
Complementation analysis, formula for
    calculating the index, 123
Congo Red Fever, *see* Fièvre rouge congolaise
Congo virus, 47–49
  in animals (1970), 48
  antibody in human, 48
  in human (1956), 47
  in mouse brain, electron microscope
    photograph, 70
Coronaviruses
  animal's response to, 225–230
  antigen, 205, 209
  assembly, 215
  bovine diarrhea virus, 225
  canine, 195
  cell culture, 204, 209, 210
  cell interaction, 225–226
  composition, chemical, 197–201
    carbohydrate, 201
    lipid, 199–201
    protein, 194
    RNA, 197–199
  defective, 211, 217
  description, 195–204
  diagnosis, 229–230
  diarrhea
    in calf, neonatal, 209, 223, 225, 229
    in human, 194, 329
  disease, 223, 225
    listed, 220
    pathogenesis, 218–231

Coronaviruses (*cont.*)
  envelope, 203
  –cell membrane fusion, 208
  feline, 195
  fusion of envelope and cell membrane, 208
  genetics, 236–237
  glycoprotein, 201
  growth
    curve, 205–207
    multiplication kinetics, 205–207
  hemagglutination, 201
  host
    cell metabolism, 216–217
    listed, 195
    range, 207
  human, 195
  infection
    intrauterine, 223
    rate, 219
    route, 219–225
  infectivity
    assay, 204–205
    modification, 207
  interference, 217–218
  intrauterine infection, 223
  kill cell, 225
  macromolecule biosynthesis, 209–215
  members, 194–195
  morphology, 195–197
  mouse hepatitis virus, *see* Mouse hepatitis
    virus
  mucosal disease virus of sheep, 225, 234
  multiplication sequence, 216
    adsorption, 207
    penetration, 208–209
    uncoating, 208–209
  neonatal calf diarrhea, 195
  nucleocapsid, 203–204, 212–213
  organ tropism, 207
  pathogenesis, 218–231
    demyelination, primary, 219
    hepatitis, 219
    immunity depressed, 219, 230
    kill cell, 230
    meningoencephalitis, human, 219
    nephritis, interstitial, 219
    organs infected, 218
      polyorgan tropism, 218
    pneumonitis, interstitial, 219
    vasculitis, 230
    viremia, 230
  peplomer, 201–203
  persistence, 231–236
  properties defined, 237

Coronaviruses (*cont.*)
 protein, 199, 214–215
  structural, listed, 200, 202
 resistance to infection, 226–229
 RNA
  double-stranded, 211
  genome, 193, 194, 209, 211
  mRNA, 209–211
  pathogenic, 193
  single-stranded, 193, 197
  species, 211–214
 route of infection, 219–225
 spike, 202
 structure, fine, 202–204
  envelope, 203
  nucleocapsid, 203–204
  peplomer, 201–203
 syncytia in organ, 226
 turkey bluecomb disease virus, 225
 vaccine, 228
 viropexis, 208, 209
Corripalta virus, 287, 298, 322–323, 327
Coxsackie B5 virus, 250
CPH, *see* Hepatitis, chronic persistent
Crimean Hemorrhagic Fever, 4, 47–49
 in animals (1970), 48
 antibody in human, neutralizing, 48
 in human (1946), 47
 in *Hyalomma plumbeum plumbeum* (1945),
  47
Culex sp., 8–10, 17–21, 25, 27, 28, 31, 34,
  36–38, 40, 41, 47, 55, 60, 63, 67
Culicoides sp., 39–41, 52, 287, 328–329
Culiseta sp., 12, 21, 22, 24
Cycloheximide, 368, 387
cyprinus carpio (*see* Carp pox virus), 403
Cytoplasmic polyhedrosis virus, 299
Cytosine arabinoside, 370

D'Aguilar virus, 327
Dahlia mosaic virus, 349
Dane particle, 476–482
 B$_e$ antigen, 486–487
  discovery (1972), 486
 and carriers of hepatitis B virus, 488
 core antigen, 485–486
  polypeptide, 486
 described (1970), 477
 DNA
  circular, 479
  polymerase, 478, 479, 481, 482, 486, 489,
   491
  sedimentation, 481
  synthesis, 482

Dane particle (*cont.*)
 is the hepatitis B virus (*see also* Hepatitis
  virus), 478
Daunomycin, 479
Didelphis sp., 18
Down's syndrome, 497
Drosophila melanogaster, 428, 429
Dugbe virus
 in *Culicoides* sp. (1970), 52
 in domestic animals (1971), 52
 in ticks (1971), 52

Eel virus disease, 446–447
 American, 426, 437, 438
 European, 418, 437, 438
 by rhabdovirus, 429–430
Egtved virus, 426
EHDV, *see* Epizootic hemorrhagic disease
  viruses
Encephalitis demyelination and coronavirus
  infection, 220–221
Endonuclease, bacterial
 *Eco*RI, 482, 483
 *Hae*III, 479–480, 482
 single strand specific, 480
Entebbe East African Virus Research Institute,
  Uganda, 8
Enteric coronavirus, human, 195
Enteritis and coronavirus, 220–221
Ependymitis and coronavirus, 220–221
Epithelioma papillosum-associated virus, 405
Epizootic hemorrhagic disease viruses
 in antelope, 326
 in *Culicoides* sp., 287
 in deer, 326
 serotype, 287
Equine encephalosis virus, 287, 331
Esox
 E. lucius, 442
 lymphosarcoma due to retrovirus, 441–442
 E. masquinongy, 442
  lymphosarcoma, 442
 retrovirus and epidermal hyperplasia, 442
 sarcoma, 441–442
Eubenangee virus, 287, 298, 322, 327
Eyach virus, 323
Eye infection by coronavirus, 220–221

Facey's Paddock virus, in *Culex* sp. (1974), 40
Feces and hepatitis A antigen, 502–504
Feline calicivirus (*see also* Calicivirus) antigen,
  254
Feline coronavirus, 195

Fièvre rouge congolaise (Congo Red Fever)
    and Tataguine virus (1969), 66
Fish viruses, 401–470
    infections, 401–470
Flavivirus, 17
Fluorophenylalanine, 377–379
5–Fluorouracil, 116, 118
Foot-and-mouth disease virus, 250
Frijoles virus, 53
Frog virus 3, 348, 349
    cell culture growth curve, 365
    cell infected with, 384
    cleavage, posttranslational, 379–380
    control
        correlations, 380–384
        quantitative, 376–379
    DNA, 357
        conversion from resistant to sensitive for
            DNase, 367, 368
    encapsidated, 384
    poly(A) lacking, 374
    polymerase, 368
    synthesis
        in nucleus, 385, 386
        prevention of, 370
    electron microscope photograph, 355, 363
    enzymes, 359
        deoxyribonuclease, 359
        nucleotide phosphohydrolase, 359
        protein kinase, 359
        protein phosphatase, 359
        ribonuclease, 359
    in fathead minnow as a model, 364
    genome, 384–385
    growth curve in cell culture, 365
    in hamster kidney as a model, 364
    inclusion body, 361
    infection, 367
    lipid
        phospholipid, 360
        sphingomyelin, 360
    modification, posttranscriptional, 369
    mutant ts, 366
    nucleic acid, viral, 385, 387
    pinocytosis, 361, 367
    protein
        modification, posttranslational, 379–380
        polypeptides, 358
        synthesis, 375–380
            qualitative control, 375–378
            quantitative control, 378
            rate of, 378–379
    purification, 359

Frog virus (cont.)
    replication, 364–385
        adsorption, 367–368
        in cytoplasm, 385
        of DNA genome, 384–385
        in nucleus, 385–390
        penetration, 367–368
        uncoating, 367–368
    RNA
        control, qualitative, 369
        modification, posttranslational, 374–375
        molecular weight, listed, 372
        polymerase, DNA-dependent, 367
        synthesis, 364, 368–375, 383
    transcription, 368–375
        control
            qualitative, 369–370
            quantitative, 370–373
            temporal, 373–374
    translation efficiency, 383
    ts mutant, 366

Gamboa virus, 44
    in Aedeomyia squamipennis, 45
    tranmission, transovarial, 45
Gan Gan virus, 4, 50–52
    in Aedes sp. (1970), 51
Ganjam virus, 49, 52
    in membrane of hepatocyte, electron
        microscope photograph, 71
    in tick (1968), 52
Germiston virus, 8, 9, 13
GFA, see Grunt fin agent
Gill necrosis of carp-associated virus, 54–55
Glomerulonephritis, membranous and
        hepatitis, 494
Glucosamine, 182
Glycolipoprotein, 199, 201
Gold shiner virus, 422
    disease, 416
Goldfish, see Carassius auratus
Golgi apparatus and Bunya virus maturation,
        75
Gonaditis and coronavirus, 220–221
Gordil virus
    in gerbil (1975), 55
    in Lemnyscomys striatus (1971), 55
Grand Arbaud virus
    in Argas reflexus (1966), 62
Grunt fin agent (GFA), 452–454
    composition, chemical, 453
    growth cycle, 453

Grunt fin agent (GFA) (*cont.*)
  morphology, 453
  properties, biological, 453
Guajara virus, 2, 32, 33
Guama group of viruses, 2, 33–35
  hemagglutination inhibition reactions, listed, 35
  members, listed, 2, 34–35
  neutralization reactions listed, 34
Guaratuba virus, 44
  in *Aedes* sp., 45
  in bird, 45
  in sentinel hamster, 45
  in sentinel mouse, 45
Guaroa virus, 8, 10, 11
  ts mutant recombination analysis, 121
Gumbaio, 294
  an infectious disease of chickens, 294
Gumbo Limbo virus, 17

Haemulon sciurus, 452
Hamster, Syrian, 160
Hazara virus
  in human, 49
  in mouse brain, electron microscope
      photograph, 70
  in tick, 49
HCV, *see* Coronavirus, human
HECV, *see* Coronavirus, human enteric
Hemagglutinating encephalomyelitis virus
      (HEV), 236
Hepatitis
  carrier state, 495–496
    in mouse model, 231
  and coronavirus, 220–221
  human, 471–526
    virus in feces (1973), 472
  mouse model of chronic, 231
  posttransfusion hepatitis and mortality in
      U.S.A., 495
  prevalence,
    in United States, 494–495
    in world, 495
  transmission, experimental
    to chimpanzee (1973), 472
    to marmoset (1969), 472
  virus A and virus B are unrelated, 472
Hepatitis A virus, 471–526
  antigen (HAAg), 502–504
    in bile (1975), 502–504
    in feces (1973), 502–504
    in liver (1975), 502–504
      synthesis in, 504–505

Hepatitis A virus (*cont.*)
  in chimpanzee, 512
  diseases associated with, 507–512
  epidemiology, 507–512
  in feces (1973), 502–504
  immunity, 507
  incidence, 508–509
  infection, 501–502
    course of, 505–506
  marker in
    blood, 506
    feces, 506
    liver, 506
  recognition, 471–473
  transmission, 509–512
    fecal-oral, 509–510
    food, 511–512
    nonfecal, 510
    percutaneous, 519–511
    water, 511–512
Hepatitis B virus, 471–526
  and acrodermatitis, infantile papular, 494
  acute disease, 492–493
  antibody, 490, 492
  antigens
    Australia, discovered (1965), 474
    core, 485–486
    HB$_c$, 485–486
    HB$_e$, 486–487
    HB$_s$, 474–477, 490
    on surface, 474–477
    synthesis in infected liver, 487–488
  Australia antigen, 474
  carrier state, 491
  chronic state
    active (CAH), 492–493
    persistent (CPH), 492–493
  core antigen, 485–486
  Dane particle
    DNA polymerase as marker of, 489, 491
    electron microscope photograph, 476
    is the virus, 478
  disease associated with, 492–494
  DNA, 477–484
    cloned, 483–484
    polymerase as marker of Dane particle,
        478–479, 482, 489, 491
    recombination experiment, 483
  epidemiology, 494–500
    persistent, 495–497
    in United States, 494–495
  gene
    map, 483

Hepatitis B virus (*cont.*)
  gene (*cont.*)
    number of, 488
  and glomerulonephritis, membranous, 494
  HB$_e$ antigen, and hepatocellular carcinoma,
      493
  incomplete form, 484–485
  infection, 473–500
    course, 489–492
    disease associated with, 492–494
    marker in blood, 489–491
    persistent, 491–492
    self-limited, 489–491
  marker in blood during infection, 489–491
  particle 22 nm, 484–485
  and polyarteritis nodosa, 494
  polypeptide, virus-specified, 484–485, 488
  recognition, 471–473
  structures found in human blood, 474
    electron microscope photograph, 475
  surface antigen (HB$_s$), 474–477
  transmission, 498–500
    experimental to ape, 473
      man, 473
      monkey, 473
Hepatocyte infection by hepatitis B virus,
      487–488
Herpesviridae of fish (*see also* Herpes virus
      salmonis, Nerka virus, Channel
      catfish virus), 401–409
  capsid, 405
  core, 405
  disease, biology of, 402–403
  envelope, 405
  size, listed, 405
Herpes virus salmonis, 401–403, 405
  cell culture, 407, 409
  DNA bands, 406
  electron microscope photograph, 404
  isolation
    from rainbow trout, 402
    from sockey salmon, 402
HEV, *see* Hemagglutinating encephalomyelitis
      virus

Ibaraki virus, 325
  RNA, double-stranded, 298
ICDV, *see* Icosahedral cytoplasmic
      deoxyriboviruses
Icosahedral cytoplasmic deoxyriboviruses,
      347–399
  in *Aedes aegypti*, 348
  in *Aedes albopictus*, 348
  antigen, 359

Icosahedral cytoplasmic deoxyriboviruses
      (*cont.*)
  catalogue of, 350–352
  classification, 348–349
  composition, chemical, 356–360
  DNA, 353, 356–358
    synthesis, 364, 389
  electron microscope photograph, 352, 354,
      355, 362, 363
  enzymes, 359–360
    deoxyribonuclease, 359
    nucleotide phosphorylase, 359
    protein kinase, 359
    protein phosphatase, 359
    ribonuclease, 359
  hosts, listed, 350–351
  lipid, 360
  members, 350–352
  molecular weight, 356–357
  morphology, 353–356
  plant- (*see also* separate plant viruses), 349
  properties
    biological, 348–349
    physical, 356
  protein, 358–359
  replication interpreted by electron
      microscopy only, 361
  RNA
    capped, 375
    methylated, 375
    modification, posttranscriptional, 374–375
  size, 349–353
  structure, 353–356
IBV, *see* Infectious bronchitis virus
Ictalurus nebulosus, 447
  I. punctatus, 402
Icoaraci virus, 53
  in mosquito, 54
  in rodent (1960), 54
  in sandfly, 54
IHN, *see* Infectious hematopoietic necrosis
Ilesha virus, 8, 9, 13
Immune complex disease, 228
Immunofluorescence, 180
Immunoglobulin
  IgA, 228
  IgG, 228
  IgM, 228
Infectious bronchitis virus, 194, 205, 209, 228,
      229, 234
  cell culture, 205, 209
  electron microscope photograph, 196
  genome, 197
  nephritis, chronic interstitial, 228, 229

Infectious bronchitis virus (*cont.*)
  organ culture, chicken tracheal ring,
    multiplication in, 205, 209
Infectious hematopoietic necrosis (IHN),
    426–427
Infectious hematopoietic necrosis virus
  biology, 430–431
  cell culture, 430, 436–438
    growth curve, 437
  defective, 431
  electron microscope photograph, 430
  envelope, 431
  interferon induced in cell culture, 440
  morphology, 430
  RNA analysis, 439
Infectious pancreatic necrosis virus, 415–426
  antigenicity, 418
  in brook trout, 415
  in carrier, lifelong, 415
  cell culture susceptibility, 423
  composition, chemical, 419–421
  defective, 416
  electron microscope photograph, 417
  growth cycle, 421–425
  interferon synthesis, 425–426
  molecular weight, 419
  morphology, 417–418
  mutant, 418
  persistence, 425–426
  polypeptide, autoradiograph of, 423
    molecular weight, listed, 422
  properties, biological, 418–419
  protein, 420–421, 424–425
  replication, 421, 422
  RNA, 420
    characteristics, 422, 425
    double-stranded, 420
    polymerase, RNA-dependent, 425
    synthesis, 425
  sedimentation coefficient, 419
  stability, 419
  structure
    of capsid, 417
    icosahedral, 417
Ingwavuma virus
  in *Culex* sp., 40
  in *Hyphanturgus ocularis*, 40
Inini virus, in *Pteroglossus* sp., 42
Inkoo virus, 19, 20, 22, 28–29
  in *Aedes* sp., 28
International Catalogur of Arboviruses (1975),
    1
Iridescent virus, *see* Mosquito iridescent virus

Iridoviridae of fish, 409–414
  disease, biology of, 409–410
  growth curve, 409
  lymphocystis (*see also* Lymphocystis virus),
    409–410, 412
  piscine erythrocytic necrosis (*see also* Piscine
    erythrocytic necrosis virus), 412
Irituia virus, 323
Itaporanga virus
  in bird, 54
  in mosquito, 54
  in sentinel mouse (1962), 54
Itaqui virus, 17, 19
Ixodes sp., 58, 59, 62, 222, 328

Jamestown Canyon virus, 20, 22, 24
  in *Aedes* sp., 24
  in *Culiseta inornata*, 24
  in *Psorophora* sp., 24
Japanaut virus, 287
Jaundice *see also* Hepatitis, history of, 471
Jerry Slough virus
  in *Culiseta inornata*, (1963), 24
JHMV, *see* Mouse hepatitis virus
Juan Diaz virus, 2, 32, 33
  in sentinel mouse (1962), 31
Junin virus, 158, 159, 169, 172, 173
  in *Akodon azarae*, 159
  in Argentine hemorrhagic fever patient
    (1958), 158
  in *Calomys* spp., 159, 160
Jurona virus, 44
  in *Hemagogus* sp., 45

Kaenf Khoi virus, 44, 46
  in bedbug (1976), 45
  in guano miners in Thailand, 45
  in *Tadaria plicata* (1969), 45
Kaikalur virus, 40
  in *Culex* sp. (1970), 40
Kairi virus, 10, 11, 13
Kaisodi virus, 4, 49–50
  in tick (1957), 49
Karimabad virus
  in bird (1975), 55
  electron microscope photograph, 72
  in sandfly (1959), 55
Kasba virus, 322
Kemerovo virus, 287
Kern County, California, 12, 20
Ketapang virus, in *Culex* sp. (1956), 47
Keystone virus, 2, 22, 27–28
  in *Aedes atlanticus-tormenta* (1962), 27, 28
  in *Anopheles* sp., 27

Keystone virus (*cont.*)
  in *Culex* sp., 27
  transmission, transovarial, 28
Khasan virus, in *Haemaphysalis longicornis*
      (1977), 64
Kongool virus, 2, 35–36
  in *Ficalbia* sp., (1975), 36
Konwanyama virus
  in *Anopheles* sp. (1963), 64
  in domestic animals (1970), 64

LAC virus, *see* LaCrosse virus
LaCrosse virus, 16, 20, 22, 24–26
  in *Aedes* sp., 24–26
  in *Anopheles* sp., 25
  antibody, 25
  base ratio of RNA, 81
  in *Culex* sp., 25
  genetic relationships, listed, 99
  in human brain tissue (1960), 24
  in *Hybomitra lasiophthalma* (horsefly), 24
  infectivity assay, 82
  molecular weight, listed, 99
  morphology, 77
  mutant *ts*, recombination
    analysis, 120
    experiment, 125
    pathogenic potential, 101
  nucleocapsid, 101
  nucleotide, terminal, 82
  oligonucleotide fingerprinting, 89
  polypeptides, listed, 99
  in *Psorophora* sp., 25
  RNA
    circular, closed, 83–85
    molecular weight, 87
    –protein mass ratio, 79
    species, listed, 99
  structure, components, listed, 99
  symptoms, 26
  transmission, transovarial, 25
  weight, 78–79
Lake Oneida, New York, 444
Lanjan virus, in tick (1967), 49
Lassa fever virus, 157, 159, 166, 172
  in *Mastomys natalensis*, 159, 160
  photograph by electron microscope, 166
Latino virus, 159
  in *Calomys callosus*, 159
Lebombo virus, 287
Lepomis macrochirus, 451
Leprosy, lepromatous type, 497
Leukemia, lymphocytic chronic, 497

Liver (*see also* Hepatitis)
  carcinoma, hepatocellular, 493
  cirrhosis, postnecrotic, 493
  and hepatitis A antigen, 502–505
Lockern virus, 11–13
Lone Star virus
  in mouse brain, electron microscope
      photograph, 71
  in tick (1967), 64
Lukuni virus, 15, 16
Lumbo, Mozambique, 23
Lumbo virus, 22–24
  in *Aedes pembaensis* (1959), 23
  RNA
    circular, closed, 83–85
    polymerase, RNA–directed, 104
    sedimentation coefficient, 85–86
Lutjanus synagris, 453
Lymphocystis disease of fish, 349
Lymphocystis virus, 354, 409, 413, 414
Lymphocytic choriomeningitis virus, (LCM),
      159, 162, 171–173, 177
  antigen in infected cell, 171
  cell culture, 167, 178, 179, 181
  complement fixation antigen in infected cell,
      171
  defective interfering, 182, 183
  fever, 157–158
  in human, 158
  interference, 182
  in monkey (1933), 158
  in mouse, 158–162
    intracerebral inoculation, 162
  polypeptide, 168, 170
Lymphoreticuloendothelial system, 160
Lymphosarcoma, 442
  experimentally transmitted, 442

Machupo virus, 158, 159, 172
  and Bolivian hemorrhagic fever, 158
  in *Calomys callosus*, 159
  in cell culture, Vero cells, 165
  electron microscope photograph, 165
  in hamster, 159
Madrid virus, 17
Maguari virus, 8, 10, 11, 13
Mahagony Hammock virus, 33
Main Drain virus, 11–13
Manawa virus
  in *Argas abdussalami* (1970), 62
  in *Rhipicephalus* sp. (1970), 62
Mansonia sp., 8, 9, 11

Manzanilla virus, 43
  in *Alouatta seniculus insularis* (1960), 41
Maprik virus, 4, 51, 52
  in *Aedes* sp. (1966), 50
Maputta group viruses, 4, 50–52
  in *Anopheles* sp. (1960), 50
  complement fixation relationships, listed, 52
  members listed, 4, 51, 52
  neutralization relationships, listed, 51
Marituba virus, 17–19
Marmosa sp., 17, 18
Mastomys natalensis, 159
Matruh virus, 42, 45
  in bird, 42
  in tick, 42
Melao virus, 2, 19, 22, 29
  in *Aedes scapularis* (1955), 29
  in *Psorophora ferox*, 29
Melajo Forest, Northeast Trinidad, 29, 34
Meningoencephalitis, acute, 24
  of adult mouse, 157
6–Mercaptopurine, 414
Mermet virus, 43, 44
  in martin (1964), 42
Mesocricetus auratus, 160
6-Methyladenosine, 375
N-Methyl-*N'*-nitro-*N*-nitrosoguanidine, 116,
    118
Minatitlan, Veracruz, Mexico, 36
Minatitlan virus
  in mosquito (1970), 36
  in sentinel hamster (1967), 36
Mirim virus, 2, 36
  in *Cebus apella* (1957), 36
Mitchell River virus, 322
MIV, *see* Mosquito iridescent virus
Moju virus
  antibody, 35
  in *Culex* sp. (1959), 34
  in *Mansonia* sp., 35
  in sentinel mouse, 35
Moriche virus, in *Culex* sp. (1964), 31
Mosquito, *see* separate genera
Mosquito iridescent virus, 353, 360
  DNA, 357
  protein, 358
Mouse heptatitis virus (MHV), 194, 195
  cell culture, 211–214, 235
  defective, 217
  demyelination of brain, 223
  genetics, 236
  immunofluorescence microassy, 205
  interference, 217

Mouse hepatitis virus (MHV) (*cont.*)
  multiplication, 214
  persistence, 231–233
    in cell culture, 235
  resistance to, 227
    located in H-2 region of mouse genome,
      227
  strain
    A59V, 211–214
    JHMV, 211–214
M'Poko virus, 4
  in *Culex* sp. (1960), 60
Mucosal disease virus, 225, 234
Mudjinbarry virus, 316, 322
Multiple sclerosis, 231
Murutucu virus, 17–19

Nairobi sheep disease virus, 49
  in goat (1958), 51
  in human (1958), 52
  isolated in Nairobi, Kenya (1910), 51
  in tick (1958), 51, 52
Naples sandfly fever virus, 53
  epidemic among U.S. troops in Italy, 55
  in *Phlebotomus papatasi*, 55
Neacomys sp., 159
Necrosis, ulcerative dermal (UDN), 454
Nectomys sp., 31
Negamer, 265
Neonatal calf diarrhea coronavirus (NCDCV),
    195
Nephritis and coronavirus, 220–221
Nepuyo virus, 17, 18
Nerka virus, 402–403, 405
Neutral red dye, 269
Nique virus, 53
Nola virus, in *Culex* sp. (1975), 41
Northern pike
  lymphoma cell, electron microscope
      photograph, 443
  lymphosarcoma, 442
  rhabdovirus (pike fry rhabdovirus), 429, 437,
      438
Northway virus, 11, 12
Norwalk virus, 253
Notemigonus crysoleucas, 415
Nucleocapsid, 196, 199, 203, 204, 404
Nyabira virus, 322, 331

Olifantsvlei, Johannesberg, South Africa, 37
Olifantsvlei group of viruses, 2, 36–37
  members listed, 36
  neutralization relationships, 37

Oncorhynchus nerka, 402
Orbivirus
  in *Aedes albopictus*, 308
  antigen, 318–325
    variation, 323–324
  in *Argas* sp., 328
  assay, 286–290
    dilution end-point, 290
    plaque, 290
  in *Boöphilus* sp., 328
  capsid, 290, 303–307, 312–315
    polypeptide, 304–306
  capsomere, 290
  cell culture, 286, 288–289, 308, 317, 318
  and cell function, 317–318
  classification, groups listed, 287
  complement fixation, 320
  composition, chemical, 296–298
  core, 292, 305–306
  cross-hybridization, 303
  in *Culicoides* sp., 328–329
  cultivation, 288–289
  cytopathology, 289–290
    in cell culture, 289
  defective interfering, 316–317
  description, 290–308
  ecology, 329
  electron microscope photograph, 293, 295
  enzyme, RNA polymerase, 307–308
  epizootiology, 325–331
  in flies, 328
  genome, 298–303
    coding relationships, 307
    homology, 302–303
    segmented, 299–302
    size of segments, 307
  hemagglutination, 321–322
  host range, 325–327
  hybrids, 303
  immunity, 324–325
  immunodiffusion, 320–321
  immunofluorescence, 321
  inoculation, intracerebral, in mouse, 286
  in insects, 286, 308, 325, 328
    transmission by, 328
  interferon, 318
  isolation, primary, 286–288
  in *Ixodes* sp., 328
  macromolecule synthesis, 317–318
  measurements, 291
  morphology, 290–294
  mutant *ts*, 316–317
  neutralization, 318–320
  in *Ornithodoros* sp., 328

Orbivirus (*cont.*)
  pathogenesis, 329–331
  polypeptide, 304–306
    serotype, specific, 303
    synthesis, 307, 312–315
  propagation, 286–290
  properties, physical, 294–296
  protein
    layer removed, 295
    synthesis, 312–316
  purification, 291
  replication, 309–318
    adsorption, 309
    penetration, 309
    site of, 309
  in *Rhipicephalus* sp., 328
  RNA
    double-stranded, 298–299, 312
    mRNA synthesis, 310
    polymerase, 307–308
      RNA-dependent, 312
    species, 315
      molecular weight listed, 311
    transcriptase, 312
  in sandfly, 328
  serology and classification, 322–323
  size, 291–292
  stability, 296–298
  structure, 292–294
    and classification, 294
    and core, 292
  transcription
    replication of, 310–311
  translation, control of, 315–316
  tubule, virus-associated, 313
    electron microscope photograph, 314
  transmission of virus
    by insect, 328
    by tick, 328
    by wind, 329
Oriboca virus, 17–19
Oropouche virus, 43, 44
  in *Culicoides* sp., 41
  in human (1955), 41
    epidemics in Brazil (1961–1975), 41
Orungo virus, 287
Orthomyxovirus-like particle, electron
      microscope photograph, 449
Oryzomys sp., 17, 159
Ossa virus, 17, 18

Pahayokee virus, 38
  in *Culex* sp. (1964), 37
Palyam virus, 287, 298, 322

Pancreatitis and coronavirus, 220–221
Papilloma
    external in flathead sole, electron microscope
        photograph, 450
    oral, 447
Papovavirus group, 447
    in eel, 447
Parana virus, 159, 173
    defective, 183
    in *Oryzomys buccinatus*, 159
Pata virus, 322
Patois virus, 2, 37–38
    antibody, 38
    in *Culex* sp., 38
    neutralization relationships, listed, 37
    in *Sigmodon hispidus* (1966), 37
Peaton virus, in *Culicoides brevitarsis* (1976),
        40
PEN, *see* Piscine erythrocytic necrosis virus
PFR, *see* Northern pike fry rhabdovirus
Phlebotomus fever group viruses (*see also*
        Sandfly), 4, 53–58
Phoniomyia sp., 10
Pichinde virus, 159, 163, 169, 170–174, 177
    cell culture, 171
    defective, 183
    glycopeptide, 168, 169
    in *Oryzomis albigularis*, 159, 160
    polypeptide, 170
    RNA, 174
Picornavirus study group, 249
Pike fry rhabdovirus, *see* Northern pike
Piscine erythrocytic necrosis virus, 409–414
    cell culture, 414
    composition, chemical, 412–413
    dimensions, listed, 412
    DNA, 413
    electron microscope photograph, 411
    growth cycle, 413–414
    lipid, 413
    lymphocystis due to, 412
    morphology, 410–412
    properties, biological, 412
Pleuronectid epidermal papilloma-associated
        virus, 449–451
Pleuronectiformes sp., 449
Pneumonitis, upper respiratory and
        coronavirus, 220–221
Polyarteritis nodosa and persistent hepatitis B
        virus, 494
Ponteves virus
    in *Argas reflexus* (1966), 62
Porcine hemagglutinating encephalitis virus,
        195

Porcine transmissible gastroenteritis virus, 195
Poxvirus, 348, 364, 366
Proflavine dye, 269
Psorophora sp., 12, 19, 21, 24, 25, 29
Punta Toro virus, 53, 55
    in human (1967), 55
    in *Lutzomyia* sp., 55
Rat
    coronavirus, 195
    sialodacryoadenitis virus, 195
Razdan virus, in *Dermacentor marginatus*, 64
Reoviridae of fish (*see also* Infectious
            pancreatic necrosis, Golden shiner
            virus disease), 414–426
    RNA, segmentation of, 299
    surface morphology, 293
Reovirus, 299
Retroviridae of fish, 440–445
    diseases listed, 441
Reverse transcriptase, 444
Rhabdoviridae of fish, 426–440
    antigenicity, 431–432
    carbohydrate, 433, 436
    cell culture, 438, 440
    composition, chemical, 433–436
    cytopathology, 440
    defective, 431
    disease of eel, 429–430
    genetics, 432
    growth cycle, 436–437
    hemagglutination, 432
    interferon, 440
    lipid, 433, 436
    morphology, 430–431
    protein
        molecular weight, listed, 435
        structural, 433, 435
        synthesis, 438
        viral, 433–436
    protein kinase, 436
    RNA
        characteristics, listed, 434
        density, 434
        genome, 433
        molecular weight, 434
        sedimentation coefficient, 434
        single-stranded, non-segmented, 433
        synthesis, 438–440
    stability, 432–433
        inactivation by solvent, 432, 436
Retrovirus, 442–445
    and Atlantic salmon fibrosarcoma, 441
Reverse transcriptase, *see* DNA polymerase,
            RNA-dependent

Rice dwarf virus, 299
Rift Valley fever virus
  in domestic animals (1931), 64
    epizootic in Egypt (1977), 65
  in human (1975), 64–65
    epidemic in Egypt (1977), 64
    symptoms, 65
  in lamb (1930) in Kenya, 64
  in mouse brain, electron microscope
    photograph, 70
Rio Grande virus
  in *Neotoma micropus* (1974), 57
RNA, *see* separate RNA-containing viruses
Rongola virus, 16
Rotavirus, surface morphology, 293
Runde tick coronavirus, 195

Sabethini sp., 11
Sabo virus, 43, 44
  in cattle, 41
  in *Culicoides* sp., 41
  in goat (1966), 41
Sacramento River chinook disease, 426
Saimiri monkey, 11
Saint Floris virus, 55
Sakhalin virus, 4, 58–59
  antibody in seabirds (1974), 59
  in *Ixodes putus* (1969), 58
Salehabad virus
  in sandfly (1959), 55
  in sheep (1975), 55
Salmo gairdneri, 402, 427
  S. salar, 441, 454
  S. trutta lacustris, 454
  S. trutta trutta, 459
  viral hemorrhagic septicemia, 427
    stages of the disease (acute, chronic,
      nervous or latent), 428
Salmon (Atlantic)
  fibrosarcoma, 441
  leiomyosarcoma, 441
Samford virus, in *Culicoides* sp. (1972), 40
San Angelo virus, 2, 22, 29
  in *Anopheles* sp. (1958), 29
  in *Psorophora confinnis*, 29
  transmission, transovarial, 29
Sandfly fever, epidemics in Greece decreasing
      after 1950, 56
  in Italy decreasing after 1950, 57
  in Turkestan (1974), 56
Sango virus, 43
  in cattle (1970), 41
  in midges, 41
  in mosquitoes, 41

Sanguinus sp., 501–502
  and transmission of hepatitis A virus,
    501–502
San Joaquin Valley California, 20
San Miguel sea lion virus (SMSV), 249,
    251–253
  antibody, 251
  antigen, 253
  lesion on flipper, 251
  polypeptide, nonstructural, 262
  radioimmune precipitation, 253
  reproductive failure, 251
  RNA, 261
  in swine, 251
  and vesicular exanthema swine virus
    antigen relationships, 252
Santa Rosa virus, 11, 100
Sathuperi virus, 43, 44
  in cattle (1972), 40, 41
  in *Culex* sp. (1957), 40
  in *Culicoides* sp. (1972), 40
Scironomus plumosus virus, 353
Scophthalmus maximus virus, 403
Semliki Forest virus, 80
Sericesthis iridescent virus, 353, 354
Serra do Navio virus, in *Aedes fulvus*, 29
Shamonda virus, 44
  in cattle, 41
  in *Culicoides* sp., 41
Shark River virus
  in *Culex* sp. (1964), 37
  in sentinel hamster (1972), 37
Shokwe virus, 9
Shuni virus
  in cattle, 41
  in *Culex* sp., 40, 41
  in *Culicoides* sp., 41
  in human, 41
  in sheep, 41
Sialodacryoadenitis in rat, 222
Sicilian sandfly fever virus, 53, 56
  in cattle (1975), 56
  in *Phlebotomus* sp. (1960), 56
  in sheep (1975), 56
Sigmodon sp., 159
Silverwater virus, in tick (1961), 49
Simbu group viruses, 2, 38–42
  in *Aedes* sp. (1955), 41
  complement fixation relationships, listed, 44
  in human, 41
  members listed, 43
  neutralization test relationships, listed, 43
SIV, *see Sericethis* iridescent virus

Snowshoe hare virus, 20, 26–27
  in *Aedes* sp., 27
  antibody, 27
  in *Citellus* sp., 27
  in *Lepus americanus* (1959), 26
  in *Marmota monax*, 27
  mutant *ts*
    complementation analysis, 124
    crosses, pairwise, 122–123
    frequency, 118
    progeny release and mutagen, 117
    recombination
      analysis, 120
      experiment, 125–127
    yield
      after mixed infection, 119
      after single infection, 119
  RNA
    base ratio, 81
    oligonucleotide fingerprinting, 89
    5′-terminal nucleotide, 82
Sororoca virus, 11, 13
South River virus, 20, 24
Spring viremia of carp (SVC), 428–429,
    437–438
  interferon is not produced, 440
Stizostedion vitreum vitreum, 442
Stomatopapilloma of eel–associated viruses,
    446–447
  cauliflower disease, 446
  electron microscope photograph, 448
  head of eel with, 446
Sunday Canyon virus, in *Argas* sp. (1969), 66
SVC, *see* Spring viremia of carp
Swine, *see* Porcine

Tacaiuma virus, 15, 16
Tacaribe virus, 158, 159, 169, 172, 177
  in *Antibesis* spp., 159
  in bat, 158
  complex, 158–161
  persistent, 161
Taggert virus
  in *Ixodes* sp. (1972), 59
  in penguin (1975), 59
Tahyna virus, 2, 19, 20, 22–24
  in *Aedes caspius* (1958), 22
  antibody, 23
Taiassui virus, 10, 11
Tamdy virus, in *Hyalomma asiaticum* (1971),
    66
Tamiami virus, 159, 169
  cell inclusion, 167

Tamiami virus (*cont.*)
  electron microscope photograph, 167
  ribosome aggregates, 167
Tataguine virus
  in *Anopheles* sp. (1966), 66
  in human (1975), 66
  and fièvre rouge congolaise (1969), 66
Tensaw virus, 8, 11–13, 16
Tete group viruses, 2, 42–45
  in bird (1959), 44
  members listed, 45
  neutralization relationships, listed, 45
Thimiri virus
  in *Ardeola grayii* (1963), 40
  in *Culicoides* sp. (1974), 40
  in *Sylvia* sp. (1969), 40
Thogoto virus, 4, 59–60
  in *Boophilus* sp. (1960), 59
  in human (1969) in Nigeria, 59
  in *Rhipicephalus* sp. (1965), 59
Tilligerry virus, 322
Tipula iridescent virus (TIV), 353
  electron microscope photograph, 354, 362
  polypeptides, 358
TIV, *see* Tipula iridescent virus
Tlacotalpan virus, 10, 11
Togavirus, 215–216
Transcriptase, RNA-dependent, viral, 438
Transmissible gastroenteritis virus (TGEV),
    porcine, 194, 198, 201, 225, 226, 236
  genome, 198
  lipid, 201
  symptoms, 226
Trichoprosopon sp., 10
Trivittatus virus, 22, 29–30
  in *Aedes* spp., 28, 30
  isolation (1948), 29
  ts mutant, recombination
    analysis, 121
    experiment, 126
Trubanaman virus, 4, 51, 52
  in *Anopheles* sp. (1966), 50
Tsuruse virus, 44, 45
Turkey bluecomb disease virus, 195
Turlock virus, 4, 60–61
  in bird (1966), 60
  in *Culex tarsalis* (1954), 60
  neutralization test relationships, listed, 61

UDN, *see* Ulcerative dermal necrosis
Ulcerative dermal necrosis–associated virus,
    454
Umatilla virus, 287

Umbre virus, 4
　in *Culex* sp. (1955), 60
Urucuri virus, in rodent (1957), 57
Utinga Forest, Belem, Brazil, 31, 54
Utinga virus, 43, 44
　in *Bradypus tridactylus*, 41
Uukuniemi virus
　in *Apodemus flavicollis* (1970), 62
　in bird (1973), 62
　composition, chemical, 79
　electron microscope photograph, 72
　in *Ixodes ricinus* (1960), 62
　morphology, 72
　phospholipid content, 80
　RNA
　　base ratio, 81
　　circular, closed, 83–85
　　　electron microscope photograph, 84
　　molecular weight, 86
　　polymerase, RNA-direct, 104
　　5′-terminal nucleotide analysis, 82

Vellore virus, 322
Vero cell, electrophoresis pattern on
　　polyacrylamide gel, 263
Vesicular exanthema of swine (VES), 250, 259
　antigen, 253–254
　electron microscope photograph, 258
　outbreak of 1956, 250
　sedimentation rate, 266
VHS, *see* Viral hemorrhagic septicemia
Vibrio cholerae enterotoxin, 226

Viral hemorrhagic septicemia (VHS), 427–428
　interferon induced in cell culture, 440
Viremia, 222
Viroplasmic focus, 257, 258

Wallal virus, 287, 298, 316
　RNA, double-stranded, 298
Walleye
　dermal sarcoma by retrovirus, 442–443
　　electron microscope photograph, 445
　epidermal hyperplasia by retrovirus, 444
　and retrovirus, 442–445
Warrego virus, 287
　in *Culicoides* sp., 287
　in kangaroo, 327
White sucker epidermal papilloma by
　　retrovirus, 444
Witwatersrand virus
　in *Culex ribinotus* (1958), 67
　in human (1960), 67
　in rodent (1975), 67
Wongal virus, 35
　in *Culex* sp. (1960), 36
Wound tumor virus, 299
Wyeomyia virus, 8, 10

Yaba-1 virus, 60–61

Zaliv Terpeniya virus, in *Ixodes putus* (1969),
　　62
Zegla virus
　antibody, 38
　in *Sigmodon hispidus* (1966), 37